W9-BQK-509

FOURTH EDITION

CASE FILES®
Emergency Medicine

Eugene C. Toy, MD
Assistant Dean for Educational Programs
Director, Doctoring Courses
Professor and Vice Chair of Medical Education
Department of Obstetrics and Gynecology
McGovern Medical School at University of
  Texas Health Science Center (UTHealth)
  at Houston
Houston, Texas

Barry C. Simon, MD
Chairman, Department of Emergency
  Medicine
Alameda Health System/Highland General
  Hospital
Oakland, California
Clinical Professor of Emergency Medicine
University of California
San Francisco, California

Katrin Y. Takenaka, MD
Associate Professor
Associate Residency Program Director
Department of Emergency Medicine
McGovern Medical School at University of
  Texas Health Science Center (UTHealth) at
  Houston
Houston, Texas

Terrence H. Liu, MD, MPH
Physician and Surgeon
Sutter East Bay Medical Group
Berkeley, California

Adam J. Rosh, MD, MS
Assistant Professor
Department of Emergency Medicine
Wayne State University School of Medicine
Detroit Receiving Hospital
Detroit, Michigan

Mc
Graw
Hill
Education

New York   Chicago   San Francisco   Athens   London   Madrid
Mexico City   Milan   New Delhi   Singapore   Sydney   Toronto

Case Files®: Emergency Medicine, Fourth Edition

3 4 5 6 7 8 9   LCR   22 21 20 19 18

ISBN 978-1-259-64082-7
MHID 1-259-64082-5

Notice

Medicine is an ever-changing science. As new research and clinical experience broaden our knowledge, changes in treatment and drug therapy are required. The authors and the publisher of this work have checked with sources believed to be reliable in their efforts to provide information that is complete and generally in accord with the standard accepted at the time of publication. However, in view of the possibility of human error or changes in medical sciences, neither the editors nor the publisher nor any other party who has been involved in the preparation or publication of this work warrants that the information contained herein is in every respect accurate or complete, and they disclaim all responsibility for any errors or omissions or for the results obtained from use of the information contained in this work. Readers are encouraged to confirm the information contained herein with other sources. For example and in particular, readers are advised to check the product information sheet included in the package of each drug they plan to administer to be certain that the information contained in this work is accurate and that changes have not been made in the recommended dose or in the contraindications for administration. This recommendation is of particular importance in connection with new or infrequently used drugs.

This book was set in Adobe Jenson Pro by Cenveo® Publisher Services.
The editors were Bob Boehringer and Cindy Yoo.
The production supervisor was Catherine H. Saggese.
Project management was provided by Anupriya Tyagi, Cenveo Publisher Services.

This book is printed on acid-free paper.

Library of Congress Cataloging-in-Publication Data

Names: Toy, Eugene C., author. | Simon, Barry C., 1954- author. | Takenaka,
    Katrin Y., author. | Liu, Terrence H., author. | Rosh, Adam J., author.
Title: Case files. Emergency medicine / Eugene C. Toy, Barry C. Simon,
    Katrin Y. Takenaka, Terrence H. Liu, Adam J. Rosh.
Other titles: Emergency medicine
Description: Fourth edition. | New York : McGraw-Hill Education, [2017] |
    Preceded by Case files. Emergency medicine / Eugene C. Toy ... [et al.].
    3rd ed. c2013. | Includes bibliographical references and index.
Identifiers: LCCN 2016045347| ISBN 9781259640827 (paperback : alk. paper) |
    ISBN 1259640825 (paperback : alk. paper)
Subjects: | MESH: Emergency Medicine—methods | Emergencies | Diagnosis,
    Differential | Problems and Exercises | Case Reports
Classification: LCC RC86.9 | NLM WB 18.2 | DDC 616.02/5—dc23 LC record available at https://lccn.loc.gov/
    2016045347

To the McGovern Medical School at the University of Texas Health Science Center (UTHealth) at Houston Class of 2020. You are the most incredibly talented, motivated, bright, compassionate, and energetic students I could ever hope to teach. Thank you for helping to restore my love for teaching.

—ECT

To my best friend and wife Zina Rosen-Simon and to my daughters Jamie and Kaylie for teaching me and always reminding me what is most important in life. I would also like to thank my faculty at Highland General Hospital and all the residents and students who have passed through our doors for helping make my career as an academic emergency physician challenging and immensely rewarding.

—BS

To my parents, who continue to be my guiding light. To my residents and colleagues, who never fail to impress me with their dedication to our profession. And to Clare, who remains my teacher and friend.

—KYT

To my wife Eileen for her continuous support, love, and friendship. To all the medical students and residents for their dedication to education and improving patient care.

—THL

A hearty thanks goes out to my family for their love and support, especially Ruby; the dedicated medical professionals of the EDs at NYU/Bellevue Hospital and Wayne State University/DRH; and my patients, who put their trust in me, and teach me something new each day.

—AR

CONTENTS

Tiffany Chioma Anaebere, MD
Resident Physician
Department of Emergency Medicine
Alameda Health System/Highland Campus
Oakland, California
Chest Pain

Mike Anana, MD
Assistant Residency Director
Department of Emergency Medicine
Rutgers New Jersey Medical School
Newark, New Jersey
Facial Laceration

Ciara J. Barclay-Buchanan, MD, FACEP
Associate Residency Program Director
Department of Emergency Medicine
Assistant Professor
University of Wisconsin School of Medicine and Public Health
Madison, Wisconsin
Altered Mental Status
Emerging Infections
Frostbite and Hypothermia

Keenan M. Bora, MD
Assistant Professor
Department of Emergency Medicine
Wayne State University School of Medicine
Toxicologist, Children's Hospital of Michigan
Regional Poison Control Center
Detroit, Michigan
Animal Bites and Snake Bites
Anti-muscarinic Toxidromes

Magdalene A. Brooke, MD
Resident
UCSF-East Bay Surgery Residency
Oakland, California
Extremity Fracture and Neck Pain
Penetrating Trauma

Andrew Coyne, MD
Emergency Medicine Physician
Houston, Texas
Bacterial Pneumonia
Congestive Heart Failure/Pulmonary Edema

David Diller, MD
Assistant Program Director
LAC+USC Emergency Medicine Residency Program
Assistant Professor of Clinical Emergency Medicine
University of Southern California Keck School of Medicine
Los Angeles, California
Pulmonary Embolism
Stroke/TIA
Syncope

David Duong, MD, MS
Assistant Clinical Professor
Department of Emergency Medicine
University of California, San Francisco
Associate Residency Director
Department of Emergency Medicine
Alameda Health System/Highland Campus
Oakland, California
Bacterial Meningitis
Fever in the Newborn

David K. English, MD, FACEP
Assistant Clinical Professor
Department of Emergency Medicine
University of California, San Francisco
Faculty
Department of Emergency Medicine
Alameda Health System/Highland Campus
Oakland, California
Diabetic Ketoacidosis
Hyperkalemia Due to Renal Failure

Bradley W. Frazee, MD
Clinical Professor
Department of Emergency Medicine
University of California, San Francisco
Faculty
Department of Emergency Medicine
Alameda Health System/Highland Campus
Oakland, California
Chest Pain/MI
Skin and Soft Tissue Infections

Jocelyn Freeman Garrick, MD, MS, FACEP
Associate Clinical Professor
Department of Emergency Medicine
University of California, San Francisco
EMS Base Director
Alameda Health System/Highland Campus
Oakland, California
Septic Arthritis (Child)

Jeffrey Glassberg, MD
Assistant Professor of Emergency Medicine
Hematology and Medical Oncology
Associate Director of The Mount Sinai Comprehensive Sickle Cell Program
Icahn School of Medicine at Mount Sinai
New York, New York
Sickle Cell Crisis

Indira Gowda, MD
Resident
Department of Emergency Medicine
Icahn School of Medicine at Mount Sinai
New York, New York
Sickle Cell Crisis

Casey Green, MD
Resident Physician
Oregon Health & Science University
Portland, Oregon
Stroke/TIA

Cherie A. Hargis, MD
Assistant Clinical Professor
Department of Emergency Medicine
University of California, San Francisco
Attending Physician
Department of Emergency Medicine
Alameda Health System/Highland Campus
Oakland, California
Red Eye

H. Gene Hern, MD, MS
Associate Clinical Professor
Department of Emergency Medicine
University of California, San Francisco
Vice Chair of Education
Department of Emergency Medicine
Alameda Health System/Highland Campus
Oakland, California
Streptococcal Pharyngitis ("Strep Throat")

Andrew A. Herring, MD
Assistant Clinical Professor of Medicine
Department of Emergency Medicine
University of California, San Francisco
Associate Director of Research
Attending Physician
Department of Emergency Medicine
Alameda Health System/Highland Campus
Oakland, California
Airway Management/Respiratory Failure

Shannon Lee, MD
Resident Physician
Oregon Health & Science University
Portland, Oregon
Syncope

Brian Lin, MD
Resident
Department of Emergency Medicine
NYU/Bellevue Emergency Medicine Residency Program
New York, New York
Hypertensive Encephalopathy

Lia I. Losonczy, MD, MPH
Critical Care Fellow
Department of Medicine
Clinical Instructor
Department of Emergency Medicine
University of Maryland Medical Center/R Adams Cowley Shock Trauma Center
Baltimore, Maryland
Noncardiac Chest Pain

Dan Mantuani, MD, MPH
Associate Director, Emergency Ultrasound
Department of Emergency Medicine
Alameda Health System/Highland Campus
Oakland, California
Seizure

Chad McCarthy, MD, MAT
Resident Physician
Department of Emergency Medicine
Alameda Health System/Highland Campus
Oakland, California
Fever in the Newborn

Omar Metwalli, MD
Administration & Quality Assurance Fellow
McGovern Medical School at University of Texas Health Science Center
    (UTHealth) at Houston
Houston, Texas
Acetaminophen Toxicity
Cocaine Intoxication
Submersion Injury

Emily Miraflor, MD
Assistant Professor of Surgery
UCSF School of Medicine
Oakland, California
Bowel Obstruction
Submersion Injury
Transfusion Complications

Michael Mirza, MD
Resident Physician
Department of Emergency Medicine
Rutgers New Jersey Medical School
Newark, New Jersey
Facial Laceration

David Mishkin, MD
Attending Physician
Department of Emergency Medicine
Baptist Hospital of Miami
Miami, Florida
Acute Pyelonephritis

Arun Nagdev, MD
Assistant Clinical Professor
Department of Emergency Medicine
University of California, San Francisco
Director, Emergency Ultrasound
Department of Emergency Medicine
Alameda Health System/Highland Campus
Oakland, California
Febrile Seizure/Otitis Media

Julie Kautz Oliva, MD
Resident Physician
Department of Emergency Medicine
Alameda Health System/Highland Campus
Oakland, California
Anaphylaxis
Bacterial Meningitis
Penetrating Trauma

Barnard JA Palmer, MD, Med
Associate Residency Director
UCSF-East Bay Surgery Residency
Assistant Professor of Surgery
UCSF School of Medicine
Oakland, California
Heat-related Injury
Lightning Injury

Berenice Perez, MD
Clinical Instructor in Medicine
University of California, San Francisco
Attending Physician and Co-Medical Director
Department of Emergency Medicine
Alameda Health System/Highland Campus
Oakland, California
Penetrating Trauma to the Chest, Abdomen, and Extremities

Heather Robinson, MD
Resident Physician
McGovern Medical School at University of Texas Health Science Center
   (UTHealth) at Houston
Houston, Texas
Ethanol Withdrawal
Headache
Rash With Fever
Scrotal Pain

Javid Sadjadi, MD
Associate Clinical Professor of Surgery
UCSF School of Medicine
Oakland, California
Abdominal Pain

Dean Sagun, MD
Resident Physician
McGovern Medical School at University of Texas Health Science Center
   (UTHealth) at Houston
Houston, Texas
Bell Palsy
Low Back Pain
Regular Rate Tachycardia
Swallowed Foreign Body

Inna Shniter, MD
Resident Physician
Oregon Health & Science University
Portland, Oregon
Pulmonary Embolism

Amandeep Singh, MD
Assistant Clinical Professor of Medicine
Department of Emergency Medicine
University of California, San Francisco
Attending Physician
Department of Emergency Medicine
Alameda Health System/Highland Campus
Oakland, California
Acute Exacerbation of Asthma
Sepsis

Eric R. Snoey, MD
Clinical Professor
Department of Emergency Medicine
University of California, San Francisco
Vice Chair
Department of Emergency Medicine
Alameda Health System/Highland Campus
Oakland, California
Atrial Fibrillation

Bryce Snow, MD
Chief Resident Physician
Department of Emergency Medicine
University of Wisconsin School of Medicine and Public Health
Madison, Wisconsin
Frostbite and Hypothermia

Aparajita Sohoni, MD
Attending Physician
Department of Emergency Medicine
Alameda Health System/Highland Campus
Oakland, California
Hemorrhagic Shock

Anand K. Swaminathan, MD, MPH
Assistant Professor of Emergency Medicine
Ronald O. Perelman Emergency Department
Assistant Residency Director
NYU/Bellevue Emergency Medicine Residency Program
New York, New York
Hypertensive Encephalopathy

David S. Tillman, MD
Education Fellow
Clinical Instructor
Department of Emergency Medicine
University of Wisconsin School of Medicine and Public Health
Madison, Wisconsin
Emerging Infections

Allison L. Toy, RN
Staff Nurse
Baylor Scott & White at Hillcrest Medical Center
Waco, Texas
Primary manuscript reviewer
Review Questions

Gregory P. Victorino, MD
Trauma Director, Highland Hospital
Professor of Clinical Surgery
UCSF School of Medicine
Oakland, California
Extremity Fracture and Neck Pain
Penetrating Trauma

Alexander Wade, MD, JD
Resident Physician
Department of Emergency Medicine
University of Wisconsin Hospitals and Clinics
Madison, Wisconsin
Altered Mental Status

Marcus L. Williams, MD
Resident Physician
Department of Emergency Medicine
Alameda Health System/Highland Campus
Oakland, California
Child with a Limp

Charlotte Page Wills, MD
Associate Clinical Professor
Department of Emergency Medicine
University of California, San Francisco
Residency Director
Department of Emergency Medicine
Alameda Health System/Highland Campus
Oakland, California
Anaphylaxis

ACKNOWLEDGMENTS

The curriculum that evolved into the ideas for this series was inspired by two talented and forthright students, Philbert Yau and Chuck Rosipal, who have since graduated from medical school. It has been a pleasure to work with Dr. Barry Simon, a wonderfully skilled and compassionate emergency room physician, and Dr. Kay Takenaka, who is as talented in her writing and teaching as she is in her clinical care. It has been excellent to have Adam Rosh join us. McGraw-Hill and I have had the fortune to work with Adam while he was a medical student, resident, and now an accomplished emergency medicine physician and educator. Likewise, I have cherished working together with my friend since medical school, Terry Liu, who initially suggested the idea of this book. I am so proud of my daughter Allison who has become an accomplished nurse, and also an expert in the "case files" format. This fourth edition has five new cases, includes updates on nearly every case, and is completely reorganized so that the cases fit into condition-based systems. I am greatly indebted to Catherine Johnson, whose exuberance, experience, and vision helped to shape this series. I appreciate McGraw-Hill's believing in the concept of teaching through clinical cases. I am also grateful to Catherine Saggese for her excellent production expertise and to Cindy Yoo for her wonderful editing and outstanding production skills. Without the support of Dr. Patricia Butler in the Office for Educational Programs, Dr. Sean Blackwell, Chair of the Department of Ob/Gyn, and Dr. John Riggs, Ob/Gyn Chief at LBJ Hospital, I would not have been able to succeed in this book. Most of all, I appreciate my everloving wife Terri, and four wonderful children, Andy and his wife Anna, Michael, Allison, and Christina, for their patience, encouragement, and understanding.

Eugene C. Toy

Mastering the cognitive knowledge within a field such as emergency medicine is a formidable task. It is even more difficult to draw on that knowledge, procure and filter through the clinical and laboratory data, develop a differential diagnosis, and finally to form a rational treatment plan. To gain these skills, the student often learns best at the bedside, guided and instructed by experienced teachers and inspired toward self-directed, diligent reading. Clearly, there is no replacement for education at the bedside. Unfortunately, clinical situations usually do not encompass the breadth of the specialty. Perhaps the best alternative is a carefully crafted patient case designed to simulate the clinical approach and decision-making. In an attempt to achieve that goal, we have constructed a collection of clinical vignettes to teach diagnostic or therapeutic approaches relevant to emergency medicine. Most importantly, the explanations for the cases emphasize the mechanisms and underlying principles, rather than merely rote questions and answers.

This book is organized for versatility: it benefits the student "in a rush" to go quickly through the scenarios and check the corresponding answers, as well as the student who wants thought-provoking explanations. The answers are arranged from simple to complex: a summary of the pertinent points, the bare answers, an analysis of the case, an approach to the topic, a comprehension test at the end for reinforcement and emphasis, and a list of resources for further reading. The clinical vignettes are purposely placed in a systematic order to allow students to compare and contrast like cases. A listing of cases is included in Section III to aid the student who desires to test his/her knowledge of a certain area or to review a topic. Finally, we intentionally did not primarily use a multiple choice question (MCQ) format because clues (or distractions) are not available in the real world. Nevertheless, several MCQs are included at the end of each scenario to reinforce concepts or introduce related topics.

HOW TO GET THE MOST OUT OF THIS BOOK

Each case is designed to simulate a patient encounter with open-ended questions. At times, the patient's complaint is different from the most concerning issue, and sometimes extraneous information is given. The answers are organized with four different parts.

PART I

1. **Summary:** The salient aspects of the case are identified, filtering out the extraneous information. The student should formulate his/her summary from the case before looking at the answers. A comparison to the summation in the answer will help to improve one's ability to focus on the important data while appropriately discarding the irrelevant information, a fundamental skill in clinical problem solving.
2. A **straightforward answer** is given to each open-ended question.
3. The **Analysis of the Case,** which is comprised of two parts:

   a. **Objectives of the Case:** A listing of the two or three main principles that are crucial for a practitioner to manage the patient. Again, the student is challenged to make educated "guesses" about the objectives of the case upon initial review of the case scenario, which will help to sharpen his/her clinical and analytical skills.
   b. **Considerations:** A discussion of the relevant points and brief approach to the **specific** patient.

PART II

Approach to the Disease Process, which has two distinct parts:
   a. **Definitions or pathophysiology:** Terminology or basic science correlates pertinent to the disease process.
   b. **Clinical Approach:** A discussion of the approach to the clinical problem in general, including tables, figures, and algorithms.

PART III

Comprehension Questions: Each case contains several multiple-choice questions that reinforce the material or introduce new and related concepts. Questions about material not found in the text will have explanations in the answers.

PART IV

Clinical Pearls: A listing of several clinically important points, which are reiterated as a summation of the text, to allow for easy review such as before an examination.

LISTING BY CASE NUMBER

LISTING BY DISORDER (ALPHABETICAL)

How to Approach Clinical Problems

Part 1. Approach to the Patient

Applying "book learning" to a specific clinical situation is one of the most challenging tasks in medicine. To do so, the clinician must not only retain information, organize facts, and recall large amounts of data, but also apply all of this to the patient. The purpose of this text is to facilitate this process.

The first step involves gathering information, also known as establishing the database. This includes taking the history, performing the physical examination, and obtaining selective laboratory examinations, special studies, and/or imaging tests. Sensitivity and respect should always be exercised during the interview of patients. **A good clinician also knows how to ask the same question in several different ways, using different terminology.** For example, patients may deny having "congestive heart failure" but will answer affirmatively to being treated for "fluid in the lungs."

CLINICAL PEARL

▶ The **history** is usually the **single most important** tool in obtaining a diagnosis. The art of seeking this information in a nonjudgmental, sensitive, and thorough manner cannot be overemphasized.

HISTORY

1. **Basic information:**
   a. **Age:** Some conditions are more common at certain ages; for instance, chest pain in an elderly patient is more worrisome for coronary artery disease than the same complaint in a teenager.
   b. **Gender:** Some disorders are more common in men such as abdominal aortic aneurysms. In contrast, women more commonly have autoimmune problems such as chronic idiopathic thrombocytopenic purpura or systemic lupus erythematosus. Also, the possibility of pregnancy must be considered in any woman of childbearing age.
   c. **Ethnicity:** Some disease processes are more common in certain ethnic groups (such as type 2 diabetes mellitus in the Hispanic population).

CLINICAL PEARL

▶ The possibility of pregnancy must be entertained in any woman of childbearing age.

2. **Chief complaint:** What is it that brought the patient into the hospital? Has there been a change in a chronic or recurring condition or is this a completely new problem? The duration and character of the complaint, associated symptoms, and exacerbating/relieving factors should be recorded. The chief complaint engenders a differential diagnosis, and the possible etiologies should be explored by further inquiry.

> **CLINICAL PEARL**

> ► The first line of any presentation should include **age, ethnicity, gender, and chief complaint.** Example: A 32-year-old white man complains of lower abdominal pain of 8-hour duration.

3. **Past medical history:**
   a. Major illnesses such as hypertension, diabetes, reactive airway disease, congestive heart failure, angina, or stroke should be detailed.
      i. Age of onset, severity, end-organ involvement.
      ii. Medications taken for the particular illness including any recent changes to medications and reason for the change(s).
      iii. Last evaluation of the condition (example: when was the last stress test or cardiac catheterization performed in the patient with angina?)
      iv. Which physician or clinic is following the patient for the disorder?
   b. Minor illnesses such as recent upper respiratory infections.
   c. Hospitalizations no matter how trivial should be queried.

4. **Past surgical history:** Date and type of procedure performed, indication, and outcome. Laparoscopy versus laparotomy should be distinguished. Surgeon and hospital name/location should be listed. This information should be correlated with the surgical scars on the patient's body. Any complications should be delineated including, for example, anesthetic complications and difficult intubations.

5. **Allergies:** Reactions to medications should be recorded, including severity and temporal relationship to the dose of medication. Immediate hypersensitivity should be distinguished from an adverse reaction.

6. **Medications:** A list of medications, dosage, route of administration and frequency, and duration of use should be developed. Prescription, over-the-counter, and herbal remedies are all relevant. If the patient is currently taking antibiotics, it is important to note what type of infection is being treated.

7. **Social history:** Occupation, marital status, family support, and tendencies toward depression or anxiety are important. Use or abuse of illicit drugs, tobacco, or alcohol should also be recorded.

8. **Family history:** Many major medical problems are genetically transmitted (eg, hemophilia, sickle cell disease). In addition, a family history of conditions such as breast cancer and ischemic heart disease can be a risk factor for the development of these diseases.

9. **Review of systems:** A systematic review should be performed but focused on the life-threatening and the more common diseases. For example, in a young man with a testicular mass, trauma to the area, weight loss, and infectious symptoms are important to note. In an elderly woman with generalized weakness,

symptoms suggestive of cardiac disease should be elicited, such as chest pain, shortness of breath, fatigue, or palpitations.

PHYSICAL EXAMINATION

1. **General appearance:** Is the patient in any acute distress? The emergency physician should focus on the **ABCs (Airway, Breathing, Circulation)**. Note cachetic versus well-nourished, anxious versus calm, alert versus obtunded.

2. **Vital signs:** Record the temperature, blood pressure, heart rate, and respiratory rate. An oxygen saturation is useful in patients with respiratory symptoms. Height, weight, and body mass index are often placed here.

3. **Head and neck examination:** Evidence of trauma, tumors, facial edema, goiter and thyroid nodules, and carotid bruits should be sought. In patients with altered mental status or a head injury, pupillary size, symmetry, and reactivity are important. Mucous membranes should be inspected for pallor, jaundice, and evidence of dehydration. Cervical and supraclavicular nodes should be palpated.

4. **Breast examination:** Inspection for symmetry and skin or nipple retraction, as well as palpation for masses. The nipple should be assessed for discharge, and the axillary and supraclavicular regions should be examined.

5. **Cardiac examination:** The *point of maximal impulse* should be ascertained, and the heart auscultated at the apex as well as the base. It is important to note whether the auscultated rhythm is regular or irregular. Heart sounds (including S_3 and S_4), murmurs, clicks, and rubs should be characterized. Systolic flow murmurs are fairly common in pregnant women because of the increased cardiac output, but significant diastolic murmurs are unusual.

6. **Pulmonary examination:** The lung fields should be examined systematically and thoroughly. Stridor, wheezes, rales, and rhonchi should be recorded. The clinician should also search for evidence of consolidation (bronchial breath sounds, egophony) and increased work of breathing (retractions, abdominal breathing, accessory muscle use).

7. **Abdominal examination:** The abdomen should be inspected for scars, distension, masses, and discoloration. For instance, the Grey Turner sign of bruising at the flank areas may indicate intra-abdominal or retroperitoneal hemorrhage. Auscultation should identify normal versus high-pitched and hyperactive versus hypoactive bowel sounds. The abdomen should be percussed for the presence of shifting dullness (indicating ascites). Then careful palpation should begin away from the area of pain and progress to include the whole abdomen to assess for tenderness, masses, organomegaly (ie, spleen or liver), and peritoneal signs. Guarding and whether it is voluntary or involuntary should be noted.

8. **Back and spine examination:** The back should be assessed for symmetry, tenderness, or masses. The flank regions particularly are important to assess for pain on percussion that may indicate renal disease.

9. **Genital examination:**
   a. **Female:** The external genitalia should be inspected and then the speculum used to visualize the cervix and vagina. A bimanual examination should attempt to elicit cervical motion tenderness, uterine size, and ovarian masses or tenderness.
   b. **Male:** The penis should be examined for hypospadias, lesions, and discharge. The scrotum should be palpated for tenderness and masses. If a mass is present, it can be transilluminated to distinguish between solid and cystic masses. The groin region should be carefully palpated for bulging (hernias) upon rest and provocation (coughing, standing).
   c. **Rectal examination:** A rectal examination will reveal masses in the posterior pelvis and may identify gross or occult blood in the stool. In females, nodularity and tenderness in the uterosacral ligament may be signs of endometriosis. The posterior uterus and palpable masses in the cul-de-sac may be identified by rectal examination. In the male, the prostate gland should be palpated for tenderness, nodularity, and enlargement.

10. **Extremities/skin:** The presence of joint effusions, tenderness, rashes, edema, and cyanosis should be recorded. It is also important to note capillary refill and peripheral pulses.

11. **Neurological examination:** Patients who present with neurological complaints require a thorough assessment including mental status, cranial nerves, strength, sensation, reflexes, and cerebellar function. In trauma patients, the Glasgow coma score is important (Table I–1).

CLINICAL PEARL

▶ A thorough understanding of anatomy is important to optimally interpret the physical examination findings.

12. Laboratory assessment depends on the circumstances:
   a. CBC (complete blood count) can assess for anemia, leukocytosis (infection), and thrombocytopenia.
   b. Basic metabolic panel: Electrolytes, glucose, blood urea nitrogen, and creatinine (renal function).
   c. Urinalysis and/or urine culture: To assess for hematuria, pyuria, or bacteruria. A pregnancy test is important in women of childbearing age.
   d. AST (aspartate aminotransferase), ALT (alanine aminotransferase), bilirubin, alkaline phosphatase for liver function; amylase and lipase to evaluate the pancreas. Glasgow coma scale score is the sum of the best responses in the three areas: eye opening, motor response, and verbal response.
   e. Cardiac markers (CK-MB [creatine kinase myocardial band], troponin, myoglobin) if coronary artery disease or other cardiac dysfunction is suspected.

Table I–1 • GLASGOW COMA SCALE	
Assessment Area	Score
Eye opening	
Spontaneous	4
To speech	3
To pain	2
None	1
Best motor response	
Obeys commands	6
Localizes pain	5
Withdraws to pain	4
Decorticate posture (abnormal flexion)	3
Decerebrate posture (extension)	2
No response	1
Verbal response	
Oriented	5
Confused conversation	4
Inappropriate words	3
Incomprehensible sounds	2
None	1

f. Drug levels such as acetaminophen level in possible overdoses.

g. Arterial blood gas measurements give information about oxygenation, but also carbon dioxide and pH readings.

13. **Diagnostic adjuncts:**

a. Electrocardiogram if cardiac ischemia, dysrhythmia, or other cardiac dysfunction is suspected.

b. Ultrasound examination useful in evaluating pelvic processes in female patients (eg, pelvic inflammatory disease, tubo-ovarian abscess) and in diagnosing gallstones and other gallbladder disease. With the addition of color-flow Doppler, deep venous thrombosis and ovarian or testicular torsion can be detected.

c. The FAST (focused assessment with sonography for trauma) examination can decrease the time to treating intra-abdominal bleeding. The examination includes views of the hepatorenal recess (Morrison pouch), the perisplenic view, subxiphoid pericardial window, and the perisplenic window (Douglas pouch). In the extended FAST (E-FAST) examination, the bilateral hemithoraces and upper anterior chest wall are also visualized.

d. Computed tomography (CT) useful in assessing the brain for masses, bleeding, strokes, and skull fractures. CTs of the chest can evaluate for masses, fluid collections, aortic dissections, and pulmonary emboli. Abdominal CTs can detect infection (abscess, appendicitis, diverticulitis), masses, aortic aneurysms, and ureteral stones.

e. Magnetic resonance imaging (MRI) helps to identify soft tissue planes very well. In the emergency department (ED) setting, this is most commonly used to rule out spinal cord compression, cauda equina syndrome, and epidural abscess or hematoma. MRI may also be useful for patients with acute strokes.

Part 2. Approach to Clinical Problem-Solving

CLASSIC CLINICAL PROBLEM-SOLVING

There are typically five distinct steps that an emergency department clinician undertakes to systematically solve most clinical problems:

1. Addressing the ABCs and other life-threatening conditions

2. Making the diagnosis

3. Assessing the severity of the disease

4. Treating based on the stage of the disease

5. Following the patient's response to the treatment

EMERGENCY ASSESSMENT AND MANAGEMENT

Patients often present to the ED with life-threatening conditions that necessitate **simultaneous evaluation and treatment.** For example, a patient who is acutely short of breath and hypoxemic requires supplemental oxygen and possibly intubation with mechanical ventilation. While addressing these needs, the clinician must also try to determine whether the patient is dyspneic because of a pneumonia, congestive heart failure, pulmonary embolus, pneumothorax, or for some other reason.

As a general rule, **the first priority is stabilization of the ABCs** (see Table I–2). For instance, a comatose multi-trauma patient first requires intubation to protect the airway. See Figures I–1 through I–3 regarding management of airway and breathing issues. Then, if the patient has a tension pneumothorax (breathing problem), (s)he needs an immediate needle thoracostomy. If (s)he is hypotensive, large-bore IV access and volume resuscitation are required for circulatory support. Pressure should be applied to any actively bleeding region. Once the ABCs and other life-threatening conditions are stabilized, a more complete history and head-to-toe physical examination should follow.

CLINICAL PEARL

▶ Because emergency physicians are faced with unexpected illness and injury, they must often perform diagnostic and therapeutic steps simultaneously. **In patients with an acutely life-threatening condition, the first and foremost priority is stabilization—the ABCs.**

Table I–2 • ASSESSMENT OF ABCS		
	Assessment	Management
Airway	Assess oral cavity, patient color (pink vs cyanotic), patency of airway (choking, aspiration, compression, foreign body, edema, blood), stridor, tracheal deviation, ease of ventilation with bag and mask	Head-tilt and chin-lift If cervical spine injury suspected, stabilize neck and use jaw thrust If obstruction, Heimlich maneuver, chest thrust, finger sweep (unconscious patient only) Temporizing airway (laryngeal mask airway) Definitive airway (intubation [nasotracheal or endotracheal], cricothyroidotomy)
Breathing	Look, listen, and feel for air movement and chest rising Respiratory rate and effort (accessory muscles, diaphoresis, fatigue) Effective ventilation (bronchospasm, chest wall deformity, pulmonary embolism)	Resuscitation (mouth-to-mouth, mouth-to-mask, bag and mask) Supplemental oxygen, chest tube (pneumothorax or hemothorax)
Circulation	Palpate carotid artery Assess pulse and blood pressure Cardiac monitor to assess rhythm Consider arterial pressure monitoring Assess capillary refill	If pulseless, chest compressions and determine cardiac rhythm (consider epinephrine, defibrillation) Intravenous access (central line) Fluids Consider 5 Hs and 5 Ts: **H**ypovolemia, **H**ypoxia, **H**ypothermia, **H**yper-/**H**ypokalemia, **H**ydrogen (acidosis); **T**ension pneumothorax, **T**amponade (cardiac), **T**hrombosis (massive pulmonary embolism), **T**hrombosis (myocardial infarction), **T**ablets (drug overdose)

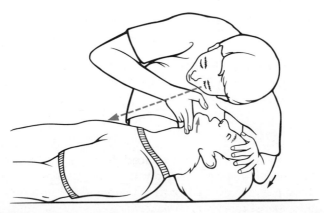

Figure I–1. **Determination of breathlessness.** The rescuer "looks, listens, and feels" for breath.

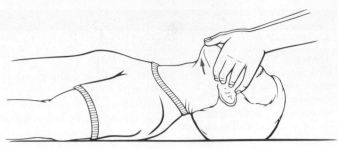

Figure I–2. **Jaw-thrust maneuver.** The rescuer lifts upward on the mandible while keeping the cervical spine in neutral position.

MAKING THE DIAGNOSIS

This is achieved by carefully evaluating the patient, analyzing the information, assessing risk factors, and developing a list of possible diagnoses (the differential). Usually a long list of possible diagnoses can be pared down to a few of the most likely or most serious ones, based on the clinician's knowledge, experience, and selective testing. For example, a patient who complains of upper abdominal pain and who has a history of nonsteroidal anti-inflammatory drug use may have peptic ulcer disease; another patient who has abdominal pain, fatty food intolerance, and abdominal bloating may have cholelithiasis. Yet another individual with a 1-day history of periumbilical pain that now localizes to the right lower quadrant may have acute appendicitis.

> **CLINICAL PEARL**
>
> ▶ The second step in clinical problem-solving is making the diagnosis.

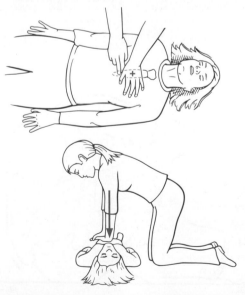

Figure I–3. **Chest compressions.** Rescuer applying chest compressions to an adult victim.

ASSESSING THE SEVERITY OF THE DISEASE

After establishing the diagnosis, the next step is to characterize the severity of the disease process; in other words, to describe "how bad" the disease is. This may be as simple as determining whether a patient is "sick" or "not sick." Is the patient with a urinary tract infection septic or stable for outpatient therapy? In other cases, a more formal staging may be used. For example, the Glasgow coma scale is used in patients with head trauma to describe the severity of their injury based on eye-opening, verbal, and motor responses.

> **CLINICAL PEARL**
>
> ▶ The third step in clinical problem-solving is to **establish the severity or stage of disease.** This usually impacts the treatment and/or prognosis.

TREATING BASED ON STAGE

Many illnesses are characterized by stage or severity because this affects prognosis and treatment. As an example, a formerly healthy young man with pneumonia and no respiratory distress may be treated with oral antibiotics at home. An older person with emphysema and pneumonia would probably be admitted to the hospital for IV antibiotics. A patient with pneumonia and respiratory failure would likely be intubated and admitted to the intensive care unit for further treatment.

> **CLINICAL PEARL**
>
> ▶ The fourth step in clinical problem-solving is **tailoring the treatment to fit the severity or "stage" of the disease.**

FOLLOWING THE RESPONSE TO TREATMENT

The final step in the approach to disease is to follow the patient's response to the therapy. Some responses are clinical such as improvement (or lack of improvement) in a patient's pain. Other responses may be followed by testing (eg, monitoring the anion gap in a patient with diabetic ketoacidosis). The clinician must be prepared to know what to do if the patient does not respond as expected. Is the next step to treat again, to reassess the diagnosis, or to follow up with another more specific test?

> **CLINICAL PEARL**
>
> ▶ The fifth step in clinical problem-solving is to **monitor treatment response or efficacy.** This may be measured in different ways—symptomatically or based on physical examination or other testing. For the emergency physician, the vital signs, oxygenation, urine output, and mental status are the key parameters.

Part 3. Approach to Reading

The clinical problem-oriented approach to reading is different from the classic "systematic" research of a disease. Patients rarely present with a clear diagnosis; hence, the student must become skilled in applying textbook information to the clinical scenario. Because reading with a purpose improves the retention of information, the student should read with the goal of answering specific questions. There are seven fundamental questions that facilitate **clinical thinking.**

1. What is the most likely diagnosis?

2. How would you confirm the diagnosis?

3. What should be your next step?

4. What is the most likely mechanism for this process?

5. What are the risk factors for this condition?

6. What are the complications associated with the disease process?

7. What is the best therapy?

CLINICAL PEARL

▶ **Reading with the purpose of answering the seven fundamental clinical questions improves retention of information** and facilitates the application of "book knowledge" to "clinical knowledge."

WHAT IS THE MOST LIKELY DIAGNOSIS?

The method of establishing the diagnosis was covered in the previous section. One way of attacking this problem is to develop standard "approaches" to common clinical problems. It is helpful to understand the most common causes of various presentations, such as "the worst headache of the patient's life is worrisome for a subarachnoid hemorrhage." (See the Clinical Pearls at end of each case.)

The clinical scenario would be something such as: "A 38-year-old woman is noted to have a 2-day history of a unilateral, throbbing headache and photophobia. What is the most likely diagnosis?"

With no other information to go on, the student would note that this woman has a unilateral headache and photophobia. Using the "most common cause" information, the student would make an educated guess that the patient has a migraine headache. If instead the patient is noted to have "the worst headache of her life," the student would use the Clinical Pearl: "The worst headache of the patient's life is worrisome for a subarachnoid hemorrhage."

> ## CLINICAL PEARL

> ▶ The more common cause of a unilateral, throbbing headache with photophobia is a migraine, but **the main concern is subarachnoid hemorrhage.** If the patient describes this as "the worst headache of her life," the concern for a subarachnoid bleed is increased.

HOW WOULD YOU CONFIRM THE DIAGNOSIS?

In the aforementioned scenario, the woman with "the worst headache" is suspected of having a subarachnoid hemorrhage. This diagnosis could be confirmed by a CT scan of the head and/or lumbar puncture. The student should learn the limitations of various diagnostic tests, especially when used early in a disease process. The lumbar puncture showing xanthochromia (red blood cells) is the "gold standard" test for diagnosing subarachnoid hemorrhage, but it may be negative early in the disease course.

WHAT SHOULD BE YOUR NEXT STEP?

This question is difficult because the next step has many possibilities; the answer may be to obtain more diagnostic information, stage the illness, or introduce therapy. It is often a more challenging question than "What is the most likely diagnosis?" because there may be insufficient information to make a diagnosis, and the next step may be to pursue more diagnostic information. Another possibility is that there is enough information for a probable diagnosis, and the next step is to stage the disease. Finally, the most appropriate answer may be to treat. Hence, from clinical data, a judgment needs to be rendered regarding how far along one is on the road of:

(1) Make a diagnosis → (2) Stage the disease →
(3) Treat based on stage → (4) Follow the response

Frequently, the student is taught "to regurgitate" the same information that someone has written about a particular disease, but is not skilled at identifying the next step. This talent is learned optimally at the bedside, in a supportive environment, with freedom to take educated guesses, and with constructive feedback. A sample scenario might describe a student's thought process as follows:

1. **Make the diagnosis:** "Based on the information I have, I believe that Mr. Smith has a small-bowel obstruction from adhesive disease *because* he presents with nausea and vomiting, abdominal distension, high-pitched hyperactive bowel sounds, and has dilated loops of small bowel on x-ray."

2. **Stage the disease:** "I don't believe that this is severe disease because he does not have fever, evidence of sepsis, intractable pain, peritoneal signs, or leukocytosis."

3. **Treat based on stage:** "Therefore, my next step is to treat with nothing per mouth, NG (nasogastric) tube drainage, IV fluids, and observation."

4. **Follow the response:** "I want to follow the treatment by assessing his pain (I will ask him to rate the pain on a scale of 1-10 every day), his bowel function (I will ask whether he has had nausea or vomiting, or passed flatus), his temperature, abdominal examination, serum bicarbonate (for metabolic acidemia), and white blood cell count, and I will reassess him in 48 hours."

In a similar patient, when the clinical presentation is unclear, perhaps the best "next step" may be diagnostic, such as an oral contrast radiological study to assess for bowel obstruction.

CLINICAL PEARL

▶ Usually, the vague query, "What is your next step?" is the most difficult question because the answer may be diagnostic, staging, or therapeutic.

WHAT IS THE LIKELY MECHANISM FOR THIS PROCESS?

This question goes further than making the diagnosis, but also requires the student to understand the underlying mechanism for the process. For example, a clinical scenario may describe a 68-year-old man who notes urinary hesitancy and retention, and has a nontender large hard mass in his left supraclavicular region. This patient has bladder neck obstruction either as a consequence of benign prostatic hypertrophy or prostatic cancer. However, the indurated mass in the left neck area is suspicious for cancer. The mechanism is metastasis occurs in the area of the thoracic duct, because the malignant cells flow in the lymph fluid, which drains into the left subclavian vein. The student is advised to learn the mechanisms for each disease process, and not merely memorize a constellation of symptoms. Furthermore, in emergency medicine, it is crucial for the student to understand anatomy, physiology, and ways that would correct the problem.

WHAT ARE THE RISK FACTORS FOR THIS PROCESS?

Understanding the risk factors helps the practitioner to establish a diagnosis and to determine how to interpret tests. For example, understanding risk factor analysis may help in the management of a 55-year-old woman with anemia. If the patient has risk factors for endometrial cancer (such as diabetes, hypertension, anovulation) and complains of postmenopausal bleeding, she likely has endometrial carcinoma and should have an endometrial biopsy. Otherwise, occult colonic bleeding is a common etiology. If she takes NSAIDs or aspirin, then peptic ulcer disease is the most likely cause.

CLINICAL PEARL

▶ Being able to assess risk factors helps to guide testing and develop the differential diagnosis.

WHAT ARE THE COMPLICATIONS TO THIS PROCESS?

Clinicians must be cognizant of the complications of a disease so that they will understand how to follow and monitor the patient. Sometimes the student will have to make the diagnosis from clinical clues and then apply his or her knowledge of the consequences of the pathological process. For example, "a 26-year-old man complains of right-lower-extremity swelling and pain after a trans-Atlantic flight" and his Doppler ultrasound reveals a deep vein thrombosis. Complications of this process include pulmonary embolism (PE). Understanding the types of consequences also helps the clinician to be aware of the dangers to a patient. If the patient has any symptoms consistent with a PE, CT angiographic imaging of the chest may be necessary.

WHAT IS THE BEST THERAPY?

To answer this question, not only does the clinician need to reach the correct diagnosis and assess the severity of the condition, but the clinician must also weigh the situation to determine the appropriate intervention. For the student, knowing exact dosages is not as important as understanding the best medication, route of delivery, mechanism of action, and possible complications. It is important for the student to be able to verbalize the diagnosis and the rationale for the therapy.

CLINICAL PEARL

▶ Therapy should be logical and based on the severity of disease and the specific diagnosis. An exception to this rule is in an emergent situation such as respiratory failure or shock when the patient needs treatment even as the etiology is being investigated.

SUMMARY

1. The first and foremost priority in addressing the emergency patient is stabilization, then assessing and treating the ABCs (airway, breathing, circulation).

2. There is no replacement for a meticulous history and physical examination.

3. There are five steps in the clinical approach to the emergency patient: addressing life-threatening conditions, making the diagnosis, assessing severity, treating based on severity, and following response.

4. There are seven questions that help to bridge the gap between the textbook and the clinical arena.

REFERENCES

Hamilton GC. Introduction to emergency medicine. In: Hamilton GC, Sanders AB, Strange GR, Trott AT, eds. *Emergency Medicine: An Approach to Clinical Problem-Solving.* Philadelphia, PA: Saunders; 2003:3-16.

Hirshop JM. Basic CPR in adults. In: Tintinalli J, Stapczynski JS, Ma OJ, Cline D, Cydulka R, Meckler G, eds. *Emergency Medicine.* 8th ed. New York, NY: McGraw-Hill; 2015.

Ornato JP. Sudden cardiac death. In: Tintinalli J, Stapczynski JS, Ma OJ, Cline D, Cydulka R, Meckler G, eds. *Emergency Medicine.* 8th ed. New York, NY: McGraw-Hill; 2015.

Shapiro ML, Angood PB. Patient safety, errors, and complications in surgery. In: Brunicardi FC, Andersen DK, Billiar TR, et al, eds. *Schwartz's Principles of Surgery.* 10th ed. New York, NY: McGraw-Hill; 2014.

Cases

An 87-year-old man is brought in by ambulance from a skilled nursing facility after being found unresponsive in bed with rapid, shallow breathing after 3 days of worsening cough. Paramedics report his room air saturation in the field was 67%. In the emergency department he is obtunded with sonorous respirations, labored breathing, and copious thick yellow secretions. His vital signs are: temperature 38.7°C, BP 90/58 mm Hg, P 118 bpm, RR 29 breaths per minute, and oxygen saturation 84% on a non-rebreather face mask.

▶ What is the immediate first step in the management of this patient?
▶ What special factors need to be considered?

ANSWERS TO CASE 1:
Airway Management/Respiratory Failure

Summary: This patient is an elderly male with a depressed level of consciousness, hypoxia, respiratory distress, and pooling secretions. He is not oxygenating well or protecting his airway from aspiration.

- **First step:** This patient needs immediate airway management and endotracheal intubation.

- **Additional factors:** As a critically ill patient, it is important to attempt to verify his code status before intubating.

ANALYSIS

Objectives

1. Learn how to evaluate the airway and indications for intervention.

2. Become more familiar with emergency airway procedures.

3. Understanding of the rationale for and the steps involved with rapid sequence intubation.

4. Recognize and anticipate the potentially difficult airway and special circumstances.

Considerations

This patient has several concerning findings indicating he will need emergent airway management. He is hypoxic, tachypneic, and with his altered mental status, he may not able to protect his airway from aspiration of secretions or emesis. Because of his depressed level of consciousness and inability to protect his airway, he is not an appropriate candidate for noninvasive positive pressure ventilation (NIPPV) (such as bi-level positive airway pressure [BiPAP]).

He likely has a pneumonia and/or aspiration event, but it is also important to consider that he may have had a separate preceding event such as a cerebral vascular accident or medication overdose which created the altered mental status before aspirating. His other vital signs indicate that he is probably septic and will need to be resuscitated after his airway is addressed.

APPROACH TO:
Airway Management

CLINICAL APPROACH

Evaluation

Begin by observing the appearance of the patient, paying particular attention to key markers of oxygenation and ventilation skin color and presence of cyanosis, evidence of severe bronchospasm such as intercostal retractions, difficulty speaking, low or falling oxygen saturation, and increased or decreased respiratory rate. Evaluation of the airway includes not just the actual structures of the head and neck but also the patient's mental status and amount of secretions or blood present in the airway.

Indications for active airway intervention:

1. Respiratory failure: persistent and or worsening hypoxia, severe hypercarbia/respiratory acidosis.

2. Airway protection: absent gag, depressed level of consciousness, excess secretions.

3. Impending or existing airway obstruction: mass, infection, angioedema, foreign matter or excess secretions, etc.

4. Facilitation of further studies or to protect the airway during transport when deterioration may be anticipated.

Airway Protection There are several signs of an inadequately protected airway that indicate need for intubation: pooling secretions (eg, gurgling sounds with respiration), an absent or weak cough reflex, and depressed mental status, often correlating with Glasgow Coma Scale (GCS) of 8 or less. In general, a patient whose level of consciousness is depressed enough to tolerate insertion of an oropharyngeal airway (OPA) is not protecting his or her airway and requires airway protection.

Reversible and/or transient causes of a decreased level of consciousness must be considered prior to active airway intervention. Treating hypoglycemia or suspected opiate overdose before intubating can save the patient a major intervention. Additionally, providers should consider that the patient may be postictal, in which case they may improve rapidly to a point where they can protect their airway.

Respiratory Failure Respiratory failure refers to either failure to oxygenate or failure to ventilate. Failure to oxygenate is reflected by hypoxia despite maximum supplemental oxygen administration. Failure to ventilate indicated by elevated levels of carbon dioxide (measured on blood gas or capnography) can be equally life-threatening. Hypercapnia may manifest as somnolence, agitation, or otherwise altered mental status.

In select patients who are awake and alert, NIPPV (BiPAP) may be an option to delay or prevent intubation in the setting of hypoxic or hypercapnic respiratory failure.

Anticipated Clinical Deterioration The emergency physician needs to anticipate the potential clinical course of a patient and may wish to "intubate early" to avoid less controlled intubation conditions later. Situations in which this may be considered include worsening airway obstruction such as in patients with anaphylaxis, angioedema, severe burns or smoke inhalation, penetrating neck trauma with an expanding neck hematoma, epiglottitis, and deep space neck infections. Clinical scenarios that require the transfer of critically ill patients to a higher level of care requires a great deal of caution. If deterioration of the mental or respiratory status is anticipated, it may be prudent to proceed with intubation prior to transfer.

Facilitation of Medical Evaluation Occasionally, patients require intubation to safely complete necessary studies or procedures. One such scenario is that of the agitated trauma patient who requires emergent CT imaging. Here, sedation and intubation may be required to allow necessary interventions and diagnostic testing. Often, these patients can be promptly extubated after completion if they are without respiratory issues.

Interventions Airway management is much more than just intubation. It can be as simple as providing supplemental oxygen or repositioning the patient. Knowledge of minimally invasive maneuvers and devices can be lifesaving.

Supplemental Oxygen Supplemental oxygen can be delivered (in order of increasing delivery) via nasal cannula, face mask, non-rebreather mask, and high-flow nasal cannula. These are appropriate first steps for patients who are hypoxic but are otherwise protecting their airway.

Airway Positioning The most common cause of airway obstruction in the semiconscious or unconscious patient is loss of muscle tone, causing the tongue and soft tissue to occlude the airway. The simplest corrective maneuver is the chin lift. This maneuver is contraindicated in patients with a suspected cervical spine injury. A jaw thrust can also be performed by placing two or three fingers behind the angle of the mandible and lifting anteriorly. Since neck manipulation is not required, this maneuver can be safely performed in the context of cervical spine injury.

Other obstructive processes such as mediastinal masses, very large tonsils, or morbid obesity may require an upright position. A patient in respiratory failure from pulmonary edema will likely not tolerate laying flat, and it is important to allow them to be upright.

Airway Adjuncts Placement of an OPA and/or nasopharyngeal airway (NPA) may be highly effective in preventing the tongue from obstructing the posterior pharynx. The OPA is only used in unconscious patients who do not have a cough or a gag reflex. Using an appropriate-sized OPA is important; a device which is too small will be ineffective, while an overly large OPA can worsen obstruction. Using an OPA when giving positive pressure ventilations (PPVs) through a bag valve mask (BVM) can reduce obstruction caused by external pressure on the patient chin.

In the semiconscious patient with an intact gag reflex, insertion of an OPA can induce vomiting and possible aspiration. An NPA is the more appropriate adjunct for the semiconscious patient, as it rarely induces gagging. The NPA functions by helping bypass tongue obstruction. It is contraindicated in patients with severe facial trauma due to the risk of brain intrusion.

Suctioning along the sides of the mouth is also important in patients with pooling secretions. The suction device should not be inserted deep into the oropharynx where it is likely to induce gagging and emesis.

Noninvasive Positive Pressure Ventilation NIPPV is often used in the emergency department. Most commonly used NIPPV are continuous positive airway pressure (CPAP) and BiPAP. A tightly secured mask is used to deliver NIPPV without an invasive airway in place such as an endotracheal tube (ETT). In some patients its use may prevent the need for intubation. Patients who are most likely to respond to NIPPV have conditions such as chronic obstructive pulmonary disease and cardiogenic pulmonary edema. Other clinical indications include severe respiratory acidosis, hypoxia, dyspnea, tachypnea, and increased work of breathing. NIPPV can also be used temporarily as a preoxygenation technique before intubation.

Absolute contraindications to NIPPV include coma, cardiac arrest, respiratory arrest, and any condition warranting immediate intubation. Relative contraindications include evidence of airway obstruction, cardiac instability (shock requiring pressors, ventricular dysrhythmias), gastrointestinal (GI) bleeding, inability to protect airway, and status epilepticus.

Intubation The need for intubation is obvious when there is clear failure to oxygenate or ventilate using less invasive means. Decision making is far more difficult when the clinical indications are less extreme.

Crash intubations are indicated in pulseless and apneic patients, often without the use of preoxygenation or medications. Urgent intubations refer to patients needing intubation within minutes rather than seconds and do allow for the use of preoxygenation and induction medication. Stable patients who are likely to require active airway protection allow for a trial of alternative treatments and careful preparation.

RAPID SEQUENCE INTUBATION — *sedate + paralyze to prepare for intubation*

What Is It?

Rapid sequence intubation (RSI) attempts to simultaneously sedate and paralyze a patient while creating optimum intubating conditions. The major goal is to leave the airway unprotected for the shortest time possible. The procedure assumes that the patient may have a full stomach and is at risk of vomiting and aspiration.

What Are the Steps of Rapid Sequence Intubation?

Step 1: Preparation

Assess the Patient Is the patient a good candidate for RSI? Remember, the patient will be paralyzed, and the physician is taking complete control over the airway. How likely is the intubation to be successful? Can the patient be ventilated with a BVM if RSI should fail? Does the patient have dentures or signs of upper airway obstruction, such as drooling or stridor, due to edema, trauma, or mass? Heavy facial hair, a short thick neck, a recessed chin, or a large tongue should all be considered as potential impediments to BVM ventilation or oral tracheal intubation. A scar from a prior cricothyroidotomy is a concerning sign. Restriction of neck mobility or cervical spine immobilization will make intubation more difficult.

There are a few rules of airway evaluation that may be helpful in alert and cooperative patients. The first is the 3-3-2 rule. The patient should be able to insert at least 3 fingers into his/her mouth in the vertical orientation, between the upper and lower front teeth; the hyomental distance (from the hyoid cartilage to the chin) should be at least 3 finger breadth; and there should be at least 2 finger breadth between the floor of the mouth and the thyroid cartilage. The Mallampati score is another means of predicting intubation difficulty. The patient is asked to stick out his/her tongue while opening the mouth wide as possible. The amount of posterior pharynx visible is divided into four classes. The best view is referred to as "class one" and includes full visibility of the tonsils, uvula, and soft palate. The more limited class-three and class-four views may be associated with difficult intubations.

Concerns that the patient is not a good candidate for RSI should prompt consultation with an anesthesiologist. A surgeon should also be consulted if a cricothyroidotomy is likely.

Prepare Materials Necessary pre-intubation equipment includes oral and nasal pharyngeal airways, suction, oxygen, and a BVM. Basic intubation equipment includes a laryngoscope handle and several blades. The most commonly used laryngoscope blades are the curved Macintosh blade and the straight Miller blade. They should be tested for adequate light function before use.

Endotracheal tubes of various sizes and stylets must also be ready for use. The ETT has a distal balloon that should be inflated and deflated before use to test for leaks. The ETT should be preloaded with an internal stylet and is typically bent in the shape of a hockey stick to allow it to pass more anteriorly. Several other ETTs, at least a 1/2 size larger and smaller, should also be available. The formula used to predict ETT size for children ages 2 and older is: (age in years + 16)/4.

Airway "rescue" devices should always be available and familiar to the provider to be used in case of unexpected difficulty during intubation. These devices include bougies, a video laryngoscope, and several sizes of supraglottic airway devices. Cricothyroidotomy materials should always be nearby.

The medications selected for induction and paralysis should be drawn up and ready. The patient should be attached to a cardiac monitor with frequently cycling blood pressure, a pulse oximeter, and an end-tidal CO_2 monitor. Importantly, the patient must have a freely flowing IV. These steps are summarized by the mnemonic SOAP ME IV (Table 1–1).

Step 2: Preoxygenation This creates a greater reservoir of oxygen in the lungs via nitrogen washout. Three to five minutes of high-flow O_2 is adequate and allows

↳ if breathing

Table 1–1 • MATERIALS FOR ENDOTRACHEAL INTUBATION	
Suction	Pharmacology *(induction + paralysis)*
Oxygen	Monitoring Equipment *(cardiac, BP, Pulse ox, Tidal*
Airway adjuncts	IV *CO₂)*

for a substantial apneic period without oxygen desaturation in otherwise healthy patients (see Figure 1–1). Preoxygenating with high-flow oxygen requires that the patient is breathing. If the patient is apneic, studies have shown that eight full-volume BVM ventilations over 1 minute are equivalent. However, BVM ventilation of the spontaneously breathing patient is contraindicated because it unnecessarily increases the risk of gastric distension and aspiration.

Step 3: Pretreatment Manipulation of the airway causes a transient increase in intracranial pressure (ICP) that may harm patients with increased ICP (eg, intracerebral hemorrhage). Several medications may be used in sequence in attempt to diminish the effect of airway manipulation on ICP. Starting a few minutes before induction, fentanyl (3-5 µg/kg) followed by lidocaine (1.5 mg/kg) may be given, as well a defasciculating dose of the paralytic agent (1/10th the treatment dose). However, there are conflicting data regarding the potential benefit with the use of these medications, and pretreatment may lead to other complications and a delay in intubation.

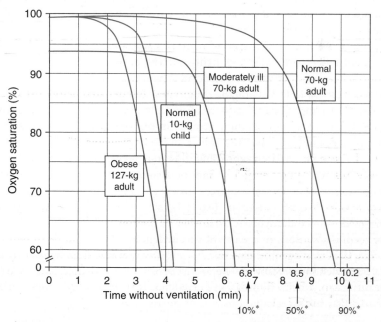

*Mean time to recovery of twitch from 1 mg/kg succinyl choline IV

Figure 1–1. **Hemoglobin desaturation curve.**

Table 1–2 • INDUCTION AGENTS					
Drug	IV Dose (mg/kg)	Class	BP	HR	Positive/Adverse Effects
Etomidate	0.3	Imidazole derivative	None	None	**Rapid onset** **Hemodynamically neutral** **cerebroprotection** Adrenal suppression → _avoid w/ sepsis_
Ketamine	1.5	Phencyclidine derivative	↑	↑	**Bronchodilator**/Increases ICP Avoid in pts with CAD✳
Propofol	1.5-2	Alkylphenol derivative	(↓↓)	None or ↑	**Rapid onset** Hypotension Egg allergy
Thiopental	3-5	Barbiturate	↓	None or ↑	**Rapid onset, short acting** Hypotension Histamine release

(handwritten margin notes: "status anaphylaxis shock" next to Ketamine; "Rapid seq. Intubation" next to Propofol)

Step 4: Induction and Paralysis (see Table 1–2) Induction involves administering a medication that will sedate the patient prior to paralysis. The induction agent most commonly used in emergency medicine is etomidate (0.3 mg/kg), as it meets these criteria well. It is rapidly sedating and hemodynamically neutral. It is also thought to be cerebroprotective. Although the clinical significance of this effect is uncertain, some physicians avoid etomidate when intubating septic patients due to concern for adrenal suppression.

Ketamine (1.5 mg/kg IV) may also be used for induction and is ideally suited for patients in status asthmaticus, anaphylactic shock, and sepsis. It has rapid onset of action and causes increases in blood pressure and heart rate through catecholamine release. It is unique in that it leaves airway reflexes protected and does not induce apnea. Additionally, it has bronchodilatory and analgesic properties. Propofol and thiopental are other fast-acting sedative agents of short duration but are less commonly used in RSI due to associated hypotension.

Paralysis (see Table 1–3) Paralytic drugs come in two basic types—depolarizing and nondepolarizing, describing their action at the neuromuscular junction. The only depolarizing agent in common clinical use is succinylcholine, which has the most rapid onset and shortest duration of all paralytics. It acts by transiently binding to acetylcholine (Ach) receptors and keeping ion channels open, leading to paralysis. Succinylcholine action at the motor endplate causes potassium efflux, elevating extracellular potassium levels, and it should be avoided in patients with recent or ongoing neuromuscular disorders, subacute burns, severe debilitation, crush injuries, or rhabdomyolysis. Acute head injury, acute burns, and acute strokes are not contraindications to the use of succinylcholine.

Nondepolarizing agents cause paralysis by competitive inhibition of the postsynaptic acetylcholine receptor. The agents most commonly used are rocuronium and vecuronium. Rocuronium is preferred for RSI among the nondepolarizing agents, as it has the most rapid onset and shortest duration.

Step 5: Positioning and Protection Patient positioning for RSI is extremely important. The proper head position in adults is the "sniffing" position, with the base

Table 1–3 • PARALYTIC AGENTS					
Drug	Dose	Class	Onset	Duration	Contraindications
Succinylcholine _binds ACh-R→ ↑K⁺ out_	1.5 mg/kg	[Depolarizing]	45-60 sec	6-10 min	Hyperkalemia, ✳ neuromuscular disorders, rhabdomyolysis
Rocuronium	1 mg/kg	Nondepolarizing	45-60 sec	30 min	Anticipated difficult airway
Vecuronium	0.01 mg/kg priming dose then 0.15 mg/kg	Nondepolarizing	2-3 min	20-40 min	Anticipated difficult airway

*handwritten annotations: "binds ACh-R→ ↑K⁺ out", "comp ⊖ of ACh-R", "*prefer w/ RSI"*

of the neck flexed forward and the head hyperextended. The patient's ear should be at the level of the sternum, and the head should be positioned at the end of the bed, which should be at an appropriate height for the operator. Once induction agents are given, firm downward pressure to the cricoid cartilage (known as the Sellick maneuver) may be considered to prevent aspiration. However, recent studies have suggested that this is likely ineffective and can worsen the view of the operator.

Step 6: Placement with Proof Once the patient is paralyzed and positioned, the ETT should be placed without delay. First, open the patient's mouth and insert the laryngoscope blade along the right side deep into the posterior oropharynx. Then move to the center, sweeping the tongue out of the way while lifting up and out to provide a view of the vocal cords. The ETT is advanced until the balloon is just beyond the vocal cords, and then the operator must **stop,** inflate the balloon, and remove the stylet.

The next step is to confirm that the ETT is in the right place. The absolute best way to do this is to watch it pass through the cords. Other confirmatory measures (end-tidal CO_2 change, fogging of the tube, and listening for breath sounds) should always be performed. However, these are nonspecific signs and can all be misleading in various circumstances.

Step 7: Postintubation Management Once placed and confirmed, the ETT must be secured. A chest x-ray is obtained to assess appropriate depth of the ETT. The chest x-ray is not useful for differentiating tracheal from esophageal intubation. Next, orders should be given for a longer-acting sedative agent as well as analgesia. Finally, ventilator settings should be established, which include the mode, respiratory rate, F_{IO_2}, tidal volume, and peak-end expiratory pressure. The seven Ps for RSI are summarized in Table 1–4.

CASE CORRELATION

- See also Case 2 (Hemorrhagic Shock), Case 3 (Sepsis), Case 4 (Resuscitation and Critical Care Medicine Practices in the Emergency Department), Case 5 (Diabetic Ketoacidosis), and Case 13 (Acute Exacerbation of Asthma).

Step	Name	Time to Intubation
Table 1–4 • THE 7 Ps FOR RSI		
1	Preparation* 332"	10 min
2	Preoxygenation high flow O₂ vs BVM	3-5 min
3	Pretreatment fent, Lidocaine	3 min
4	Paralysis with induction Eto, Ket→	1 min Succ, Rocuronium
5	Positioning and protection	45 sec
6	Placement with proof R→sweep middle	Time 0 *visualize vocal cords
7	Postintubation management αR	+ 1 min

COMPREHENSION QUESTIONS

1.1 You are evaluating a 34-year-old asthmatic patient for possible need for rapid sequence endotracheal intubation. How would you quickly judge the patient's mouth to assess airway and ease of intubation?

  A. Able to insert four fingers horizontally in the mouth

  B. Able to insert three fingers vertically between the front teeth

  C. 90-degree opening of the TMJ

  D. Able to jut the lower teeth and jaw at least 2 cm in front of the upper teeth

1.2 Which of the following is a contraindication to succinylcholine?

  A. Acute burns

  B. Acute renal failure

  C. History of coronary artery disease

  D. Sepsis

1.3 A 20-year-old man presents to the emergency department after being stung by a bee. His skin is red and covered with welts. He has obvious swelling of his lips and tongue but no wheezes, and he is able to open his mouth without difficulty. After treatment with appropriate medications, he complains of throat swelling, and his voice is hoarse. He has stridorous inspirations but a normal respiratory rate and effort and oxygen saturation. What is the most appropriate management of this patient's airway?

  A. Continued observation as long as oxygen saturation remains normal.

  B. Prepare for RSI.

  C. Begin high-dose nebulized albuterol and continue to observe.

  D. Cricothyroidotomy.

1.4 You are the first person on scene to a code blue in your hospital. You arrive to find an elderly woman who is unconscious, has a weak pulse, and does not appear to be breathing. Your first steps are:

A. Wait for the code cart to arrive and then intubate the patient.

B. Begin chest compressions and mouth-to-mouth resuscitation.

C. Attempt to remove any foreign body from the mouth and reposition the airway with chin lift or jaw thrust.

D. Begin bagging the patient immediately.

ANSWERS

1.1 **B.** In using the 3-3-2 rule, the first assessment is to judge the ability of the patient to open the mouth wide enough. Being able to insert three fingers between the front teeth is a good rough evaluation.

1.2 **B.** Succinylcholine transiently increases serum potassium levels. It is presumptively contraindicated in renal failure patients who often have elevated potassium levels. Acute burns are not a contraindication. Beginning 2 to 3 days after a burn, acetylcholine receptor upregulation can lead to hyperkalemia. Neither coronary artery disease nor sepsis is a contraindication to the use of succinylcholine.

1.3 **B.** This patient displays signs of impending airway obstruction. His worsening airway edema, despite appropriate medical therapy, dictates that intubation should be performed quickly before complete airway occlusion. There is no wheezing to suggest bronchoconstriction that could be treated with a bronchodilator such as albuterol. Stridor is a worrisome sign of upper airway obstruction. Normal respiratory rate and oxygen saturation should not delay intubation, as falling oxygen saturation is a late sign of respiratory failure. Cricothyroidotomy is only indicated after all other measures have failed, or if there is such upper airway edema and distortion that intubation would be impossible. For instance, findings of tachypnea, use of accessory muscles, and drooling may indicate the need for cricothyroidotomy.

1.4 **C.** The most common cause of airway obstruction is the tongue and/or soft tissues of the upper airway. No other adjuncts may be necessary for initial management except relieving the obstruction with airway repositioning. This should certainly be the first step, and there is no need to wait for the code cart before performing this maneuver. There is no indication for chest compressions in a patient with palpable pulses. The patient will require BVM ventilation after airway repositioning and placement of an oral airway. If the patient is easy to ventilate, reversible causes of respiratory depression, such as a narcotic overdose, should be investigated and may eliminate the need for RSI.

CLINICAL PEARLS

▶ Remember the noninvasive maneuvers and interventions that may eliminate the need for intubation: nasopharyngeal airways, chin lift, suction, BiPAP.

▶ Always have suction available.

▶ Bag-valve-mask ventilation is a lifesaving intervention for almost all patients with respiratory failure—know how to do it!

▶ Use an oral airway when bagging a patient.

▶ Head position is key for both basic and advanced airway management.

▶ Take time to thoroughly prepare for RSI. Poor preparation should never be the reason for a failed airway.

▶ Call anesthesia and/or surgery early if a difficult airway is anticipated.✶

▶ Always anticipate the difficult airway and have backup airway devices immediately available.

REFERENCES

Apfelbaum JL, Hagberg CA, Caplan RA, et al. Practice Guidelines for Management of the Difficult Airway: an Updated Report by the American Society of Anesthesiologists Task Force on Management of the Difficult Airway. *Anesthesiology.* 2013;118(2):251-270.

Brown CA, Bair AE, Pallin DJ, et al. Techniques, success, and adverse events of emergency department adult intubations. *Ann Emerg Med.* 2010;65(4):363-370.

Bruder EA, Ball IM, Ridi S, et al. Single induction dose of etomidate versus other induction agents for endotracheal intubation in critically ill patients. *Cochrane Database Syst Rev.* 2015;1:CD010225.

Delay JM, Sebbane M, Jung B, et al. The effectiveness of noninvasive positive pressure ventilation to enhance preoxygenation in morbidly obese patients: a randomized controlled study. *Anesth Analg.* 2008;107(5):1707-1713.

El-Orbany M, Connolly LA. Rapid sequence induction and intubation: current controversy. *Anesth Analg.* 2010;110(5):1318-1325.

Ellis DY, Harris T, Zideman D. Cricoid pressure in emergency department rapid sequence intubations: a risk-benefit analysis. *Ann Emerg Med.* 2007;50(6):653-665.

Hayes-Bradley C, Lewis A, Burns B, et al. Efficacy of Nasal Cannula Oxygen as a Preoxygenation Adjunct in Emergency Airway Management. *Ann Emerg Med.* 2016;68(2):174-180.

Kory P, Guevarra K, Mathew JP, et al. The impact of video laryngoscopy use during urgent endotracheal intubation in the critically ill. *Anesth Analg.* 2013;117(1):144-149.

Sakles JC, Javedani PP, Chase E, et al. The use of a video laryngoscope by emergency medicine residents is associated with a reduction in esophageal intubations in the emergency department. *Acad Emerg Med.* 2015;22(6):700-707.

Scherzer D, Leder M, Tobias JD. Pro-con debate: etomidate or ketamine for rapid sequence intubation in pediatric patients. *J Pediatr Pharmacol Ther.* 2012;17(2):142-149.

Upadhye S, Cyganik O. Is single-dose etomidate induction safe in emergency intubation of critically ill patients? *Ann Emerg Med*. 2016;67(3):399-400.

Walls RM. *Rapid Sequence Intubation in Manual of Emergency Airway Management*. 4th ed. Philadelphia, PA: Lippincott Williams & Wilkens; 2012.

Weingart SD, Trueger NS, Wong N, et al. Delayed sequence intubation: a prospective observational study. *Ann Emerg Med*. 2015;65(4):349-355.

A 23-year-old man is transported to your emergency department (ED) from the scene of a rollover motor vehicle collision (MVC). He was found approximately 1 hour after the accident occurred. At the scene, the patient was awake and complained of pain in his back and legs. In the ED, he is awake, his speech is clear and appropriate, and he has normal breath sounds over bilateral lung fields. He has palpable, equal bilateral femoral pulses. His temperature is 35.6°C (96.1°F) (rectally), pulse rate is 106 beats per minute, blood pressure is 110/88 mm Hg, respiratory rate is 24 breaths per minute, and Glasgow coma scale is 15. Multiple abrasions are noted over the neck, shoulders, abdomen, and legs. His chest wall is nontender. His abdomen is mildly tender. The pelvis is stable, but he has extensive swelling and tenderness of the right thigh. He has a deep scalp laceration over his right temporal area that continues to ooze. A focused abdominal sonography for trauma (FAST) examination is performed, revealing free fluid in Morison pouch and no other abnormalities. The patient's initial complete blood count (CBC) reveals a white blood cell count (WBC) of 14,800 cells/mm³, hemoglobin of 11.2 g/dL, and hematocrit of 34.4%.

► What is the next step in the evaluation of this patient?
► If this patient becomes hypotensive, what is the most likely cause?

ANSWERS TO CASE 2:

Hemorrhagic Shock

Summary: A healthy 23-year-old man presents following a motor vehicle accident with mild tachycardia, scalp laceration, femur fracture, and a tender abdomen with a positive FAST examination.

- **Next step: The Emergency Medicine approach to every critically ill patient begins with evaluation and stabilization of the airway, breathing, and circulation (ABC).** This approach is also advocated by Advanced Trauma Life Support (ATLS) guidelines. Once the ABCs are stabilized, a thorough secondary survey, consisting of a detailed physical examination, should follow. In this patient, the ABCs are stable, and the secondary survey reveals abdominal pain and a likely right femur fracture with intact pulses. Immediately subsequent to the secondary survey, the ultrasound examination demonstrates free fluid in the hepatorenal potential space known as Morison pouch. Presence of fluid in the hepatorenal space indicates intra-abdominal hemorrhage likely secondary to solid organ injury. Since this patient is hemodynamically stable, a computed tomography (CT) scan of the abdomen and pelvis should be done to identify and grade the severity of the injuries. In addition to estimating the amount of intraperitoneal free fluid, the CT scan can aid in identifying the source of bleeding and the presence of other injuries that may not have been appreciated on clinical examination. The limitations of CT scans in blunt trauma—mainly the lower sensitivity for hollow organ injuries and bowel wall hematomas—should be kept in mind when reviewing a CT scan in this setting.

- **Most likely cause of hypotension:** Hemorrhagic shock. The probable sources of blood loss in this patient are thigh, abdomen, and scalp laceration. Other possible causes or contributors to his hypotension are cardiogenic shock secondary to myocardial contusion or spinal shock secondary to injury to the spinal cord. The latter can easily be ruled out by performing a neurologic examination during the secondary survey, or even as part of the disability evaluation during the primary survey.

ANALYSIS

Objectives

1. Learn the basics of initial assessment of a trauma patient (Figure 2–1).

2. Learn the definitions and pathophysiology of shock and hemorrhagic shock.

3. Learn the advantages and disadvantages of base deficit, serum lactate, hemoglobin/hematocrit, and pulmonary artery catheter application for shock identification and patient resuscitation.

4. Learn the initial approach to managing and treating the patient with hemorrhagic shock.

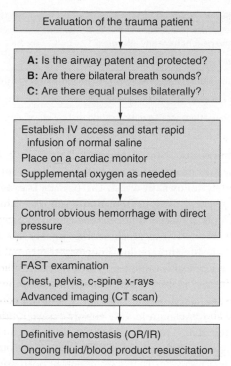

Figure 2–1. Algorithm for assessment/management of the trauma patient.

Initial Assessment of the Trauma Patient

The **first priorities in the evaluation of any trauma patient are the ABCs.** Airway is assessed by asking the patient to state his or her name, followed by noting the presence or absence of tracheal deviation. If the patient is unable to protect his airway because of confusion, loss of consciousness, or an extrinsic threat to the airway (ie, expanding neck hematoma), the patient should be intubated with an endotracheal tube. Next, breathing is assessed by listening to the chest for the presence of equal bilateral breath sounds and by observing the symmetry of chest wall expansion. The **unstable patient with clinical signs of pneumothorax or tension pneumothorax should be treated with immediate needle decompression** followed by placement of a chest tube. Finally, circulation is assessed via the vital signs and by palpation of bilateral femoral, radial, or pedal pulses. Any suggestion of cardiovascular instability requires immediate crystalloid or colloid resuscitation through two large bore peripheral IVs.

Next, the patient's ability to follow commands should be evaluated, and an overall assessment of his/her level of functioning should be made. This consists of assigning a score on the Glasgow coma scale, ranging from 3 to 15 (see also Table I–1 in Section I). Subsequently, a focused history should be quickly elicited. The **mnemonic "AMPLE"** is useful for guiding the history taking (Table 2–1).

Based on the capability of your hospital and trauma or emergency services, bedside ultrasound can be incorporated into the initial evaluation of the trauma patient. Aside from the FAST examination (assessment for free fluid in Morison pouch, splenorenal and supra-splenic space, pelvis, and pericardial space), ultrasound can be used for rapid

Table 2–1 • "AMPLE" GUIDE TO HISTORY-TAKING IN THE TRAUMA PATIENT	
A	Does the patient have any **allergies?**
M	Does the patient take any **medications?**
P	Does the patient have any significant **past medical history?**
L	When was the patient's **last meal?**
E	Does the patient recall **events** leading up to, or involving, the accident?

identification of pneumothorax, hemothorax, cardiac activity, and central line placement if needed. The use of ultrasound in the trauma patient is operator-dependent.

The secondary survey follows, in which the patient is examined from head to toe. In the presence of severe, obvious injuries, it is appropriate to start the examination at the affected sites. However, one must be cautious and diligent to complete a thorough physical examination to preclude missing any less obvious but equally important or potentially life-threatening injuries. Additional history from paramedics and emergency medical technicians (EMTs) should also be elicited.

In this patient, the entire history is very concerning. In addition to being ejected from a vehicle involved in a collision at high speed and therefore at risk for multisystem injuries secondary to a high kinetic energy transfer, the patient was found 1 hour following the incident. The risk for hypothermia and a diminished ability to respond to hemorrhagic shock is great.

APPROACH TO:
Hemorrhagic Shock

DEFINITIONS

SHOCK: Insufficient cellular perfusion/inability to deliver sufficient oxygen to the tissues.

HEMORRHAGIC SHOCK: Inadequate tissue oxygenation resulting from a blood volume deficit. In this situation, the loss of blood volume decreases venous return, cardiac filling pressures, and cardiac output. End-organ perfusion is subsequently decreased, as blood flow is preferentially preserved to the brain and heart.

CLINICAL APPROACH

In shock, the lack of oxygen available to cells results in an inability of mitochondria to generate adequate ATP. Instead, anaerobic metabolism dominates, leading to an accumulation of pyruvate that is converted to lactate.

Shock is divided into three stages: compensated, progressive, and irreversible. Shock is initially compensated by control mechanisms that return cardiac output and arterial pressure back to normal levels. Within seconds, baroreceptors and chemoreceptors elicit powerful sympathetic stimulation that vasoconstricts arterioles and increases heart rate and cardiac contractility. After minutes to hours, angiotensin constricts the peripheral arteries while vasopressin constricts the veins to maintain arterial pressures and improve blood return to the heart. Angiotensin and vasopressin also increase water retention, thereby improving cardiac filling pressures. Locally, vascular control preferentially dilates vessels around the hypoxic tissues to increase blood flow to injured areas. The **normal manifestations of shock do not apply** to pregnant women, athletes, and individuals with altered autonomic nervous systems (older patients, those taking β-blockers).

As shock evolves into the *progressive stage*, **arterial pressure falls.** This leads to cardiac depression from decreased coronary blood flow and in turn further decreases arterial pressure. The result is a feedback loop that becomes a vicious cycle toward uncontrolled deterioration. Inadequate blood flow to the nervous system eventually results in complete inactivation of sympathetic stimulation. In the microvasculature, low blood flow causes the blood to sludge, amplifying the inadequate delivery of oxygen to the tissues. This ischemia results in increased microvascular permeability, and large quantities of fluid and protein move from the intravascular space to the extravascular compartment, which exacerbates the already decreased intravascular volume. The **systemic inflammatory response syndrome caused by severe injury and shock may progress to multiorgan failure.** Pulmonary edema, acute respiratory distress syndrome (ARDS), poor cardiac contractility, loss of electrolyte and fluid control, and inability to metabolize toxins and waste products set in. Cells lose the ability to maintain electrolyte balance, metabolize glucose, maintain mitochondrial activity, and prevent lysosomal release of hydrolases. Resuscitation during this progressive stage of tissue ischemia can cause reperfusion injury from the burst of oxygen-free radicals.

Finally, the patient enters the *irreversible stage* of shock, and any therapeutic efforts become futile. Despite transiently elevated arterial pressures and cardiac output, the body is unable to recover, and death becomes inevitable.

Pathophysiology and Stages of Hemorrhagic Shock

Hemorrhagic shock is the most common cause of death in trauma patients aside from traumatic brain injury. A high level of suspicion for hemorrhage and hemorrhagic shock should dominate evaluation of a trauma patient, especially as vital signs may not become abnormal until a significant amount of hemorrhage has occurred. Hemorrhagic shock is classified by the ATLS into four categories to further emphasize the progression of vital sign instability in response to blood loss (Table 2–2).

Table 2–2 • ATLS CLASSIFICATION OF HEMORRHAGE				
Class of Hemorrhage	Class I	Class II	Class III	Class IV
Blood loss (mL)	<750	750-1500	1500-2000	>2000
Pulse (beats/min)	<100	>100	>120	>140
Blood pressure	Normal	Normal	Decreased	Decreased
Pulse pressure (mm Hg)	Normal	Decreased	Decreased	Decreased
Respiratory rate (breaths/min)	14-20	20-30	30-40	>40
Urine output (mL/h)	>30	20-30	5-15	Negligible
Central nervous system (mental status)	Slightly anxious	Mildly anxious	Anxious, confused	Lethargic

Additional clinical signs that indicate hemorrhagic shock include skin pallor/coolness, delayed capillary refill, weak distal pulses, and anxiety.

As demonstrated by the ATLS classification of stages of hemorrhagic shock, the clinician must not rely solely on vital signs for determination of extent of hemorrhage. This patient obviously has had some blood loss from his femur fracture, and the **FAST examination suggests intra-abdominal solid organ injury associated with additional hemorrhage.** Additionally, his scalp laceration must be evaluated as a potential source for serious exsanguination. Despite these multiple sources of hemorrhage, our patient has a normal blood pressure and only a slightly elevated heart rate, which places him in Class II hemorrhagic shock.

DIAGNOSTIC APPROACH

Identify the Source of Bleeding

A trauma patient should be carefully screened to locate the source of blood loss. The possibility of bleeding should be assessed in **five areas:** (1) **external bleeding** (eg, scalp/extremity lacerations); (2) **thorax** (eg, hemothorax and aortic injury); (3) **peritoneal cavity** (eg, solid organ lacerations and large vessel injury); (4) **pelvis/retroperitoneum** (eg, pelvic fracture); and (5) **soft-tissue compartments** (eg, long-bone fractures). Adjunctive studies that should be obtained in blunt trauma patients early during their evaluation include chest and pelvic roentgenograms and CT scans of the head, chest, abdomen, and pelvis. Chest roentgenograms can identify a hemothorax and potential mediastinal bleeding. Pelvic films can demonstrate pelvic fractures as a source of pelvic blood loss. Films of any affected extremity, in this case the femur, should also be obtained. Fractures are not only associated with blood loss from the bone and adjacent soft tissue, but their presence indicates significant energy transfer (often referred to as a significant mechanism of injury) and should increase the clinical suspicion for intra-abdominal and retroperitoneal bleeding. Typically, tibial or humeral fractures can be associated with 750 mL of blood loss (1.5 units of blood), whereas femur fractures can be associated with up to 1500 mL of blood (3 units of blood) in the thigh. Pelvic fractures may result in even more blood loss; up to several liters can be lost into a retroperitoneal hematoma.

Laboratory Evaluation

Laboratory studies that aid (but are not necessary) in evaluating acute blood loss are hemoglobin, hematocrit, base deficit, and lactate levels. In the setting of **acute hemorrhage hemoglobin and hematocrit levels may or may not be decreased.** These values measure concentration, not absolute amounts. Hemoglobin is measured in grams of red blood cells per deciliter of blood; hematocrit is the percentage of blood volume that is red blood cells. Loss of whole blood will not decrease the red blood cell concentration or the percentage of red cells in blood. The initial minor drops in hemoglobin and hematocrit levels are the result of mechanisms that compensate for blood loss by drawing fluid into the vascular space. To see significant decreases in these values, blood loss must be replaced with crystalloid solution; therefore, most decreases in hemoglobin and hematocrit values are not seen until patients have received large volumes of crystalloid fluid for resuscitation.

With the ongoing metabolic acidosis of hemorrhagic shock, an increased base deficit and lactate level will be seen. **Both lactate and base deficit levels are laboratory values that indicate systemic acidosis, not local tissue ischemia.** They are global indices of tissue perfusion, and normal values may mask areas of under-perfusion as a consequence of normal blood flow to the remainder of the body. These laboratory tests are not true representations of tissue hypoxia. It is, therefore, not surprising that **lactate and base deficit are poor prognostic indicators of survival in patients with shock.** Although absolute values of these laboratory results are not predictors of survival in patients with shock, the baseline value and trends can be used to determine the extent of tissue hypoxia and adequacy of resuscitation. **Normalization of base deficit and serum lactate within 24 hours after resuscitation is a good prognostic indicator of survival.** Of note, because lactate is metabolized in the liver, it is not a reliable value in patients with liver dysfunction.

Central Monitoring

The approach to central monitoring in the trauma patient has changed dramatically. The biggest benefit of central monitoring is to accurately determine cardiac preload, given that preload, or end-diastolic sarcomere length, is the driving force behind the cardiac output as defined by the Starling Curve. Previously, placement of a pulmonary artery (PA) catheter was used to measure the pulmonary capillary occlusion (wedge) pressure. This number was used as an approximation of left atrial pressure, which in turn was an indirect measurement of left ventricular end-diastolic pressure and volume. **Left-ventricular end-diastolic volume is considered the best clinical estimate of preload.** However, in recent years the invasive nature and complications associated with PA catheters has raised concern about their placement. Clinical practice varies, but in general it has shifted toward the use of central venous catheters recording central venous pressure (CVP) to estimate volume status. Even more recently, ultrasound has been used to assess intravascular volume status by examining the respiratory variation of the inferior vena cava (more variation signifying low intravascular volume) or by calculating a ratio of the diameter of the IVC to the aorta. The adoption of these techniques is highly institution-specific.

Management of Hemorrhagic Shock

Resuscitation The **most common and easily available fluid replacements are isotonic crystalloid solutions,** such as normal saline or lactated Ringer solution. For each liter of these solutions that is infused, approximately 300 mL stays in the intravascular space, while the remainder leaks into the interstitial space. This distribution has led to the guideline of **3 mL crystalloid replacement for each 1 mL of blood loss.** A blood transfusion is indicated if the patient persists in shock despite the rapid infusion of 2 to 3 L of crystalloid solution or if the patient has had such severe blood loss that cardiovascular collapse is imminent. When possible, typed and cross-matched blood is optimal; however, in the acute setting, this is often unfeasible. Type-specific unmatched blood is the next best option, followed by O-negative blood in females and O-positive blood in males. Blood is generally administered as packed erythrocytes or packed red blood cells (PRBCs). Crystalloids, fresh-frozen plasma (FFP), and/or platelets may need to be transfused if massive blood volumes have been given. Transfusion protocols differ by institution regarding the ratio of FFP to platelets to PRBCs that should be administered. Colloid solutions such as albumin and hetastarch or dextran are not superior to crystalloid replacement in the acute setting and have the potential for large fluid shifts and pulmonary or bowel wall edema. Hypertonic solutions such as 7.5% saline have the advantage of retaining as much as 500 mL in the intravascular space and may be useful in trauma situations with no access to blood products, such as in military settings.

The concept of permissive hypotension is now more widely accepted in trauma care. The central tenet is that patients suffering from hemorrhagic shock (excluding intracranial hemorrhages) may benefit from judicious fluid administration. In permissive hypotension, the patient's blood pressure is not resuscitated to their normal blood pressure, or to what physicians consider a normal blood pressure. Instead, the blood pressure is allowed to remain low (mean arterial pressures of 60-70 mm Hg or a systolic blood pressure of 80-90 mm Hg). Permissive hypotension is thought to be effective in hemorrhagic shock because it is theorized that post-hemorrhage, the artificially increased blood pressure by aggressive fluid resuscitation may disrupt endogenous clot formation and promote further bleeding. Also, crystalloid is often administered at room temperature, which is actually colder than the body temperature and can result in hypothermia following excessive administration. Crystalloid can also dilute the endogenous clotting factors and erythrocyte concentration, resulting in poorer control of bleeding and also diminished oxygen carrying capacity. Though shown to have great benefits in animal models, permissive hypotension studies in humans are few. However, this concept is becoming more accepted in trauma centers. Patients who are not candidates for permissive hypotension are: (1) those with traumatic brain injuries who require maintenance of their cerebral perfusion pressure; and (2) those with a history of hypertension, congestive heart failure, or coronary artery disease, since these individuals may not tolerate hypotension, leading to stroke or myocardial infarction.

Controlling Hemorrhage Achieving hemostasis is paramount in managing the trauma patient with hemorrhagic shock. Wounds amenable to local tamponade with direct pressure, dressings, or tourniquet application should be managed as such. For other injuries that require operative repair, such as intra-abdominal injuries or pelvic fractures that require advanced therapies such as interventional radiology (IR)-guided embolization, the appropriate specialists should be contacted immediately. While contacting and arranging for further definitive care, appropriate resuscitation of the patient should be initiated.

CASE CORRELATION

- See also Case 1 (Advanced Airway Management/Respiratory Failure), Case 3 (Sepsis), Case 4 (Resuscitation and Critical Care Medicine Practices in the Emergency Department), Case 17 (GI Bleeding), Case 43 (Penetrating Trauma), and Case 45 (Trauma at Extremes of Age).

COMPREHENSION QUESTIONS

2.1 A 32-year-old man was involved in a knife fight and had stab injuries to his abdomen, though it is unclear how deep these injuries are. He is brought into the emergency room with a heart rate of 110 beats per minute and blood pressure of 84/50 mm Hg. Based on the clinical assessment, which of the following is the amount of acute blood loss he has experienced?

    A. 250 mL

    B. 500 mL

    C. 1000 mL

    D. 1500 mL

2.2 Which of the following is an advantage of the FAST examination in a patient with hemorrhagic shock?

    A. Can identify retroperitoneal hematomas

    B. Can be performed quickly at bedside

    C. Can identify the specific site of injury

    D. Can quantify the exact amount of blood loss

2.3 A 20-year-old man involved in a motor vehicle accident is brought into the emergency room having lost much blood at the accident scene. His initial blood pressure is 80/40 mm Hg and heart rate 130 beats per minute. He is given 3 L of normal saline intravenously and is still hypotensive. Which of these statements most accurately describes the pathophysiology of his condition?

    A. Insufficient cardiac preload

    B. Insufficient myocardial contractility

    C. Excessive systemic vascular resistance

    D. Excessive IL-6 and leukotrienes

2.4 A 35-year-old man has been involved in a motor vehicle accident and is found to be hypotensive. Which of the following locations of bleeding can cause significant complications but does not explain the hypotension?

    A. Chest and abdomen

    B. Pelvic girdle and soft-tissue compartments

    C. External bleeding

    D. Intracranial bleeding

ANSWERS

2.1 **D.** Blood pressure at rest typically does not decrease until class III hemorrhagic shock, when 1500 to 2000 mL of blood is lost (30%-40% of blood volume). Class I hemorrhagic shock is well compensated associated with 750 mL estimated blood loss (EBL) or less, with no effect on blood pressure and minimal effect on heart rate. Class II shock, associated with 750 to 1500 mL EBL, is associated with tachycardia but normal blood pressure at rest, and low urine output.

2.2 **B.** DPL and FAST cannot rule out retroperitoneal injury or identify the specific site of injury, but they can be performed quickly at bedside on unstable trauma patients. To find the specific site of injury and rule out retroperitoneal injury, a CT scan can be done; however, the trauma patient must be hemodynamically stable to be transported to the CT scan suite.

2.3 **A.** In situations of trauma and hemorrhage, persistent hypotension is caused by blood loss unless otherwise proven, leading to reduced preload. Preload is end-diastolic sarcomere length, and insufficient circulating volume does not allow for sufficient venous return or cardiac output.

2.4 **D.** It is important to systematically check for bleeding sources in the chest, abdomen, pelvic girdle, soft-tissue compartments (long-bone fractures), and external bleeding. Intracranial bleeding, although a significant injury, is usually not the cause of hypotension. The exception to this is the patient who is moribund secondary to a head injury.

CLINICAL PEARLS

▶ Evaluation of a trauma patient begins with assessment and stabilization of the ABCs.

▶ Hypotension in a trauma patient is hemorrhage until proven otherwise.

▶ A trauma patient should be assessed systematically for the source of hemorrhage.

▶ Laboratory evaluation is not as sensitive as the combination of history, clinical examination, physical examination findings, and vital sign abnormalities for the diagnosis of hemorrhagic shock.

▶ Therapy must be initiated promptly with blood product administration or with fluids if blood products are not immediately available.

▶ Definitive therapy for control of hemorrhage should be arranged as soon as possible.

REFERENCES

Ali J. Priorities in multisystem trauma. In: Hall JB, Schmidt GA, Kress JP, eds. *Principles of Critical Care.* 4th ed. New York, NY: McGraw-Hill; 2015:1116-1121.

Holcroft JW. Shock—approach to the treatment of shock. In: Wilmore DW, Cheung LY, Harken AH, et al, eds. *ACS Surgery.* New York, NY: Webmed Professional Publishers; 2003:61-74.

Peck G, Buchman TG. Initial assessment and resuscitation of the trauma patient. In: Cameron JL, Cameron AM, eds. *Current Surgical Therapy.* New York, NY: Elsevier Saunders; 2014:981-984.

Wilson M, Davis DP, Coimbra R. Diagnosis and monitoring of hemorrhagic shock during the initial resuscitation of multiple trauma patients: a review. *J Emerg Med.* 2003;24(4):413-422.

A 73-year-old woman is brought to the emergency center from an assisted-living facility. The patient has a history of dementia, hypertension, and type II diabetes mellitus. By report, she has had chills and a productive cough for several days. In the past 24 hours she has become weaker and does not want to get out of bed. The physical examination reveals a thin, elderly woman who is somnolent but arousable. Her rectal temperature is 38.2°C (100.8°F), pulse rate is 118 beats per minute, blood pressure is 84/50 mm Hg, and respiratory rate is 22 breaths per minute. Her mucous membranes are dry. Her heart is tachycardic but regular. She has crackles at her right lung base with a scant wheeze. Her abdomen is soft and nontender. The extremities feel cool, and her pulses are rapid and thready. The patient is moving all extremities without focal deficits.

▶ What is the most likely diagnosis?
▶ What is the most likely etiology for this condition?

ANSWERS TO CASE 3:

Sepsis

Summary: A 73-year-old woman presents from an assisted-living facility with cough, lethargy and hypotension of unknown etiology.

- **Most likely diagnosis:** Sepsis.
- **Most likely etiology:** Pneumonia (Health-Care Associated).

ANALYSIS

Objectives

1. Learn to recognize the clinical presentations of sepsis.

2. Learn the pathophysiology, systemic effects, and management of sepsis and its common complications.

3. Become familiar with the initial Emergency Department therapy for the treatment of sepsis and septic shock.

Considerations

This woman appears to be suffering from sepsis, a clinical entity on the continuum from mild infection to septic shock with multiorgan system failure. In her case, the etiology is likely pneumonia, an extremely common cause of sepsis in elderly patients, and given her residence in a nursing home, she is by definition a patient with Health Care-Associated Pneumonia (HCAP). The current focus on emergency department care is on rapid recognition and treatment of these patients. Rapid assessment of sepsis severity involves using the **quick SOFA (sequential organ failure assessment) score and lactate assessment.** See below for details. Early antibiotics and appropriate fluid administration should be initiated **within 3 hours** of arrival at the Emergency Department.

APPROACH TO:

Sepsis

PATHOPHYSIOLOGY

Sepsis occurs when a generalized proinflammatory response results from an infectious trigger. Typically, a bacterial pathogen enters a sterile site and initiates a localized host response. Immune cells, particularly macrophages, recognize and bind microbial components, setting off a series of reactions that result in bacterial lysis with phagocytosis of bacterial components and injured cells/tissue. This process can be associated with the production and release of a range of proinflammatory cytokines (eg, tumor necrosis factor-alpha, interleukin-1) resulting in additional inflammatory cell recruitment. When the response becomes generalized, a systemic inflammatory response and sepsis can be recognized. Continued cellular injury leads to tissue ischemia, cytopathic injury, and alteration in apoptosis. The mechanism of organ failure may relate to decreased oxygen delivery and utilization, imbalance in the coagulation and fibrinolytic system, and cytopathic injury.

DIAGNOSIS

The systemic inflammatory response syndrome (SIRS) criteria was previously used as the cornerstone to establish the diagnosis of the host response to infection. These criteria consisted of:

1. Temperature >38°C or <36°C

2. Heart rate >90 beats per minute

3. Tachypnea or hyperventilation (respiratory rate >20 breaths per minute or $PaCO_2$ <32 mm Hg)

4. White blood cell count >12,000 cells/mL or <4000 cells/mL, or >10% bands.

A patient with **two out of four of these criteria** who was also confirmed to have, or was suspected of having, an infection was considered to have the **diagnosis of sepsis.** A patient with sepsis-related organ failure or lactate >4 mmol/L was classified as **severe sepsis. Septic shock** was defined as sepsis with **hypotension** (SBP < 90 mm Hg or MAP < 70 mm Hg) **after** 30 mL/kg crystalloid fluid bolus.

In 2016, The Third International Consensus Definitions for Sepsis and Septic Shock (Sepsis-3) redefined the term **sepsis as life-threatening organ dysfunction due to a dysregulated host response secondary to an infection.** Retrospective studies of patients with confirmed sepsis have demonstrated that the SIRS criteria lack adequate sensitivity and specificity for the diagnosis of sepsis, and thus the inclusion of these variables as part of the new definition for sepsis have been removed. Per Sepsis-3 recommendations, sepsis clinical criteria should be defined by an increase of 2 points or more in the **Sequential Organ Failure Assessment (SOFA) score.** Patients with suspected infection who are likely to have a prolonged ICU stay or die in the hospital can be promptly identified at the bedside with a quick SOFA (qSOFA) score of 2 or more. The qSOFA score assigns one point to each of the following: (1) hypotension (SBP ≤ 100 mm Hg), (2) altered mental status (any GCS < 15), and (3) tachypnea (RR ≥ 22/min). The mnemonic **HAT** has been proposed to assist in remembering these elements (H—hypotension, A—altered mental status, T—tachypnea). The Sepsis-3 group considered the term severe sepsis redundant, and this terminology has been removed. Septic shock is a subset of sepsis in which the underlying circulatory and cellular/metabolic abnormalities are significant enough to substantially worsen mortality. Patients who, after adequate volume resuscitation, have persistent hypotension requiring vasopressors to maintain MAP greater than or equal to 65 mm Hg and also have a lactate greater than or equal to 2 mmol/L are categorized as having septic shock.

CLINICAL PRESENTATION

The clinical manifestations of sepsis depend on the initial site of infection, the causative organism, the pattern of acute organ dysfunction, the underlying health status of the patient, and the interval before initiation of treatment. Sepsis begins with signs of an inflammatory response (eg, fever, tachycardia, tachypnea, and leukocytosis) and can progress to hypotension and organ dysfunction. It is important to remember that, especially in **infants and the elderly,** initial presentation may lack some of the more salient features—that is, they may present with **hypothermia** rather than hyperthermia, leukopenia rather than leukocytosis, and they may not be able to mount a tachycardia (as in elderly patients on beta- or calcium channel-blockers) or they may have a tachycardia attributed to other causes (as in anxious infants). In a patient at the extremes of age, any nonspecific systemic complaint—vomiting, fatigue, behavioral changes—should prompt concern for infection, with a low threshold to obtain a chest radiograph and urinalysis.

EVALUATION AND MANAGEMENT

Like many severe acute illnesses, treatment of sepsis must start at the first suspicion of the diagnosis, and thereafter evaluation and treatment should proceed simultaneously.

Initial Treatment Considerations

Any critically ill patient should immediately be placed on continuous cardiac and pulse-oxygenation monitoring with automated manual blood pressure checks. Supplemental oxygen by nasal cannula or facemask should be titrated to keep oxygen saturation greater than 93%, two large bore, peripheral IVs should rapidly be inserted, and in the absence of a fluid overload condition (eg, congestive heart failure and advanced renal failure), a fluid bolus of 30 mL/kg (2-4 L in adults) crystalloid administered. Intubation with mechanical ventilation should be initiated for a patient who is unable to adequately protect their airway.

Blood should be drawn for a complete blood count (with differential), comprehensive metabolic panel, blood cultures (two sets), and **lactic acid level.** A urinalysis with culture (and urine pregnancy test in a woman of child-bearing age) and chest x-ray should be obtained expeditiously. An ECG should also be ordered early in the work-up to evaluate for cardiac ischemia secondary to hypoperfusion (see Table 3–1).

A smaller fluid bolus may be appropriate for patients with significant underlying fluid overload conditions (eg, congestive heart failure and advanced renal failure).

Intravenous antibiotics should be started rapidly—ideally after the cultures have been drawn and **within 3 hours of presentation** to the Emergency Department. Initial broad-spectrum therapy against both gram-positive and gram-negative bacteria is recommended, as there is evidence that inappropriate antibiotic selection is associated with worsened mortality. Table 3–2 has a list of suggested antibiotics based on suspected source of the infection. Consult with your local

Table 3–1 • INITIAL MANAGEMENT OF PATIENT WITH SUSPECTED SEPSIS
Two large bore IVs
Lactic acid
Initial fluid bolus of 30 mL/kg over the first 3 hours of treatment*
CBC
CMP
Blood cultures (2 sets)
Urinalysis with culture
Pregnancy test in women of childbearing age
Chest radiograph
Consider lumbar puncture (LP) if meningitis is suspected
Empiric antibiotics (ideally after blood cultures obtained)

hospital's antibiotic guide or Infectious Disease specialist for clarification of antibiotic choice.

If the patients (or caretakers) are able to report any preceding symptoms that hint at other sources, or your examination leads you to consider a source other than the lungs or urine, it should be immediately investigated, with a low threshold for ordering imaging studies. If a source is found and is amenable to an intervention (eg, laparotomy for a perforated appendicitis, dilation and curettage for retained products of conception, or removal of an infected intravenous catheter), such measures should be taken as soon as the patient is stable enough to undergo the procedure.

SUBSEQUENT PRIORITIES

Frequent reassessment is key to good patient care of critically ill patients. Immediately upon conclusion of the 30 mL/kg crystalloid fluid bolus, the patient should be reassessed by repeat focused examination (including vital signs, cardiopulmonary exam,

Table 3–2 • ANTIBIOTIC SELECTION RECOMMENDATIONS	
Location	Antibiotcics
Sepsis, source unclear	Pip/tazo + vancomycin + amikacin (1 dose)
Suspected Pulmonary source	CAP: Pip/tazo + levofloxacin HCAP: Pip/tazo + vancomycin + amikacin (1 dose)
Suspected Urinary source	Levofloxacin (or Ceftazadime for severe infections)+ amikacin (1 dose)
Suspected Intra-abdominal source	Pip/tazo (or Cefoxitin for perforated appendicitis or cholecystitis; or levofloxacin ± PO vancomycin for colitis)
Suspected Pelvic infection	Cefoxitin + doxycycline
Suspected Skin/Soft tissue source	Cefazolin ± vancomycin
Suspected CNS source	Vancomycin + Ceftriaxone ± Ampicillin
Suspected Cardiac infection	Pip/tazo + vancomycin + amikacin (1 dose)
Suspected Line-associated	Vancomycin

capillary refill, pulse, and skin findings), central venous pressure monitoring, central venous oxygen saturation assessment, bedside cardiovascular ultrasound, and/or dynamic assessment of fluid responsiveness to passive leg raise or fluid challenge. Additionally, a repeat lactate is often obtained at this stage to monitor the response to the initial therapy. **If the patient continues to be hypotensive *or* has a repeat lactate level greater than 2 mmol/dL, the patient falls into the category of septic shock and additional interventions, specifically vasopressor use, should be initiated.**

In 2001, a standardized early-goal directed treatment (EGDT) protocol that consisted of (1) crystalloid or colloid fluid boluses to maintain a central venous pressure of 8 to 12 mm Hg, (2) maintaining a mean arterial pressure of greater than 65 mm Hg with the use of vasopressors, and (3) using packed red blood cell transfusions, a positive inotrope such as dobutamine, and intubation/mechanical ventilation to ensure central venous oxygen saturation greater than 70%, resulted in a significant mortality reduction in patients with sepsis and septic shock. Since that time three large, well-done, multicenter, randomized controlled trials have concluded that the **early use of antibiotics, adequate crystalloid fluid resuscitation, and vasopressors constitute the foundation of good sepsis care in the Emergency Department.** The use of additional therapies, such as inotropic therapy or red blood cell transfusion, are typically reserved for patients with refractory shock (ie, MAP < 65 mm Hg) in whom the $ScvO_2$ remains less than 70% after optimization of intravenous fluid and vasopressor therapy. Additional therapies are listed in Table 3–3.

Table 3–3 • ADDITIONAL THERAPIES FOR SEPTIC SHOCK	
Therapy	**Rationale/Current Status**
Glucocorticoids	Evidence from randomized trials suggests that corticosteroid therapy is most likely to be beneficial in patients who have severe septic shock unresponsive to adequate fluid resuscitation and vasopressor administration.
Intensive insulin therapy	The optimal blood glucose range is controversial. Most clinicians target blood glucose levels between 140 and 180 mg/dL (7.7 to 10 mmol/L).
External cooling	Evidence from single randomized controlled trial supports use of external cooling in febrile patients with septic shock requiring vasopressors, mechanical ventilation, and sedation. Additional trials are needed before this intervention can be recommended.
Antipyretics for fever control	The role of antipyretics for fever control in critically ill patients is of uncertain benefit.
Venous thromboembolism prophylaxis	Patients with sepsis and septic shock are at increased risk for venous thromboembolism such that patients should receive thromboprophylaxis.
Gastric ulcer prophylaxis	Indicated to protect against formation of gastric ulcer in critically ill patients.

COMPLICATIONS

Acute Lung Injury (ALI) and Acute Respiratory Distress Syndrome (ARDS): The diagnostic criteria for acute lung injury and acute respiratory distress syndrome include: (1) acute onset, (2) presence of bilateral infiltrates on chest radiography consistent with pulmonary edema, (3) pulmonary artery wedge pressure less than 18 mm Hg or clinical absence of left atrial hypertension, and (4) hypoxemia with PaO_2/FiO_2 less than or equal to 300 mm Hg for ALI or less than or equal to 200 mm Hg for ARDS. Specific ventilator strategies (eg, ARDS-Net low tidal volume ventilation strategy and ventilation in prone position) have been shown to improve mortality in patients with ALI and ARDS.

Disseminated Intravascular Coagulation (DIC): Disseminated intravascular coagulation is a syndrome characterized by a systemic activation of coagulation leading to the intravascular deposition of fibrin in the microvasculature and the simultaneous consumption of coagulation factors and platelets. Physical examination signs may reveal petechiae, ecchymosis, gangrene, mental disorientation, hypoxia, hypotension, and GI bleeding. The diagnosis is established by abnormalities in coagulation tests, including decreased platelet count, increased prothrombin time, elevated fibrin-related markers (D-dimer/fibrin degradation), and decreased fibrinogen level. DIC can lead to life-threatening hemorrhage, acute renal failure, and gangrene with loss of digits.

CASE CORRELATION

- See also Case 2 (Hemorrhagic Shock), Case 5 (Diabetic Ketoacidosis), Case 15 (Bacterial Pneumonia), Case 20 (Acute Diarrhea), Case 24 (Acute Pyelonephritis), Case 35 (Acute PID), Case 39 (Bacterial Meningitis), and Case 40 (Skin/Soft Tissue Infections).

COMPREHENSION QUESTIONS

3.1 A 32-year-old woman is noted to have a MAP < 65 mm Hg from suspected sepsis despite 4 L of IV normal saline. Which of the following is the best next step?

    A. Use colloid (albumin) for the next bolus.

     B. Initiate norepinephrine infusion.

    C. Administer corticosteroid therapy.

    D. Transfuse with fresh-frozen plasma.

    E. Administer activated protein C.

3.2 An 84-year-old woman is transferred from a nursing home with confusion, fever, and abnormal smelling urine. A lactate is noted to be 4.5 mmol/L. What are your initial priorities for this patient?

A. Order an intravenous pyelogram.

B. Rapid administration a 30 mL/kg fluid bolus and broad-spectrum antibiotics directed at urinary pathogens.

C. Initiate a workup for fictitious fever.

D. Consult a surgeon for possible appendicitis.

E. Discharge the patient back to the nursing home.

3.3 A 66-year-old woman is noted to have acute severe pneumonia and has been treated with adequate fluid, antibiotics, and vasopressors. Which of the following is a sign that the patient is going into septic shock?

A. Urine output of >1 mL/kg/h

B. Mean arterial blood pressure of 80 mm Hg

C. Lactic acid level of 6 mmol/dL

D. Serum bicarbonate level of 22 mEq/L

E. Hematocrit 35%

ANSWERS

3.1 **B.** A vasopressor agent such as norepinephrine (or dopamine) is the treatment of choice for hypotension that is unresponsive to intravenous saline infusion. The use of colloids during resuscitation has not been shown to improve outcome compared to crystalloids. Fresh-frozen plasma and activated protein C are not indicated.

3.2 **B.** The patient has a severe urinary infection. The initial priorities in this patient are to rapidly administer a 30 mL/kg fluid bolus (to assist in perfusion and support BP) and broad-spectrum antibiotics directed at urinary pathogens. Option E (Discharge back to the nursing home is inappropriate). Answer C (factitious fever) is unlikely with the patient's global manifestations of infection. Specific management such as surgery consult is warranted after stabilization.

3.3 **C.** The abnormal lactate level despite adequate fluid resuscitation is a sign that this patient is in septic shock. The patient's MAP of 80 mm Hg is adequate for perfusion. The other variables are not part of the new definition of septic shock.

CLINICAL PEARLS

▶ Sepsis is defined as a life-threatening organ dysfunction due to a dysregulated host response secondary to an infection.

▶ The qSOFA score has been developed to rapidly identify patients at increased risk for death secondary to sepsis.

▶ Patients are categorized as having septic shock if after adequate volume resuscitation, they have persistent hypotension requiring vasopressors to maintain MAP greater than or equal to 65 mm Hg and also have a lactate greater than or equal to 2 mmol/L.

▶ Patients with septic shock should be reassessed by repeat focused examination (including vital signs, cardiopulmonary exam, capillary refill, pulse, and skin findings), central venous pressure monitoring, central venous oxygen saturation assessment, bedside cardiovascular ultrasound, and/or dynamic assessment of fluid responsiveness to passive leg raise or fluid challenge.

▶ Rapid administration of 30 mL/kg crystalloid fluids and broad-spectrum antibiotics are the cornerstone of ED therapy for patients with sepsis.

REFERENCES

Kaukonen KM, Bailey M, Pilcher D, Cooper DJ, Bellomo R. Systemic inflammatory response syndrome criteria in defining severe sepsis. *N Engl J Med*. 2015;372(17):1629-1638. doi: 10.1056/NEJMoa1415236. Epub 2015 Mar 17.

Seymour CW, Liu VX, Iwashyna TJ, et al. Assessment of clinical criteria for sepsis: for the Third International Consensus Definitions for Sepsis and Septic Shock (Sepsis-3). *JAMA*. 2016; 315(8):762-774. doi: 10.1001/jama.2016.0288.

Seymour CW, Rosengart MR. Septic shock: advances in diagnosis and treatment. *JAMA*. 2015;314(7):708-717. doi: 10.1001/jama.2015.7885.

Shankar-Hari M, Phillips GS, Levy ML, et al; Sepsis Definitions Task Force. Developing a new definition and assessing new clinical criteria for septic shock: for the Third International Consensus Definitions for Sepsis and Septic Shock (Sepsis-3). *JAMA*. 2016;315(8):775-787. doi: 10.1001/jama.2016.0289.

Singer M, Deutschman CS, Seymour CW, et al. The Third International Consensus Definitions for Sepsis and Septic Shock (Sepsis-3). *JAMA*. 2016;315(8):801-810. doi: 10.1001/jama.2016.0287.

CASE 4

A middle-age man had a witnessed collapse in a busy coffee shop. He was immediately assessed by bystanders and found to be pulseless and apneic. Cardiopulmonary resuscitation was initiated immediately by bystanders and continued by EMS personnel during his transport to the hospital emergency department. According to the report from the prehospital providers, the patient has been in and out of ventricular fibrillation. He received cardioversion and cardiopulmonary resuscitation (CPR) during his transport to your facility. The patient remained in pulseless ventricular fibrillation at the time of his arrival to the resuscitation room of the hospital. After endotracheal intubation, several rounds of medication administration and cardioversions, the patient had return of a faint pulse, blood pressure of 96/60 mm Hg, and was noted to be in sinus tachycardia on the monitor with a heart rate of 115 beats per minute.

▶ What additional treatments should be provided at this time?
▶ What process implementations and culture changes are associated with improvements in the outcome of critically ill patients treated in the emergency department?

ANSWERS TO CASE 4:

Resuscitation and Critical Care Medicine Practices in the Emergency Department

Summary: A middle-aged man had a witnessed out-of-hospital cardiac arrest. He received immediate CPR and was transported to the emergency department. He is noted to be in ventricular fibrillation. His ventricular fibrillation was successfully converted to an organized rhythm with a pulse following the administration of medications and cardioversion.

- **Additional treatments:** Coronary angiography with percutaneous interventions and cardiac electrophysiology evaluations have been shown to improve survival, as cardiac ischemia is the cause for the ventricular fibrillation in the majority of patients with out-of-hospital cardiac sudden death. Hypothermia therapy has been demonstrated to improve the neurologic outcomes in post-cardiac arrest survivors.

- **Process Implementation and Culture Change to Improve Outcome:** The implementation of post-cardiac arrest consult teams has been demonstrated to improve patient outcome in a recent Canadian multicenter study. The acceptance of critical care medicine and increased emphasis in critical care medicine training during emergency medicine residency training, along with increasing critical care medicine expertise through critical care fellowship training, are expected to improve the care and outcome of critically ill patients in the emergency department.

ANALYSIS

Objectives

1. Learn the recent trends in patient resuscitation.

2. Learn the factors promoting critical care medicine emphasis in emergency medicine.

Considerations

A middle-aged man is brought to the hospital following witnessed out-of-the-hospital cardiac arrest. He is found to be in ventricular fibrillation. With CPR, pharmacologic therapy, and cardioversion, he now has sinus tachycardia and a blood pressure of 96/60 mm Hg. Important considerations for this patient at this juncture include early arrangement for coronary angiography with percutaneous intervention, cardiac electrophysiology studies, rapid cooling to reduce his core temperature to 32-34°C, and maintaining the hypothermia for 24-48 hours to help decrease the neurological sequelae associated with cardiac arrest. The infectious complication and bleeding complications are slightly increased in patients who receive therapeutic hypothermia; however, the neurologic benefits far outweigh the complications. **Roughly 50% of patients with cardiac arrest who arrive to the ICU will survive to hospital discharge; therefore, it is critical for early implementation of strategies that will lead to improved functional outcomes and survival.** The benefit of hypothermia therapy for post-cardiac arrest patients is mainly to improve neurological outcomes, but there is emerging evidence to suggest that this treatment strategy may also play a role in reducing the post-arrest cardiomyopathy. Management of a post-cardiac arrest patient by a multidisciplinary consult team has been demonstrated to be associated with decreased likelihood in withdrawing of life-sustaining therapy. A team approach also has been shown to improve the process: early and appropriate hypothermia therapy, coronary angiography/percutaneous intervention and cardiac electrophysiology interventions to identify and address the underlying cardiac disease.

APPROACH TO:
Resuscitation and Critical Care Patients in the Emergency Department

DEFINITIONS

THERAPEUTIC HYPOTHERMIA: Rapid cooling strategy to reduce core temperature to 32-34°C and maintaining the temperature for 24-48 hours to help improve neurologic outcomes in patients following resuscitation from cardiac arrest.

SURVIVING SEPSIS CAMPAIGN: An international collaborative effort design to improve outcomes associated with septic shock management. The treatment approach has been validated to improve patient outcomes in a variety of hospital settings worldwide.

PERMISSIVE HYPOTENSION OR HYPOTENSIVE RESUSCITATION: An approach toward the resuscitation of trauma patients with hemorrhagic shock. This approach is based on the concept that when the blood pressure goes up, the patient bleeds more. This approach to the hypotensive trauma patient without concomitant traumatic brain injuries is to limit treatments that would contribute to more bleeding. This begins with limiting resuscitation to a systolic blood pressure of 80-90 mm Hg until bleeding sources are identified and can be addressed by surgery or percutaneous treatments. Resuscitation approaches that are believed to contribute to increase in bleeding include crystalloid administration that leads to hypothermia, dilution of clotting factors, and induction of hypothermia. Concurrently, it is generally believed that the best way to minimize on-going bleeding in these individuals is to address the blood loss with the administration of blood products (packed cell, fresh frozen plasma, and platelets) in a 1:1:1 ratio.

PRINCIPLES OF RESUSCITATION

There have been major paradigm shifts in the approach to patient resuscitation. In the past, the goals or end-points of resuscitation were to restore normal vital signs and/or to restore laboratory measurements to normal in patients who present with signs and symptoms of shock. The current goal of resuscitation is not the restoration of normal vital signs, but the provision of sufficient MAP for perfusion of vital organs.

RESUSCITATION APPROACHES DIRECTED AT VARIOUS PATIENT GROUPS

Trauma Patients

For trauma patients with hemorrhagic shock, the concept of permissive hypotension has been shown to reduce transfusion requirements and improve outcome. For approach to hemorrhaging trauma patients without traumatic brain injuries, the strategy is to minimize crystalloid fluid administration and to resuscitate primarily with blood products in a 1:1:1 ratio (packed rbc cells: fresh frozen plasma: platelets); these products are given to improve the patient's systolic blood pressure to the 85-90 mm Hg range to preserve perfusion to the brain and vital organs. With this approach, there are also simultaneous arrangements made to establish source control to stop the bleeding; these can be done by surgery or catheter-based therapy, depending on the situation. Observations from the recent military conflicts in the Middle East showed that this management strategy was associated with reduced transfusion-related coagulopathy, transfusion requirements, and injury related mortality.

Acute Upper GI Bleeding Patients

The resuscitation goal for patients with acute GI hemorrhage has recently been modified based on observations from a randomized-controlled clinical trial. In the past, massive GI bleeding patients were often resuscitated to target Hgb values of 9-10 g/dL. The multicenter randomized controlled trial reported by Villanueva et al in the *New England Journal of Medicine* in 2013 showed that patients with acute upper GI hemorrhage randomized to a restricted transfusion strategy with a target Hgb of 7 g/dL had lower transfusion requirements, fewer complications, and increased survival when compared to patients randomized to a liberal transfusion strategy with a target Hgb of 9 g/dL. All of the study patients appeared to have benefited from a restrictive strategy, and patients with acute variceal bleeding were observed to have derived the greatest benefits from the restrictive transfusion approach.

Patients with Septic Shock

The Surviving Sepsis Campaign is an international initiative that has provided specific guidelines regarding the early care of septic shock patients. The implementation of these practices has been observed to improve patient outcomes and survival in a variety of practice settings internationally. The guidelines stressed the importance of early source control that includes appropriate antimicrobial therapy within 1 hour of diagnosis. Several resuscitation endpoints are outlined in the early management of the adult patient with septic shock. These include resuscitation to a target mean arterial pressure greater than 65 mm Hg, urine output of greater than 0.5 mL/kg/h, and CVP targets of 8-12 mm Hg. In individuals who remain in shock despite having normalized CVP targets, the use of norepinephrine (Levophed) drip should be initiated. When the patients remain hypotensive despite volume repletion and norepinephrine administration, vasopressin administration at a constant rate of 0.03 unit/min can be helpful to improve the patient's cellular response to catecholamine administration. If the patients remain hypotensive despite sufficient fluid repletion, norepinephrine administration, and vasopressin administration, corticosteroid replacement may be considered based on observations from the CORTICUS trial.

CRITICAL CARE IN THE EMERGENCY CENTER

The need for critical care medicine delivery in the emergency department has steadily increased over time in the United States, and this trend is largely due to the increased disease acuity and severity in most hospitals. Another contributor to the increasing delivery of critical care services to patients in the emergency department is the hospital bed shortage, which has contributed to increased length of emergency department stays for critically ill patients. The increased need for the care of ICU patients in the emergency department is being addressed in a number of ways in different hospital settings. One approach is the increase in critical care medicine training and exposure during residency training in emergency medicine. To address the increasing need for critical care expertise among emergency medicine physicians, there has been increased emphasis on critical medicine training during EM residency training. In addition, there has been an increasing number of EM Critical Care fellowship training programs established for the training of postgraduate emergency medicine physicians. Based on a recent survey, emergency medicine providers who have completed their critical care medicine fellowships generally will combine emergency medicine and critical medicine practices in their professional activities.

Other ways to address the EM critical care provider shortage is through the introduction of "rapid response" or consultation teams; these teams are made up of intensivists and ICU nurses who are mobilized to respond to critical care patient care needs during patients' emergency department stays. It remains unclear at this point how best to address the increasing critical care needs of the emergency department patients. The important issue remaining is that medical care providers in emergency medicine should become very familiar with the evolving practices in resuscitation care and the delivery of medical care that have been traditionally delivered in the ICU settings.

CASE CORRELATION

- See also Case 1 (Advanced Airway Management/Respiratory Failure), Case 2 (Hemorrhagic Shock), Case 3 (Sepsis), Case 5 (Diabetic Ketoacidosis), and Case 6 (Anaphylaxis).

COMPREHENSION QUESTIONS

4.1 Which of the following treatment approaches is a recommendation based on the Surviving Sepsis Campaign?

A. Mean arterial target goal of 75 mm Hg

B. CVP target goal of 12-16 mm Hg

C. Norepinephrine for patients with refractory hypotension following volume repletion

D. Vasopressin drip titration to achieve a mean arterial pressure of 65 mm Hg when patients do not respond to norepinephrine drip

E. Physiologic doses of corticosteroid administration for septic shock patients irregardless of clinical responses to norepinephrine

4.2 Which of the following is NOT an accurate description of hypothermia therapy for post-cardiac arrest patients?

A. Rapid cooling to reduce core temperature to 32-34°C for 24-48 hours

B. Therapeutic hypothermia has a proven effect in reducing the rate of recurrent ventricular fibrillation

C. Therapeutic hypothermia is associated with increased infections and bleeding complications

D. Therapeutic hypothermia is associated with some improved recovery of myocardial functions

E. The primary benefit of therapeutic hypothermia in the post-arrest patient is improved neurologic recovery

4.3 Which of the following resuscitation strategies is associated with increased adverse outcomes?

A. Correction of hypotension with volume resuscitation prior to definitive operative treatment for traumatic injuries from gunshot wound to the abdomen

B. Fluid restriction to target a CVP of 4 mm Hg in patients within 4 hours after successful resuscitation from septic shock

C. Substituting norepinephrine drip with dobutamine drip in the resuscitation of patients with hypotension related to ischemic cardiomyopathy

D. Rapid cooling of core temperature of post-cardiac arrest patients to 32-34°C for 24-48 hours

E. Coronary angiography in patients following successful resuscitation from ventricular fibrillation arrests

ANSWERS

4.1 **C.** Norepinephrine administration to improve the blood pressure in patients with adequate volume resuscitation is a strategy advocated by the Surviving Sepsis Campaign. Other important recommendations are early source control (of infection) including appropriate antimicrobial therapy within 1 hour of diagnosis of septic shock, volume resuscitation to achieve a CVP of 8-12 mm Hg, resuscitation to achieve a mean arterial pressure of 65 mm Hg and urine output of >0.5 mL/kg/h.

4.2 **B.** Therapeutic hypothermia describes the practice of rapid cooling of patients to core temperatures of 32-42°C for 24-48 hours. This treatment approach has been shown to reduce the neurologic sequelae in the post-arrest patients. The treatment has also been suggested to improve the myocardial dysfunction associated with post-cardiac arrest patients. Therapeutic hypothermia has not been shown to reduce the recurrence of ventricular arrhythmia in post-arrest patients. Early coronary angiography and percutaneous coronary interventions have been demonstrated to prevent recurrent cardiac arrhythmias and sudden cardiac death.

4.3 **A.** The correction of hypotension in patients with abdominal gunshot wounds prior to the initiation of operative treatment to address the intra-abdominal injuries will contribute increased bleeding, increased transfusion requirements, and worse treatment outcomes. The use of dobutamine instead of norepinephrine for blood pressure support in patients with hypotension due to ischemic cardiomyopathy is usually associated with decreased myocardial oxygen demand and improved myocardial performance. Appropriated limitation of fluid administration to target a CVP of 4 has been demonstrated to improve outcomes in patients successfully resuscitated from septic shock. Systemic hypothermia is associated with improvement in neurologic outcomes in the post-cardiac arrest patients.

CLINICAL PEARLS

► The goals of patient resuscitation are not normalization of vital signs and laboratory parameters but to sufficiently perfuse key organs.

► Trauma patients who are hypotensive and resuscitated to normal blood pressures are likely to have a greater amount of bleeding and increased transfusion requirements.

► Permissive hypotension should not be applied in the treatment of hypotensive trauma patients who also have moderate or severe traumatic brain injuries because low blood pressures can contribute to secondary brain injuries.

► Each organization and practice facility should identify workable approaches to address the increased critical care medicine needs of patients encountered in the emergency department.

► Introduction of a post-cardiac arrest consult team has led to improvements in outcomes in post-cardiac arrest patients.

REFERENCES

Abella BS, Leary M. Therapeutic hypothermia. In: Hall JB, Schmdt GA, Kress JP, eds. *Principles of Critical Care*. 4th edn. New York, NY: McGraw Hill Medical; 2015: 174-179.

Brooks SC, Scales Dc, Pinto R, et al. The post cardiac arrest consult team: impact on hospital care process for out-of-hospital cardiac arrest patients. *Critical Care Med*. August 2016. DOI: 10.1097/ CCM00000000000001863.

Cotton B, Reddy N, Quiton A, et al. Damage control resuscitation is associated with a reduction in resuscitation volume and improvement in survival in 390 damage control laparotomy patients. *Ann Surg*. 2011;254;1-15.

Dellinger RP, Levy MM, Rhodes A, et al. Surviving sepsis campaign: international guidelines for management of severe sepsis and septic shock. *Critical Care Med*. 2013;41:580-637.

Holcomb J, Tilley B, Barniuk S, et al. Transfusion of plasma, platelets, and red blood cells in a 1:1:1 vs a 1:1:2 ratio and mortality in patients with severe trauma: the PROPPR randomized clinical trial. *JAMA*. 2015;313:471-482.

A 19-year-old man is brought to the emergency department (ED) with altered level of consciousness. Family reports that he has had diffuse abdominal pain and vomiting. The patient's symptoms began several days ago, when he complained of "the flu." His symptoms at onset included profound fatigue, nausea, mild abdominal discomfort, and some urinary frequency. Today he was found in bed moaning, but otherwise he is unresponsive. His past medical history is unremarkable, and he is currently taking no medications. On examination, the patient appears pale and ill. His temperature is 36.0°C (96.8°F), pulse rate is 140 beats per minute, blood pressure is 82/40 mm Hg, and respiratory rate is 32 breaths per minute. He has dry mucous membranes and sunken eyes; there is an unusual odor to his breath. Lungs are clear bilaterally with irregular, deep respirations. Cardiac examination reveals tachycardia, no murmurs, rubs, or gallops. The abdomen is diffusely tender to palpation, with hypoactive bowel sounds and involuntary guarding. Rectal examination is normal. Skin is cool and dry with decreased turgor. On neurologic examination, the patient moans and localizes pain but does not speak coherently. Laboratory studies: the leukocyte count is 16,000 cells/uL, and the hemoglobin and hematocrit levels are normal. Electrolytes reveal a sodium of 124 mEq/L, potassium 3.4 mEq/L, chloride 98 mEq/L, and bicarbonate 6 mEq/L. BUN and creatinine are mildly elevated. Serum glucose is 740 mg/dL (41.1 mmol/L). The lipase, bilirubin, AST, ALT, and alkaline phosphatase are within normal limits. A 12-lead ECG shows only sinus tachycardia. His CXR is normal.

▶ What is the most likely diagnosis?
▶ What are the next steps?

ANSWERS TO CASE 5:
Diabetic Ketoacidosis

Summary: This is a 19-year-old man with acute diabetic ketoacidosis (DKA). He has new-onset diabetes mellitus. The constellation of severe hyperglycemia and anion-gap acidosis makes DKA likely, and the additional finding of ketosis (manifested by the breath odor, soon proven by testing for serum ketones) is diagnostic. The other findings of dehydration, hyponatremia, hypotension, altered level of consciousness, and diffuse abdominal pain are typical of a particularly severe episode of DKA. Initial episodes are often quite severe because without a known history of diabetes the diagnosis is not suspected until symptoms are advanced.

- **Most likely diagnosis:** Diabetic ketoacidosis.

- **Next steps:** Management of the ABCs, including fluid resuscitation, the initiation of insulin therapy, and a careful search for any precipitating or concomitant illness.

ANALYSIS

Objectives

1. Recognize the clinical settings, signs and symptoms, and complications of DKA.

2. Understand the diagnostic and therapeutic approach to suspected DKA.

Considerations

This patient's clinical presentation is typical for diabetic ketoacidosis. Morbidity may result either from underlying precipitating conditions or from delayed or inadequate treatment. Prompt recognition, effective resuscitation, and diligent attention to fluid, electrolyte, and insulin replacement are essential. (Table 5–1 lists typical laboratory values in DKA.) A comprehensive and thoughtful search for

Table 5–1 • TYPICAL LABORATORY VALUES IN DIABETIC KETOACIDOSIS		
	Moderate	Severe
Glucose (mg/dL)	<500-700	≥900
Sodium (mEq/L)	130	125
Potassium (mEq/L)	4-6	5-7
HCO_3 (mEq/L)	6-10	<5
BUN (mg/dL)	20-30	30+
pH	7.1	6.9
PcO_2 (mm Hg)	15-20	>20 (respiratory failure)

associated illnesses, along with frequent reassessment of the patient, will lead to the best outcome.

APPROACH TO:
Suspected Diabetic Ketoacidosis

CLINICAL APPROACH

Diabetic ketoacidosis is a metabolic emergency. A delay in treatment leads to increased morbidity and mortality. In up to one-quarter of patients, DKA is the initial presentation of type I diabetes, so lack of a diabetic history cannot exclude the diagnosis. Most cases occur in patients with type I diabetes, though a substantial portion of patients with type II diabetes may develop DKA during severe physiologic stress. Some patients will present with the classical symptoms of diabetes, such as polyuria, polydipsia, and fatigue. Others will complain more of dyspnea related to the metabolic acidosis or of the idiopathic but often severe abdominal pain that frequently accompanies DKA. Patients with an underlying infection or other precipitating illness may have symptoms predominantly from that process. As in our case presentation, some patients have such an altered sensorium that a good history is unobtainable.

DKA results from an absolute or severe relative lack of insulin, leading to a starvation state at the cellular level. Gluconeogenesis is stimulated even as glucose utilization falls. Hyperglycemia and ketoacidosis cause profound osmotic diuresis and massive fluid shifts. The diuresis and acidosis cause severe electrolyte disturbances, with wasting of sodium, potassium, magnesium, and phosphate. Acidosis, dehydration, hyperosmolality, and insulin deficiency can lead to potassium shifts into the extracellular space, **so patients may have significant serum hyperkalemia at presentation, even with massive total body deficits of potassium.** Nausea and vomiting can be severe and further cloud the clinical picture with variable superimposed acid-base and electrolyte disturbances.

Diagnosis is based on the triad of hyperglycemia, ketosis, and anion-gap metabolic acidosis. The major differential diagnosis is hyperosmolar hyperglycemic state (HHS), which can present with very high glucose, but slight or no acidosis. Starvation, pregnancy, alcoholic ketoacidosis, and various toxic ingestions can present with elevated serum ketones, but the glucose is usually normal or low. Patients can be rapidly screened for DKA with a point-of-care blood glucose measurement and a dipstick urinalysis. Except for the rare anuric patient, the absence of ketones in the urine reliably excludes the diagnosis of DKA. Serum ketones are commonly measured to confirm the diagnosis, but the absolute value is not as helpful because most labs measure only one of several ketone bodies that may be present. Table 5–2 is a guide to the differential diagnosis of DKA.

Patients with first-time DKA may not have any illness other than new diabetes, but most patients with recurrent DKA have an underlying cause of the episode. All symptoms require a thorough investigation. In some studies, more than 90% of episodes were associated with an underlying illness. Infection is the most

Table 5–2 • DIFFERENTIAL DIAGNOSIS OF DIABETIC KETOACIDOSIS		
Hyperglycemia	Acidosis	Ketosis
Diabetes	Hyperchloremic acidosis	Starvation
Stress hyperglycemia	Salicylate poisoning	Pregnancy
Nonketotic hyperosmolar coma	Uremia	Alcoholic ketoacidosis
Impaired glucose tolerance	Lactic acidosis	Isopropyl alcohol ingestion
Dextrose infusion	Other drugs	
DKA	DKA	DKA

frequent trigger of DKA, but it has also resulted from pancreatitis, myocardial infarction, stroke, pregnancy, and many drugs including corticosteroids, thiazides, sympathomimetics such as cocaine, and some antipsychotic drugs. In children and adolescents, voluntary cessation of insulin for psychosocial reasons is a frequent and serious cause of DKA.

Patients in DKA can have massive fluid deficits, sometimes as much as 5-10 L. Shock is common and must be promptly treated with crystalloid infusion to prevent further organ damage. Adults with clinical shock should receive an initial 2 L bolus of normal saline with frequent reassessment. In children, shock is treated with boluses of 10-20 mL/kg of normal saline. Although overaggressive hydration can present substantial complications later in the course of treatment, this concern takes a back seat to the early reversal of shock. Untreated shock promotes multiple-organ dysfunction and contributes further to the severe acidosis seen in DKA.

Insulin is required to reverse the ketoacidosis. Most institutions will have a regimented protocol or order set for insulin dosing, fluids, electrolyte replacement, and frequent retesting; such order sets reduce errors in management. Short-acting ("regular") insulin is usually given by continuous IV infusion, though frequent IV boluses may be nearly as effective. IM injections are painful and less reliably absorbed when the patient is in shock. There is no role for long-acting insulin until the ketoacidotic state has resolved. (There are proposed protocols for treating *mild* and *recurrent* episodes of DKA with subcutaneous short-acting insulin, but those protocols have not yet been universally adopted.) The combination of rehydration and insulin will usually lower the serum glucose much faster than ketones are cleared. **Regardless of the glucose level, insulin infusion should continue until the anion gap has returned to normal. Dextrose should be added to the IV infusion when the serum glucose falls to 200-300 mg/dL** (11.1-16.7 mmol/L) to prevent hypoglycemia, a common complication of treatment.

An insulin dose of 0.1 U/kg/h (5-10 U/h in the adult) is adequate for almost all clinical situations. Higher doses are no more effective and do cause a higher rate of hypoglycemia. An initial bolus of insulin, equal to a 1-hour infusion, is commonly given but has not been shown to hasten recovery or provide any other benefit. Insulin boluses are not recommended in pediatric patients. Insulin does bind readily to common medical plastics, so IV tubing should be thoroughly flushed with the drip solution at the start of therapy.

Patients in DKA generally have massive total body deficits of water, sodium, potassium, magnesium, phosphate, and other electrolytes. Specific laboratory values may vary widely depending on the patient's intake, gastrointestinal and other losses, medications, and comorbid illnesses. It is not usually necessary to calculate exact sodium and water deficits and replacements, except in cases of severe renal failure. Simply reverse shock with normal saline, and then continue an infusion of half-normal saline at two to three times maintenance. Remember that glucose should be added *before* the serum glucose falls to the normal range, usually when the glucose level reaches 250 mg/dL.

Potassium deficits are usually quite large, yet the serum potassium at presentation may be low, normal, or even high. If the potassium is elevated initially, look for and treat any hyperkalemic changes on the ECG. Give fluids without potassium until the serum K reaches the normal range, and then add potassium to the IV infusion. If the initial serum K is normal or low, potassium replacement can be started immediately. Magnesium supplementation may be necessary to help the patient retain potassium. Phosphate replacement has not been shown to improve clinical outcomes, but extremely low phosphate levels (<1.0 mg/dL) are known to cause muscle weakness and possibly rhabdomyolysis. For such patients, some of the potassium can be given in the form of potassium phosphate.

Because metabolic acidosis is such a prominent feature in DKA, some clinicians have administered substantial doses of sodium bicarbonate. Many studies have failed to demonstrate any improvement from this treatment even at surprisingly low serum pH values, but even skeptical physicians sometimes encounter a patient who is so acidotic that they feel compelled to give bicarbonate. There are multiple theoretical and observed complications from bicarbonate, including hypernatremia, hypokalemia, paradoxical CSF acidosis, and residual systemic alkalosis. Of course, in the case of severe hyperkalemia, bicarbonate might be a useful antidote and should not be withheld.

Cerebral edema is a rare but devastating complication of DKA, seen most often and most severely in children. It almost always occurs during treatment and is a leading cause of morbidity and mortality in pediatric DKA. It has been ascribed to the development of cryptogenic osmoles in the CNS to counter dehydration, which then draw water intracellularly during treatment, but this remains unproven. It has been variously associated with overhydration and vigorous insulin therapy, leading many pediatric centers to use extremely conservative, slow and low-dose treatment protocols for DKA. However, at least one large well-controlled study showed that the only reliable predictor of cerebral edema was the severity of metabolic derangements at presentation. Concern for cerebral edema should not be used as an excuse for the undertreatment of clinical shock. Once shock is reversed, pediatric DKA patients should be managed in consultation with an experienced pediatric endocrinologist or intensivist.

CASE CORRELATION

- See also Case 2 (Hemorrhagic Shock), Case 3 (Sepsis), and Case 6 (Anaphylaxis).

COMPREHENSION QUESTIONS

5.1 A 17-year-old adolescent boy who is a type I diabetic is brought in by his parents with concern for DKA. He has had several prior episodes of DKA. Which of the following is most diagnostic of DKA?

A. Polyuria, polydipsia, fatigue

B. Hypotension, dehydration, fruity breath odor

C. Hyperglycemia, ketosis, metabolic acidosis

D. Serum blood sugar of 600 mg/dL in the face of high concentrations of insulin

E. Elevated HCO_3 and elevated glucose

5.2 A 28-year-old insulin-requiring woman is found at home by her husband. She is stuporous and cannot provide any history. She is brought to the ED, and a diagnosis of severe DKA is made. Her blood pressure is 78/40 mm Hg and heart rate 140 beats per minute. The glucose level is 950 mg/dL, potassium level 6 mEq/L, and HCO_3 4 mEq/L. Which of the following is the most appropriate initial treatment?

A. Administer 20 units regular insulin intramuscularly, and normal saline at 250 mL/h.

B. Begin intravenous pressors to raise BP above 90, then insulin at 10 U/h.

C. Initiate normal saline 2 L with KCl 20 mEq/L and insulin 10 U/h.

D. Provide an intravenous normal saline 2 L bolus, then start an insulin drip at 10 U/h.

5.3 The patient in Question 5.2 is undergoing therapy. Which of the following principles is most accurate in the treatment of DKA?

A. Isotonic saline with no dextrose should be used during the hospitalization because the patient is diabetic.

B. Insulin and dextrose solution will need to be continued until the acidosis has resolved.

C. Since the patient is hyperkalemic, potassium replacement will not be necessary.

D. Sodium bicarbonate is helpful to resolve the anion gap more quickly.

5.4 Patients in DKA often have other illnesses or precipitating factors that initiated the ketoacidosis. Which one of the following is unlikely to precipitate DKA?

A. Asthmatic exacerbation

B. Cocaine use

C. Cholecystitis

D. Missed insulin doses

E. Urinary tract infection

ANSWERS

5.1 **C.** The triad of hyperglycemia, ketosis, and acidosis is diagnostic of DKA. Many other conditions cause one or two of the triad, but not all three. Although a fruity breath odor may suggest acetone, it is not reliably present, and not all clinicians can distinguish it.

5.2 **D.** Fluid resuscitation via isotonic crystalloid solution to reverse shock, and IV insulin to reverse ketoacidosis, are the mainstays of therapy. Though most patients will require potassium, it should not be given while the serum K is elevated, and typically not until urine output is seen. Pressors have a limited role until the intravascular volume is restored.

5.3 **B.** The serum glucose often drops much more rapidly than the ketoacidosis resolves; insulin is necessary to metabolize the ketone bodies but dextrose prevents hypoglycemia. Potassium replacement is usually necessary but should wait until hyperkalemia is excluded or has resolved. Bicarbonate does not hasten resolution of DKA.

5.4 **A.** Many serious illnesses can precipitate an episode of DKA in the susceptible patient, including infection, stroke, myocardial infarction, pancreatitis, trauma, and surgery. Associated or precipitating illness should always be sought diligently. In most studies, infection is the single most common underlying cause. Noncompliance with insulin therapy is also a very common cause. Asthma exacerbation is not strongly associated with DKA.

CLINICAL PEARLS

▶ Hyperglycemia, ketosis, and acidosis confirm the diagnosis of DKA and are enough reason to start fluids. Some providers prefer to wait for a potassium level before starting insulin.

▶ Patients in DKA are almost always dehydrated and have significant sodium and potassium deficits, regardless of their specific laboratory values.

▶ Abdominal pain is a common feature in DKA and is usually idiopathic, especially in younger patients.

▶ Most morbidity in DKA is iatrogenic.

REFERENCES

Charfen MA, Fernández-Frackelton M. Diabetic ketoacidosis. *Emerg Med Clin North Am.* 2005; 23(3):609-628, vii.

Chua HR, Schneider A, Bellomo R. Bicarbonate in diabetic ketoacidosis—a systematic review. *Annals of Intensive Care.* 2011;1:23. doi:10.1186/2110-5820-1-23.

Gosmanov AR, Gosmanova EO, Kitabchi AE. Hyperglycemic crises: diabetic ketoacidosis (dka), and hyperglycemic hyperosmolar state (HHS) [Updated 2015 May 19]. In: De Groot LJ, Beck-Peccoz P, Chrousos G, et al., eds. *Endotext [Internet]*. South Dartmouth (MA): MDText.com, Inc.; 2000. Available from: http://www.ncbi.nlm.nih.gov/books/NBK279052/

Kitabchi AE, Umpierrez GE, Murphy MB, et al. Hyperglycemic crises in adult patients with diabetes: a consensus statement from the American Diabetes Association. *Diabetes Care*. 2006;29(12): 2739-2748.

Levin DL. Cerebral edema in diabetic ketoacidosis. *Pediatr Crit Care Med*. 2008;9(3):320-329.

Marcin JP, Glaser N, Barnett P, et al; American Academy of Pediatrics. Factors associated with adverse outcomes in children with diabetic ketoacidosis-related cerebral edema. *J Pediatr*. 2002;141(6): 793-797.

Mazer M, Chen E. Is subcutaneous administration of rapid-acting insulin as effective as intravenous insulin for treating diabetic ketoacidosis? *Ann Emerg Med*. 2009;53(2):259-263.

Wolfsdorf J, Craig ME, Daneman D, et al; International Society for Pediatric and Adolescent Diabetes. Diabetic ketoacidosis. *Pediatr Diabetes*. 2007;8(1):28-43.

A 20-year-old woman is brought to the emergency department (ED) by ambulance after collapsing at home. She was seen by her regular doctor earlier in the day and prescribed penicillin for bacterial pharyngitis. Paramedics report field vital signs remarkable for a blood pressure of 70/30 mm Hg, heart rate of 140 beats per minute, respiratory rate of 40 breaths per minute, and an oxygen saturation of 76%. Intravenous fluids and oxygen were administered during transport. Paramedics are assisting the patient's breathing with bag-valve mask ventilation, but oxygen saturations remains low. On physical examination, the patient is obtunded with perioral cyanosis, tongue swelling, stridor, wheezing, and labored breathing. Her skin is cool and clammy with large urticarial lesions.

▶ What are the next steps?
▶ What treatments should be instituted?

ANSWERS TO CASE 6:
Anaphylaxis

Summary: This 20-year-old woman is demonstrating signs and symptoms of ana-phylaxis. Anaphylaxis is a rapidly progressive, life-threatening, severe allergic reac-tion that can compromise airway, breathing, and circulation. Successful treatment of anaphylaxis requires early recognition of the symptoms of anaphylaxis, airway support, and rapid epinephrine administration.

- **Next steps:** A **definitive airway** will need to be immediately established in the face of impending airway obstruction (see Cases 1 and 48), and the patient's cardiovascular compromise must be treated with epinephrine. Consider the emergent approach to anaphylaxis by adding "DE" to the traditional ABCs of emergency medicine. ABCDE: Airway, Breathing, Circulation, "Deliver Epinephrine." The first dose of epinephrine should be administered intramus-cularly in the anterolateral thigh. In the setting of a severe reaction like the one described earlier, moving quickly to intravenous infusion of epinephrine is recommended.

- **Further treatments:** This patient requires rapid resuscitation and stabilization. While preparing for intubation, high-flow oxygen therapy should be admin-istered. Her lower extremities should be elevated to improve venous return. Additional therapies include volume resuscitation with crystalloid, nebu-lized beta agonists, corticosteroids, antihistamines (H_1 and H_2 blockers), and removal of any remaining antigen (ie, bee stinger in applicable cases). Patients who are taking β-blockers may be less responsive to standard therapy and therefore also require administration of glucagon.

ANALYSIS

Objectives

1. Rapidly recognize the characteristic clinical features of anaphylaxis.

2. Understand the underlying pathophysiology of anaphylaxis.

3. Become familiar with the available treatment options, including the correct administration of epinephrine.

Considerations

This 20-year-old woman is brought into the ED with swelling of the tongue and labored breathing. The perioral cyanosis, diffuse wheezing, stridor, and hypoxia all indicate **impending airway obstruction and respiratory failure.** After recognizing this presentation as anaphylaxis, the most critical intervention is the administration of epinephrine. This patient likely has edema of the pharynx and larynx making intu-bation technically difficult. Airway management in a patient like this may require a **cricothyroidotomy** if endotracheal intubation fails.

APPROACH TO:
Anaphylaxis

CLINICAL APPROACH

Epidemiology

Millions of people present to emergency departments every year with allergic symptoms ranging from minor rashes to multi-organ system anaphylaxis. Most of the time, it is difficult if not impossible to identify the trigger. Because the spectrum of allergic responses is so broad, anaphylaxis is under recognized. As a result, it is difficult to calculate a precise incidence of this disease. For instance, there are an estimated 30,000 ED visits every year for adverse food reactions, some of which may be anaphylactic in nature. In the United States, the number of admissions for anaphylactic reactions has slowly increased, but mortality rates have remained low, with only 0.3% of patients who were hospitalized for anaphylaxis dying during their hospital stay. Risk factors for severe anaphylaxis and a poor outcome include peanut and tree allergy, pre-existing cardiovascular disease, asthma, advanced age, pregnancy, taking β-blockers and ACE inhibitors, and **delayed administration of epinephrine.**

Pathophysiology

True anaphylaxis is a **type 1 hypersensitivity** reaction occurring after a previous sensitizing exposure. In its purest form, this is an IgE immune-mediated **activation of basophils and mast cells with subsequent release of prostaglandins, leukotrienes,** and **histamine.** An anaphylactoid reaction also includes release of these compounds but through non–immune-mediated pathways. The only clinical significance of this difference is that anaphylactoid reactions can occur without prior sensitization. Regardless of the underlying mechanism, their effects are similar, and early recognition will determine successful clinical management in these patients (see Table 6–1 for pitfalls in management).

When a patient is first exposed to a substance, binding antibodies trigger class switching and regulatory changes in gene expression, effectively priming the immune system for its next encounter with the offending agent. In certain cases, this leads to **immunoglobulin (IgE) binding to mast cells and basophils. In** the classic anaphylactic reaction, the antigen again encounters the immune system, binds to the IgE on the mast cells and basophils, and releases a flood of cytokines that set the clinical response in motion. In an anaphylactoid reaction, the antigen causes

Table 6–1 • PITFALLS IN ANAPHYLAXIS MANAGEMENT
Failure to recognize the symptoms of anaphylaxis
Underestimating the severity of laryngeal edema and failure to secure the airway early
Reluctance to administer epinephrine early in the course of illness
Forgetting to remove the allergen; eg, the IV drip of penicillin or bee stinger
Lack of appropriate patient education
Failure to prescribe an epinephrine auto-injector prior to discharge

direct release of cytokines by mast cells and basophils, without need for prior sensitization. In both cases, the end result is the same and is clinically indistinguishable.

The early stages of some anaphylactic reactions involve increased secretion by mucous membranes. In addition to **watery eyes and rhinorrhea, increased bronchial secretions and increased smooth muscle tone cause wheezing** and increase the work of breathing. Decreased vascular tone and **increased capillary permeability** lead to **cardiovascular compromise and hypotension.** Patients may lose over 30% of their blood volume to extravasation in the first 10 minutes of their allergic reaction. Other cytokines, specifically histamine, can cause **urticaria and angioedema.** There are numerous cytokines involved in the immunologic cascade following exposure, and no one major substance is felt to be primarily responsible. Leukotriene C_4, prostaglandin D_2, histamine, and tryptase are known key components in the reaction.

Causes

The most common causes of anaphylaxis are medications, insect bites, and food allergies. Culprit medications include antibiotics (especially penicillins), NSAIDs, and biological agents (chemotherapy and monoclonal antibodies). Some studies suggest as many as 1 in 500 exposures to penicillin will result in anaphylaxis. Radiographic intravenous contrast agents can also cause an anaphylactoid response. Overall, there are an estimated 0.9 fatal reactions per 100,000 patients exposed to intravenous contrast. The incidence of serious reaction skyrockets to 60% in patients who have had a prior exposure and reaction.

Hymenoptera (bee and wasp) stings are another cause of anaphylaxis. Anaphylaxis from stings results in an average of 50 deaths per year in the United States. Overall, the number of cases of arthropod anaphylaxis seen by physicians is small compared to the number of iatrogenic cases, but because exposures often occur miles from medical treatment, they can have serious outcomes.

Food sources round out the major causes of serious allergic reactions. Food allergies are the most common cause of anaphylaxis in children. **Peanuts** and other tree nuts are the **most common cause of serious allergic reactions.** Other food allergens include milk, eggs, shellfish, fish, soybean, sesame, and mangos, but any food can be responsible.

Diagnosis

The diagnosis of anaphylaxis is made clinically. The most commonly affected system is the skin, which manifests with **angioedema, urticaria, erythema, and pruritus** in 80% to 90% of patients with anaphylaxis. The cardiovascular system is also affected, primarily as a result of decreased vasomotor tone and capillary leakage. This leads to **hypotension and tachycardia.** Respiratory compromise of both the upper and lower airways is common, associated with rhinorrhea, sneezing, throat tightness, stridor, tachypnea, dyspnea, **bronchospasm, bronchorrhea, and wheezing.** Lower respiratory tract symptoms in combination with edema of the upper respiratory tract are the most feared and difficult to manage aspects of anaphylaxis. After administration of epinephrine, control of the airway is the most important therapeutic intervention, as **nearly all deaths caused by anaphylaxis are a result of airway compromise.** Gastrointestinal symptoms including nausea, vomiting, cramping, and diarrhea may be seen and are associated with particularly severe anaphylactic reactions. It is critical to recognize that patients can manifest systemic symptoms of anaphylaxis WITHOUT mucosal and skin involvement. In addition, central nervous system symptoms may include a sense of impending doom, headache, dizziness, confusion, and altered mental status.

Clinical Criteria for Diagnosis of Anaphylaxis

Clinical criteria were developed from a multidisciplinary consortium to best identify anaphylaxis early and accurately. Anaphylaxis is highly likely if any one of the following three diagnostic criteria exist.

1. **Acute onset** (minutes to hours) with reaction of the skin and/or mucosal tissue **in addition** to **respiratory symptoms or hypotension.** Skin symptoms include itching, redness, hives, generalized urticaria, and mucosal edema. Respiratory manifestations include laryngeal stridor, bronchospasm, bronchorrhea, and hypoxia. Hypotension results from extravasation of fluid from the vasculature and loss of vasomotor tone.

2. Two or more of the following occurring rapidly (minutes to hours) **after exposure to a likely allergen:** involvement of the **skin-mucosal** tissue, **respiratory symptoms, hypotension,** or **gastrointestinal symptoms** (abdominal pain, cramping, or diarrhea).

3. **Hypotension occurring rapidly (minutes to hours)** after exposure to a known allergen for that patient. Hypotension may present as faintness or altered mental status.

Treatment

The primary initial therapy for anaphylaxis is **epinephrine** (Table 6–2). Epinephrine acts as a vasopressor for hemodynamic support, a bronchodilator to relieve wheezing, and it also counteracts released mediators to prevent their further release. Epinephrine can be dosed intramuscularly or intravenously. **Subcutaneous administration of epinephrine is no longer recommended** as it has been proven less effective than intramuscular administration. Initial administration is intramuscular in the anterior thigh with the more concentrated 1:1000 dose at 0.01 mg/kg, generally 0.3-0.5 mg every 5 minutes for up to a total of 3 doses. If there is no response or if the patient is already demonstrating cardiovascular compromise, intravenous administration should be started immediately at a dose of 2-10 µg/min (pediatric dosing: 0.1-0.3 µg/kg/min). Although there are NO absolute contraindications to epinephrine administration in suspected anaphylaxis, intravenous administration of epinephrine can cause hypertension, tachycardia, dysrhythmias, and myocardial ischemia. Extra caution must be taken in patients with known coronary artery disease.

Inhaled beta agonists are indicated for wheezing, and nebulized racemic epinephrine has been hypothesized to decrease laryngeal edema. Other adjuvants include systemic **steroids,** specifically methylprednisolone and prednisone. Steroids will not take action for at least 6 hours but will blunt further immune responses. Steroids should be continued for days after the reaction and may or may not be tapered. H_1 and H_2 blockers should also be administered to blunt histamine release

Table 6–2 • TREATMENT FOR ANAPHYLAXIS		
Drug	Adult Dose	Pediatric Dose
Epinephrine	IV single dose: 100 µg over 5-10 min IV infusion: 2-10 µg/min IM: 0.3-0.5 mg	IV infusion: 0.1-0.3 µg/kg/min; maximum 1.5 µg/kg/min IM: 0.01 mg/kg (max 0.3 mg)
IV fluids: NS or LR	1-2-L bolus	10-15 mL/kg bolus
Diphenhydramine	25-50 mg q6h IV, IM, or PO	1 mg/kg q6h IV, IM, or PO (max 50 mg)
Ranitidine	50 mg IV over 5 min	0.5 mg/kg IV over 5 min
Cimetidine	300 mg IV	4-8 mg/kg IV
Hydrocortisone	250-500 mg IV	5-10 mg/kg IV (max 500 mg)
Methylprednisolone	125 mg IV	1-2 mg/kg IV (max 50 mg)
Albuterol	Single treatment: 2.5-5.0 mg nebulized Continuous nebulization: 5-10 mg/h	Single treatment: 1.25-2.5 mg nebulized Continuous nebulization: 3-5 mg/h
Ipratropium bromide	Single treatment: 250-500 µg nebulized	Single treatment: 125-250 µg nebulized
Magnesium sulfate	2 g IV over 20 min	25-50 mg/kg IV over 20 min (max 2 g)
Glucagon	1 mg IV q5min until hypotension resolves, followed by 5-15 µg/min infusion	50 µg/kg q5min
Prednisone	40-60 mg/day PO divided bid or qd (for outpatients: 3-5 days; tapering not required)	1-2 mg/day PO divided bid or qd (for outpatients: 3-5 days; tapering not required)

Source: Reprinted, with permission, Tintinalli JE, Kelen GD, Stapczynski JS. Emergency Medicine. 6th ed. New York, NY: McGraw-Hill Education; 2004:250.

and systemic response. Diphenhydramine and ranitidine are the most commonly employed agents. It should be remembered that these other medications, while safe and easy to administer, are not first-line agents and will not counteract immediate respiratory and cardiovascular compromise.

Intravenous glucagon has been proposed for individuals on β-blockers since the response to epinephrine may be blunted. Glucagon may overcome hypotension by activating adenyl cyclase independent of the beta adrenergic receptor. In patients taking ACE inhibitors presenting with angioedema, **icatibant** has shown promise for treatment. This novel medication is a **bradykinin receptor antagonist** and reduces inflammation.

> ## CASE CORRELATION
> - See also Case 13 (Asthma), Case 14 (Pulmonary Embolism), Case 40 (Soft Tissue Infection), and Case 41 (Rash with Fever).

COMPREHENSION QUESTIONS

6.1 An 18-year-old woman is brought to the ED with suspected anaphylaxis. Which of the following symptoms is most specific for anaphylaxis rather than a simple allergic reaction?

    A. Itching

    B. Watery eyes

    C. Blood pressure of 80/40 mm Hg

    D. Hives

    E. Headache

6.2 A 26-year-old woman with a known peanut allergy is brought to the ED after accidentally consuming salad with a peanut dressing. She is wheezing and reports abdominal cramping. Which of the following should be the first intervention?

    A. Endotracheal intubation

    B. Normal saline 20 cc/kg IV

    C. Examination of the skin

    D. Epinephrine 0.3 mg intramuscular

    E. Nebulized epinephrine

6.3 Risk factors for severe anaphylaxis include:

    A. Heavy consumption of nuts

    B. Well-controlled asthma

    C. Extremely young age

    D. Prior antibiotic use

    E. Pregnancy

6.4 A 65-year-old man collapsed in a park and is brought to the ED by paramedics. He was stung by a bee and known to be highly allergic. He appears cyanotic and had extreme stridor in the ambulance. Severe laryngeal edema is notable. Which of the following is the best treatment?

    A. Nebulized albuterol, H_1 and H_2 antagonists, corticosteroids, and crystalloids.

    B. Intramuscular epinephrine, H_1 and H_2 antagonists, and corticosteroids.

    C. Rapid sequence intubation, intramuscular epinephrine, and corticosteroids.

    D. Intramuscular epinephrine, rapid sequence intubation, and corticosteroids.

    E. Nebulized albuterol, H_1 and H_2 antagonists, IV fluid resuscitation, and reassessment for improvement.

ANSWERS

6.1 **C.** Hypotension indicates a systemic reaction and cardiovascular compromise, thereby classifying this allergic reaction as anaphylaxis. The other options may all be part of an anaphylactic response but may also just be simple allergic reactions.

6.2 **D.** Intramuscular epinephrine should be administered immediately. If there is significant respiratory or airway compromise, then the patient's airway should be controlled. Subsequent interventions include fluid resuscitation for hypotension, as well as H_2 blockers and systemic steroids to mitigate further histamine and cytokine release.

6.3 **E.** Risk factors for severe anaphylaxis include a history of poorly controlled asthma or other chronic lung disease (eg, COPD), advanced age, pregnancy, and taking β-blockers and ACE inhibitors. Each subsequent exposure to an allergen may be worse than the prior allergic reaction.

6.4 **D.** This patient has severe anaphylaxis, and epinephrine should be administered immediately. If intravenous dosing is not immediately available, then intramuscular epinephrine should be given. One caution is that dosing errors have been noted with IV epinephrine and delay in getting IV access and equipment tubing etc; for this reason, some centers only use IM epinephrine to treat anaphylaxis. Attention should then be turned to managing the airway. Because of the significant laryngeal edema, endotracheal intubation will be nearly impossible; hence, cricothyroidotomy may be required. After securing the airway, fluids, steroids, beta agonists, and H_1 and H_2 antagonists should be administered.

CLINICAL PEARLS

▶ The airway should be secured early and often. It is much easier to extubate a patient without severe laryngeal edema than to intubate a patient with an occluded posterior oropharynx.

▶ Epinephrine should be given at the first sign of respiratory distress or cardiovascular compromise.

▶ Look for causes of anaphylaxis after you have started your initial resuscitation.

▶ Steroids, antihistamines, and beta agonists are all helpful pharmacologic adjuvants for managing the many symptoms of anaphylaxis.

REFERENCES

Campbell RL, Li JTC, Nicklas RA, et al. Emergency department diagnosis and treatment of anaphylaxis: a practice parameter. *Ann Allergy Asthma Immunol.* 2014:113:599-608.

deShazo R. Anaphylaxis: my "top 10" list. *South Med J.* 2007;100(3):233-234.

Ma L, Danoff TM, Borish L. Case fatality and population mortality associated with anaphylaxis in the United States. *J Allergy Clin Immunol.* 2014;133(4):1075-1083.

Sampson HA, Munoz-Furlong A, Campbell RL, et al. Second symposium on the definition and management of anaphylaxis: summary report—Second National Institute of Allergy and Anaphylaxis Network Symposium. *J Allergy Clin Immunol.* 2006;117(2):391-397.

Simons FE, Ardusso L, Bilo M, et al. World Allergy Organization Guidelines for the Assessment and Management of Anaphylaxis. *World Allergy Organ J.* 2011;4(2):13-37.

Simons FE, Ebisawa M, Sanchez-Borges M, et al. 2015 update of the evidence base: World Allergy Organization Anaphylaxis Guidelines. *World Allergy Organ J.* 2015;8(1):32.

Soar J, Pumphrey R, Cant A, et al. Emergency treatment of anaphylactic reaction: guidelines for healthcare providers. *Resuscitation.* 2008;77:157-169.

A 61-year-old man arrives at the emergency department (ED) complaining of chest pain. The pain began 45 minutes ago while watching television and is described as severe and pressure-like. It is substernal in location, radiates to the jaw and left shoulder, and is associated with shortness of breath. The patient has hyperlipidemia and hypertension and takes simvastatin and hydrochlorothiazide. His blood pressure is 160/110 mm Hg, pulse rate is 93 beats per minute, respiration rate is 22 breaths per minute, temperature is 37.1°C, and oxygen saturation is 97%. The patient appears anxious, is diaphoretic and vomited once. On auscultation, faint crackles are heard at both lung bases. The cardiac and abdominal examinations are unremarkable.

▶ What is the most likely diagnosis?
▶ What are the next diagnostic steps?
▶ What therapies should be instituted immediately?

ANSWERS TO CASE 7

Myocardial Infarction, Acute

Summary: This is a 61-year-old man presenting with acute severe chest pain, diaphoresis, dyspnea, and emesis. The patient has a number of risk factors for underlying coronary artery disease, and the history and physical examination are typical of an **acute coronary syndrome.**

- **Most likely diagnosis:** Acute myocardial infarction.

- **Next diagnostic steps:** Place the patient on a cardiac monitor, establish IV access, and obtain an electrocardiogram (ECG) immediately. A chest x-ray and serum levels of cardiac markers should be obtained as soon as possible.

- **Immediate therapies:** Aspirin is the most important immediate therapy. Oxygen and sublingual nitroglycerin are also standard early therapies. Depending on the result of the ECG, emergency reperfusion therapy, such as a percutaneous coronary intervention (PCI), may be indicated. Intravenous beta-blockers, IV nitroglycerin, low-molecular-weight heparin, and additional antiplatelet agents, such as clopidogrel, might also be indicated.

ANALYSIS

Objectives

1. Recognize acute myocardial infarction (MI) and the spectrum of acute coronary syndromes (ACSs).

2. Know the appropriate diagnostic tests and their limitations.

3. Understand the therapeutic approach to ACS.

Considerations

Coronary heart disease (CHD) is the leading cause of death in adults in the United States. Chest pain accounts for more than 8 million visits every year to EDs in the United States. Of these 8 million visits, nearly 400,000 will end with a diagnosis of ST elevation MI (STEMI), and 2 million will be given the diagnoses of unstable angina (UA) or non-ST elevation myocardial infarction (NSTEMI). Emergency physicians should be very familiar with this problem since ACS is common and treatable, and **missed MI accounts for the most money paid in malpractice claims in emergency medicine.**

   Acute coronary syndrome, which encompasses the spectrum of STEMI, NSTEMI, and UA, involves a dynamic process of inflammation and intravascular thrombosis, beginning with coronary artery plaque rupture. The fate of this plaque, in terms of its location, extent of thrombosis, and subsequent heart muscle damage, determines the clinical presentation and correlates with the subdivisions of ACS. The concept of fixed coronary artery narrowing explains only stable angina brought on by increased myocardial demand.

STEMI occurs when total occlusion of an epicardial vessel causes transmural infarction, classically presenting as unremitting chest pain and ST segment elevation on the ECG. It is treated with immediate reperfusion therapy such as thrombolysis or PCI. NSTEMI and UA, in contrast, are caused by subendocardial infarction or ischemia, respectively. Chest pain often comes and goes. ECG changes such as ST segment depression or T-wave inversion may be present. Elevation in cardiac markers eventually distinguishes NSTEMI from UA. Immediate therapy for both NSTEMI and UA focuses on halting ongoing thrombosis and reducing myocardial demand. Many patients go on to have PCI directed at the unstable plaque.

APPROACH TO:
Suspected Myocardial Infarction

DEFINITIONS

MYOCARDIAL INFARCTION: Myocardial cell death caused by ischemia, evidenced by a rise and fall in cardiac biomarkers.

ACUTE CORONARY SYNDROME: An ischemic chest pain syndrome usually associated with coronary artery plaque rupture. Encompasses STEMI, NSTEMI, and UA.

UNSTABLE ANGINA: An acute coronary syndrome in which chest pain is of new onset, increasing severity, or occurs at rest, and cardiac biomarkers are not elevated.

NON-ST ELEVATION MYOCARDIAL INFARCTION: An acute coronary syndrome in which cardiac biomarkers are eventually elevated but which lacks new ST elevation on ECG.

ST ELEVATION MYOCARDIAL INFARCTION: An acute coronary syndrome in which significant ST elevation is found in two or more contiguous ECG leads. It is typically associated with epicardial coronary artery occlusion and transmural infarction, resulting in myocardial cell death evidenced by Q waves if perfusion is not soon restored.

CLINICAL APPROACH

Evaluation

The cornerstone of diagnosis of acute coronary syndromes is the **ECG.** Findings on the initial ECG present a **critical branch point in therapy,** and patients presenting to the ED with chest pain suggestive of ACS should have an ECG within 10 minutes of arrival. **Identifying STEMI by ECG as soon as possible is the first step** toward rapidly establishing reperfusion and reducing mortality (Table 7–1). In NSTEMI and UA, ECG findings range from subtle or absent to ST segment depression or T-wave inversion; however, these are not required for diagnosis or initiation of therapy. In patients eventually diagnosed with MI, the initial ECG is non-diagnostic in about 50% and completely normal in up to 8%. Changes may be appreciated

Table 7–1 • KEY ECG FINDINGS IN ACS
STEMI: indications for immediate reperfusion therapy
• ST elevation >1 mV (1 mm) in two contiguous leads and <12 h since pain onset • Left bundle-branch block not known to be old with a history suggestive of acute MI • ST elevations in posterior leads (V7, V8, and V9) or ST depression in V1-V3 with a prominent R wave and upright T-wave suggestive of posterior STEMI
Typical ECG findings in NSTEMI and UA
• Horizontal ST-segment depression • ECG findings change in accord with symptoms • Deep T-wave inversions

Source: Data from Hollander JE, Diercks DB. Intervention strategies for acute coronary syndromes. In: Tintinalli JE, Kelen GD, Stapczynski JS, eds. Emergency Medicine. 6th ed. New York, NY: McGraw-Hill; 2004:108-124.

when the current ECG is compared to old tracings. Serial ECGs performed at 15- to 30-minute intervals may reveal subtle dynamic changes of UA or those of an evolving MI (Table 7–2 lists the anatomical locations of MI). Leaving the ECG leads on the patient is helpful when comparing one ECG with the next.

In the face of a normal or non-diagnostic ECG, the decision whether to evaluate further for ACS depends on the patient's overall risk profile and likelihood that the pain is of cardiac origin. Inquiring about risk factors for CHD remains standard in evaluating chest pain. CHD risk factors are listed in Table 7–3. High risk is easily established if there is a prior history of definite CHD, such as prior MI or abnormal stress testing or coronary angiogram. Characteristics of the history and physical examination that alter the likelihood that the pain is of cardiac origin are listed in Table 7–4. Patients with an atypical story, few to no risk factors and a non-diagnostic ECG can usually be safely discharged without further evaluation for ACS. Clinical decision rules such as the history, ECG, age, risk factor, and troponin (**HEART**) score have been developed to help classify patients with undifferentiated chest pain with regard to their risk for ACS. For patients with known or suspected UA or NSTEMI, short-term prognosis and mortality can be calculated using the thrombolytics in myocardial infarction (**TIMI**) score (Table 7–5).

Table 7–2 • FINDINGS AND ANATOMICAL CORRELATION		
Coronary Artery	**Location**	**ECG Leads**
LAD	Anteroseptal	V1, V2, V3
LAD	Anterior	V2-V4
LCA	Lateral	I, aVL, V4-V6
RCA	Inferior	II, III, aVF
RCA	Right ventricular	V4R (also II, III, and aVF)
RCA, LCA	Posterior	R waves in V1, V2

Abbreviations: LAD = left anterior descending artery; LCA = left circumflex artery; RCA = right circumflex artery; V4R = right-sided lead which should be placed any time an inferior MI is suspected.
Source: Data from Hollander JE, Diercks DB. Intervention strategies for acute coronary syndromes. In: Tintinalli JE, Kelen GD, Stapczynski JS, eds. Emergency Medicine. 6th ed. New York, NY: McGraw-Hill; 2004:108-124.

Table 7–3 • RISK FACTORS FOR CORONARY HEART DISEASE
Diabetes mellitus
Hypercholesterolemia; high-density lipoprotein (HDL) cholesterol <40 mg/dL
Current tobacco use
Hypertension
Age (male ≥45 years; female ≥55 years or premature menopause)
Family history of premature CHD (MI or sudden death before age 55 years in male first-degree relative; before 65 years in female first-degree relative)
Sympathomimetics (cocaine and amphetamines)
Rheumatologic conditions (rheumatoid arthritis and systemic lupus erythematous)

Source: Data from Hollander JE, Diercks DB. Intervention strategies for acute coronary syndromes. In: Tintinalli JE, Kelen GD, Stapczynski JS, eds. Emergency Medicine. 6th ed. New York, NY: McGraw-Hill; 2004:108-124.

Serum cardiac markers are used to confirm or exclude myocardial cell death and are **the gold standard for the diagnosis of MI.** There are a number of markers currently in wide use, including myoglobin, CKMB and troponin. While algorithms vary, serum levels of one or more cardiac markers should be obtained initially and 3-6 hours after symptom onset. Troponin I is extremely sensitive and specific for cardiac damage; thus, an elevated level confirms infarction, whereas a normal level at 8-12 hours after the onset of pain excludes infarction. Cardiac markers have limitations since their levels remain normal in UA, serum elevations are often delayed until 4-12 hours after infarction and mild elevations can be seen in other conditions such as heart failure and renal failure.

Other studies that are routinely obtained in the workup of ACS include a **chest radiograph** (CXR), complete blood count, chemistries, and coagulation studies. The CXR serves to identify pulmonary edema and to assess for other causes of chest pain, such as aortic dissection and pneumonia.

Treatment

When ACS is suspected based on history, treatment should be started immediately. The patient should be placed on a cardiac monitor, IV access established, and an ECG obtained. Unless allergic, patients should immediately be given **aspirin to chew** (162 mg dose is common). Aspirin is remarkably beneficial across the entire spectrum of ACS. For example, in the setting of STEMI, the survival benefit from a single dose of aspirin is roughly equal to that of thrombolytic therapy but with

Table 7–4 • HISTORY AND PHYSICAL IN THE EVALUATION OF POSSIBLE ACS	
Increases Likelihood That Chest Pain Is from CHD	Decreases Likelihood That Chest Pain Is from CHD
Pressure-like quality	Pleuritic quality
Radiation to either arm, neck, or jaw	Constant pain for days
Diaphoresis	Pain lasting <2 min
Third heart sound	Discomfort localized with one finger
Pain that is similar to prior MI pain	Discomfort reproduced by movement or palpation

Table 7–5 • TIMI RISK SCORE[a]
Age >65 years
Prior documented coronary artery stenosis >50%
Three or more CHD risk factors
Use of aspirin in the preceding 7 days
Two or more anginal events in the preceding 24 hours
ST-segment deviation (transient elevation or persistent depression)
Increased cardiac markers

Abbreviation: TIMI = thrombolysis in myocardial infarction.
[a]One point is assigned to each of the seven components. Risk of death, MI, or revascularization at 2 week by score: 1, 5%; 2, 8%; 3, 13%; 4, 20%; 5, 26%; 6, 41%.
Source: Data from Antman EM, Cohen M, Bernink PJ, et al. The TIMI risk score for UA/NSTEMI. JAMA. 2000;284(7):835-842.

negligible risk or cost. Other mainstays of initial treatment are **oxygen** if the patient is in respiratory distress, pulse oximetry if saturation levels are 90% or less and sublingual **nitroglycerin**, which can decrease wall tension and myocardial oxygen demand. **Morphine** is the analgesic of choice for ischemic chest pain. These therapies make up the mnemonic **"MONA"** (morphine, oxygen, nitroglycerin, aspirin), though one should note the therapies are not given in the order listed in the mnemonic. Based on the initial ECG results, therapy then progresses in one of two directions.

ST Elevation MI

When the ECG reveals **STEMI** and symptoms have been present for less than 12 hours, **immediate reperfusion therapy** is indicated. Optimally, total ischemic time should be limited to less than 120 minutes. There are two ways to achieve reperfusion: primary PCI (angioplasty, or stent placement) and thrombolysis.

PCI is the treatment of choice when it can be performed rapidly by an experienced cardiologist. The standard "door-to-balloon time" goal is 90 minutes, although benefit extends to 12 hours from time of pain onset. In patients with severe heart failure or cardiogenic shock, PCI may still be indicated irrespective of the time delay from symptom onset.

Recent studies suggest that if a patient presents to a hospital that does not offer PCI, transfer to a neighboring facility for primary PCI is superior to thrombolysis if transfer can be accomplished within **120 minutes.** However, when PCI is not an option within this time frame, intravenous thrombolytic agents may be used to achieve reperfusion. Though the benefit of thrombolysis extends out to 12 hours, it is **greatest when begun within 4 hours** and approaches that of primary PCI when started within **30 minutes.** Adjunctive antithrombotic therapy with unfractionated or low-molecular-weight heparin is required with most thrombolytic agents. Patients receiving thrombolytic agents should then be transferred immediately to a PCI center. If there is no reperfusion with thrombolytics, rescue PCI can be performed. Even if there is evidence of successful reperfusion, PCI should generally be performed within 24 hours of thrombolytic therapy.

Table 7–6 lists other measures, in addition to aspirin and reperfusion therapy, that reduce mortality after MI.

Table 7–6 • THERAPIES OF PROVEN BENEFIT FOR MI
Aspirin (162 mg, chewed immediately, then continued daily for life)
Primary percutaneous coronary intervention (angioplasty or stenting the blocked artery)
Thrombolysis (if primary PCI not available; most regimens require heparin therapy)
β-blockers (immediate IV use and started orally within 24 hours; if no contraindications then continued daily)
Angiotensin-converting enzyme inhibitor (started within 1-3 days and continued for life)
Cholesterol-lowering drugs (started within 1-3 days and continued daily for life)
Enoxaparin (dosage given prior to thrombolysis or PCI, for patients <75 years of age)
Clopidogrel (75 mg daily with or without reperfusion therapy)

Source: Data from American College of Cardiologists. Guidelines for managing patients with AMI, UA, and NSTEMI. J Am Coll Cardiol. 2002;40:1366-1374.

Unstable Angina/Non-ST Elevation MI

Cases of ACS lacking ECG criteria for reperfusion fall into the UA/NSTEMI category. The approach to therapy for UA/NSTEMI tends to be graded based on ECG findings, cardiac marker results, TIMI risk score, and whether the patient is likely to undergo early angiography and PCI. **Aspirin and nitroglycerin constitute the minimum therapy.** Morphine is added when chest discomfort continues despite nitroglycerin therapy. Beta-blockers, such as IV metoprolol, may be added in cases presenting with hypertension or tachycardia; however, they should be used with caution. Mortality benefit of chronic beta-blocker therapy after MI is well established, but in the acute setting, this can put patients at risk for cardiogenic shock.

In high-risk patients, such as those with ischemic ECG changes, elevated cardiac markers and TIMI risk score 3 or greater, adding **low-molecular-weight heparin** and **oral clopidogrel,** an antiplatelet agent, may work to halt the thrombotic process. Intravenous glycoprotein IIB/IIIA inhibitors, such as abciximab, or direct thrombin inhibitors, such as bivalirudin, are often used in patients undergoing early angiography and PCI.

Recent studies show that an **early invasive strategy,** where high-risk patients with UA and NSTEMI are taken for angiography and PCI within 24-36 hours, has slightly superior efficacy to medical therapy and delayed angiography. Early PCI is strongly indicated for any of the following: refractory angina; hemodynamic instability; signs of heart failure; ventricular tachycardia; ST depressions on ECG; or elevated cardiac enzymes.

Complications

Several life-threatening complications of acute MI may arise at any time after presentation (Table 7–7). Serious complications occur most often in the setting of anterior STEMI. MI-associated **ventricular tachycardia** and **ventricular fibrillation** (sudden death) are the most frequently encountered complications in the ED and prehospital setting, occurring in approximately 10% of cases. **Bradyarrhythmias,** including heart block from irreversible damage to the His-Purkinje system after an anterior MI or arteriovenous (AV) node dysfunction from an inferior MI, may also occur.

Table 7–7 • POTENTIAL COMPLICATIONS FROM ACUTE MI	
Ventricular fibrillation	Cardiogenic pulmonary edema
Ventricular tachycardia	Ventricular septal defect
Heart block	Cardiogenic shock
Right ventricular infarction	Mitral regurgitation
Free wall rupture	Pericarditis
Ventricular aneurysm	Thromboembolism
Hemorrhage secondary to therapy	

Data from Hollander JE, Diercks DB. Intervention strategies for acute coronary syndromes. In: Tintinalli JE, Kelen GD, Stapczynski JS, eds. Emergency Medicine. 6th ed. New York, NY: McGraw-Hill; 2004:108-124.

Left ventricular dysfunction that occurs with anterior MI usually causes **pulmonary edema or cardiogenic shock.** A new systolic murmur may be heard if cardiogenic pulmonary edema is caused by papillary muscle dysfunction and acute mitral regurgitation. Signs of cardiogenic shock range from frank hypotension to indicators of impaired perfusion such as cool moist skin, oliguria, and confusion. Treatment includes emergent PCI, pressor agents, and, if necessary, an intra-aortic balloon pump. **Right ventricular infarction** from an inferior MI usually presents as hypotension without pulmonary congestion. Treatment is aggressive volume loading. Nitroglycerine will decrease preload and must be avoided in patients with right ventricular infarction.

Late complications of MI that tend to occur several hours to days after presentation include left ventricular free wall rupture causing tamponade, ventricular septal defect, pericarditis, left ventricular aneurysm, and thromboembolism. Finally, iatrogenic complications of MI therapy can occur. Heparin and antiplatelet therapies lead to significant bleeding in up to 10% of patients. Intracranial hemorrhage occurs in 0.5% to 0.7% of patients who receive thrombolytics for STEMI. These bleeds are usually fatal.

CASE CORRELATION

- See also Case 8 (Noncardiac Chest Pain), Case 11 (Congestive Heart Failure/Pulmonary Edema), Case 14 (Pulmonary Embolism), and Case 15 (Bacterial Pneumonia).

COMPREHENSION QUESTIONS

7.1 A 65-year-old man with history of diabetes presents to the Emergency Department stating he has had substernal chest pain and diaphoresis for 45 minutes. Which is the most important next step in management?

    A. Sublingual nitroglycerin

    B. Oxygen

    C. Placement of defibrillator pads

    D. Aspirin to chew

    E. Morphine sulfate

7.2 In the initial evaluation of a patient with chest pain, which is the most important diagnostic test?

A. Treadmill stress test

B. PT

C. Chest x-ray

D. Troponin

E. ECG

7.3 A 54-year-old man is seen at a rural ED with 1 hour of nausea and substernal chest pain radiating to his jaw. The ECG shows STEMI. PCI is not performed at this hospital and only performed at a hospital $2\,^1/_2$ hours away. Which of the following statements is most accurate?

A. Obtain a repeat ECG to assess if the patient truly has a STEMI.

B. Transfer the patient now for emergent PCI.

C. Administer thrombolytics, then transfer to PCI center.

D. Give aspirin, start heparin, and obtain a thallium stress test.

ANSWERS

7.1 **D.** While all of these interventions may be useful, aspirin significantly decreases mortality, with almost no downside in non-allergic patients, and it should be given immediately. Thus, aspirin is the first intervention.

7.2 **E.** The history of chest pain is important to obtain. The ECG is the crucial first diagnostic test in the evaluation of chest pain. Presence versus absence of ST elevation represents a major branch point in deciding treatment. Serum cardiac levels take time and sometimes are not elevated at the time of patient encounter.

7.3 **C.** PCI is the treatment of choice when it can be performed rapidly by an experienced cardiologist. However, if a patient presents to a hospital that does not offer PCI and cannot be transferred to one within 120 minutes, administration of thrombolytics, preferably within 30 minutes of arrival, is indicated. The patient should then be transferred to the nearest PCI center.

CLINICAL PEARLS

▶ MONA greets chest pain at the door (morphine, oxygen, nitroglycerin, and, most importantly, aspirin).

▶ An ECG should be performed immediately in all patients with chest pain concerning for ACS.

▶ The ECG will dictate the next step in management; new ST elevation generally requires immediate reperfusion therapy. "Time is myocardium."

REFERENCES

Amsterdam EA, Wenger NK, Brindis RG, et al. 2014 AHA/ACC guideline for the management of patients with non–ST-elevation acute coronary syndromes: executive summary. *Circulation.* 2014;130:2354-2394.

O'Gara PT, Kushner FG, Ascheim DD, et al. 2013 ACCF/AHA guideline for the management of ST-elevation myocardial infarction: executive summary. *Circulation.* 2013;127:529-555.

Panju AA, Hemmelgarn BR. Is this patient having a myocardial infarction? *JAMA.* 1998;280: 1256-1263.

Reeder et al. Initial evaluation and management of suspected acute coronary syndrome (myocardial infarction, unstable angina) in the emergency department. Available at· www.uptodate.com. Accessed Oct 03, 2016.

A 28-year-old man arrives at the emergency department (ED) complaining of 1 day of chest pain (CP) beginning suddenly after multiple episodes of retching and vomiting following a night of heavy drinking. Since the pain began, he has had subjective fevers, feels very weak, is unable to tolerate any food or water, and has urinated only once. He describes lower anterior CP that is non-radiating and of moderately severe intensity, aggravated by swallowing. While he is speaking in full sentences, he states that he has to control his breathing to avoid a "tight feeling in his throat," and he is concerned that his voice sounds "different." The review of systems is otherwise negative. His temperature is 38°C, hear rate is 132 beats per minute, blood pressure is 148/74 mm Hg, and respiration rate is 22 breaths per minute with an O_2 saturation of 98% on room air. Physical examination shows an ill and uncomfortable appearing man who is tachycardic, diaphoretic, and borderline febrile. He has dry mucous membranes and faint bibasilar crackles. He has no past medical history and is taking no medications.

▶ What is the most likely diagnosis?
▶ What are the next steps in management?
▶ What therapies should be instituted immediately?

ANSWERS TO CASE 8:
Noncardiac Chest Pain

Summary: This is a 28-year-old man presenting with acute severe CP, diaphoresis, and dyspnea after multiple episodes of vomiting.

- **Most likely diagnosis:** Spontaneous esophageal perforation or Boerhaave syndrome.

- **Next management steps:** Place the patient on a cardiac monitor, establish IV access and obtain an electrocardiogram (ECG) immediately. A chest x-ray (CXR) should be obtained as soon as possible.

- **Immediate therapies:** Nil per os (NPO), nasogastric tube (NGT), IV resuscitation with isotonic fluids, broad spectrum antibiotics, pain management, and urgent surgical consultation.

ANALYSIS

Objectives

1. Become familiar with the serious causes of noncardiac chest pain (NCCP).

2. Consider spontaneous esophageal perforation in the differential diagnosis of CP and recognize the key signs and symptoms of Boerhaave syndrome.

3. Understand the approach to evaluating and treating NCCP in general and Boerhaave syndrome in particular.

Considerations

CP is one of the most common reasons patients come to the ED. The role of the emergency provider (EP) is to differentiate the life threatening presentations of CP from those that are benign and to quickly and appropriately treat patients who present with an emergent condition. In order to identify dangerous presentations, EPs must consider and exclude (or diagnose) the causes of NCCP in all patients who present with CP. The differential for dangerous causes of CP includes immediate life threatening causes such as aortic dissection, pulmonary embolism, tension pneumothorax, esophageal perforation, and pericardial effusion with tamponade. It also includes still concerning but less time sensitive diagnoses such as pneumonia, pneumothorax or hemothorax, myocarditis, pericarditis, multiple rib fractures, esophageal spasm, and gastrointestinal causes such as pancreatitis, hepatitis, biliary disease, or severe peptic ulcer disease (PUD). More benign causes include chest wall contusion, costochondritis, muscular strain, gastroesophageal reflux disease (GERD), or anxiety. In the case presented, this young man presents with a dangerous cause of CP, Boerhaave syndrome related to alcohol-induced repetitive vomiting. There are several clues to the diagnosis, as we will discuss in the following text.

APPROACH TO:
Noncardiac Chest Pain

DEFINITIONS

BOERHAAVE SYNDROME: Barotrauma induced rupture of the esophagus, usually caused by vomiting.

GASTROGRAFIN: Water-soluble iodinated radiographic contrast agent.

BARIUM: Water insoluble radiographic contrast agent composed of a particulate suspension of barium sulfate.

APPROACH TO SUSPECTED BOERHAAVE SYNDROME

Pathophysiology

Boerhaave syndrome is esophageal perforation that results from an abrupt increase of intraluminal pressure in the esophagus. While usually due to vomiting, there are rare cases reported after prolonged labor, laughing, seizures, and even defecation. The esophagus is especially vulnerable to rupture because it lacks the serosal layer present in more distal portions of the GI tract. In most cases, the tear occurs along the left posterolateral aspect of the distal intrathoracic esophagus, where the support structures are weakest. However, cervical or intra-abdominal esophageal perforation may also occur.

Esophageal rupture can occur from other causes, such as trauma, ingestion of a caustic substance or foreign body, and surgical procedures near or on the esophagus. The majority of esophageal ruptures are iatrogenic due to endoscopy. However, these ruptures are distinct from the effort-related rupture known as Boerhaave syndrome.

Morbidity and mortality associated with Boerhaave syndrome are due in part to the overwhelming inflammatory response to gastric contents and oropharyngeal bacteria being introduced into the mediastinum and the resultant infections. Contamination of the mediastinal and pleural spaces can result in pneumonia, mediastinitis, empyema, sepsis, and multi-organ failure. Untreated Boerhaave syndrome has a 100% case fatality rate. When treated quickly and appropriately, mortality is still as high as 20%.

Evaluation

Mackler triad consists of vomiting, lower CP, and subcutaneous emphysema. Though these symptoms are classically described in Boerhaave syndrome, they are seen in only a minority of cases. Important potential signs and symptoms include fever, CP, back pain, tachypnea, tachycardia, dyspnea, subcutaneous emphysema, and Hamman sign (a "mediastinal crunch" heard with each heart beat due to the surrounding air). Breath sounds may be decreased on the side of perforation due to pleural effusion.

If **esophageal perforation** is suspected, a CT scan of the chest should be ordered promptly. A CXR will likely be the initial study performed and may show pleural effusion, pneumomediastinum, widened mediastinum, or pneumothorax. It should be noted that early in the presentation, the CXR can be negative. CT scan is far more sensitive and may show esophageal wall thickening, periesophageal fluid, extraesophageal air, and/or air and fluid in pleural spaces. Contrast radiographic studies of the esophagus may be necessary to localize the perforation. Gastrografin or other water soluble contrast should be used instead of barium contrast to avoid barium-related inflammation of the mediastinum if there is indeed perforation. Small esophageal perforations are frequently missed by both contrast modalities. If a thoracentesis is performed, pleural fluid typically will reveal pH <6 and elevated amylase, and it can possibly contain food particles. Endoscopy has no role in the evaluation of Boerhaave syndrome and may exacerbate the perforation due to air insufflation during the procedure.

Treatment

An immediate surgical consult should be obtained. **Definitive treatment will depend on the size and location of the perforation, whether or not it is contained,** and the presence of preexisting disease. If the CT scan shows containment, treatment initially consists of NPO status, NGT placement with suction to remove gastric fluids and prevent further contamination, broad spectrum IV antibiotics, and parenteral nutrition. If the perforation is not contained, surgical repair is indicated. Some esophageal tears may be amenable to endoscopic stenting. Pain control and antiemetics to prevent additional valsalva-induced barotrauma should be given as early as possible in the course of treatment.

Complications

Any delay in diagnosis or treatment will result in increased morbidity and mortality. Death due to spontaneous esophageal rupture may be as high as 20% to 40% of treated cases. Complications of surgical repair include mediastinitis, sepsis, and persistent esophageal leaks.

CLINICAL APPROACH TO NONCARDIAC CHEST PAIN

Chest pain is responsible for more than 6 million visits per year to the ED in the United States. The evaluation of acute CP should always begin with a complete history focusing on quality, radiation of pain, context of onset, duration, risk factors, and exacerbating factors.

Due to the high morbidity and mortality of myocardial infarction, an ECG should be obtained immediately upon presentation to assess the possibility of acute myocardial ischemia. Even when NCCP is suspected, reevaluation may be necessary if traditional cardiac risk factors suggest a high pretest probability of cardiac disease. The pretest probability of a cardiac etiology for an episode of CP increases with the patient age and positive risk factor profile.

Although often helpful, a single ECG does not always demonstrate evidence of a cardiac cause of CP when it is cardiac in nature. A meta-analysis of exercise treadmill stress test results reported a sensitivity of 68% and a specificity of 77% for cardiac ischemia. Unless the patient is having an acute ST elevation myocardial infarction, a single ECG will likely not be any more sensitive or specific than this result.

However, repeat ECGs with changes over time may increase the diagnostic certainty. Thus for any patient initially presenting with moderate or greater pretest probability of cardiac disease, a workup including **serial ECGs and cardiac enzymes** is indicated before diagnosing them with NCCP.

NCCP is generally defined as CP occurring in the presence of normal coronary artery anatomy and thus not related to myocardial ischemia. A small percentage of these patients may have ischemia due to vasospasm or isolated distal arterial disease, but this does not change the general approach or differential diagnosis.

Differential Diagnosis of Noncardiac Chest Pain

The differential for NCCP is wide and includes both dangerous and benign causes. The majority of NCCP is due to musculoskeletal etiologies, esophageal/GI, psychiatric, and pulmonary causes, and the most common cause of NCCP seen in the ED is GERD. The etiology behind many cases of atypical NCCP is never found.

Musculoskeletal Chest Pain Musculoskeletal CP is usually associated with a history of trauma, specific injury, or repetitive use. This kind of CP should be **reproducible on careful examination by palpation or through specific motions or movements** of the involved anatomic structures. The pain may also be pleuritic, or associated with deep breathing. Correlation with the muscular and boney anatomy of the neck, thorax, and upper abdomen can further solidify the cause of NCCP. Frequently, the only evaluation needed will be a careful and complete history and physical examination. Nonetheless, CXR is appropriate if boney or pulmonary disease is being considered. Bedside ultrasound or formal echocardiography may be used to rule out pneumothorax, pericarditis, structural heart disease, or aortic pathology. Liberal utilization of ECG is indicated and appropriate. Keep in mind, while having tenderness to palpation along the chest wall may make acute coronary syndrome less likely, it does not rule it out, so close attention must still be paid to the history of the pain and risk factors of the patient. Localized, well circumscribed, discrete tenderness is more consistent with NCCP. Once the diagnosis of musculoskeletal CP has been made, appropriate care includes reassurance, analgesics, nonsteroidal anti-inflammatory drugs (NSAIDs), and temporary behavioral restrictions to minimize reinjury. Follow-up examination in 1-2 weeks is recommended with their primary care physician.

Esophageal and Gastrointestinal Causes of Chest Pain Multiple pathologies of the esophagus may result in CP. These include reflux and esophagitis, esophageal ulceration, foreign body, perforation, and spasm. Esophageal perforation is discussed previously. Esophageal foreign body is usually obvious from the patient history, except in young children and the elderly. CXR and neck films will identify radiopaque foreign bodies, while other objects require upper endoscopy for further evaluation. Many patients suffer from GERD. The history in patients with GERD may include epigastric pain at night or when laying supine and a correlation with large meals near bedtime. Some will describe a foul taste in their mouth, especially in the morning. Caffeine, alcohol, and tobacco use all decrease lower esophageal sphincter pressure and increase the likelihood of reflux. NSAIDs and alcohol may also injure the esophageal mucosa. **Long-term reflux and**

esophagitis can result in histologic changes in the distal esophageal mucosa (Barrett esophagus) that can lead to adenocarcinoma. Physical examination is nonspecific and may show only subxiphoid or epigastric tenderness. Acute treatments are not helpful from the standpoint of narrowing the differential and can lead to errors in diagnosis. Nitroglycerin has been shown to relieve GERD-associated esophageal spasm but also relieves cardiac CP. The classic "GI cocktail" of antacid, lidocaine, and H2 blocker relieves GERD pain, but relief from these medications is not a reliable indicator that the pain was not cardiac in origin. Thus, neither of these treatments should ever be used to rule out or rule in any single diagnosis. Long-term management of esophageal disorders includes various medications (PPI, H2 blocker, and mucosal protectants) to allow healing of the esophageal mucosa. Additionally, behavior modification to prevent nocturnal reflux may be helpful. Peptic ulcer disease is frequently associated with GERD. Triple therapy with PPI, H2 blockers, and antibiotics for eradication of *Helicobacter pylori* have resulted in more than 90% PUD healing rate. Referral to a gastroenterologist for ongoing management is appropriate in more complicated cases.

Diseases of the upper abdominal organs may also cause NCCP. **Hepatitis** can cause pain that radiates into the upper right chest due to inflammation of the right hemidiaphragm. **Cholecystitis** can result in substernal CP and subxiphoid epigastric pain. **Pancreatitis** can cause pain that radiates from the epigastrum into the back or into the left chest in association with a transudative pulmonary effusion. Splenic hematoma or infarction can result in CP that radiates to the left upper chest due to inflammation of the left hemidiaphragm.

Psychiatric Causes of Chest Pain Depression and anxiety frequently result in complaints of chest or abdominal pain. The patient may or may not be aware of the depression. Patients complaining of CP should be questioned about symptoms of depression such as anhedonia, early morning awakening, insomnia, and loss of interest or pleasure in normal activities. Physical examination in the organically depressed patient may reveal emotional lability, flattened affect, suicidal ideation, or psychomotor retardation, but it is generally negative for specific findings associated with other physical causes of CP. Somatization refers to a physical symptom that a patient feels as the manifestation of their depression or anxiety. The patient may be fixated on the presenting physical complaint and unaware of the depressive component to their complaint. Diagnostic workup of this type of patient should be guided by a careful history and physical examination. A reasonably extensive initial diagnostic workup is indicated since a psychiatric etiology for CP must be a diagnosis of exclusion. Recent meta-analysis has revealed a potential association between the diagnoses of panic attack/anxiety with CP and CAD in the primary care and ED settings. The care provider should also keep in mind that depression may coexist with other organic causes of CP and that this risk increases with age. Also to be kept in mind is that depression alone may have lethal consequences and requires accurate diagnosis and aggressive therapy by a mental healthcare professional.

Pulmonary Causes of Chest Pain The lungs, air passages, and pleura can all cause chest discomfort. Irritation of the pleura can be caused by: inflammation from infectious causes such as pneumonia, ischemia due to pulmonary embolism or infarction, and mechanical irritation due to pneumothorax, pneumomediastinum, exudative effusions and some cancers. **If fever and hypoxia are present, infectious causes of CP should be suspected.** Pneumothorax or pulmonary embolism should be suspected when the patient has acute unilateral pleuritic pain and risk factors for venous thromboembolism. Unilateral pleuritic CP ipsilateral to blunt chest trauma strongly suggests pneumothorax or hemothorax. **Tracheal deviation, hypoxia, hypotension, and hyperresonance of the hemithorax contralateral to the tracheal deviation indicate the presence of tension pneumothorax.** This is an immediately life-threatening condition that requires emergency needle decompression of the hyper-resonant hemithorax with a large gauge needle or angiocath. If available, bedside ultrasound (US) may rapidly diagnose pneumothorax. In the unstable patient, treatment of tension pneumothorax should never be delayed for radiographic confirmation. Occult hypoxia may be uncovered by obtaining ambulatory pulse oximetry. Physical examination of the chest may reveal rales, rhonchi, wheezing, decreased breath sounds, signs of consolidation or effusion, and/or abnormalities of the chest wall. These findings may occur together or in isolation and should be correlated with the history and a two view CXR to accurately determine the cause and scope of the patient pathology. If an infectious etiology is suspected in a patient, antibiotics should be administered, and the patient may require admission to the hospital.

Other Causes of Chest Pain Pericarditis is a non-ischemic cause of cardiac CP that results from inflammation of the pericardium, the connective tissue sack which envelops the heart. The pain associated with this entity is worse when supine and improves with erect posture or sitting up. **Auscultation of the heart may reveal a rough scratchy sound known as a pericardial friction rub.** ECG findings vary over the course of the illness but initially include diffuse concave ST elevations associated with PR depression, and isolated PR elevation in avR. Many causes of pericarditis exist. These include but are not limited to autoimmune, infectious (viral, bacterial, and fungal), postinfarction (Dressler syndrome), and traumatic. Viral infection is the most common non-infarction cause. **Evaluation should include ECG and serial cardiac enzymes since cardiac ischemia should remain high in the differential.** A troponin can be sent to evaluate for involvement of the myocardium, known as myocarditis. Echocardiography can be used to evaluate for a pericardial effusion and to rule out the potentially lethal complication of pericardial tamponade. Tamponade may develop if pressure from the effusion is great enough to significantly impair cardiac filling. Emergent treatment of cardiac tamponade consists of pericardial drainage by needle aspiration. Treatment of uncomplicated pericarditis consists of analgesics, NSAIDs, colchicine, and frequent follow-up until improvement is achieved.

A **high suspicion must always be maintained for aortic dissection and pulmonary embolism** to avoid missing these difficult to make but life threatening diagnoses. In both diseases, the onset of CP can be sudden and associated with syncope and dyspnea. Aortic dissection can be very difficult to diagnose, as it presents in many different ways. The classic presentation is a patient complaining of CP radiating to the back. However, according to the IRAD (International Registry of Acute Aortic Dissections) database, only 75% of patients complain of CP, 50% complain of back pain, and only 30% report radiation. If the dissection involves the root of the aorta and thus the coronary arteries, the patient may also have CP due to cardiac ischemia. Patients can also develop pericardial tamponade from the dissection. Early echocardiography and/or CT imaging will result in timely diagnosis.

Pulmonary embolism is a blockage of an artery in the lung from a substance, usually a blood clot that has traveled from elsewhere in the body. The most common origin for blood clots is the deep veins of the lower extremities. If one or both of the main pulmonary arteries are blocked, shock and even death can ensue. Patients typically present with sudden onset of pleuritic CP and shortness of breath. Risk factor assessment has an important role to play in diagnosing pulmonary embolism. Those associated with pulmonary embolism include recent surgery or immobilization, exogenous hormone use, and active cancer. A CT angiogram is the diagnostic test of choice. Treatment of pulmonary embolism is controversial and will depend on the size, location, and extent of hemodynamic compromise due to the clot burden. Thrombolytic therapy with TPA is the treatment for cardiac arrest due to pulmonary embolism.

Another consideration in a vomiting patient with CP is the less serious but still potentially life threatening **Mallory-Weiss tear**. This entity involves a traumatic mucosal disruption usually located either at the gastroesophageal junction or gastric cardia. These esophageal tears may result in significant GI hemorrhage and can perforate if intense vomiting or retching continues. Deeper tears of the esophageal mucosa may manifest as intramural esophageal hematomas, which can develop into full esophageal perforations with delayed rupture during the inflammatory weakening that accompanies healing.

Spontaneous pneumomediastinum without evidence of gastrointestinal or pleural source has been reported. It is usually seen in patients undergoing a vigorous valsalva episode against a closed glottis, which may occur in cases like powerful coughing. This CP is universal, and on examination a loud crunching sound may be heard as mediastinal air is squeezed by the beating heart (Hamman crunch). Crack cocaine smokers appear to be at particular risk. Despite the ominous CXR findings, this entity has a generally benign course. Nonetheless, the diagnosis of pneumomediastinum requires a diligent and exhaustive search for both pulmonary and gastrointestinal sources.

Breast pathology should be considered in the differential of NCCP in women presenting to the ED. Causes of breast pain include infectious etiologies, mastitis or abscess, benign lumps, cysts, or inflammatory carcinoma. Physical examination may reveal an asymmetric breast mass with or without signs of significant local induration, erythema, and tenderness. The patient with more serious pathology is often febrile. Intravenous analgesics, antibiotics, and early surgical consultation are appropriate if an infectious cause is suspected.

The preceding list is not exhaustive, and difficult clinical cases may require evaluation for more esoteric causes of NCCP. In the geriatric population, many patients may have more than one diagnosis causing their NCCP. As such, it is imperative that early primary care follow-up be arranged for these patients.

Presentation of Boerhaave Syndrome (Pressure Induced Esophageal Rupture)

The classical presentation of Boerhaave syndrome follows an episode of forceful retching and vomiting and includes retrosternal CP and/or epigastric pain. Odynophagia, dyspnea, tachypnea, cyanosis, fever, and shock may all develop thereafter. In one review, 40% of patients had a history of heavy drinking, 41% suffered from PUD, 83% complained of pain, 79% had a history of vomiting, 32% presented with shock, and 39% had dyspnea. The diagnosis of Boerhaave syndrome may be delayed because the clinical presentation may not be typical, and causes are broad: childbirth, defecation, seizures, and heavy lifting. Common misdiagnoses include: myocardial infarction, pancreatitis, lung abscess, pericarditis, and spontaneous pneumothorax. Concurrent alcohol intoxication may also delay diagnosis.

CASE CORRELATION

- See also Case 7 (Acute Coronary Syndrome), Case 14 (Pulmonary Embolism), and Case 15 (Bacterial Pneumonia).

COMPREHENSION QUESTIONS

8.1 A 45-year-old man presents to the ED with the acute onset of CP. Which of the following would point to a non-life threatening etiology of CP?

    A. Shortness of breath

    B. Worse when laying down and after large meals

    C. Diffuse ST segment elevation

    D. Cervical subcutaneous emphysema

    E. Unilateral pleuritic CP

8.2 A 35-year-old woman presents to her physician's office with CP of 1 week's duration. The physician suspects possible musculoskeletal etiology. Which of the following would be the best evidence to confirm this diagnosis?

    A. Relief with nitroglycerin

    B. Tracheal deviation

    C. Radiation down the left arm

    D. Reproduced with palpation

8.3 Which test will best help you identify CP of cardiac origin?

    A. ECG

    B. CXR

    C. CT thorax

    D. Barium esophagram

ANSWERS

8.1 **B. Pain that worsens with lying down and after a large meal is more suggestive of GERD.** While GERD is a cause of pain that may eventually lead to esophagitis or even malignancy, it is not an immediate life threatening cause of CP. Aortic dissection, pulmonary embolism, cardiac tamponade, pneumothorax, and acute myocardial infarction can all lead to imminent death and therefore must be diagnosed and intervened upon immediately if found.

8.2 **D.** Musculoskeletal causes are the most common etiologies of NCCP. The best way to confirm the diagnosis is to reproduce the pain with palpation in the anatomical region or with movement. Nitroglycerin is a treatment of CAD. Tracheal deviation suggests tension pneumothorax. Radiation down the left arm may be associated with angina.

8.3 **A.** ECG is the best initial test for cardiac CP since it is easy to obtain, is not invasive, and can be specific for ischemia. A CXR, CT of the thorax, and barium esophagram all evaluate for other causes of CP.

CLINICAL PEARLS

▶ Boerhaave syndrome should always be considered in the differential diagnosis of acute CP, especially if the patient has been vomiting or performing any activity where barotrauma may have been sustained due to valsalva maneuver.

▶ When doing contrast studies to locate the site of esophageal perforation, Gastrografin should be used instead of barium to avoid severe mediastinal and intra-pleural inflammatory reactions.

▶ GI Cocktail cannot be used to reliably rule out a cardiac etiology for an episode of CP.

▶ Response to a trial of sublingual nitroglycerin does not distinguish between coronary artery disease and GERD induced esophageal spasm.

▶ A single normal ECG cannot be used to make the diagnosis of NCCP.

▶ A significant percentage of patients (2%-3%) labeled with a diagnosis of NCCP will have an adverse cardiac event within 30 days.

REFERENCES

Chambers J, Bass C, Mayou R. Non-cardiac chest pain: assessment and management. *Heart.* 1999;82:656-657.

Dumville JC, MacPherson H, Griffith K, Miles JN, Lewin RJ. Non-cardiac chest pain: a retrospective cohort study of patients who attended a Rapid Access Chest Pain Clinic. *Fam Pract.* 2007;24(2): 152-157.

Glombiewski JA, Rief W, Bösner S, Keller H, Martin A, Donner-Banzhoff N. The course of non-specific chest pain in primary care: symptom persistence and health care usage. *Arch Intern Med.* 2010;170(3):251-255.

Gräni C, Senn O, Bischof M, et al. Diagnostic performance of reproducible chest wall tenderness to rule out acute coronary syndrome in acute chest pain: a prospective diagnostic study. *BMJ Open.* 2015;5(1):e007442 doi:10.1136/bmjopen-2014-007442.

Herring N, Paterson DJ. ECG diagnosis of acute ischaemia and infarction: past, present and future. *QJM.* 2006;99(4):219-230.

Katerndahl DA. Chest pain and its importance in patients with panic disorder: an updated literature review. *Prim Care Companion J Clin Psychiatry.* 2008;10(5):376-383.

Kiev J, Amendola M. A management algorithm for esophageal perforation. *Am J Surg.* 2007;194: 103-106.

Klinkman MS, Stevens D, Gorenflo DW. Episodes of care for chest pain: a preliminary report from MIRNET. *J Fam Pract.* 1994;38(4):345-352.

Long CM, Ezenkwele UA. Esophageal perforation, rupture and tears. Available at: www.emedicine.com. Accessed June, 2010.

Martina B, Bucheli B, Stotz M, Battegay E, Gyr N. First clinical judgment by primary care physicians distinguishes well between nonorganic and organic causes of abdominal or chest pain. *J Gen Intern Med.* 1997;12(8):459-465.

Mayou RA, Bass C, Hart G, Tyndel S, Bryant B. Can clinical assessment of chest pain be made more therapeutic? *QJM.* 2000;93(12):805-811.

Mayou RA, Bass CM, Bryant BM. Management of non-cardiac chest pain: from research to clinical practice. *Heart.* 1999;81(4):387-392.

Newby DE, Fox KA, Flint LL, Boon NA. A 'same day' direct-access chest pain clinic: improved management and reduced hospitalization. *QJM.* 1998;91(5):333-337.

Svavarsdóttir AE, Jónasson MR, Gudmundsson GH, Fjeldsted K. Chest pain in family practice. Diagnosis and long-term outcome in a community setting. *Can Fam Physician.* 1996;42:1122-1128. Erratum in: *Can Fam Physician.* 1996;42:1672.

Triadafilopoulos G, LaMont JT. Boerhaave syndrome: effort rupture of the esophagus. Available at: www.uptodate.com. Accessed June, 2010.

Verdon F, Herzig L, Burnand B, et al. Chest pain in daily practice: occurrence, causes and management. *Swiss Med Wkly.* 2008;138(23-24):340-347.

A 73-year-old woman presents to the emergency department complaining of palpitations and new shortness of breath with minor exertion for the past 2 weeks. Previously, she could walk everywhere, but now she becomes fatigued climbing the stairs of her home. Occasionally, she has felt her heart racing even when she is at rest. Her past medical history is notable for diet controlled diabetes and hypertension, for which she takes hydrochlorothiazide and amlodipine. On physical examination, she appears comfortable and speaks in full sentences without difficulty. Her blood pressure is 130/90 mm Hg, heart rate is 144 beats per minute, respiratory rate is 18 breaths per minute, oxygen saturation is 98% on room air, and temperature is 37°C (98.6°F). The head and neck examination is unremarkable. Her lungs are clear to auscultation. Her heartbeat is irregular and rapid, without murmurs, rubs, or gallops. She has no extremity edema or jugular venous distension. Her abdomen is soft and nontender, without masses. Labs show a normal complete blood count (CBC), normal electrolytes, blood urea nitrogen (BUN), creatinine, troponin, brain natriuretic peptide (BNP), and thyroid stimulating hormone. A chest x-ray reveals a normal cardiac silhouette with no pulmonary edema. The ECG is shown below (Figure 9–1).

▶ What is the most likely diagnosis?
▶ What are some of the common contributing factors?
▶ What are some of the complications to this condition?

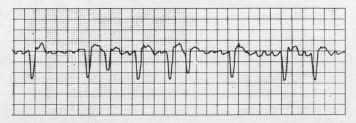

Figure 9–1. Electrocardiogram. *(Reproduced with permission from Tintinalli JE, Kelen GD, Stapczynski JS. Emergency Medicine. 6th ed. New York, NY: McGraw-Hill Education; 2004:185.)*

ANSWERS TO CASE 9:
Atrial Fibrillation

Summary: A 72-year-old woman presents with mild dyspnea on exertion and palpitations. The physical examination reveals a heartbeat that is irregular and rapid at a rate of 144 beats per minute.

- **Most likely diagnosis:** Atrial fibrillation (AF) with rapid ventricular response (RVR).

- **Common contributing factors:** Increasing age, underlying cardiopulmonary disease (such as hypertension, heart failure, valvular disease, and chronic obstructive pulmonary disease [COPD]), hyperthyroidism, sepsis, pulmonary embolism, and electrolyte abnormalities.

- **Complications:** Early—diminished cardiac output (CO) and hypotension. Late—thromboembolism and cardiomyopathy.

ANALYSIS

Objectives

1. Know that AF rarely exists in isolation and is typically a manifestation of other underlying disease processes.

2. Be able to recognize AF on ECG.

3. Understand the approach to rate control versus rhythm control of AF.

4. Understand the role of antithrombotic therapy in both the acute and the chronic management of AF.

5. Be familiar with the various options for anticoagulation, including the newer antithrombin and anti-Xa agents.

Considerations

This individual is a 72-year-old woman of fairly high function who is brought into the emergency department because of dyspnea and palpitations. The initial approach should begin with ABCs (airway, breathing, and circulation) and an assessment of any life-threatening concerns. **Upon arrival, this patient should get an IV and be placed on cardiac and pulse oximetry monitors.** The history and physical examination should focus on the patient's cardiac and pulmonary status. Her pulse and the rhythm on the cardiac monitor will both reveal an irregular tachycardia, which should prompt an immediate ECG. The ECG shows an irregularly irregular tachycardia consistent with the diagnosis of AF with RVR.

In this patient with symptomatic AF with RVR, an **early priority in management will be to slow the ventricular rate.** For most patients with AF, the typical symptoms of palpitations and dyspnea can be alleviated through simple rate control. In rare cases, tachycardia and loss of the "atrial kick" can lead to diminished CO,

Table 9–1 • DISEASES ASSOCIATED WITH ATRIAL FIBRILLATION	
Cardiac	Hypertension (approximately 80% of cases), coronary artery disease, cardiomyopathy, valvular heart disease, rheumatic heart disease, congenital heart disease, myocardial infarction, pericarditis, myocarditis
Pulmonary	Pulmonary embolism, chronic obstructive pulmonary disease (COPD), obstructive sleep apnea
Systemic disease	Hyperthyroidism, obesity, metabolic syndrome, inflammation
Postoperative	Cardiac surgery, any surgery
Binge alcohol drinking	"Holiday heart syndrome"
Lone AF	Associated with approximately 10% of AF

hypotension, or congestive heart failure. In those cases, if the arrhythmia is thought to be the primary cause of the patient's instability, emergent electrical cardioversion is indicated. In more stable patients, the decision of whether to convert the rhythm depends on a number of factors, including risk of thromboembolism, need for anticoagulation, and odds of recurrent AF. In all patients, a search for the underlying etiology should be undertaken because AF is often best managed by treating the underlying cause of the rhythm rather than the rhythm itself (Table 9–1).

APPROACH TO:
Atrial Fibrillation

DEFINITIONS

DYSPNEA: Difficult or labored breathing, shortness of breath, or a sensation of breathlessness.

THROMBOEMBOLISM: The passage of a blood clot through the vascular system from one part of the body to another—for example, in the setting of AF, a clot forms in the heart and then embolizes through the arterial circulation to the brain, mesentery, or extremities.

CARDIOMYOPATHY: Damage to heart muscle as the result of a number of various insults causing diminished contractility, which can eventually lead to heart failure, arrhythmia, and sudden death.

CLINICAL APPROACH

AF affects 1% of the general population and is the most common treatable arrhythmia seen in the emergency department. The prevalence of AF increases with age. In adults younger than 55 years old, the prevalence is only 0.1%, whereas in adults greater than 80 years old the prevalence is greater than 10%. AF is more common in men than in women and more common in whites than in blacks. Among patients with AF, 80% have cardiovascular disease, most commonly hypertension, coronary artery disease (CAD), valvular heart disease, and cardiomyopathy. The remaining common underlying causes include pulmonary diseases such as pulmonary embolism, COPD, and obstructive sleep apnea and systemic diseases such as hyperthyroidism, obesity, and diabetes (see Table 9–1). The exception is lone AF, which is a term used to describe AF in patients younger than 60 years old who have no obvious underlying cardiopulmonary disease process.

Pathophysiology

It is theorized that AF is caused by a complex interaction between triggers for AF and abnormal atrial myocardium that has multiple reentrant circuits or automatic foci outside the sinoatrial (SA) node. This interplay leads to rapid electrical activity in the atria, which can supersede the SA node and produce the disorganized and ineffective atrial contractions typical of AF. The rapid atrial electrical activity is also conducted through the atrioventricular (AV) node, leading to an irregular ventricular response. On ECG, AF looks like an irregularly irregular, usually narrow-complex, tachycardia without associated P-waves.

AF has a number of clinical implications, most important of which are cardiomyopathy and thromboembolism. Acutely, the loss of the "atrial kick" leads to a reduction in CO by as much as 15%. Together with the RVR shortening the diastolic filling time, CO may be significantly reduced, especially in patients with already poor left ventricular function. This reduction in CO can result in hypotension and symptoms of heart failure, including dyspnea and fatigue. Over the long term, AF causes progressive structural and electrophysiologic changes in the atria that promote more frequent and sustained episodes of AF. Additionally, chronic low levels of tachycardia lead to global cardiomyopathy, which in turn predisposes to more AF. For this reason it is said that AF "begets" more AF.

In addition to heart failure and cardiomyopathy, another important clinical implication of AF is thromboembolism. The disorganized, ineffective atrial contractions caused by AF lead to areas of blood stasis in the left atria, especially in the left atrial appendage. **This stasis promotes the formation of a thrombus,** which can then dislodge and embolize through the arterial circulation, causing strokes and mesenteric and limb ischemia. Patients with AF have two- to threefold higher risk of stroke compared to the general population.

Treatment

The management of AF is challenging because AF is often merely a manifestation of some underlying cardiac, pulmonary, endocrine, or toxicological pathology. Successful management begins by **initially addressing the patient's overall clinical status,** searching for treatable contributing factors, controlling the heart rate, and preventing thromboembolism (Figure 9–2).

In stable patients with AF, the treatment options include **rate control and/or rhythm control,** with or without anticoagulation. In the **acute setting, such as the emergency department, ventricular rate control is usually the first priority.** Slowing the ventricular response to AF has a number of positive hemodynamic effects, including increasing diastolic filling time, improving stroke volume and CO, and stabilizing blood pressure. Drugs used to control the ventricular rate work by slowing conduction through the AV node (see Table 9–2).

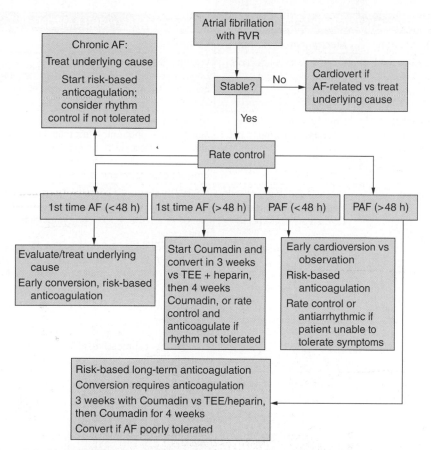

Figure 9–2. Algorithm for management of atrial fibrillation. PAF = paroxysmal atrial fibrillation.

There are two groups of patients with AF who should not receive rate controlling agents: (1) unstable patients in whom the instability is presumed to be caused by the rhythm, (2) patients with Wolff-Parkinson-White (WPW) syndrome (Figure 9–3). **Patients who are hemodynamically unstable should get immediate electrical cardioversion** to restore sinus rhythm. This approach assumes that the instability is rhythm-related. In most patients, however, the instability will be caused by other disease processes (MI, GI bleed, pulmonary embolism, etc.), with AF representing merely a potentially distracting side effect. Patients with WPW should not receive any AV nodal blocking agents since they can lead to accelerated conduction down the accessory pathway and potentially induce ventricular fibrillation and cardiac arrest. Patients with WPW and AF should instead get either pharmacologic or electrical cardioversion depending on the clinical picture.

Cardioversion

In order to cardiovert AF, several issues must first be addressed: the need for **anticoagulation** and the **timing and method of cardioversion.** During AF, uncoordinated atrial contractions lead to intra-atrial thrombus formation. The longer the duration

Table 9–2 • THERAPIES FOR RATE CONTROL OF ATRIAL FIBRILLATION		
Medication	Mechanism of Action	Comment
Calcium channel blockers (verapamil, diltiazem)	Slow AV node conduction by blocking calcium channels	Very effective Diltiazem carries the lowest risk of hypotension because it has least negative inotropic effect
β-blockers (metoprolol, propranolol, esmolol, atenolol)	Slow AV node conduction by decreasing sympathetic tone	Very effective More negative inotropic effect than diltiazem and carry a greater risk for hypotension, particularly in patients with borderline low blood pressure or poor LV function
Digoxin	Slows AV node conduction by increasing parasympathetic tone via the vagus nerve	Limited role in the ED because of its slow onset of action, long half-life, and ineffectiveness at rate control in the typical high-sympathetic tone ED patient Has a role in rate control in sedentary patients or those with chronic CHF. May be used in association with above meds when initial rate control is unsuccessful
Amiodarone, (oral or IV) **Dronedarone** (oral only)	Antiarrhythmics that have some beta-blocking activity	Less effective than the pure rate control agents listed earlier If cardioversion is the goal, these drugs may be a single-agent approach to maintaining NSR and rate control

Abbreviations: AV = atrioventricular; CHF = congestive heart failure; ED = emergency department; LV = left ventricle; NSR = normal sinus rhythm.

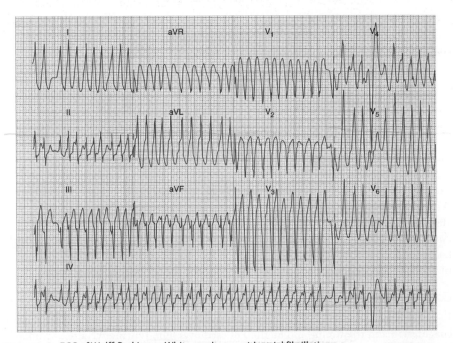

Figure 9–3. ECG of Wolff-Parkinson-White syndrome with atrial fibrillation.

of AF, the greater is the likelihood of clot formation. Furthermore, following cardioversion, the period of "atrial stunning" (the delayed onset of atrial contractility after cardioversion lasting several weeks) can also lead to thrombogenesis. Without anticoagulation, up to 6% of patients will have a thromboembolic event in the first week following cardioversion, either from the dislodging of an existing clot or from the formation of new clot caused by the "atrial stunning." This risk increases with the duration of the AF and the underlying disease processes.

Many practitioners use **the "48-hour rule"** to guide **anticoagulation:** AF of less than 48 hours duration does not generally require acute anticoagulation, conferring an embolic risk of ~0.6%, which is similar to that of a fully anticoagulated patient. Exceptions to the 48-hour rule include patients with mitral valve disease, severe left ventricle dysfunction, or prior history of embolic stroke, in which case no duration of AF, no matter how short, is safe. Several recent studies have shown that it is both safe and cost-effective for patients with an uncomplicated clinical status who present to the emergency department with AF for less than 48 hours to be cardioverted and discharged directly from the emergency room.

Conversely, patients presenting with AF of greater than 48 hours duration should be anticoagulated *prior to* cardioversion. The two main approaches for pre-cardioversion anticoagulation are warfarin (Coumadin) or the combination of heparin/enoxaparin (LMWH) plus a screening transesophageal echocardiography (TEE). The conventional approach is to give warfarin therapy with an INR goal of 2 to 3 for 3 to 4 weeks before cardioversion. The alternative approach is quicker and consists of doing a TEE and, if no clot is seen, administering heparin or enoxaparin and proceeding immediately to cardioversion (Table 9 3). In both approaches, warfarin therapy (with an INR goal of 2-3) must be continued for at least 3 to 4 weeks post-cardioversion in order to prevent new clot formation during the "atrial stunning window." Both approaches reduce the risk of thromboembolism to less than 1% over 8 weeks.

The two methods of cardioversion are direct current (DC) cardioversion and pharmacologic cardioversion, with DC cardioversion being the more effective

Table 9–3 • ANTICOAGULATION APPROACHES FOR CARDIOVERSION		
	Conventional Warfarin	**TEE plus Heparin/Enoxaparin**
Pre-cardioversion	Warfarin for 3-4 weeks	If no clot on TEE, administer heparin or enoxaparin and proceed with immediate cardioversion
Post-cardioversion	Warfarin for 3-4 weeks	Warfarin for 3-4 weeks
Advantages	Withstood the "test of time"	Shortens period of anticoagulation, reducing the risk of bleeding complications Reduces the time in AF, increasing the chance of successful conversion to sinus rhythm
Disadvantages	Prolongs period of anticoagulation Delays cardioversion	Requires a TEE to be performed

Table 9–4 • DC CARDIOVERSION	
Preparation	IV, O$_2$, cardiac, and pulse oximetry monitors—following standard procedural sedation protocols, advanced cardiac life support/airway material ready and available
Synchronized DC Cardioversion	100-200 Joules, best success when starting with 200 Joules
Success rate	75%-93%
Complications	15% have complications including: bradycardia, ventricular tachycardia, ventricular stunning with hypotension

approach (see Tables 9–4 and 9–5). The risk of thromboembolism is similar, regardless of which method is chosen. The **likelihood of a successful cardioversion for either method** depends on the **characteristics of the patient,** the **etiology** of the AF and, most importantly, the **duration** of the AF. New-onset AF will spontaneously convert in about 70% of cases, whereas cases of AF with a longer duration and dilated atria may prove refractory to all attempts at cardioversion. The success rate for electrical cardioversion is between 75% and 93% but is only about 50% if the AF has been present for more than 1 year. The success rate of pharmacological cardioversion, regardless of the drug used, is between 50% and 70% for recent onset AF and about 30% for chronic AF.

Following cardioversion for first time AF, it is estimated that up to 30% of patients will remain in normal sinus rhythm (NSR) for life. This fact underlies the adage that every AF patient deserves at least one shot at cardioversion and potentially lifelong sinus rhythm. In truth, most patients will have a recurrence of AF, especially those with a history of hypertension, enlarged left atrium, heart failure,

Table 9–5 • DRUGS FOR PHARMACOLOGIC CARDIOVERSION			
Drug Class	**Agent**	**Adverse Effects**	**Comment**
Ic	Flecainide (oral)	Dizziness, dyspnea	Contraindicated in CAD
Ic	Propafenone (oral)	Dizziness, VT	Contraindicated in CAD
III	Dofetilide (oral)	VT, torsade de pointes	Preferred if any structural heart disease is present, especially LV dysfunction
III	Amiodarone (oral or IV)	Hypotension, bradycardia, pulmonary toxicity, hepatotoxity, hyper-/hypothyroidism, photosensitivity, ataxia, peripheral neuropathy, blurry vision	Preferred if any structural heart disease is present, especially LV dysfunction
III	Ibutilide (IV)	VT, torsade de pointes	Specifically for AF and atrial flutter
III	Vernakalant (IV)	Hypotension, bradycardia	Rapid conversion, low proarrhythmic risk

Abbreviations: AF = atrial fibrillation; CAD = coronary artery disease; IV = intravenous; LV = left ventricle; VT = ventricular tachycardia.

or AF for more than a year. While the risk of recurrence can be mitigated some-what by antiarrhythmic agents, it is generally thought that the risk of toxicity and proarrhythmia of these agents outweighs their benefits, especially in patients with no prior episodes of AF. However, in some patients who have persistent symptoms despite adequate rate control or who are unable to maintain adequate rate con-trol, a rhythm control strategy may be chosen. Amiodarone and propafenone are commonly used agents to maintain sinus rhythm.

An alternative method for maintaining sinus rhythm that has had increasing interest and investigation is radiofrequency catheter ablation. Ablation is recom-mended for a select patient population with symptomatic AF and mild or no left atrial enlargement in whom a rhythm control strategy has been chosen but who have failed treatment with one or more antiarrhythmic drugs. Given the shortcom-ings of chronic antiarrhythmic therapy, in terms of side effects and recidivism rates, electrophysiologic interventions are likely to become more widespread.

Thromboembolic Risk Reduction

Patients with AF have a two- to threefold higher risk of stroke than the general popu-lation. The risk is the same for patients with paroxysmal, persistent or chronic AF. It was previously thought that the use of cardioversion or antiarrhythmic agents to reestablish and maintain a sinus rhythm reduced this risk. The Atrial Fibrillation Follow-up Investigation of Rhythm Management (AFFIRM) trial, which compared rhythm control to rate control plus or minus warfarin in 4060 patients, showed that **the rate control group had a trend toward better survival, fewer hospitalizations, and better quality of life scores.** Interestingly, an analysis of rhythm control patients found that risk of stroke was independent of the time spent in sinus rhythm. Risk of stroke appeared closely linked to the presence of certain comorbidities (see CHADS score in the following text) and whether the patients were anticoagulated. These data suggest that even patients with rare or intermittent AF can benefit from antithrombotic therapy, depending on their risk profile.

The type of antithrombotic therapy (either anticoagulation or antiplatelet therapy) used to prevent thromboembolism depends on the patient's individual risk of hav-ing a thromboembolic event and the risk of bleeding on antithrombotic therapy. **The most validated and clinically useful risk stratification models for determining stroke risk are the CHADS2 and CHADS-VASc Score (Table 9–6).**

Table 9–6 • CHADS2	
Parameters	**Points**
Congestive heart failure	1
Hypertension	1
Age ≥75 years	1
Diabetes	1
Stroke or transient ischemic attack	2

Note: CHADS vasc score takes into account the higher stroke rate seen in patients who are female, aged >65 and have known vascular disease.

Table 9–7 • NOVEL ORAL ANTICOAGULATION AGENTS (NOAC's)				
	Dosing	Onset of Action (hours)	Half-life (hours)	Antidote
Dabigatran	BID	1-3	12-17	Idarucizumab
Rivaroxaban	Once daily	2-4	5-12	Andexanet
Apixaban	BID	3-4	12	Andexanet
Edoxaban	Once daily	1-2	9-11	Andexanet
Warfarin	Once daily	72-96	48-72	Vit K, FFP, PCC

Anticoagulation therapy traditionally consists of warfarin with an INR goal between 2 and 3. Antithrombin and anti-Xa agents, collectively called NOACs (Novel Oral Anticoagulation agents) are a class of new oral anticoagulation drugs shown to be superior to warfarin in stroke prevention for non-vavular AF (Table 9–7). In general, NOACs reduce the rate of ischemic and hemorrhagic strokes, major bleeding, and overall mortality compared to warfarin. In addition to being safer and more effective, NOACs do not require INR monitoring, are less susceptible to diet and drug interactions, and do not have warfarin's narrow therapeutic window. However, the drawbacks to the NOACs are higher cost and the need for adjustment in patients with renal failure. When the NOACs were first introduced, the lack of an antidote in case of bleeding or trauma was a major concern for clinicians. Recently, reversal agents covering both the antithrombin and anti-Xa agents were approved (Table 9–7). A single dose is capable of nearly 100% reversal in a matter of minutes. NOACs are now expanding their clinical profile to include anticoagulation in deep vein thrombosis (DVT), pulmonary embolism, and acute coronary syndromes.

Antiplatelet therapy consists of aspirin 75 to 325 mg daily, clopidogrel 75 mg daily, or both together. Aspirin has only a limited ability to reduce stroke risk, estimated to be ~1/3 that of warfarin. For patients with no risk factors for stroke, the current evidence shows that the risk of bleeding from aspirin likely exceeds the small benefit of decreased stroke risk. For patients who need anticoagulation but cannot take warfarin or a NOAC, the combination of clopidogrel plus aspirin is more effective than aspirin alone. However, this combination carries similar bleeding risks to formal anticoagulation (Table 9–8).

Table 9–8 • CHADS2 SCORE AND ANTITHROMBOTIC THERAPY CHOICE			
CHADS2 Score	Stroke Risk	Stroke Risk/Year	Preferred Therapy (in Order of Preference)
0	Low	0.5%-1.7%	No therapy > aspirin
1	Intermediate	2%	Warfarin or NOAC[a] > aspirin
2-6	High	>4%	Warfarin or NOAC
Prior stoke or TIA or thromboembolic event	High	10%	Warfarin or NOAC

[a]Annual bleeding risk on NOAC or warfarin therapy is about 2%.

> **CASE CORRELATION**
>
> - See also Case 7 (Acute Coronary Syndrome), Case 10 (Regular Rate Tachycardia), and Case 11 (Congestive Heart Failure/Pulmonary Edema).

COMPREHENSION QUESTIONS

9.1 A 75-year-old man is found to have asymptomatic AF. Which of the following is the most common complication of his AF long term?

A. Myocardial infarction

B. Stroke

C. Hypotension

D. Cardiomyopathy

9.2 An 83-year-old woman with a history of hypertension presents to the emergency department with bright red blood per rectum and a blood pressure of 85/50 mm Hg. Her pulse is 160 beats per minute and irregular. An ECG confirms she is in new onset AF. Which of the following is the best treatment for this patient?

A. Diltiazem

B. Amiodarone

C. DC Cardioversion

D. Transfusion and IV fluids

9.3 A 72-year-old woman with history of HTN and non-insulin dependent diabetes mellitus (NIDDM) is seen in the emergency department for knee pain after tripping and falling. On examination, she has an abrasion and contusion to her knee with negative x-rays. However, her heart rate is 80 beats per minute and irregular to palpation. On ECG, she is diagnosed with AF. She does not recall ever being told about this condition. Which of the following is the best initial treatment for this patient's AF?

A. Diltiazem

B. DC cardioversion

C. Oral anticoagulation

D. IV anticoagulation

E. No further therapy

ANSWERS

9.1 **B.** The two complications associated with AF are stroke and cardiomyopathy. Stroke is two to three times more likely in patients with AF than in the general population. While cardiomyopathy is also a complication of AF, it is far less common than thromboembolism.

9.2 **D.** AF is commonly related to underlying disease processes. When an AF patient presents as unstable, the clinician must determine which process (AF or something else) is the culprit. It is rare for patient with AF RVR to have rhythm-related instability, and in the setting of an obvious lower GI bleed, management with blood and fluids should take precedent over rhythm/rate control.

9.3 **C.** The patient has asymptomatic AF that appears well rate controlled. With a CHADS-VASc score of 4, she has a ~4% annual risk of thromboembolism. While many ED physicians will defer anticoagulation decisions to a PMD, starting warfarin or a NOAC in the ED is justifiable and appropriate. Bridging with heparin or low molecular weight heparin is not required when starting warfarin in patients with AF.

CLINICAL PEARLS

▶ Treatment of atrial fibrillation (AF) begins with a search for any underlying reversible causes of the arrhythmia.

▶ In the acute setting, the initial management of AF is typically directed toward ventricular rate control through the use of AV nodal blocking drugs.

▶ Unstable patients with AF or Wolff-Parkinson-White tachyarrhythmia with AF should undergo immediate electrical cardioversion.

▶ Stable patients with AF for less than 48 hours can be cardioverted in the ED without anticoagulation provided they have no prior history of thromboembolism, mitral valve disease, or LV dysfunction. Long-term anticoagulation is based on the CHADs/CHADS-VASc score and risk of bleeding.

▶ Stable patients with AF of greater than 48 hours or unknown duration can be cardioverted in two ways: (1) anticoagulation for 3 to 4 weeks prior to, and following cardioversion, or (2) imaging by TEE and, if no intracardiac thrombus is seen, acute anticoagulation with heparin/LMWH, followed by cardioversion, and anticoagulation for 3 to 4 weeks.

▶ The rate of success of cardioversion is closely linked to the duration of the AF. Up to 70% of new onset AF will spontaneously convert.

▶ Patients with AF have a two to three times higher risk of stroke than the general population. Risk mitigation for stroke begins in the ED with an assessment of CHADS/CHADS-VASc scores and possible initiation of anticoagulation.

▶ Anticoagulation with either warfarin (INR goal of 2-3) or NOAC reduces the risk of thromboembolism.

REFERENCES

Connolly SJ, Ezekowitz MD, Yusuf S, et al. Dabigatran versus warfarin in patients with atrial fibrillation. *N Engl J Med*. 2009;361(12):1139-1151.

Connolly SJ, Pogue J, Hart R, et al. Clopidogrel plus aspirin versus oral anticoagulation for atrial fibrillation in the Atrial fibrillation Clopidogrel Trial with Irbesartan for prevention of Vascular Events (ACTIVE W): a randomised controlled trial. *Lancet*. 2006;367(9526):1903-1912.

Fuster V, Rydén LE, Cannom DS, et al. 2011 ACCF/AHA/HRS Focused Updates Incorporated Into the ACC/AHA/ESC 2006 Guidelines for the Management of Patients With Atrial Fibrillation. A Report of the American College of Cardiology Foundation/American Heart Association Task Force on Practice Guidelines. Developed in partnership with the European Society of Cardiology and in collaboration with the European Heart Rhythm Association and the Heart Rhythm Society. *J Am Coll Cardiol*. 2011;57(11):e101-e198.

Gallagher MM, Hennessy BJ, Edvardsson H, et al. Embolic complications of direct current cardioversion of atrial arrhythmias: association with low intensity of anticoagulation at the time of cardioversion. *J Am Coll Cardiol*. 2002;40:926-933.

Granger CB, Alexander JH, McMurray JJ, et al. Apixaban versus warfarin in patients with atrial fibrillation. *N Engl J Med*. 2011;365:981-992.

Giugliano RP, Ruff CT, Braunwald E, et al. Edoxaban versus warfarin in patients with atrial fibrillation. *N Engl J Med*. 2013;369:2093-2104.

Manning W, Singer E, Lip G, et al. Antithrombotic therapy to prevent embolization in nonvalvular atrial fibrillation. Available at: http://www.uptodate.com. Accessed October 31, 2016.

Michael JA, Stiell IG, Agarwal S, Mandavia DP. Cardioversion of paroxysmal atrial fibrillation in the emergency department. *Ann Emerg Med*. 1999;33(4):379-387.

Patel MR, Mahaffey KW, Garg J, et al. Rivaroxaban versus warfarin in nonvalvular atrial fibrillation. *N Engl J Med*. 2011;365:883-891.

Pollack CV Jr, Reilly PA, Eikelboom J, et al. Idarucizumab for Dabigatran Reversal. *N Engl J Med*. 2015;373:511-520.

Siegal DM, Curnutte JT, Connolly SJ, et al. Andexanet Alfa for the Reversal of Factor Xa Inhibitor Activity. *N Engl J Med*. 2015;373:2413-2424.

Stewart S, Hart CL, Hole DJ, McMurray JJ. A population-based study of the long-term risks associated with atrial fibrillation: 20 year follow-up of the Renfrew/Paisley study. *Am J Med*. 2002;113:359-364.

Stiell IG, Dickinson G, Butterfield NN, et al. Vernakalant hydrochloride: a novel atrial-selective agent for the cardioversion of recent-onset atrial fibrillation in the emergency department. *Acad Emerg Med*. 2010;17(11):1175-1182.

Wyse DG, Waldo AL, DiMarco JP, et al. A comparison of rate control and rhythm control in patients with atrial fibrillation. *N Engl J Med*. 2002;347:1825-1833.

Xavier Scheuermeyer F, Grafstein E, Stenstrom R, Innes G, Poureslami I, Sighary M. Thirty-day outcomes of emergency department patients undergoing electrical cardioversion for atrial fibrillation or flutter. *Acad Emerg Med*. 2010;17(4):408-115.

You JJ, Singer DE, Howard PA, et al. Antithrombotic therapy for atrial fibrillation: Antithrombotic Therapy and Prevention of Thrombosis, 9th ed. American College of Chest Physicians Evidence-Based Clinical Practice Guidelines. *Chest*. 2012;141(2 Suppl):e531S-575S.

A 25-year-old man presents to the emergency department (ED) with palpitations and lightheadedness. These symptoms started acutely about 1 hour prior to arrival while he was watching television. The patient does not have any chest pain or shortness of breath. He also denies any recent fever, upper respiratory symptoms, and hemoptysis. He does not have any significant past medical history or family history. He is not taking any medications, does not smoke, and has never used any illicit drugs.

On examination, his temperature is 98.2°F, blood pressure is 88/46 mm Hg, heart rate is 186 beats per minute, respiratory rate is 22 breaths per minute, and oxygen saturation is 97% on room air. He is mildly anxious but otherwise in no acute distress. He does not have any jugular venous distention. His lungs are clear to auscultation, and his heart sounds are regular without any murmurs, rubs, or gallops. There is no lower extremity edema, and peripheral pulses are equal in all four extremities. The cardiac monitor reveals a regular rhythm with narrow-QRS complexes at a rate of 180 to190 beats per minute.

▶ What is the most likely diagnosis?
▶ What is the most appropriate next step?

ANSWERS TO CASE 10:

Regular Rate Tachycardia

Summary: This is a 25-year-old man with acute onset of palpitations and dizziness. He is hypotensive and has a narrow-QRS complex tachycardia at a rate of 180 to 190 beats per minute.

- **Most likely diagnosis:** Supraventricular tachycardia (SVT).

- **Most appropriate next step:** Obtain IV access and a 12-lead ECG. Prepare for synchronized cardioversion of this unstable patient with a tachyarrhythmia.

ANALYSIS

Objectives

1. Learn the differential diagnosis for regular rate tachycardias.

2. Recognize the clinical signs and symptoms to differentiate between stable and unstable patients with regular rate tachycardias.

3. Understand the diagnostic and therapeutic approach to regular rate tachycardias.

Considerations

When evaluating a patient with a tachyarrhythmia, assessment of the patient's stability is paramount. Unstable patients will require immediate synchronized cardioversion. Stable patients may be able to be managed medically. All patients will require continuous cardiac monitoring, intravenous (IV) access, and a 12-lead ECG. Regular rate tachycardias include several types of SVTs and VTs (Table 10–1). As a general rule, narrow-QRS complex tachycardias arise from above the ventricles, while wide-QRS complex ones may be supraventricular or ventricular in origin.

Table 10–1 • VARIOUS TYPES OF TACHYARRHYTHMIAS		
Regular	Narrow-QRS complex	Sinus tachycardia Atrial tachycardia Atrioventricular nodal reentrant tachycardia (AVNRT) Atrioventricular reentrant tachycardia (AVRT) Junctional tachycardia Atrial flutter
	Wide-QRS complex	Ventricular tachycardia Antidromic AVRT Narrow complex tachycardia with aberrancy
Irregular	Narrow-QRS complex	Atrial flutter with variable block Atrial fibrillation Multifocal atrial tachycardia
	Wide-QRS complex	Polymorphic ventricular tachycardia Narrow complex tachycardia with aberrancy

APPROACH TO:
Regular Rate Tachycardia

CLINICAL APPROACH

Patients with tachyarrhythmias may present with a host of complaints, including palpitations, fatigue, and weakness. Other symptoms may suggest a component of hypoperfusion (dizziness, near syncope, or syncope) or cardiac ischemia (chest pain and dyspnea). If the patient is stable enough for a complete history to be performed, the history should also include information about the time and circumstances surrounding symptom onset, duration of symptoms, past medical history (eg, history of coronary artery disease, congestive heart failure, dysrhythmia, valvular disease, and thyroid disease), current medications (including herbal or homeopathic regimens, over-the-counter medicines, and illicit drugs), and family history (eg, sudden cardiac death, dysrhythmia, and other types of heart diseases).

The physical examination will initially focus on assessing the patient's stability and adequacy of the airway, breathing, and circulation (ABCs). Any evidence of hypotension, pulmonary edema, acutely altered mental status, or ischemic chest pain indicates that the patient is unstable and that treatment must be initiated immediately (see treatment section later in chapter). Once the patient is stabilized, a complete head-to-toe examination can be performed. Special consideration should be given to the cardiovascular and pulmonary components of the examination: auscultating heart sounds for gallops, murmurs, and rubs; palpating for the point of maximal impulse and any heaves; inspecting for jugular venous distention; listening for any rales or other findings of volume overload; assessing the quality of peripheral pulses. The examination may also reveal clues regarding underlying causes of tachycardia (eg, pale mucous membranes with anemia; thyromegaly or goiter with thyrotoxicosis; barrel chest or nail clubbing with chronic lung disease).

A 12-lead ECG is ostensibly the most useful diagnostic test when evaluating a patient with a tachyarrhythmia (Figures 10–1 and 10–2). **These arrhythmias may be separated into regular and irregular rate tachycardias as well as narrow- (≤ 0.12 sec), or wide-QRS** (>0.12 second) complexes (see Table 10–1). As a general rule, narrow-QRS complex tachycardias arise from above the ventricles, while wide-QRS complex ones may be supraventricular or ventricular in origin.

Table 10–2 lists the distinguishing ECG characteristics of the various types of regular rate tachycardias.

VT may be difficult to differentiate from SVT with aberrant conduction. Certain factors favor VT, including age above 50, history of coronary artery disease or congestive heart failure, history of VT, atrioventricular dissociation, fusion beats, QRS >0.14 second, extreme left axis deviation, and precordial concordance (QRS complexes either all positive or all negative). In contrast, age less than or equal to 35, history of SVT, preceding ectopic P waves with QRS complexes, QRS <0.14 second, normal or almost normal axis, and slowing or cessation of the arrhythmia with vagal maneuvers suggest SVT with aberrancy. If the provider cannot distinguish between VT and SVT with aberrancy with certainty, the patient should be treated as if VT is present.

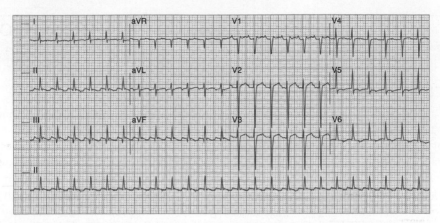

Figure 10–1. Atrial flutter with 2:1 conduction. *(Reproduced, with permission, from Longo DL, Fauci AS, Kasper DL, et al. Harrison's Principles of Internal Medicine. 18th ed. New York, NY: McGraw-Hill Education, 2011 (Figure e30-14).)*

Chest x-rays may be useful to assess for chamber enlargement, cardiomegaly, pulmonary congestion or edema. A basic metabolic panel can rule out electrolyte abnormalities that predispose to tachyarrhythmias (eg, hypokalemia, hypocalcemia, and hypomagnesemia). If the clinical scenario is suggestive, thyroid function studies (for hyperthyroidism), drug levels (eg, digoxin), or urine drug screen (for cocaine, methamphetamines, and other stimulants) may be warranted.

Treatment

All patients with tachyarrhythmias require monitoring of vital signs (blood pressure, oxygen saturation, and continuous cardiac monitoring) and **IV access.** If the patient

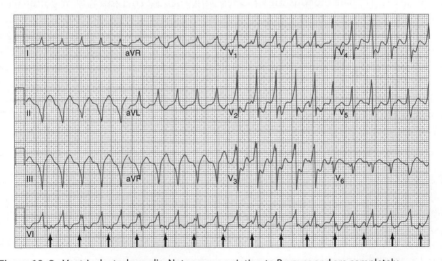

Figure 10–2. Ventricular tachycardia. Note arrows pointing to P waves and are completely dissociated from the QRS complexes. *(Reproduced, with permission, from Longo DL, Fauci AS, Kasper DL, et al. Harrison's Principles of Internal Medicine. 18th ed. New York, NY: McGraw-Hill Education, 2011 (Figure 233-10).)*

Table 10–2 • REGULAR RATE TACHYCARDIAS

Narrow-QRS complex

Sinus tachycardia	Atrial rate 100-160 beats per minute 1:1 conduction Normal sinus P waves and PR intervals	Similar to normal sinus rhythm except >100 beats per minute Treat underlying cause
Atrial tachycardia	P wave morphologically different from sinus P wave 1:1 conduction	Will not convert to sinus with vagal maneuvers or adenosine If stable, consider diltiazem, β-blockers Treat underlying cause
Atrioventricular nodal reentrant tachycardia (AVNRT)	P wave usually buried in QRS complex 1:1 conduction Often preceded by premature junctional or atrial contraction Rarely >225 beats per minute	Reentry within AV node If stable, consider vagal maneuvers, adenosine, calcium-channel blockers or β-blockers
Atrioventricular reentrant tachycardia (AVRT)	Inverted retrograde P waves after QRS complex	Retrograde reentry involving bypass tract If stable, consider vagal maneuvers, adenosine, calcium-channel blockers or β-blockers
Junctional tachycardia	Inverted P wave before or after QRS or buried in QRS complex Rate >100 beats per minute	Will not convert to sinus with vagal maneuvers or adenosine If stable, consider diltiazem, β-blockers Treat underlying cause
Atrial flutter	Atrial rate 250-350 beats per minute "Sawtooth" flutter wave (best seen in II, III, aVF, V1-V2) 2:1 conduction common (although may be any ratio)	Will not convert to sinus with vagal maneuvers or adenosine If stable, consider calcium-channel blockers, β-blockers Treat underlying cause

Wide-QRS complex

Ventricular tachycardia	Dissociated P wave (if present) 100-250 beats per minute	If stable, consider amiodarone, procainamide, or sotalol Lidocaine as second-line agent
Antidromic AVRT	Retrograde P waves may or may not be visible	Anterograde conduction through bypass tract, retrograde through AV node Avoid β-blockers, calcium-channel blockers, and adenosine
Narrow complex tachycardia with aberrancy	Preceding ectopic P waves with QRS complexes QRS usually <0.14 s. Axis normal or almost normal	If stable, adenosine

is hypoxic or in respiratory distress, supplemental oxygen and airway support are indicated. If the patient is unstable (as evidenced by hypotension, pulmonary edema, altered mental status, or ischemic chest pain), **synchronized cardioversion** should be performed immediately. If time allows, sedation should be given prior to cardioversion.

In stable patients, a 12-lead ECG should be obtained, and medical therapy can be initiated. Potential interventions for regular narrow-complex tachyarrhythmias include vagal maneuvers (such as carotid massage and valsalva), adenosine, β-blockers, and calcium-channel blockers. Although vagal maneuvers will not terminate tachyarrhythmias that do not involve the AV node, they may slow the rate enough to unmask the underlying rhythm abnormality. Stable patients with regular wide-complex tachycardias may benefit from amiodarone, procainamide, or sotalol. Adenosine may be considered for regular monomorphic wide-complex tachycardias.

CASE CORRELATION

- See also Case 2 (Hemorrhagic Shock), Case 3 (Sepsis), and Case 9 (Atrial Fibrillation).

COMPREHENSION QUESTIONS

10.1 A 22-year-old baseball player comes into the ED complaining of 12 hours of intermittent chest pain and a pounding heartbeat. He denies a history of trauma. On examination, he is tachycardic. Which of the following is the best next step?

A. Synchronized cardioversion

B. Valsalva maneuver

C. Discharge home and follow-up within the next 48 hours

D. Obtain an ECG

10.2 A 52-year-old healthy jogger is brought to the ED following a syncopal episode. A diagnosis of ventricular tachycardia is made, and the patient is cardioverted. She states that she has had prior episodes of VT lasting less than 30 seconds each. What is the most appropriate treatment at this time?

A. No further therapy at this time

B. Amiodarone

C. β-blocker

D. Procainamide

10.3 All of these are AV nodal blocking maneuvers *except*:

A. Diving reflex

B. Carotid massage

C. Valsalva maneuver

D. Holding one's breath at the end of expiration

10.4 An 87-year-old woman presents with chest pain and shortness of breath. The 12-lead ECG shows a "sawtooth" pattern with a heart rate of 150 beats per minute. What is the most likely diagnosis?

   A. AVNRT
   B. VT
   C. Atrial flutter
   D. Atrial fibrillation with rapid ventricular rate

10.5 A 37-year-old woman presents with chest pain after smoking crack cocaine 2 hours ago. What are you most likely to see on the ECG?

   A. Sinus tachycardia
   B. SVT
   C. VT
   D. Atrial fibrillation

ANSWERS

10.1 **D.** One must characterize the rhythm before initiating treatment, which is why ECG is important to obtain. Answer C (discharge home) is not prudent since the patient has a tachycardia and it has not been diagnosed and may be dangerous. Therapy such as cardioversion or Valsalva requires a diagnosis first.

10.2 **A.** Nonsustained VT is by definition a self-terminating event, and therefore usually no specific treatment is indicated at this time in the ED. Rather, treatment is directed at any existing heart condition. Thus, it is important for the patient to have a thorough evaluation by a cardiologist to assess the risk of recurrence and danger.

10.3 **D.** AV nodal blocking maneuvers include Valsalva, diving reflex, and carotid massage. They act through the parasympathetic nervous system. If an SVT involves the AV node, slowing conduction through the node can terminate the arrhythmia. SVTs that do not involve the AV node will not usually be terminated by AV nodal blocking maneuvers. However, these maneuvers may still cause a transient AV block and unmask the underlying rhythm abnormality.

10.4 **C.** Classically, atrial flutter presents with a saw tooth pattern on ECG. The rate of 150 beats per minute denotes that it's likely a 2:1 conduction block.

10.5 **A. Although cocaine intoxication can cause multiple tachycardias,** the most common regular rate tachycardia is sinus tachycardia. Thus, although it is most likely to be a sinus tachycardia, an ECG is important to obtain to ensure that there is not a more concerning rhythm.

CLINICAL PEARLS

▶ Regular rate tachycardias include several types of supraventricular tachycardias and ventricular tachycardias. As a general rule, narrow-QRS complex tachycardias arise from above the ventricles, while wide-QRS complex ones may be supraventricular or ventricular in origin.

▶ If the patient is unstable (as evidenced by hypotension, pulmonary edema, altered mental status, or ischemic chest pain), synchronized cardioversion should be performed immediately. In stable patients, a 12-lead ECG should be obtained, and medical therapy can be initiated.

▶ If the provider cannot distinguish between VT and SVT with aberrancy with certainty, the patient should be treated as if VT is present.

▶ *Always* order an ECG in a patient with suspected tachyarrhythmia.

REFERENCES

Brugada P, Brugada J, Mont L, Smeets J, Andries EW. A new approach to the differential diagnosis of a regular tachycardia with a wide QRS complex. *Circulation.* 1991;83(5):1649-1659.

Lau EW, Ng GA. Comparison of the performance of three diagnostic algorithms for regular broad complex tachycardia in practical application. Pacing and clinical electrophysiology. *PACE.* 2002;25(5):822-827.

Marill KA, deSouza IS, Jisijima DK, et al. Amiodarone or procainamide for the termination of sustained stable ventricular tachycardia: a historical multicenter comparison. *Acad Emerg Med.* 2010;17(3):297-306.

Marx JA, Hockberger RS, Walls RM, eds. *Rosen's Emergency Medicine: Concepts and Clinical Practice.* 8th ed. Philadelphia, PA: Saunders; 2014.

Mathew PK. Diving reflex. Another method of treating paroxysmal supraventricular tachycardia. *Arch Intern Med.* 1981;141(1):22-23.

Stewart RB, Bardy GH, Greene HL. Wide complex tachycardia: misdiagnosis and outcome after emergent therapy. *Ann Intern Med.* 1986;104 (6):766-771.

Tintinalli JE, Stapczynski JS, Ma OJ, et al, eds. *Emergency Medicine: A Comprehensive Study Guide.* 8th ed. New York, NY: McGraw-Hill; 2016.

Wellens HJ, Bar FW, Lie KI. The value of the electrocardiogram in the differential diagnosis of a tachycardia with a widened QRS complex. *Am J Med.* 1978;64(1):27-33.

Zipes DP, Camm AJ, Borggrefe, et al. ACC/AHA/ESC 2006 guidelines for management of patients with ventricular arrhythmias and the prevention of sudden cardiac death. *J Am Coll Cardiol.* 2006;48(5):e247-346.

A 63-year-old woman arrives in the emergency department (ED) in respiratory distress. The paramedics who transported her were not able to obtain any information about her past medical history but did bring her bag of medications, which included furosemide.

On examination, her temperature is 37.5°C (99.5°F), blood pressure is 220/112 mm Hg, heart rate is 130 beats per minute, respiratory rate is 36 breaths per minute, and oxygen saturation is 93% on a non-rebreather mask. The patient's skin is cool, clammy, and diaphoretic. She is alert but can only answer yes-or-no questions because of dyspnea. She has jugular venous distention to the angle of the jaw, rales in both lung fields, and +2 pretibial edema bilaterally. Her heart sounds are regular but tachycardic, with an S_3/S_4 gallop.

▶ What is the most likely diagnosis?
▶ What is the most appropriate next step?

ANSWERS TO CASE 11:

Congestive Heart Failure/Pulmonary Edema

Summary: This is a 63-year-old woman in respiratory distress with signs of heart failure (HF) and fluid overload.

- **Most likely diagnosis:** Congestive heart failure (CHF) and cardiogenic acute pulmonary edema.

- **Most appropriate next step:** Management of the ABCs (airway, breathing, circulation), preload and afterload reduction, and eventual diuresis.

ANALYSIS

Objectives

1. Recognize the clinical presentation and complications of CHF.

2. Understand the diagnostic and therapeutic approach to suspected CHF.

Considerations

This 63-year-old woman is brought into the ED with signs of severe CHF: dyspnea, tachypnea, hypoxia, hypertension, and tachycardia. Her medications include furosemide, strongly suggesting a history of CHF. This clinical presentation is classic for a CHF exacerbation. Rapid assessment of the ABCs, IV access, and prompt initiation of preload and afterload reduction are the mainstays of therapy. Supplemental oxygen should be administered. Non-invasive positive pressure ventilation (NIPPV) or endotracheal intubation may be necessary for severe cases. Once the patient is stabilized, it is important to try to identify any precipitants of the exacerbation. Diagnostic tests should be directed at excluding myocardial infarction, a common cause of worsening CHF.

APPROACH TO:

Congestive Heart Failure/Pulmonary Edema

CLINICAL APPROACH

Emergency physicians must be comfortable identifying and treating patients with HF, as it is associated with significant morbidity and mortality (50% mortality rate at 4 years after the onset of symptoms). HF can be due to dysfunction of normal relaxation and filling (diastolic HF) or contractile ability (systolic HF) of the ventricles. The term "congestive" refers to abnormal fluid retention resulting from this loss of relaxation/contractility. There are many causes of HF, the most common of which are coronary artery disease (ischemic) and hypertension (non-ischemic). HF can involve one or both sides of the heart. Right-sided failure results in increased systemic venous pressures and subsequent peripheral edema, while left-sided

Table 11–1 • COMMON PRESENTATIONS OF HEART FAILURE		
Type of Failure	**Symptoms**	**Examination Findings**
Right sided	Peripheral edema, right upper quadrant pain, no pulmonary symptoms	Dependent edema, right-upper-quadrant tenderness, hepatomegaly, hepatojugular reflex, jugular venous distention
Left sided	Dyspnea, orthopnea, paroxysmal nocturnal dyspnea, fatigue, weakness, cough	Tachypnea, pulmonary crackles or wheezes, S_3 or S_4

failure causes increased pulmonary venous pressures and subsequent pulmonary edema. Each has different symptoms and physical findings (Table 11–1).

Clinical Evaluation

During the evaluation, the clinician must be able to distinguish patients with CHF from those with other conditions with similar clinical presentations, such as acute respiratory distress syndrome (ARDS), pneumonia, pneumothorax, pulmonary embolus, and exacerbation of chronic obstructive pulmonary disease (COPD) (Table 11–2). In addition, the clinician must try to determine what caused the patient's condition to decompensate. **The most common precipitants of acute exacerbations are ischemia/infarction and noncompliance with medications, dialysis, or dietary restrictions.** Sympathetic crisis with hypertension (increased afterload) can lead to acute left-sided failure, while a pulmonary embolus can lead to acute right-sided failure. Other causes of right- and left-sided failure include valvular dysfunction, arrhythmia, volume overload, kidney injury, and iatrogenic etiologies. Thyrotoxicosis, anemia, and AV fistulas can lead to high output HF.

The sequence of the clinical evaluation depends on the patient's clinical status. If the patient is stable, a more detailed history can be obtained. Important historical

Table 11–2 • DIFFERENTIAL DIAGNOSES OF HEART FAILURE
Dyspnea
• Asthma or chronic obstructive pulmonary disease exacerbation
• Pneumonia or ARDS
• Pneumothorax
• Pulmonary embolus
• Pleural effusion
• Physical deconditioning or obesity
Peripheral edema
• Deep venous thrombosis
• Hypoproteinemia (liver failure, nephrotic syndrome, and renal failure)
Decreased cardiac output
• Acute myocardial infarction
• Drug effect
• Pericardial tamponade
• Valvular insufficiency
• Dysrhythmia
• Tension hydro- or pneumothorax

points include the onset, duration, and character of respiratory complaints; any associated symptoms (such as chest pain or fever); past medical history (including prior heart disease and cardiac workup); and current medications (including recent changes in doses and any missed doses).

On examination, **patients with CHF may show signs of hypoperfusion: clammy skin, diaphoresis, delayed capillary refill, and thready pulses.** If the patient is hypotensive, intra-arterial blood pressure monitoring is important because noninvasive measurements are often inaccurate in vasoconstricted individuals. Patients may have crackles, rales, or wheezes on auscultation. **An S_3 or S_4 is common but may be difficult to hear in a busy ED.** The cardiac examination may also reveal the murmur of a ventricular septal defect or acute mitral regurgitation or the irregularly irregular rhythm of atrial fibrillation—all of which can precipitate acute pulmonary edema. The ED physician should also note any jugular venous distention or peripheral edema.

Electrocardiograms (ECGs) and ultrasonography are diagnostic tools immediately available at the bedside. ECGs are helpful in detecting evidence of cardiac ischemia or infarction and arrhythmias. Beside ultrasonography can be used to assess for systolic and diastolic cardiac dysfunction, along with the rapid identification of pathologic B-lines ("lung rockets") signifying pulmonary edema.

Although **x-ray findings may lag behind clinical symptoms by up to 6 hours,** chest radiography still provides valuable information for the clinician. As the pulmonary congestion increases, interstitial edema and Kerley B-lines become prominent, followed by opacification of the air spaces with alveolar edema. Other findings may include cardiomegaly, upper zone vascular redistribution (cephalization), and pleural effusions. The x-ray may also help exclude other causes of dyspnea and respiratory distress (eg, pneumothorax or pneumonia).

Laboratory studies should include complete blood count, electrolytes, blood urea nitrogen/creatinine, cardiac biomarkers, and urinalysis. If there is diagnostic uncertainty (eg, a patient with CHF and COPD), a **B-type natriuretic peptide (BNP)** level can be checked. BNP is a hormone released from the ventricles in response to stretch. Levels less than 100 pg/mL make HF unlikely, and those greater than 500 pg/mL make it highly likely. Levels between these two extremes are indeterminate. The BNP level also has prognostic significance and can be used to monitor response to therapy. Liver enzymes may be of use in patients with hepatomegaly, and lactate levels to assess perfusion in suspected cardiogenic shock.

Treatment

Treatment of CHF depends on the clinical presentation and etiology. A mild CHF exacerbation with trace pulmonary edema and fluid overload from medication or dietary noncompliance may only require diuresis. A patient with **hypotension and poor perfusion (cardiogenic shock) may require inotropic support** (dobutamine or milrinone to enhance myocardial contractility), **vasopressor support** (norepinephrine to increase coronary diastolic perfusion), and **possibly a small fluid bolus** to increase preload. An unstable patient with ischemia may need to undergo cardiac catheterization for emergent reperfusion, while the unstable patient with a new murmur (concern for valvular disruption) may need to go to the operating room for definitive care.

The patient in the case presentation has cardiogenic pulmonary edema secondary to catecholamine surge (hypertensive emergency). These patients are often euvolemic, and the goal of therapy is fluid redistribution from the pulmonary circulation to the rest of the body. The **treatment consists of oxygenation, preload and afterload reduction, and eventual diuresis.** Any patient in respiratory distress should be considered for high-flow oxygen via noninvasive positive-pressure ventilation (NIPPV) with continuous or biphasic positive airway pressure. This will lead to decreased work of breathing, increased oxygenation, and decreased preload and afterload. Ultimately, the patient may require intubation if refractory to NIPPV. Nitroglycerin (via sublingual, topical, or intravenous routes) is also critical in reducing preload and afterload. In the critically ill patient, high-dose intravenous nitroglycerin is best since it is rapid-acting and titratable. In addition, angiotensin-converting enzyme (ACE) inhibitors may play a role in afterload reduction. Diuresis with furosemide or bumetanide should only be considered after adequate afterload reduction if the patient is clinically volume overloaded. **Morphine is no longer recommended as standard therapy for CHF** due to an association with increased rates of intubation and ICU admission.

CASE CORRELATION

- See also Case 7 (Acute Coronary Syndrome), Case 9 (Atrial Fibrillation), Case 10 (Regular Rate Tachycardia), Case 13 (Asthma), Case 14 (Pulmonary Embolism), and Case 15 (Bacterial Pneumonia).

COMPREHENSION QUESTIONS

11.1 A 62-year-old woman is sent to the ED from her primary physician's office with worsening HF. The patient has had CHF, previously controlled with oral digoxin and furosemide. Which of the following is the most likely reason for the exacerbation of her CHF?

A. Valvular dysfunction

B. Arrhythmia

C. Myocardial ischemia and infarction

D. Thyrotoxicosis

11.2 A 55-year-old man has symptoms of worsening orthopnea, tachypnea, and rales on pulmonary examination. He has 2+ pitting edema in both lower extremities and jugular vein distention (JVD). Which of the following is the best description of this patient's disease process?

A. Right-sided HF

B. Left-sided HF

C. Biventricular HF

D. Acute respiratory distress syndrome

11.3　A 58-year-old man is brought into the ED by paramedics because of worsening dyspnea. He has CHF due to cardiovascular disease. On examination, his blood pressure is 150/100 mm Hg and heart rate is 104 beats per minute. He has jugular venous distention and rales in both lung fields. Which of the following is the most effective and most rapid method of reducing preload and afterload in this patient?

A.　Diuretics

B.　Nitroglycerin

C.　Dobutamine

D.　Morphine

11.4　A 54-year-old man complains of acute onset of worsening fatigue and dyspnea. He has alcohol-induced cardiomyopathy and CHF. Which of the following is the best workup for his CHF exacerbation?

A.　Chest x-ray, cardiac biomarkers, ECG

B.　Computed tomography (CT) scan of the chest, ECG, D-dimer test

C.　Echocardiogram, ECG, thallium stress test

D.　Arterial blood gas, cardiac biomarkers, pulmonary angiography

ANSWERS

11.1　**C.** Myocardial ischemia and infarction is one of the most common precipitants of a CHF exacerbation (as well as noncompliance with medications). The other answer choices can also cause exacerbation of CHF but are less common.

11.2　**C.** Left-sided HF will eventually progress to biventricular failure due to fluid overload of the right heart. This patient has evidence of both left and right HF: signs and symptoms of pulmonary edema (left), peripheral edema (right), and JVD (right). ARDS is caused by pulmonary capillary damage, allowing leakage of fluid into the interstitium of the lung; causes include sepsis, trauma, or critical illness. In contrast, pulmonary edema results from the increased hydrostatic pressure in the pulmonary capillaries, which is due to increased left atrial (left ventricular end diastolic) pressure.

11.3　**B.** Nitroglycerin is the most effective and most rapid means of reducing preload and afterload in a patient with CHF. Diuretics (especially loop diuretics) would reduce preload only. Morphine sulfate is avoided in CHF patients due to the respiratory depression that can ensue. Dobutamine is a beta-1 adrenergic agonist and is used to increase cardiac contractility.

11.4 **A.** The workup of a CHF exacerbation includes chest x-ray, ECG, electro-lytes, BUN/creatinine, and cardiac biomarkers. A BNP level may also be sent. This is because cardiac ischemia/infarction is a common cause of worsening CHF. Answer B (Computed tomography [CT] scan of the chest, ECG, D-dimer test) is an assessment of possible thromboemboli, Answer C (Echocardiogram, ECG, thallium stress test) is more of a workup for a more stable patient, and Answer D (Arterial blood gas, cardiac biomarkers, pulmonary angiography) is a workup for possible pulmonary embolism.

CLINICAL PEARLS

▶ The most common causes of CHF include coronary artery disease and hypertension, while the most common causes of an acute exacerbation are myocardial ischemia or infarct and noncompliance.

▶ BNP is a hormone released by the ventricles in response to stretch. It can be useful as a diagnostic marker for HF.

▶ Treatment of CHF includes oxygenation, correction of the underlying cause, and relief of symptoms by preload and afterload reduction, diuresis, and possibly inotropic support.

REFERENCES

Collins SP, Ronan-Bentle S, Storrow AB. Diagnostic and prognostic usefulness of natriuretic peptides in emergency department patients with dyspnea. *Ann Emerg Med.* 2003;41:532-544.

Levy P, Compton S, Welch R, et al. Treatment of severe decompensated heart failure with high-dose intravenous nitroglycerin: a feasibility and outcome analysis. *Ann Emerg Med.* 2007;50(2):144-152.

Maisel AS, Krishnaswamy P, Nowak RM, et al. Rapid measurement of B-type natriuretic peptide in the emergency diagnosis of heart failure. *N Engl J Med.* 2002;347:161-167.

Marik, PE, Flemmer M. Narrative review: the management of acute decompensated heart failure. *J Intensive Care Med.* 2012;27(6):343-353.

O'Brien JF, Falk JL. Heart failure. In: Marx JA, Hockberger RS, Walls RM, eds. *Rosen's Emergency Medicine: Concepts and Clinical Practice.* 7th ed. Philadelphia, PA: Mosby Elsevier; 2009: Chapter 79.

Thiele H, Ohman EM, Desch S, Eitel I, de Waha S. Management of cardiogenic shock. *Eur Heart J.* 2015;36(20):1223-1230.

Tintinalli JE, Stapczynski JS, Ma OJ, et al., eds. *Emergency Medicine: A Comprehensive Study Guide.* 8th ed. New York, NY: McGraw-Hill; 2016.

A 55-year-old man is brought into the emergency department (ED) by his wife for altered mental status (AMS). She states that for the past day, he has been confused and unsteady when he walks. The patient has a history of hypertension (HTN) and hyperlipidemia. He complains of headache and blurry vision. On examination, he is alert and oriented to person only. On fundoscopy, the optic discs appear hyperemic and swollen, with a loss of sharp margins. His neurological examination is nonfocal, and he otherwise has a normal physical examination. The patient's vital signs are a blood pressure of 245/140 mm Hg, heart rate of 95 beats per minute, respiratory rate of 18 breaths per minute, and oxygen saturation of 98% on room air, and he is afebrile.

▶ What is the most likely diagnosis?
▶ What is the best management?

ANSWERS TO CASE 12:

Hypertensive Encephalopathy

Summary: A 55-year-old man with a history of HTN presents with AMS, headache, and blurry vision with a blood pressure of 245/140 mm Hg. His physical examination is significant for bilateral papilledema and AMS.

- **Most likely diagnosis:** Hypertensive encephalopathy.

- **Best management:** Confirm the diagnosis by ruling out ischemic or hemorrhagic stroke, infection, and mass lesion. Lower blood pressure with intravenous (IV) medications and check for other evidence of end-organ damage.

ANALYSIS

Objectives

1. Identify the presentation of various hypertensive emergencies.

2. Recognize the difference between a hypertensive urgency and emergency.

3. Understand how to manage blood pressure in hypertensive emergencies.

Considerations

This is a 55-year-old man with AMS, papilledema, and severe HTN. This presentation is most likely hypertensive encephalopathy, which is defined as the presence of neurologic abnormalities secondary to an acute elevation in blood pressure. Hypertensive encephalopathy is one of the many forms of hypertensive emergency. The American Heart Association defines hypertensive emergency as the point at which blood pressure levels damage organs. While it is generally associated with levels exceeding 180 systolic or 120 diastolic, it can occur at lower levels in previously normotensive patients. Evidence of end-organ damage is a critical differentiating point between hypertensive emergency and hypertensive urgency, which is an elevated blood pressure with no associated organ damage. It is essential for the provider to identify and differentiate between the two, as it determines blood pressure management strategies.

Once this patient's airway, breathing, and circulation (ABCs) are addressed, the first step in management is to **obtain a non-contrast head computed tomography (NCHCT)** to rule out the presence of a mass lesion and hemorrhagic or ischemic stroke. Laboratory examinations should also be sent to aid in excluding possible metabolic or infectious causes. Once these diagnoses are eliminated and the diagnosis of hypertensive encephalopathy is established, the focus should turn to lowering the blood pressure. **Intravenous antihypertensives should be administered to lower the patient's blood pressure.** The **goal is not to normalize the blood pressure** because this can lead to cerebral ischemia secondary to hypoperfusion. Instead, the **goal is to reduce the MAP by 20% to 25% over the first hour. Various antihypertensive agents are available to manage this disorder.** This is in contrast to typical blood pressure management in patients with long-standing HTN who do not have acute end-organ damage. **Nicardipine and labetalol are potential first-line agents** for lowering blood pressure in the setting of hypertensive encephalopathy. Labetalol is administered as an IV bolus of 20 mg, which can be repeated. It can also be administered as an IV infusion at a rate of 0.5-2.0 mg/min. Nicardipine is administered at 5 mg/h and can be increased by 2.5 mg/h every 5 minutes to a maximum of 30 mg/h. Another option that was classically taught as first line but has fallen out of favor is sodium nitroprusside. This agent is administered as an IV infusion, starting at a rate of 0.25 µg/kg/min and can be increased to a maximum of 10 µg/kg/min.

APPROACH TO:
Hypertensive Emergencies

DEFINITIONS

HYPERTENSION: Blood pressure greater than or equal to 140/90 mm Hg.

HYPERTENSIVE EMERGENCY: The presence of acute end-organ damage in the setting of elevated blood pressure.

HYPERTENSIVE URGENCY: The presence of elevated blood pressure, without evidence of acute, ongoing end-organ damage.

HYPERTENSIVE ENCEPHALOPATHY: A type of hypertensive emergency characterized by neurologic symptoms associated with elevated blood pressure.

CLINICAL APPROACH

Hypertension is found in 20% to 30% of adults in developed countries. It is more common in men than in women, and blood pressure seems to increase with age. The incidence of HTN is 1.5-2.0 times greater in African Americans than in Caucasians. HTN is defined as two readings of greater than 140/90 mm Hg on two different occasions. Hypertensive emergencies will occur in approximately 1% of these individuals and account for approximately 2% to 3% of all ED visits. The most common risk factor in hypertensive emergencies is a history of HTN.

Hypertensive urgencies are acute elevations in blood pressure **without** the **signs or symptoms of acute end-organ damage.** Previously, it was believed that hypertensive urgencies required immediate, aggressive blood pressure reduction. However, no studies demonstrated a benefit of this management. Additionally, **potential harm exists, as an excessive drop in blood pressure can also lead to ischemic complications such as stroke, myocardial infarction, and blindness.** Elevated blood pressures in this circumstance should be reduced over days to weeks, and the patient can be discharged from the ED and followed up in 24-48 hours as an outpatient. The pathophysiology of hypertensive end-organ damage is not completely understood. Current theory holds that the acute rise in blood pressure leads to a series of vascular events, which causes end-organ damage. In hypertensive encephalopathy it is believed that the **acute rise in blood pressure causes endothelial cell dysfunction in the brain's vascular supply, leading to cerebral edema.** Hypertensive encephalopathy can manifest clinically as visual changes, papilledema, focal neurologic deficits, and seizure. Hypertensive encephalopathy is an uncommon clinical entity. In order to establish the diagnosis, **more common causes of AMS must be ruled out,** including, but not limited to, meningitis, encephalitis, ischemic or hemorrhagic stroke, mass lesion, and toxic ingestion.

The diagnosis of **hypertensive emergency requires evidence of acute end-organ dysfunction that is attributable to an elevation in blood pressure.** This dysfunction can manifest through **multiple organ systems** and includes **acute myocardial infarction, aortic dissection, acute left ventricular failure, acute pulmonary edema (APE), cerebral infarction or hemorrhage, acute renal failure, preeclampsia/eclampsia, symptomatic microangiopathic hemolytic anemia, and hypertensive encephalopathy.**

It is critical to differentiate a hypertensive emergency from urgency. This is accomplished through a focused history, physical examination, and appropriate ancillary tests. A detailed medical history must be obtained to determine if the patient has **underlying renal, cardiac, or endocrine manifestations.** The patient's current medications must be known and the possibility of ingestion of illicit drugs or other substances must be considered. In particular, obtaining history about the use of cocaine or other sympathomimetic substances (phenylephrine and monoamine oxidase inhibitors) is crucial, as it significantly alters the treatment regimen (beta-blockers must be avoided in the setting of sympathomimetic use). Elucidate any symptoms related to end-organ damage, such as chest pain (myocardial infarction and aortic dissection), dyspnea (congestive heart failure and pulmonary edema), anuria (renal failure), visual changes (papilledema and retinal hemorrhages), AMS, and seizures. For patients more than 20 weeks pregnant or who recently gave birth, investigate symptoms of preeclampsia.

The physical examination should also assess for signs of end-organ damage. Fundoscopy can reveal papilledema, retinal hemorrhages, and exudates. Cardiovascular examination can identify signs of heart failure, such as jugular venous distension, an S_3 gallop, pulmonary rales, and extremity edema. Neurologic examination should evaluate the mental status and signs of focal deficits.

Ancillary testing varies in the patient with hypertensive emergency depending on the patient's symptoms and which end-organ is affected. An ECG and cardiac enzymes should be obtained in patients suspected of having a myocardial infarction. Electrolytes, including creatinine (Cr) and blood urea nitrogen (BUN), hemoglobin, and proteinuria and red blood cell casts on urinalysis may point toward renal failure or glomerulonephritis. A chest radiograph may aid in the diagnosis of congestive heart failure, pulmonary edema, and aortic dissection. A head CT scan should be obtained in all patients who present with AMS or a focal neurologic deficit in order to rule out a mass lesion and ischemic or hemorrhagic stroke.

Management of Hypertensive Emergencies

Hypertensive emergency is a true medical emergency. Immediate evaluation and management is critical to limit morbidity and mortality. The patient should be placed on a cardiac monitor, and an intravenous line should be started. After the ABCs are assessed and stabilized, treatment begins by making the patient comfortable, consequently eliminating contributing factors that may exacerbate HTN such as pain, urinary retention, and hypoxia. Patients require immediate administration of antihypertensive medications to prevent irreversible end-organ damage (except in the case of acute ischemic stroke). As the elevation in blood pressure is being addressed, definitive measures should be taken to address any complications.

Understanding the concept of autoregulation is essential in the management of hypertensive emergencies. **Autoregulation** serves to maintain a constant, effective blood flow and perfusion to end organs, despite large variations in pressure. In the brain, autoregulation acts by adjusting cerebral blood flow (CBF) within the brain microcirculation. Extensive studies of cerebral circulation demonstrate that CBF is maintained across wide variations of systemic blood pressure by vasoconstriction and vasodilatation in normotensive patients. Because it is difficult to measure CBF accurately, especially regional differences and requirements, the cerebral perfusion pressure (CPP) is used as a surrogate indicator for monitoring. The CPP is the pressure gradient required to perfuse the cerebral tissue. CPP is calculated as the difference between the mean arterial pressure (MAP) and the intracranial pressure (ICP):

$$MAP - ICP = CPP$$

where MAP can be approximated as: $([2 \times$ diastolic blood pressure $+$ systolic blood pressure$] / 3)$. Local cellular oxygen demands can be met and regional CBF maintained over a wide range of CPP (between 50 and 150 mm Hg in a normally functioning system).

In individuals with chronic HTN, the CBF remains constant at higher CPP. However, if MAP, and thus CPP, drops into normal ranges, CBF precipitously declines, leading to cerebral hypoperfusion. Although not as well studied, it is theorized that rapid, large declines in blood pressure in chronically hypertensive patients would lead to hypoperfusion of other end organs as well.

Common Antihypertensive Agents Used in Hypertensive Emergencies (See Table 12–1)

Sodium nitroprusside: This is a potent peripheral vasodilator that decreases preload and afterload by dilating both arteries and veins, causing an immediate decrease in blood pressure. The recommended starting IV dose is 0.25 µg/kg/min and then titration to the desired clinical response and blood pressure. Because of its rapid action and potency, intraarterial monitoring is recommended when starting an infusion. Some drawbacks to this medication include its metabolism to a toxic cyanide compound. It is also associated with reflex tachycardia and coronary steal in the setting of acute coronary syndrome.

Labetalol: It is a selective alpha-1 adrenergic and nonselective beta-adrenergic blocker. It lowers systemic vascular resistance while maintaining renal, coronary, and CBF. Unlike other vasodilators, labetalol causes minimal reflex tachycardia.

Table 12–1 • COMMON ANTIHYPERTENSIVE AGENTS			
Antihypertensive	Preferred Use in	Recommended Starting Dose	Side Effects and Contraindications
Sodium nitroprusside	Hypertensive encephalopathy, aortic dissection*	0.25-10 µg/kg/min IV gtt	Reflex tachycardia, coronary steal, methemoglobinemia, metabolized to cyanide
Nitroglycerin	Myocardial infarction, congestive heart failure, left ventricular dysfunction	5-100 µg/min IV gtt	Hypotension: contraindicated in severe aortic stenosis, left ventricular outflow obstruction and inferior myocardial infarction
Nicardipine	Hypertensive encephalopathy, myocardial infarction, congestive heart failure, cerebral infarction/ hemorrhage	5 mg/h IV gtt, increasing by 2.5 mg/h IV every 5 minutes to a max of 30 mg/h IV gtt	Hypotension: contraindicated in severe aortic stenosis Reflex tachycardia
Labetalol	Hypertensive encephalopathy, myocardial infarction, preeclampsia/ eclampsia, cerebral infarction/hemorrhage	20-80 mg IV bolus every 10 minutes, 0.5-2 mg/min IV gtt	Hypotension: contraindicated in acute asthma, COPD, acute CHF, heart block, and sympathomimetic intoxication (eg, cocaine)
Esmolol	Hypertensive encephalopathy, myocardial infarction, eclampsia, cerebral infarction/hemorrhage	Loading dose 500 µg/kg IV over 1 min, 25-50 µg/kg/ min IV gtt titrated every 10-20 min	See labetalol
Fenoldopam	Acute renal failure, congestive heart failure	0.1-0.6 µg/kg/min IV gtt	Contraindicated in increased intraocular pressure
Enalaprilat	Congestive heart failure, active renin-angiotensin system	1.25-5 mg IV every 6 h	Contraindicated in pregnancy and ACE I-related angioedema
Hydralazine	Preeclampsia/eclampsia	5-10 mg IV bolus can be repeated every 10-15 min	Reflex tachycardia, CNS and myocardial ischemia

*Should be administered with a β-blocker to avoid reflex tachycardia.

It is contraindicated in patients with acute asthma, COPD, heart failure, heart block, and sympathomimetic drug abuse (eg, cocaine). Intravenous boluses of labetalol require 2-5 minutes to begin lowering the blood pressure. If a single bolus of 20 mg does not achieve the desired blood pressure reduction after 10 minutes, either repeated boluses at twice the original dosage can be given or an IV infusion can be started and titrated to the desired blood pressure.

Esmolol: Esmolol is a short-acting selective beta-1 adrenergic blocker. It has a rapid onset and short duration of action. These properties make it easy to titrate. Esmolol is effective in blunting the reflex tachycardia induced by nitroprusside. It carries the same contraindications as other beta-blockers (see Labetalol). Standard dosing is an IV bolus of 500 µg/kg followed by a continuous infusion of 50 µg/kg/min, which can be increased by 50 µg/kg/min every 4-5 minutes until the desired blood pressure is obtained.

Nicardipine: It is a dihydropyridine calcium channel blocker (CCB). It may have unique benefits in hypertensive encephalopathy since it crosses the blood-brain barrier (BBB) to vasorelax cerebrovascular smooth muscle and minimizes vasospasm, especially in subarachnoid hemorrhage. Nicardipine is contraindicated in patients with advanced aortic stenosis. The main adverse effect is abrupt reduction in blood pressure and reflex tachycardia, which can be harmful in patients with coronary heart disease. The initial infusion rate is 5 mg/h, increasing by 2.5 mg/h every 5 minutes to a maximum of 30 mg/h. Once the target BP is reached, downward adjustment by 3 mg/h should be attempted as tolerated.

Nitroglycerin: It is a potent vasodilator that acts mainly on the venous system. It decreases preload and also increases coronary blood flow to the subendocardium. Nitroglycerin can be administered as a paste, sublingual spray, dissolvable tablet, or infusion. It has a rapid onset and is considered the drug of choice in hypertensive emergencies in patients with cardiac ischemia, left ventricular dysfunction, and pulmonary edema. The recommended starting IV infusion dose is 5-15 µg/min and is titrated to desired clinical response. It is not recommended in patients with severe aortic stenosis, left ventricular outflow obstruction, or inferior wall myocardial infarction because of the chance of precipitating cardiovascular collapse.

Fenoldopam: This is a selective peripheral dopamine type 1 (D_1) agonist that has recently been added to the list of medications used in the treatment of hypertensive emergencies. It causes both vasodilation and natriuresis. Fenoldopam is administered as an IV infusion with a starting dose of 0.1-0.3 µg/kg/min and can be increased in increments of 0.05-0.1 µg/kg/min every 15 minutes to targeted effect. It has the advantage of increasing renal blood flow and improving creatinine clearance. As a result, fenoldopam may be the drug of choice in treating hypertensive emergencies in the setting of impaired renal function. It is contraindicated in patients with increased intraocular pressure.

Hydralazine: Hydralazine lowers blood pressure by a direct vasodilatory effect on arteriolar smooth muscle. The exact mechanism of this effect is unknown. It has been the preferred treatment by obstetricians in treating preeclampsia/eclampsia for decades but has fallen out of favor for treatment of HTN in other conditions. Hydralazine can cause reflex tachycardia and CNS and myocardial ischemia. Another downside of hydralazine is that while the half-life is 3-6 hours, the total duration of effect is up to 36 hours and can be unpredictable. The recommended starting dose is 5-10 mg IV bolus, which can be repeated every 10-15 minutes.

Enalaprilat: It is the active IV form of enalapril, an angiotensin converting enzyme (ACE) inhibitor. Enalaprilat lowers systemic vascular resistance, pulmonary capillary pressure, and heart rate while increasing coronary vasodilation. It has minimal effect on CPP. Some studies have found enalaprilat to be particularly useful in hypertensive emergency with APE. ACE inhibitors are contraindicated in pregnancy. The dose of enalaprilat is 1.25 mg IV bolus over 5 minutes and can be repeated every 6 hours. Enalaprilat cannot be titrated to effect.

Conditions Associated with Hypertensive Emergencies

Hypertensive encephalopathy: The **initial goal** is to rapidly lower the blood pressure **by 10% to 15% of the MAP in the first hour,** and by no more than 20% to 25% by the end of the first day. **More aggressive lowering of the blood pressure can lower the CPP and lead to cerebral hypoperfusion and ischemic events.** It is highly recommended to place an **arterial line** for more accurate monitoring of the patient's pressure. These patients should be watched closely in an intensive care setting. After a suitable period of targeted blood pressure control, oral medications can be started with a gradual tapering of the IV infusion. Preferred medications include labetalol and nicardipine.

Acute cerebral infarction: Elevated blood pressures are commonly seen in patients with acute stroke. This may be secondary to chronic HTN or as an acute sympathetic response. **Often, the acutely elevated blood pressure is necessary to maintain perfusion in watershed areas.** Thus, there is continued controversy as to when and how much elevated blood pressure should be lowered in patients with ischemic stroke. In fact, a recent multicenter, randomized control trial in Europe failed to demonstrate any benefit of lowering blood pressure in acute stroke and showed a trend toward harm. A special consideration is made for patients who are candidates for thrombolytic therapy; blood pressure should be lowered to below 185/110 mm Hg and maintained below 180/105 mm Hg for the next 24 hours. Otherwise, for patients who are not thrombolytic candidates, cautious lowering of pressure greater than 220/120 mm Hg is generally accepted, being careful to avoid lowering it too much or too rapidly as to induce drops in cerebral perfusion and cause greater ischemia. The preferred medications include labetalol, nitroprusside, and nicardipine.

Acute myocardial infarction: The goal in lowering the blood pressure in these cases is to decrease cardiac work by decreasing afterload and increasing coronary perfusion pressure. The preferred medications include nitroglycerin and beta-blockers. Nitroglycerin (sublingual or intravenous) reduces both LV filling pressure and systemic vascular resistance, thereby decreasing both myocardial oxygen demand and likelihood of ischemia. Higher doses of nitroglycerin produce coronary artery vasodilation. Beta-blockers are beneficial for both blood pressure reduction and prevention of ventricular dysrhythmias in ACS. While certain agents like esmolol have a more favorable profile because they have a rapid onset, shorter half-life and are easily titratable, beta-blockers should be used with caution since they can exacerbate LV failure. It is recommended to administer beta-blocker therapy only after a patient's hemodynamic condition has stabilized.

Aortic dissection: It is critical to lower blood pressure rapidly in this condition to limit progression of the dissection. Acute aortic dissection represents **the only**

hypertensive emergency where rapid, aggressive blood pressure reduction is indicated. The goal of emergency management is to control both blood pressure and heart rate in order to reduce the shear forces of LV ejection. Elevated shear forces result in a forceful flow of blood that can cause a dissection to extend. Recommended target systolic pressure is 100-110 mm Hg and heart rate less than 60 beats per minute. First-line agents are beta-blockers, as they have the ability to both simultaneously lower heart rate and blood pressure. While there is no consensus on preferred agent, esmolol is associated with a more rapid onset and is more easily titratable than labetalol. If beta-blockers are contraindicated, CCBs are acceptable alternatives.

CASE CORRELATION

- See also Case 25 (Altered Mental Status), Case 26 (Syncope), Case 28 (Stroke/TIA), and Case 29 (Headache).

COMPREHENSION QUESTIONS

12.1 A 55-year-old man presents to the ED with complaints of a severe headache, diplopia, and vomiting. His blood pressure is 210/120 mm Hg upon arrival. Which of the following is the best next step?

   A. Observe the blood pressure and recheck in 1 hour, and supportive measures for the headache and vomiting.

   B. Obtain a head CT scan, give an antihypertensive such as nicardipine, and admit to the intensive care unit.

   C. Give intravenous furosemide to decrease the blood pressure.

   D. Give lorazepam to help the patient relax.

12.2 A 54-year-old woman presents to the ED requesting medication refills on her antihypertensive medications. She has been out of her medications for 2 weeks and cannot get an appointment with her private physician until next week. She normally takes atenolol and hydrochlorothiazide. Her blood pressure is 190/100 mm Hg. The patient has no complaints. She has been waiting for 4 hours and is in a hurry to get back to work. Which of the following is the most appropriate next step?

   A. Change her medications to a CCB.

   B. Admit to the intensive care unit and initiate intravenous nitroprusside.

   C. Give her a prescription for her medications, instruct her to take them immediately and have her follow-up in 48 hours.

   D. Counsel the patient on the dangers of her noncompliance, admit to the hospital, and begin the patient on intravenous labetalol.

12.3 A 38-year-old man presents to the ED after a motor vehicle collision. After complete evaluation it is determined that he sustained a fracture of the right tibia. The patient has a history of HTN, for which he is on pharmacological treatment. The patient is writhing on the gurney in pain. His blood pressure is 210/104 mm Hg. The patient has no complaints except for right leg pain. Which of the following is the most appropriate next step in management?

A. Pain control and monitor the patient's blood pressure.

B. Start a beta-blocker and monitor the patient's blood pressure.

C. Call a social worker because of suspected drug or alcohol abuse.

D. Admit the patient to the hospital to get his blood pressure under control.

ANSWERS

12.1 **B.** This man likely has hypertensive encephalopathy, which is a medical emergency. He has symptomatic HTN causing end-organ damage. A head CT scan should be obtained prior to starting treatment to rule out any intracranial pathology. The appropriate treatment is IV antihypertensive medications to decrease his MAP by 20% to 25% over 1 hour.

12.2 **C.** This patient has hypertensive urgency. She has no symptoms related to her elevated blood pressure and no signs of end-organ damage. The patient should restart her medications and have her blood pressure reassessed in 48 hours.

12.3 **A.** Although this man has a history of HTN, he is in excruciating pain, which could be causing his elevated blood pressure. The appropriate treatment is to control the pain, have the leg set back into place, and to monitor his blood pressure. The blood pressure should decrease once his pain is controlled.

CLINICAL PEARLS

▶ Hypertensive emergency is defined as markedly elevated blood pressure in the presence of end-organ damage, whereas hypertensive urgency is markedly elevated blood pressure without end-organ effects.

▶ One of the most common reasons for hypertensive emergency is patient noncompliance with antihypertensive medication.

▶ It is critical to cautiously lower blood pressure to avoid inducing a hypoperfusion state that leads to cerebral ischemia.

▶ Patients with hypertensive emergency should be admitted to a monitored setting, preferably an intensive care unit.

REFERENCES

Amin A. Parenteral medication for hypertension with symptoms. *Ann Emerg Med.* 2008; 51(3 Suppl):S10-5. Epub 2008 Jan 11.

Blumenfeld JD, Laragh JH. Management of hypertensive crises: the scientific basis for treatment decisions. *Am J Hypertens.* 2001;14(11 Pt 1):1154-1167.

Chobanian AV, Bakris GL, Cushman WC, et al. The seventh report of the Joint National Committee on Prevention, Detection and Evaluation, and Treatment of High Blood Pressure, The JNC 7 Report. NIH Publication No. 04-5230. August 2004.

Cotton DB, Gonik B, Dorman KF. Cardiovascular alterations in severe pregnancy induced hypertension: acute effects of intravenous magnesium sulfate. *Am J Obstet Gynecol.* 1984;148:162-165.

De Gaudio AR, Chelazzi C, Villa G, Cavaliere F. Acute severe arterial hypertension: therapeutic options. *Curr Drug Targets.* 2009;10(8):788-798.

Fisher ND, Williams GH. Hypertensive vascular disease. In: Kasper DL, Braunwald E, Fauci AS, Hauser Sl, Longo DL, Jameson JL, eds. *Harrison's Principles of Internal Medicine.* 19th ed. New York, NY: McGraw-Hill; 2015: 1463-1481.

Flanigan JS, Vitberg D. Hypertensive emergency and severe hypertension: what to treat, who to treat, and how to treat. *Med Clin North Am.* 2006;90(3):439-451.

Frakes MA, Richardson LE. Magnesium sulfate therapy in certain emergency conditions. *Am J Emerg Med.* 1997;15:182-187.

Lipstein H, Lee CC, Crupi RS. A current concept of eclampsia. *Am J Emerg Med.* 2003;21:223-226.

Marik PE, Varon J. Hypertensive crises: challenges and management. *Chest.* 2007;131(6):1949-1962.

McCoy S, Baldwin K. Pharmacotherapeutic options for the treatment of preeclampsia. *Am J Health Sys Pharm.* 2009;66(4):337-344.

Pancioli AM. Hypertension management in neurologic emergencies. *Ann Emerg Med.* 2008; 51(3 Suppl):S24-27. Epub 2008 Jan 11.

Powers DR, Papadakos PJ, Wallin JD. Parenteral hydralazine revisited. *J Emerg Med.* 1998;16(2): 191-196.

Rhoney D, Peacock WF. Intravenous therapy for hypertensive emergencies, part 1. *Am J Health Sys Pharm.* 2009;66(15):1343-1352.

Rhoney D, Peacock WF. Intravenous therapy for hypertensive emergencies, part 2. *Am J Health Sys Pharm.* 2009;66(16):1448-1457.

Sandset EC, Bath PM, Boysen G, et al. The angiotensin-receptor blocker candesartan for treatment of acute stroke (SCAST): a randomised, placebo-controlled, double-blind trial. *Lancet.* 2011;377: 741-750.

Selvidge R, Dart R. Emergencies in the second and third trimesters: hypertensive disorders and antepartum hemorrhage. *Emerg Med Pract.* 2004;6(12):1-20.

Sibai B, Dekker G, Kupfemine M. Preelampsia. *Lancet.* 2005;365:785-799.

Varon J. Treatment of acute severe hypertension: current and newer agents. *Drugs.* 2008;68(3):283-297.

Varon J, Marik PE. The diagnosis and management of hypertensive crises. *Chest.* 2000;118:214-227.

Vaughan CJ, Norman D. Hypertensive emergencies. *Lancet.* 2000;356:411-417.

Vidt DG. Current concepts in treatment of hypertensive emergencies. *Am Heart J.* 1986;111:220-225.

At 3 AM the paramedics call to inform you that they are en route to the emergency department with a 33-year-old woman with a history of asthma. As she is brought in, you identify she is in severe respiratory distress. Sweat pours from her face and body as her neck and chest heave in an attempt to inhale another breath. Her efforts are ultimately futile as her consciousness slips away and she becomes apneic.

▶ What are your initial priorities in the management of this patient?
▶ What are your treatment options in managing her emergency medical condition?

ANSWERS TO CASE 13:

Acute Exacerbation of Asthma

Summary: This is a case of a 33-year-old woman experiencing a severe asthma attack who has now lost consciousness due to respiratory failure.

- **Initial priorities:** The first priority in this patient's management is addressing the ABCs (airway, breathing, circulation). Based on this presentation, immediate protection of her airway with rapid-sequence endotracheal intubation is indicated. While setting up for urgent intubation, two provider bag-valve-mask ventilation should be attempted. Her lungs should be auscultated to assess for air movement and her pulses assessed for quality and strength. Simultaneously, this patient should be placed on a cardiac monitor with automated blood pressure measurement, establishment of IV access, and continuous pulse oximetry.

- **Treatment options:** Treatment options include adrenergic agonists (eg, albuterol and terbutaline), anticholinergic agents, and corticosteroids. Intravenous magnesium sulfate is often given to patients with severe asthma exacerbations; however, its efficacy and routine administration is being challenged.

ANALYSIS

Objectives

1. Understand the pathophysiology of respiratory distress caused by acute asthma exacerbation.

2. Describe the key historical and physical examination features.

3. Be able to discuss treatment options for the patient with acute bronchospasm caused by asthma.

Considerations

This 33-year-old asthmatic patient has progressive respiratory difficulty until she becomes apneic. Regardless of the underlying etiology, airway, breathing, and an assessment of circulation are the most important initial concerns in any patient. This patient needs to have a secure airway established immediately. Administration of nebulized beta-agonist agents, nebulized anticholinergic agents, oral or parenteral corticosteroids, and search for the trigger are important issues for this patient.

> ## APPROACH TO:
> ### Asthma

CLINICAL APPROACH

Epidemiology and Pathophysiology

Asthma affects approximately 4% to 5% of the population in the United States. This disease disproportionally affects the pediatric and geriatric populations at about twice the rate of adults, and it is also seen more frequently in Hispanics and African Americans. Asthma exacerbations account for approximately 2 million Emergency Department visits, 484,000 hospitalizations, and more than 4000 deaths per year. Asthma results in more than 10 million lost school- and work-days per year, with an annual estimated disease cost of $14.5 billion.

Asthma is considered a chronic inflammatory disorder of the airways. It consists of a narrowing of the airway leading to reduced airflow, and it can be induced by smooth muscle contraction, thickening of the airway wall, and the presence of secretions within the airway lumen in response to an inciting allergen. In susceptible individuals, these changes result in recurrent episodes of wheezing, breathlessness, chest tightness, and cough.

Two distinct phases of asthma have been described. The **early (or immediate) phase** of asthma consists of acute airway hyper-responsiveness and reversible bronchoconstriction. Following allergen challenge, the lungs begin to constrict within 10 minutes. Peak bronchoconstriction occurs at 30 minutes and resolves within 1-3 hours, either spontaneously or with treatment. With continued allergen challenge or with refractory bronchoconstriction, this initial phase can progress into the late phase of asthma. This **late (or delayed) phase of asthma** begins 3-4 hours after the allergen challenge and constitutes the inflammatory component seen with acute asthma. Inflammatory cell recruitment, bronchial edema, mucoserous secretion, and further bronchoconstriction all play key roles in the development and propagation of late-phase asthma. This delayed phase of asthma can be targeted by corticosteroids, while the immediate phase is targeted by Beta-2 agonists.

Diagnosis

The history and physical examination of a patient with suspected asthma exacerbation should focus on excluding other diagnoses while evaluating the severity of the current asthma exacerbation. Key features to elicit are the nature and time course of the symptoms, precipitating triggers (Table 13–1), use of medication prior to arrival, and any highrisk historical features (Table 13–2).

A detailed history is often unobtainable in the patient presenting with a moderate-to-severe asthma attack. In these patients, treatment with a short acting bronchodilator and early consideration of steroids should be initiated after a brief history and focused physical examination. A comprehensive history can be deferred until treatment is underway.

Atypical asthma symptoms and signs include chest pain, stridor on examination, pulmonary rales, unilateral or bilateral leg edema, and fever. The presence

Table 13–1 • ASTHMA TRIGGERS
Exercise
Cold air
Smoke, Pollution
Emotional stress
Allergen exposure (dust, mold, pollen, pets/animal exposure, chemical fumes, etc)
Infection (primarily viral)
Gastro-Esophageal Reflux Disease
Hormonal fluctuations

of any of these symptoms or signs should prompt a workup for an alternative diagnosis.

Routine laboratory investigations, blood gas analysis, chest radiography, and electrocardiography are not required in the uncomplicated asthmatic. Table 13–3 suggests indications for each of these modalities.

MANAGEMENT

Immediate priorities in the management of all asthma patients include an initial assessment of the patient's airway, breathing, and circulation status. Patients in extremis require placement of peripheral intravenous lines, continuous supplemental oxygen therapy, and cardiac monitoring. While these interventions are underway, the physician should ascertain a history, perform a physical examination, and initiate appropriate therapy.

Oxygen, Compressed Air, and Heliox

Oxygen should be provided to maintain a pulse oximetry reading of at least 90% in adults and at least 95% in infants, pregnant women, and patients with coexisting heart disease. Oxygen is often used as the delivery vehicle for nebulized medications, although compressed air and helium:oxygen mixtures (heliox) can also be used. Heliox mixtures produce a more laminar airflow and potentially

Table 13–2 • HIGH RISK HISTORICAL FACTORS
Prior use of positive pressure ventilation for asthma (eg, intubation, bi-level positive pressure ventilation)
Prior hospitalization or intensive care unit admission
Frequent emergency department visits
Frequent albuterol metered-dose inhaler use
Current use or recent withdrawal of inhaled or oral corticosteroids
Comorbid medical or psychiatric conditions
Low socioeconomic status
Illicit drug use, especially inhaled cocaine

Table 13–3 • SUGGESTED INDICATIONS FOR ANCILLARY TESTING
Venous Blood Gas or Arterial Blood Gas
• To determine degree of hypercapnia or assess degree of deterioration in tiring patient not yet sick enough to warrant endotracheal intubation
Chest Radiography
• Temp >38°C
• Unexplained chest pain
• Hypoxemia
• Comorbidities/alternative diagnosis
Electrocardiogram
• Persistent tachycardia
• Comorbidities/alternative diagnosis

deliver nebulized particles to more distal airways, but they have not been shown to consistently lead to improved emergency department outcomes for all asthmatic patients. A Cochrane Database systematic review concluded that heliox may be beneficial only in patients who present with severe asthma that is refractory to initial treatment.

Adrenergic Agents

Inhaled albuterol, through nebulization or metered dose inhaler (MDI) with spacer device, is the mainstay of treatment for acute asthma. Typically 2.5-5 mg of albuterol is nebulized every 15-20 minutes for the first hour of therapy and then repeated every 30 minutes thereafter for 1-2 more hours (or, if MDI/spacer used: 4-8 puffs every 15-20 minutes for the first hour of therapy and then every 30 minutes thereafter for 1-2 more hours). Continuous nebulization with higher doses (10-20 mg/h) of albuterol benefits severe asthmatics. Beta-2 agonists bind pulmonary receptors and activate adenyl cyclase, which results in an increase in intracellular cyclic adenosine monophosphate (cAMP). This results in a drop in myoplasmic calcium and subsequent bronchial smooth-muscle relaxation. Side effects of these agents are generally mild and include tachycardia, nervousness, and shakiness or jitteriness.

Although inhalation therapy is optimal, occasionally patients with severe obstruction or those who cannot tolerate inhalation therapy are given subcutaneous administration of epinephrine or terbutaline. Epinephrine is given in a dose of 0.3-0.5 mg subcutaneously every 20 minutes to a maximal combined total dose of 1 mg. Terbutaline is given 0.25 mg subcutaneously every 20 minutes up to a maximum of three doses. Generally, terbutaline is preferable because of its beta-2 selectivity and fewer cardiac side effects.

Levalbuterol, the R-isomer of racemic albuterol, was developed because in vitro studies suggested that the S-isomer may have deleterious effects on airway smooth muscle. However, randomized trials have not shown a significant clinical advantage of levalbuterol over racemic albuterol for the treatment of acute asthma in the emergency department. National asthma treatment guidelines currently consider levalbuterol equally safe and effective to racemic albuterol and endorse its use for the treatment of acute asthma exacerbations.

Anticholinergic Agents

When added to albuterol, anticholinergic agents lead to a modest improvement in pulmonary function and decrease the admission rate in patients with moderate-to-severe asthma exacerbations. Anticholinergics decrease intracellular cyclic guanosine monophosphate (cGMP) concentrations, which reduce vagal nerve-mediated bronchoconstriction on medium- and larger-sized airways. The typical dose for ipratropium bromide is two puffs from an MDI with spacer device, or 0.5 mL of the 0.02% solution. Since there is little systemic absorption, inhaled anticholinergics are associated with few side effects.

Corticosteroids

Corticosteroids have been used to treat acute asthma exacerbations for over 50 years. Corticosteroids have a role in both acute and chronic asthma and should be initiated early in the treatment of the following cases:

- Acute asthma in patients with moderate or severe asthma attacks
- Worsening asthma over many days (>3 days)
- Mild asthma not responding to initial bronchodilator therapy or asthma that develops despite daily inhaled corticosteroid use.

Some physicians believe that more liberal use of corticosteroids is warranted and advocate steroids for any patient who presents to the Emergency Department or whose symptoms fail to resolve with a single albuterol treatment.

Steroids act on the delayed phase of asthma and modulate the inflammatory response. They have been shown to improve pulmonary function, decrease the rate of hospital admission, and decrease the rate of relapse in patients who receive them early in their ED treatment course. Oral administration of prednisone (dose 40-60 mg) is usually preferred to intravenous methylprednisolone (dose 125 mg) because it is less invasive and the effects are equivalent. Intravenous steroids, however, should be administered to patients with severe respiratory distress who are too dyspneic to swallow, patients who are vomiting, or those who are agitated or drowsy. For patients suitable for discharge from the Emergency Department, a 2-day course of oral dexamethasone (0.6 mg/kg; max dose 16 mg) or a single dose of dexamethasone (0.6 mg/kg; max dose 15 mg) has been shown to be equivalent to 5 days of prednisone in both pediatric and adult patients.

Leukotriene Antagonists

The development of leukotriene antagonists represents an important advancement in the treatment of chronic asthma. Studies involving zileuton (Zyflo Filmtab), zafirlukast (Accolate), and montelukast (Singulair) demonstrate that their daily use over the course of several months can lead to improvement in pulmonary function and decrease in asthma symptomatology. However, the role of leukotriene antagonists in the treatment of acute asthma exacerbations remains unclear.

Magnesium

Although no benefit has been shown in mild to moderate asthmatics, magnesium sulfate given intravenously at dosages of 2-4 g (or nebulized at standard nebulization doses) may benefit asthmatics with severe airway obstruction; however, recently even this has been brought into question. Magnesium is thought to compete with calcium for entry into smooth muscle, inhibit the release of calcium from the sarcoplasmic reticulum, prevent acetylcholine release from nerve endings, and inhibit mast cell release of histamine. The recently released "3Mg trial" was a multicenter, double-blind, placebo-controlled, three arm trial that randomized patients with severe acute asthma to IV magnesium, nebulized magnesium, and placebo. Despite enrolling over 1000 patients, the research group was unable to demonstrate a clinically worthwhile benefit to either IV or nebulized magnesium in acute severe asthma. Notably, patients with life-threatening asthma were not enrolled in this trial, leaving the option for treating this group with magnesium up to the medical professional. The most commonly reported side effects of magnesium therapy are hypotension, a flushing sensation, and malaise. It is contraindicated in renal failure and in cases of hypermagnesemia, as it can cause significant muscle weakness.

Other Agents—Methylxanthines, Antibiotics

The marginal benefit, significant side effects, and difficulty achieving a therapeutic dose of methylxanthines such as theophylline argue against its routine use in acute asthma. A systematic review concluded that the addition of the methylxanthine aminophylline to treatment with beta-agonists and glucocorticoids improved lung function but did not significantly reduce symptoms or length of hospital stay. Therefore, methylxanthines are not recommended in the treatment of acute asthma exacerbations.

The routine administration of antibiotics has not been shown to decrease symptomatology in asthma patients without concurrent bacterial lower respiratory infection or sinusitis.

Positive Pressure Ventilation

Positive pressure ventilation (PPV), with either invasive (IPPV, ie, use of endotracheal tube) or noninvasive methods (NIPPV, ie, continuous or bi-level PPV), is indicated for patients with respiratory failure or impending failure who are not responsive to therapy. The benefit of NIPPV in acute severe asthma is supported by evidence that PPV may have a direct bronchodilator effect, offset intrinsic PEEP, recruit collapsed alveoli, improve ventilation/perfusion mismatch, and reduce the work of breathing.

If using bi-level positive airway pressure (BiPAP), the ventilator should be set at inspiratory pressure 8-15 cm H_2O and expiratory pressure 3-5 cm H_2O. Patients who fail to improve over 30-60 minutes will likely require intubation. Obtaining blood gas values in these cases may aid in this assessment. Furthermore, contrary to prior teaching, a short trial (30 minutes) of BiPAP is considered acceptable for mild-to-moderate altered level of consciousness attributed to hypercapnia. For patients with severe asthma who are too agitated to tolerate PPV, ketamine may be given to relax and possibly bronchodilate the patient. Ketamine can be given as an intravenous bolus of 1 mg/kg, followed by a continuous infusion of 0.5-2 mg/kg/h.

Immediate rapid-sequence endotracheal intubation should be reserved for patients with respiratory failure. In awake patients, an appropriate induction agent (eg, ketamine) and paralytic agent (eg, rocuronium) should be used prior to intubation. Ketamine is the induction agent of choice because it stimulates the release of catecholamines and is believed to cause relaxation of bronchial smooth muscles, leading to bronchodilation.

Once an asthmatic patient is intubated, the ventilator should be set to promote the goal of permissive hypercapnia, which aims at minimizing dynamic hyperinflation (ie, breath stacking or auto-PEEP) with low respiratory rates and tidal volumes and increased time for expiration while limiting plateau pressures. It is critical to recognize that mechanically ventilated asthmatic patients are at high risk for hyperinflation and auto-PEEP, which can result in life-threatening complications, such as tension pneumothorax or cardiac arrest. Suggested initial settings are Assist Control (AC) mode at a respiratory rate of 8-10 breaths per minute, tidal volume 6-8 mL/kg, no extrinsic PEEP, inspiratory-to-expiratory (I/E) ratio of 1:4, and an inspiratory flow rate of 80-100 L/min.

ADMISSION/DISCHARGE CRITERIA

Acute asthma is a heterogeneous condition, and as such patients should be individualized when it comes to disposition decisions. Patients who respond well to therapy by improved subjective and objective criteria (eg, symptoms resolved, normal or near-normal pulmonary examination) are suitable candidates for discharge. Patients should be on room air (or on their baseline oxygen requirement) and moving about the emergency department before finalizing the decision to discharge the patient. Hospital admission should be considered in patients who fail to respond to therapy after 4-6 hours of treatment.

Asthmatics who are discharged from the ED should receive albuterol, an MDI spacer device, and a 3- to 10-day course of oral steroids. Most patients are typically treated for at least 5 days but can stop their oral steroids based on resolution of their symptoms and self-monitored peak flow values. Tapering is not necessary if the duration of steroid treatment is less than 3 weeks, if inhaled steroids are concomitantly prescribed for preventative ongoing therapy, or as long as the patient has not recently been on steroid therapy.

Inhaled corticosteroids (ICS) should be prescribed to anyone with frequent beta-agonist MDI use and who is symptomatic enough to warrant urgent medical evaluation. Several studies have demonstrated that ICS improve lung function, diminish symptoms, and decrease "rescue use" of beta agonists. Beneficial effects of ICS can be observed after a single dose, and therapeutic effects are achieved with chronic administration. Furthermore, one can initiate treatment alongside oral steroids without fear of added systemic toxicity.

For patients who continue to have poorly controlled asthma and recurrent exacerbations despite maximal therapy, other medications may be added, such as long-acting inhaled beta agonists, oral leukotriene antagonists, and omalizumab (a monoclonal anti-IgE antibody). A meta-analysis showed that patients with moderate-to-severe persistent allergic asthma who were treated with omalizumab experienced less asthma exacerbations and were more likely to taper off corticosteroids.

While awaiting discharge, MDI with spacer device technique should be reviewed with the patient, and the patient should be instructed on how to monitor peak flow readings at home. Additionally, patients should be educated about the common asthma precipitants and how to avoid them, as well as receive written and verbal instructions on when to return to the ED. Finally, patients should be referred for a follow-up medical appointment in a timely manner. Arranging ongoing care with an asthma specialist or a clinic focusing on asthma patients is more likely to reduce subsequent emergency department visits. Patients who are unable to follow up with their primary physician can be instructed to return to the ED for a recheck of their symptoms.

> ## CASE CORRELATION
>
> - See also Case 1 (Airway Management/Respiratory Failure), Case 11 (Congestive Heart Failure/Pulmonary Edema), Case 14 (Pulmonary Embolism), and Case 15 (Bacterial Pneumonia).

COMPREHENSION QUESTIONS

13.1 A 24-year-old man is brought into the ED complaining of an exacerbation of his asthma. Which of the following is the most appropriate method of assessing the severity of his disease?

A. Spirometry

B. Measurement of the diffusion capacity of the lungs

C. History and physical and peak expiratory flow

D. Measurement of the alveoli oxygen tension

13.2 A 19-year-old woman is admitted to the hospital for an exacerbation of asthma likely precipitated by pollen and colder weather. Her inpatient regimen includes both intravenous and inhalant medications. Which of the following medications is most likely to be used as part of her discharge plan?

A. Theophylline

B. Antibiotics

C. Magnesium

D. Histamines

E. Corticosteroids

13.3 Which of the following initial ventilator settings is appropriate for intubated asthmatics?

A. IMV mode, rate 16, tidal volume 6-8 mL/kg

B. IMV mode, rate 16, tidal volume 10-12 mL/kg

C. AC mode, rate 8-10, tidal volume 6-8 mL/kg

D. AC mode, rate 8-10, tidal volume 10-12 mL/kg

E. AC mode, rate 16, tidal volume 6-8 mL/kg

13.4 Which of the following is a benefit of using PPV in acute severe asthma?

A. Recruits collapsed alveoli

B. Improves ventilation/perfusion mismatch

C. Reduces the work of breathing

D. All of the above

ANSWERS

13.1 **C.** History and physical examination, along with peak expiratory flow, if needed, are a reliable and fairly accurate method of assessing asthma severity. Spirometry, although providing important information, is very cumbersome and rarely available in the ED.

13.2 **E.** Corticosteroids are often used after a hospitalization to treat the inflammatory component. Other standard medications include beta-agonists and oral leukotriene antagonists. None of the other medications listed as answer choices are used routinely for discharged asthma patients.

13.3 **C.** The initial settings for patients with obstructive lung disease should be AC mode, rate 8-10, tidal volume 6-8 mL/kg. Low rates and small tidal volumes are used to prevent air stacking and barotrauma.

13.4 **D.** All of the answers are believed to be benefits provided by PPV in acute severe asthma.

CLINICAL PEARLS

▶ Initiate therapy with albuterol while obtaining history and performing a physical examination for patients with significant asthma.

▶ Glucocorticosteroids should be administered early for asthmatic exacerbations and continued for at least 3-10 days.

▶ Measure peak flow to help assess asthma severity and monitor progression during treatment.

▶ Use lower than traditional ventilator settings to prevent barotrauma in the intubated asthmatic.

▶ Most moderate or severe asthmatics should be discharged with ICS for ongoing preventative therapy.

▶ The individual who presents with an initial episode of "wheezing" may have etiologies other than asthma, such as a foreign body, pneumonia, or congestive heart failure.

▶ Absence of wheezing can sometimes be misleading in the individual in extremis because of very little air movement in the airways.

REFERENCES

Akinbami LJ, Moorman JE, Liu X. Asthma prevalence, health care use, and mortality: United States, 2005-2009. National Health Statistics Reports No. 32, January 2011.

Camargo CA, Rachelefsky G, Schatz M. Managing asthma exacerbations in the emergency department: summary of the National Asthma Education and Prevention Program Expert Panel Report 3 guidelines for the management of asthma exacerbations. *J Allergy Clin Immunol.* 2009;124:S5-14.

Goodacre S, Cohen J, Bradburn M, et al. Intravenous or nebulized magnesium sulphate versus standard therapy for severe acute asthma (3 Mg trial): a double-blind, randomized controlled trial. *Lancet Respir Med.* 2013;1:293-300.

Goyal S, Agrawal A. Ketamine in status asthmaticus: a review. *Indian J Crit Care Med.* 2013;17(3): 154-161.

Keenan SP, Sinuff T, Cook DJ, Hill NS. Does noninvasive positive pressure ventilation improve outcome in acute hypoxemia respiratory failure? A systematic review. *Crit Care Med.* 2004;32(12): 2516-2523.

Krishnan JA, Davis SQ, Naureckas ET, Gibson P, Rowe BH. An umbrella review: corticosteroid therapy for adults with acute asthma. *Am J Med.* 2009;122(11):977-991.

Schatz M, Rachelefsky G, Krishnan JA. Follow-up after acute asthma episodes: what improves future outcomes? *J Emerg Med.* 2009;37:S42-S50.

A 34-year-old man presents to the emergency department (ED) complaining of shortness of breath and right-sided chest pain that increases with deep breathing. He states it started suddenly when he woke up and was worse with activity. He denies fever, chills, nausea, vomiting, or cough. He has a recent history of multiple gunshot wounds, resulting in ongoing pain in his upper back and T-10 paraplegia. One week ago, he was discharged from the hospital to a rehabilitation facility. He is currently taking acetaminophen/hydrocodone and ibuprofen for his pain, which has increased with his physical therapy and occupational therapy. He is also taking hydrochlorothiazide and lisinopril for hypertension and fluoxetine for depression. He recently quit smoking tobacco since he was hospitalized and denies any alcohol or illicit drug use. On physical examination, he is an otherwise fit young man who appears slightly short of breath and uncomfortable. His heart rate is 101 beats per minute, his blood pressure is 110/78 mm Hg, and his respiratory rate is 26 breaths per minute. His pulse oximetry is 96% on 2 L of O_2 by nasal canula. His lungs are clear to auscultation. There is mild swelling of his left calf. He has no sensation in his lower extremities. Laboratory studies reveal a white blood cell (WBC) count of 10,000/mm³. Hemoglobin, hematocrit, electrolytes, and renal function are all within normal limits. A 12-lead electrocardiogram (ECG) reveals a sinus rhythm at a rate of 103 beats per minute. His chest radiograph reveals minimal bibasilar atelectasis but no evidence of infiltrates or effusions.

► What is the most likely diagnosis?
► What are your next diagnostic steps?

ANSWERS TO CASE 14:
Pulmonary Embolism

Summary: A 34-year-old man with hypertension, depression, and recent gunshot wounds resulting in T-10 paraplegia presents with dyspnea, pleuritic right-sided chest pain, tachypnea, tachycardia, left calf swelling, and bibasilar atelectasis on chest radiography.

- **Most likely diagnosis:** Pulmonary embolism (PE) secondary to deep venous thrombosis (DVT) in the left lower extremity.

- **Next diagnostic steps:** For evaluation of PE/DVT, D-dimer level, venous duplex ultrasonography, ventilation-perfusion scan (V/Q scan), pulmonary CT angiography, and catheter pulmonary angiography are available and may be applied on a selective basis.

ANALYSIS

Objectives

1. Learn the clinical presentations of PE.

2. Learn to formulate a reasonable diagnostic strategy for the diagnosis of pulmonary embolism in the ED setting.

3. Learn the sensitivity, specificity, and limitations of the D-dimer test and the contrast-enhanced helical computed tomography angiogram for the diagnosis of DVT and PE.

Considerations

This 34-year-old patient who has been immobilized in the setting of recent trauma has a primary risk factor for venous thromboembolism. The presentation of acute dyspnea, chest pain, borderline tachycardia, and unilateral lower extremity swelling in the absence of identifiable alternative cardiopulmonary disease places him in the high-risk category for a PE. Patients with suspected PE should get an ECG and a chest x-ray as part of the initial workup. An ECG in patients with suspected PE is most helpful for identifying other etiologies of his symptoms, such as ischemic heart disease, pericarditis, and dysrhythmias, as most findings are not specific for a PE. Chest x-rays also lack specificity; in this case, however, a normal film is valuable in eliminating alternative diagnoses, such as pneumonia, pneumothorax, and congestive heart failure.

An arterial or venous blood gas can be used to assess patients with shortness of breath, but again these tests are non-specific in the diagnosis of PE. Taking into consideration the clinical, radiographic, and ECG data, a presumptive diagnosis of PE can be made. The next steps in management include maintenance of cardiopulmonary stability, consideration of empiric anticoagulation therapy, and confirmation of the diagnosis.

APPROACH TO:
DVT and PE

DEFINITIONS

DEEP VENOUS THROMBOSIS (DVT): Formation of clot (thrombus) in a deep vein (a vein that accompanies an artery). Eighty to ninety percent of diagnosed PEs arise from a DVT of the lower extremity. Thrombi of deep veins in the calf (tibial veins) are not only difficult to detect but are also much less likely to embolize than more proximal thrombi. Risk factors for thrombosis are related to the Virchow triad of hypercoagulability, venous stasis, and venous injury.

PULMONARY EMBOLISM (PE): Blockages of the pulmonary arteries, most often caused by blood clots originating from deep veins in the legs or pelvis. In rare circumstances, air bubbles, fat droplets, amniotic fluid, clumps of parasites, or tumor cells may also cause a PE.

D-DIMER ASSAY: Fibrin D-dimer is a small protein fragment present in blood after clot degradation by fibrinolysis. Multiple commercial assays are available that use a monoclonal antibody to detect the D-dimer fragment. The two most commonly used assays are the whole blood immunoagglutination test (less sensitive) and the quantitative plasma ELISA assay (more sensitive). The high-sensitivity assays can be used to rule out PE in both low and intermediate probability cases. Elevated D-dimer levels may indicate the presence of concurrent thrombus formation and degradation. Other conditions in which D-dimer elevation occurs include sepsis, recent myocardial infarction or stroke (<10 days), recent surgery or trauma, disseminated intravascular coagulation, collagen vascular disease, metastatic cancer, pregnancy, aortic dissection, sickle cell disease, superficial thrombophlebitis, hospitalized patients, and liver disease. The D-dimer may be falsely negative if clot formation is greater than 72 hours before the blood is assayed or if there is a small clot burden. Conversely, it may be falsely positive since levels may remain elevated for as long as 2 years. The generally accepted upper limit of normal is 500 ng/mL. Recent practice guidelines suggest using an age-adjusted threshold for patients over 50 years old (age x 10 ng/mL). In pregnancy, the upper limits of normal can be increased with each trimester; however, there are not any validated studies using adjusted D-dimer cutoffs or decision instruments.

VENOUS DUPLEX ULTRASONOGRAPHY: Ultrasound imaging modality combining direct visualization of veins with Doppler flow signal to assess luminal patency and compressibility of the deep venous system in the extremities and the presence of thrombosis. This imaging modality is most accurate for assessment of the iliac, femoral, and popliteal veins.

VENTILATION AND PERFUSION (V/Q) SCAN: Imaging study using radioisotopes to determine the V/Q ratio and identify ventilation-perfusion mismatches. Results are categorized into probability-ranked groups after taking into account any pulmonary comorbidities and the patient's overall clinical picture.

Radiologists interpret V/Q scans as normal, low, intermediate, or high probability for V/Q mismatch or PE in the right clinical setting. Unfortunately, **many patients with PE have nondiagnostic V/Q scans,** and because interpretations of these low-to-intermediate probability scans are subjective, there is significant inconsistency among interpreters. **V/Q scans are most beneficial in patients with renal failure who are deemed to be at risk of developing contrast-induced nephropathy from a CT scan and also for patients with contrast allergies.** V/Q scans may also be the test of choice for pregnant patients. It is reported that MDCT scanning has higher radiation exposure for the mother but lower fetal radiation exposure, whereas V/Q scan has lower maternal and higher fetal radiation exposure.

COMPUTED TOMOGRAPHY PULMONARY ANGIOGRAPHY (CTPA): Magnified CT imaging of the pulmonary vasculature obtained during the arterial phases of venous contrast injection. The introduction of multidetector CT (MDCT) scanning has greatly improved imaging of central, segmental, and subsegmental arteries. The Prospective Investigation of Pulmonary Embolism Diagnosis II (PIOPED II) study suggests that CTPA identifies more PE than V/Q scanning, but these may be false-positives or clots that may not require anticoagulation. In routine clinical practice, PEs identified by CTPA are frequently over diagnosed, as interobserver agreement for subsegmental clots is poor.

PULMONARY ANGIOGRAPHY: Imaging involving intravascular contrast injection and fluoroscopy to determine patency of the pulmonary arterial vasculature. Although once considered the gold standard for diagnosing PE, this test has largely been replaced by pulmonary CT angiography (CTA). Pulmonary angiography is invasive and is associated with increased morbidity and mortality when compared to CTA, which is comparable in its ability to detect a PE.

CLINICAL APPROACH

Deep Venous Thrombosis

Up to **60% of patients with untreated proximal DVT will develop PE. Unfortunately, the clinical features of DVT are frequently nonspecific** and may include pain, tenderness, swelling, edema, and erythema. The physical examination and the patient's risk factors for developing a clot (Table 14–1) should be considered when estimating the pretest probability of DVT, which can then be applied to a diagnostic algorithm (Figure 14–1).

   Duplex ultrasound is the most common test used to evaluate for the presence of DVT. When performed by an experienced operator, its accuracy approaches 98% for proximal DVT detection. Emergency providers can achieve comparable accuracy in detecting popliteal or femoral DVTs when performing two-point compression bedside ultrasonography. ELISA D-dimer can serve as a screening tool for DVT. Due to its high sensitivity, **a negative ELISA D-dimer suggests the absence of an acute thrombus.** Thus, in patients with low-pretest probability and a negative ELISA D-dimer, the diagnosis of DVT can be ruled out. Patients with intermediate- or high-pretest probability should get an ultrasound as the first line test (Figure 14–1). **Venography** is the traditional gold standard for DVT. However, due to its invasiveness, risk of reaction to contrast dye, and the advent

Table 14–1 • RISK FACTORS FOR VENOUS THROMBOEMBOLISM DISEASE		
Acquired Disorders	**Medical Conditions**	**Inherited Disorders**
Prior history of venous thromboembolism Immobilization Malignancy—active Obesity Trauma Surgery—recent <4 week Pregnancy Smoking Central venous catheters Estrogen use Lupus anticoagulant	Congestive heart failure Nephrotic syndrome Myocardial infarction Stroke Hyperviscosity syndrome Crohn disease	Factor V Leiden Protein C and S deficiency Antithrombin III deficiency Other blood factor deficiencies

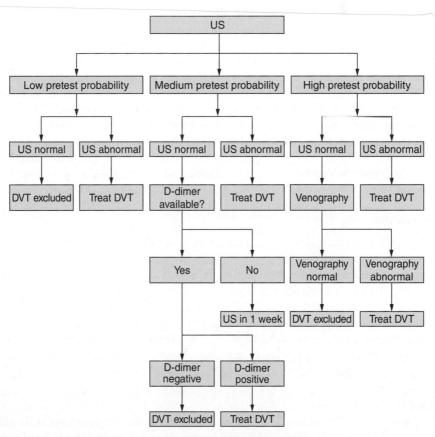

Figure 14–1. Algorithm for diagnosis of suspected lower extremity DVT.

of newer technologies that are just as accurate, venography is now rarely used in clinical practice.

All patients diagnosed with a DVT at or above the level of the popliteal vein should be treated with anticoagulation. Treatment goals are directed toward the prevention of thrombus propagation and embolization. In patients with extensive DVT involving the iliac and femoral veins, thrombolytic therapy should be considered to help minimize the postphlebitic sequelae. There are no universally accepted treatment guidelines for isolated calf vein DVTs, although many providers will recommend 3 months of anticoagulation. Alternatively, the patient can defer treatment and have a repeat ultrasound in 1 week to assess progression of the clot. Patients with isolated calf vein DVTs who have a history of DVT or significant risk factors should be anticoagulated.

For most patients, acute management consists of anticoagulation with unfractionated heparin (UFH) or low-molecular-weight heparin (LMWH). **Enoxaparin is a commonly used LMWH** and is the preferred initial medication, as it is a self-administered subcutaneous injection that patients can use at home. Additionally, it confers lower risk of major bleeding and heparin-induced thrombocytopenia (HIT). Fondaparinux is another LMWH. Patients with significant renal insufficiency should receive heparin. These medications are intended to be a bridge to warfarin and should be administered in conjunction with warfarin until a therapeutic INR is achieved. Warfarin should not be administered by itself, as it can paradoxically cause hypercoagulability when treatment is first begun. Rivaroxaban, dabigatran, and apixaban are novel oral anticoagulants approved for use in both DVT and PE; these do not require monitoring of INR levels (Table 14–2).

Patients developing recurrent DVT during optimal anticoagulation therapy should undergo evaluation for hypercoagulability conditions and be considered for inferior vena cava (IVC) filter placement (eg, Greenfield filter). **IVC filters are also useful for individuals with contraindications to anticoagulation. However, these filters present their own risks for developing thrombosis and PE and have limited effect over time.**

Pulmonary Embolism

Few common medical conditions are as elusive and difficult to diagnose as PE, as its presentation can be variable and at times vague, and it can mimic many other acute cardiopulmonary conditions. The majority of patients have dyspnea and pleuritic chest pain at presentation, whereas cardiovascular collapse is observed in 10% of the patients. Other signs and symptoms of PE include tachypnea, tachycardia, hypoxia, cough, anxiety, and low-grade fever. Hemoptysis secondary to PE is due to pulmonary infarction and is an uncommon and late finding. The classic findings—or triad—of dyspnea, pleuritic chest pain, and tachycardia can be found in up to 95% of patients with confirmed PE.

Diagnosis

The diagnosis of PE remains a difficult task despite the multitude of tests and imaging modalities available in the ED. Patients who present with signs or symptoms concerning for PE, namely chest pain, dyspnea, tachypnea, and hypoxia, should get an ECG and a chest x-ray as part of the workup. However, these are of limited

Table 14–2 • TREATMENT OPTIONS FOR DVT/PE			
Agent	**Loading Dose**	**Maintenance Dose**	**Monitoring of Levels**
Unfractionated Heparin (UFH)	5000 units (80 U/kg)	1000 units/h (18 U/kg/h)	Yes target PTT 50-90
Low-Molecular-Weight Heparins (LMWH)			
Enoxaparin	None	1.5 mg/kg SQ qd or 1 mg/kg SQ bid	None
Dalteparin	None	200 IU/kg SQ qd or 100 IU/kg SQ bid	None
Fondaparinux	None	<100 lbs 5 mg daily 110-220 lb 7.5 mg daily >220 lb 10 mg daily	None
Long-Term Oral Therapy			
Warfarin[a]	5 mg PO qd	Varies	INR 2-3
Rivaroxaban	15 mg PO BID × 21 days	20 mg PO qd	None
Dabigatran	10 mg PO BID × 7 days	5 mg PO BID	None
Apixaban	150 mg PO BID (after 5 to 10 days of parenteral anticoagulation)	150 mg PO BID (110 mg PO BID if increased risk of bleeding)	None

[a]Warfarin should always be administered in conjunction with either unfractionated or low-molecular-weight heparin until a therapeutic INR level is achieved.

utility, as they provide non-specific information and are more useful for ruling out other diagnoses.

Most patients with PE have a chest x-ray with one or more abnormalities, including cardiomegaly, basilar atelectasis, infiltrate, or pleural effusion. However, there is no one diagnostic finding that is specific for PE. In severe PE, dilation of proximal pulmonary vessels with collapse of distal vasculature is noted (**Westermark sign**). Twenty-four to seventy-two hours after a PE, atelectasis and a focal infiltrate may be seen as a consequence of loss of surfactant. Pleural effusions may be noted, and rarely, a triangular or rounded pleural-based infiltrate with its apex pointed to the hilum (**Hampton hump**) may be seen in the case of an infarction. However, these classic signs are rarely seen.

In some instances, the ECG may reveal right-heart strain patterns that are more specific for the diagnosis of PE, such as T-wave inversion in leads V_1 to V_4, incomplete or complete right bundle-branch block, and the classic but uncommon S_1-Q_3-T_3 pattern. Although nonspecific, sinus tachycardia is still the most frequent presenting ECG finding among patients with PE. However, 25% of patients with identified PE may have a normal ECG.

The most important first step in diagnosis when PE is suspected is risk stratification, or determining pretest probability. There are multiple scoring systems available that attempt to classify patients into low-, intermediate-, and high-risk

Table 14–3 • WELLS CRITERIA FOR ASSESSMENT OF PRETEST PROBABILITY OF PULMONARY EMBOLISM		
Criterion	**Points**	
Suspected DVT	3	
An alternate diagnosis is less likely than PE	3	
HR >100 beats/min	1.5	
Immobilization or surgery in the previous 4 weeks	1.5	
Previous DVT/PE	1.5	
Hemoptysis	1	
Malignancy (being treated currently or in the last 6 months)	1	
Score Range (Points)	**Mean Probability of PE**	**Interpretation of Risk**
0-2	4%	Low
3-6	21%	Moderate
>6	67%	High

Data from Wells PS, Anderson DR, Rodger M, et al. Derivation of a simple clinical model to categorize patient's probability of pulmonary embolism: increasing the model's utility with the simpliRED D-dimer. Thromb Haemost. 2000;83:416-420.

categories. A commonly used scoring system is the **Wells criteria** (Table 14–3). Overall accuracy of an experienced clinician's gestalt seems to be similar to that of structured clinical decision instruments.

The Pulmonary Embolism Rule-Out Criteria (PERC) is another commonly used clinical decision rule (Table 14–4). This rule only applies to those who are low risk for PE. If eight of the clinical criteria are met, the pretest probability that the patient has a PE is less than 1% and no further workup is needed, as the risk for PE is lower than the risk of testing. Because **clinical variables alone lack power to permit treatment decisions,** patients with intermediate-to-high probability must undergo further testing until the diagnosis is proven, ruled out, or an alternative diagnosis is identified.

As with DVT, many recent investigations have focused on the use of the highly sensitive D-dimer assay for PE diagnosis. **The power of the D-dimer test is in its negative predictive value rather than its positive predictive value, provided a highly sensitive assay is chosen.** A normal D-dimer value is helpful for the exclusion of PE in patients

Table 14–4 • PERC RULE OUT CRITERIA
Age <50 years
Pulse >100 bpm
Sao_2 >94%
No unilateral leg swelling
No hemoptysis
No recent trauma or surgery
No prior PE or DVT
No hormone use

with low pretest probability who do not meet the PERC rule out criteria. A normal D-dimer can also be used to rule out PE in patients with intermediate pretest probability. However, because intravascular thrombosis may occur in conditions other than PE and DVT, the specificity of elevated D-dimer is limited and imaging studies should be performed in these cases. **In high-risk individuals, negative D-dimer assay alone cannot effectively rule out PE, so this test should not be obtained because a negative value will not preclude the need for imaging.** CTPA is the preferred imaging study if there is no contraindication to contrast dye. V/Q scanning should be used when CTPA is unavailable or contraindicated. For patients who are hemodynamically unstable and in whom definitive imaging is unsafe, bedside echocardiography may be used to look for signs of right heart strain and obtain a presumptive diagnosis of PE to justify the administration of potentially life-saving therapies.

Interpretation of nuclear scintigraphic **ventilation-perfusion scanning (V/Q scan)** may **group patients into four result types: normal, low probability, indeterminate, and**

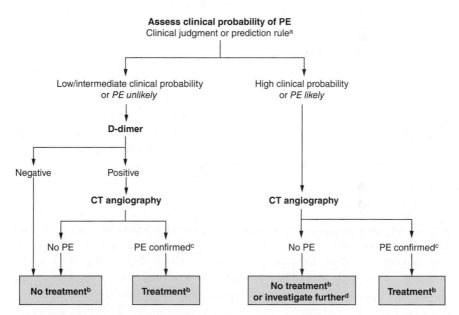

CT = computed tomographic; PE = pulmonary embolism.
[a]Two alternative classification schemes may be used for clinical probability assessment, ie, a three-level scheme (clinical probability defined as low, intermediate, or high or a two-level scheme (PE unlikely or PE likely). When using a moderately sensitive assay, D-dimer measurement should be restricted to patients with low clinical probability or a PE-unlikely classification, while highly sensitive assays may also be used in patients with intermediate clinical probability of PE. Note that plasma D-dimer measurement is of limited use in suspected PE occurring in hospitalized patients.
[b]Treatment refers to anticoagulation treatment for PE.
[c]CT angiogram is considered to be diagnostic of PE if it shows PE at the segmental or more proximal level.
[d]In case of a negative CT angiogram in patients with high clinical probability, further investigation may be considered before withholding PE-specific treatment.

Figure 14–2. Algorithm for the diagnosis of suspected acute pulmonary embolism. Source: Reproduced, with permission, from Konstantinides S, Torbicki A, Agnelli G, et al. 2014 ESC guidelines on the diagnosis and management of acute pulmonary embolism. *Eur heart J.* 2014;35(43):3033-69, 3069a-3069k.

high probability. Similar to the diagnosis of DVT, the clinical suspicion determines the pretest probability and the accuracy of V/Q scans. Therefore, the subsequent management following V/Q scans should be formulated on the basis of clinical impression and V/Q scan interpretations. One study reported that V/Q scan combined with chest radiography had the same diagnostic accuracy as pulmonary CTA and V/Q scanning.

High-resolution CT angiography has become the standard initial diagnostic test for the evaluation of high-risk patients for PE (Figure 14–2). Additionally, MDCTA has largely replaced single-detector CT scanners. MDCTA, according to PIOPED II, has a sensitivity of 83% and a specificity of 96% for diagnosing PE. A negative pulmonary MDCTA can safely exclude a PE. It has a positive predictive value of 86% and a negative predictive value of 95%. Due to limitations of PIOPED II, these results may not apply to patients with renal failure, pregnant women, and critically ill patients.

The addition of **indirect CT venography (CTV)** was also investigated in PIOPED II. Although they reported a statistically insignificant increase in sensitivity (83%-90%), specificity was not changed. CTV increases the radiation exposure and has the equivalent diagnostic results of lower-extremity sonography. It should be used with **caution in younger patients**, who have the greatest long-term risk of radiation exposure. The advantage is gaining information on both the pulmonary and venous systems through one test. Remy-Jardin reported that the greatest benefit from the addition of CTV to CTA has been shown in sicker patients, in centers with less experience, and with older equipment.

In high-pretest clinical probability patients who have a negative MDCTA test for PE, further testing is recommended. These patients represent a discordant group—high risk but with a negative test. Options include repeat pulmonary MDCTA if there were technical problems with the first test, pulmonary angiography, V/Q scan, or lower extremity venous sonography.

Laboratory Tests

The D-dimer test is best utilized for its negative predictive value. Pulse oximetry and ABG measurements are insensitive in identifying PE and should never be used to direct diagnostic workup. Despite the common practice of obtaining ABGs in the workup of PE, multiple studies demonstrate that a normal Pao_2, normal Pco_2, and normal A-a oxygen gradient does not exclude the diagnosis of PE.

Clinical Decision Making

Ultimately, it is the clinician's burden to combine the imaging and laboratory test results with clinical impression to determine whether treatment for DVT/PE is indicated. The treatment for PE in stable patients is generally the same as for DVT (see Table 14–2). **Thrombolytic therapy and/or catheter based therapies** have been advocated for those individuals with a massive PE (causing significant hemodynamic compromise) **for whom mortality is as high as 20% to 30%.** There are no conclusive studies that prove a long-term survival advantage for thrombolytic therapy in PE. However, some literature suggests a reduction in morbidity (ie, pulmonary hypertension) in patients who received half-dose thrombolytics in the setting of a submassive PE.

> **CASE CORRELATION**
>
> • See also Case 1 (Airway Management/Respiratory Failure), Case 13 (Asthma), and Case 15 (Bacterial Pneumonia).

COMPREHENSION QUESTIONS

14.1 Which of the following statements regarding DVT is most accurate?

A. A patient with thrombosis of the superficial femoral vein is never at risk for PE.

B. Venography is the definitive test for the diagnosis of DVT.

C. Thrombosis of the vena cava, subclavian veins, and right atrium are frequent sources of PE.

D. Venous duplex ultrasonography is most useful in diagnosing DVT in the pelvic veins.

E. Cancer successfully treated 5 years ago is associated with a higher risk for DVT.

14.2 A 52-year-old healthy man presents with a 3-day history of a pleuritic chest pain and SOB. He has normal vital signs and physical examination. Which test is most useful in ruling out pulmonary emboli in this patient?

A. Electrocardiogram (ECG)

B. Chest x-ray

C. Arterial blood gas (ABG)

D. D-dimer level

E. Oxygen saturation

14.3 Which of the following patients with shortness of breath has the lowest clinical probability for PE?

A. A 67-year-old man who underwent bilateral total knee replacements 2 weeks ago.

B. A 38-year-old man who underwent an uncomplicated open appendectomy 3 weeks ago.

C. A 35-year-old woman undergoing treatment for ovarian cancer.

D. A 35-year-old man with a history of a DVT 15 years ago, which occurred after an accident.

E. A 26-year-old woman who had an uncomplicated vaginal delivery 10 days ago.

14.4 A 57-year-old man presents to the ED complaining of sudden onset of short-ness of breath with pleuritic chest pain. He was recently released from the hospital after being diagnosed with lymphoma. He had an indwelling catheter placed in his left subclavian vein the day before for chemotherapy administra-tion. He was previously healthy without significant medical history. His vital signs are heart rate of 105 beats per minute, blood pressure of 126/86 mm Hg, respiratory rate of 28 breaths per minute, and O_2 saturation of 100% on room air. The breath sounds are clear bilaterally. His heart sounds are normal without an S_3 or S_4 gallop. His left arm is mildly edematous but otherwise painless, with a normal pulse examination. There is no swelling of his lower extremities, and he has no pain with palpation of his calves. His catheter inci-sion site is clean and intact. Which of the following studies is inappropriate for this patient?

A. Chest x-ray

B. ECG

C. Contrast CT scan of the chest

D. D-dimer assay

E. Duplex ultrasonography of the deep veins of the upper and lower extremities

ANSWERS

14.1 **B.** Venography is the gold standard for diagnosing thromboses of the deep veins of the extremities and is useful when duplex studies are inconclusive in high-risk, high-probability patients. Duplex ultrasonography combines direct visualization of the vein with Doppler flow signals. Part of the study relies on the examiner's ability to visualize compression of the veins to rule out an occluding thrombus. Because intra-abdominal and pelvic veins are dif-ficult to compress, their evaluation by this method is limited. Most clinically significant PE derives from the large veins of the lower extremity, especially the iliofemoral veins that can embolize large clots to the pulmonary vascula-ture with disastrous hemodynamic consequences. Infrequent sources of PE can be central veins of the upper extremity, the vena cava, or even the right atrium. Despite its name, the superficial femoral vein is considered a deep vein (it accompanies the superficial femoral artery) and can be the source of clinically significant thromboemboli. Active cancer, rather than a history of treated cancer (>5 years), is associated with a higher risk of DVT.

14.2 **D.** ECG findings are often normal or nonspecific in patients with PE and thus are not the most useful in ruling out PE in this patient. Chest radio-graphs are also usually normal, though the Westermark sign or Hampton Hump may be noted. ABG findings are often confusing, and abnormalities are usually a result of underlying pathology such as chronic obstructive pul-monary disease (COPD) or pneumonia. A low Po_2 in an otherwise healthy patient at risk for DVT/PE is more useful. O_2 saturation is rarely depressed and not very useful in the workup of PE. High-sensitivity D-dimer levels are most useful for their negative predictive value in helping to rule out PE in low-to-moderate pretest-probability patients. It is a very sensitive but non-specific test. A normal high-sensitivity D-dimer level in a low-to-moderate pretest probability patient makes PE unlikely, and further diagnostic workup is not indicated.

14.3 **B.** Malignancy, acquired or inherited hypercoagulable states, previous DVT or PE, immobility, and pregnancy are all risk factors for DVT and PE. Although surgery is a known risk factor, the length of the operation and time of postoperative immobility are factors that contribute to thrombosis. The patient who underwent an uncomplicated appendectomy is at minimal risk for a DVT. The patient with the bilateral knee replacement would have very limited mobility for a long period time, putting him at risk for DVT and PE. The patient with ovarian cancer is at risk because of her malignancy. A patient with a previous DVT certainly has a greater lifetime risk for recurrence of a DVT. The patient with a normal vaginal delivery 10 days previously would have a higher risk of DVT than the general population.

14.4 **D.** This patient may very well have a PE, but other sources of his chest pain and shortness of breath must also be considered. A chest x-ray will show other possible pulmonary processes, including pneumonia or a pneumothorax from the central line placement (as well as confirm the position of the line). An ECG will aid in the diagnosis of cardiac etiologies, including heart attacks or arrhythmias. CTA would be appropriate, as it can diagnose a PE as well as other etiologies of his symptoms. A D-dimer assay is not useful in this patient because he is a high-probability patient, and this test should only be ordered in low-probability patients. Duplex ultrasonography will help examine the venous system for thromboses and possible sources of PE, including the deep veins of the upper extremity, because this patient now has an indwelling catheter that can be a source of thrombus formation.

CLINICAL PEARLS

▶ High clinical suspicion is the most important factor in determining the workup of PE, as its presentation is often elusive.

▶ High-sensitive D-dimer study is useful for its negative predictive value in excluding DVT and PE.

▶ V/Q scan is useful in risk-stratifying patients with renal failure and possibly pregnant patients with suspected PE.

▶ MDCTA has become the initial test of choice for patients with a high-pretest probability for PE and no contraindications.

▶ Eighty percent of PEs develop from DVTs involving the iliac, femoral, or popliteal veins.

REFERENCES

Anderson DR, Kahn SR, Rodger MA, et al. Computed tomographic pulmonary angiography vs. ventilation perfusion lung scanning in patients with suspected pulmonary embolism: a randomized controlled trial. *JAMA*. 2007;298(23):2743-2753.

Baile EM, King GG, Muller NL, et al. Spiral computed tomography is comparable to angiography for the diagnosis of pulmonary embolism. *Am J Respir Crit Care Med*. 2000;161(3 Pt 1):1010-1015.

Courtney M, Kline J, et al. Clinical features from the history and physical examination that predict the presence of absence of pulmonary embolism in symptomatic emergency department patients: results of a prospective, multi-center study. *Ann Emerg Med*. 2010;55(4):307-315.

Crisp JG, Lovato LM, Jang TB. Compression ultrasonography of the lower extremity with portable vascular ultrasonography can accurately detect deep venous thrombosis in the emergency department. *Ann Emerg Med*. 2010;56:601-610.

Dupras D, Bluhm J, Felty C, et al. Institute for Clinical Systems Improvement. Venous Thromboembolism Diagnosis and Treatment. Available at: http://bit.ly/VTE0113. Updated January 2013.

Kline, JA. Venous thromboembolism. In: Tintinalli JE, Stapczynski J, Ma O, Yealy DM, Meckler GD, Cline DM, eds. *Tintinalli's Emergency Medicine: A Comprehensive Study Guide*. 8th ed. New York, NY: McGraw-Hill; 2016.

Kline JA, Courtney DM, Kabrhel C, et al. Prospective multicenter evaluation of the pulmonary embolism rule-out criteria. *J Thromb Haemost*. 2008;6:772-780.

Konstantinides S, Torbicki A, Agnelli G, et al. 2014 ESC guidelines on the diagnosis and management of acute pulmonary embolism. *Eur Heart J*. 2014;35(43):3033-3073.

Raja AS, Greenberg JO, Qaseem A, et al. Evaluation of Patients With Suspected Acute Pulmonary Embolism: Best Practice Advice From the Clinical Guidelines Committee of the American College of Physicians. *Ann Intern Med*. 2015;163(9):701-711.

Rogers RL, Winters M, Mayo D. Pulmonary embolism: remember that patient you saw last night? *Emerg Med Pract*. 2004;6(6):1-20.

Sadigh G, Kelly A, Cronin P. Challenges, controversies, and hot topics in pulmonary embolism imaging. *AJR*. 2011;196(3):497-515.

Sadosty AT, Boie ET, Stead LG. Pulmonary embolism. *Emerg Med Clin North Am*. 2003;21(2):363-384.

Stein PD, Fowler SE, Goodman LR, et al. Multi-detector computed tomography for acute pulmonary embolism. *N Engl J Med*. 2006;354(22):2317-2327.

Wells PS, Anderson DR, Rodger M, et al. Excluding pulmonary embolism at the bedside without diagnostic imaging: management of patients with suspected pulmonary embolism presenting to the emergency department by using a simple clinical model and D-dimer. *Ann Intern Med*. 2001;135(2):98-107.

A 70-year-old woman is transferred from a nursing home to the emergency department (ED) due to fever and shortness of breath. As per her daughter, the patient has had a productive cough for 2 days and became more short of breath and less responsive earlier today. The patient's past medical history is significant for diabetes mellitus, hypertension, and high cholesterol. Her vital signs include: temperature 38.9°C (102.1°F), heart rate 104 beats per minute, blood pressure 130/85 mm Hg, respiratory rate 28 breaths per minute, and room air oxygen saturation 87% (96% with 3L oxygen by nasal cannula). On examination, she is awake but slow to answer questions. The daughter states that her mother is usually more alert than this. Her skin is dry and warm to touch. Her heart sounds are regular and mildly tachycardic without any S_3 or S_4. On auscultation, she has rhonchi at the right lung base. She does not have any Jugular venous distention, lower extremity edema, or calf tenderness.

▶ What is the most likely diagnosis?
▶ How should this patient be managed?

ANSWERS TO CASE 15:

Bacterial Pneumonia

Summary: A 70-year-old woman is sent to the ED from a nursing home due to fever, productive cough, and shortness of breath. On examination, she is febrile, mildly tachycardic, tachypneic, and hypoxic on room air. She has rhonchi in the right lung base but does not have any signs of congestive heart failure or peripheral deep venous thrombosis.

- **Most likely diagnosis:** Healthcare-associated pneumonia.

- **Management:** Supplemental oxygen, intravenous antibiotics, blood and sputum cultures, and admission.

ANALYSIS

Objectives

1. Define community-acquired versus hospital-acquired versus healthcare-associated pneumonia.

2. Describe the various clinical presentations of pneumonia.

3. Learn the management of pneumonia, including the best choices for empiric antibiotic administration.

Considerations

This 70-year-old woman presents with history and physical examination findings consistent with pneumonia. **Pneumonia is the most common cause of death from infectious disease and the eighth leading cause of death overall in the United States.** Clinical presentations and common etiologic organisms vary among different patient populations. Because this patient is a nursing home resident, she is at risk for infection with multidrug-resistant bacteria. Pneumonia may be associated with significant morbidity and mortality, especially among immunocompromised and elderly patients. However, prompt initiation of therapy can result in improved patient outcomes. Treatment includes appropriate empiric antibiotics, disease assessment, and respiratory support.

APPROACH TO:

Bacterial Pneumonia

DEFINITIONS

COMMUNITY-ACQUIRED PNEUMONIA (CAP): Pneumonia that occurs in a patient living in the general population or community.

HOSPITAL-ACQUIRED PNEUMONIA (HAP): Pneumonia that arises 48 hours or more after hospital admission. HAP includes ventilator-associated pneumonia (VAP), which is infection that develops more than 48 to 72 hours after intubation.

HEALTHCARE-ASSOCIATED PNEUMONIA (HCAP): Pneumonia that occurs in a patient with substantial healthcare contact (intravenous antibiotics, chemotherapy, or wound care within the past 30 days; nursing home or long-term care facility resident; hospitalization for 2 or more days within the past 90 days; hemodialysis in the past 30 days).

CLINICAL APPROACH

Pneumonia is caused by aspiration or inhalation of pathogenic organisms into the lungs or, less commonly, by hematogenous spread. Thus patients with impaired host defenses (mucociliary clearance or overall immune system) and those with an increased risk of bacteremia or aspiration are at higher risk for developing pneumonia. These higher-risk patients include the elderly, smokers, those with an impaired gag reflex or alcoholism, and HIV-positive patients. Viral respiratory infections can also lead to the development of a superimposed bacterial pneumonia.

The most common causes of CAP are *Streptococcus pneumoniae*, *Mycoplasma pneumonia*, *Chlamydia pneumoniae*, and respiratory viruses. HAP and HCAP are most commonly due to gram-negative bacilli such as *Pseudomonas aeruginosa*, *Escherichia coli*, *Klebsiella pneumoniae*, and *Acinetobacter*. Aspiration pneumonias are often polymicrobial, including anaerobic organisms. Immunocompromised patients are at risk for infection with uncommon bacterial, fungal, and viral pathogens (eg, *Aspergillus*, cytomegalovirus, tuberculosis, and *Pneumocystis jirovecii*). Although the specific etiologic organism cannot be identified with certainty without serologic or microbiologic confirmation, historical information may help narrow the list of likely pathogens based on clinical symptomatology and risk factors for specific infections (Table 15–1).

The typical presentation of bacterial pneumonia includes fever, productive cough with purulent sputum, dyspnea, and pleuritic chest pain. However, patients at the extremes of age may have minimal or no respiratory symptoms. The **elderly may present with altered mental status or a decline in baseline function.**

The physical examination may reveal fever, tachypnea, tachycardia, or hypoxia. Severe illness may be heralded by severe respiratory distress, marked hypoxia, cyanosis, altered mental status, or hypotension. On auscultation, wheezes, rhonchi, rales, or bronchial breath sounds may be appreciated. Decreased breath sounds and dullness to percussion suggest the presence of a pleural effusion. Patients at the extremes of age and those who are immunosuppressed may have atypical examination findings. For example, the elderly are often afebrile (or even hypothermic). In these patients, tachypnea may be the most sensitive sign of pneumonia.

A demonstrable infiltrate on imaging is required for the diagnosis of pneumonia. In some cases, a patient with an initial negative chest radiograph may have infiltrates that "blossom" after rehydration or that are visualized using other types of imaging (eg, computed tomography is more sensitive than plain x-ray). The radiographic appearance of the infiltrates may suggest (but not definitively identify) a

Table 15–1 • SPECIFIC ORGANISMS, RISK FACTORS, AND CLASSIC PRESENTATIONS

Organism	Risk Factors	Classic Clinical Presentation
Chlamydia	Exposure to infected individuals	Mild subacute illness; fever, sore throat, nonproductive cough
Haemophilus influenzae	Diabetes, chronic obstructive pulmonary disease, malignancy, alcoholism, malnutrition, sickle cell disease, immunocompromise	Insidious worsening of chronic cough and sputum production (acute onset less common)
Klebsiella pneumoniae	Diabetes, alcoholism, chronic debilitating illness, aspiration risk	Acute onset of fever, rigors, chest pain, "currant jelly" sputum
Legionella	Smokers, transplant patients, immunocompromise, chronic lung disease	Severe illness with high fever, lethargy, cough. May have associated gastrointestinal symptoms (abdominal pain, vomiting, diarrhea), myocarditis, pancreatitis, pyelonephritis, sinusitis
Mycoplasma	Exposure to infected individuals	Subacute illness; sore throat, cough, headache, fever, malaise; may have associated bullous myringitis, rash, arthritis
Pseudomonas aeruginosa	Prolonged hospitalization, nursing home resident, high-dose steroids, structural lung disease	Severe pneumonia, cyanosis, confusion
Staphylococcus aureus	Intravenous drug abuse, recent influenza infection, chronic lung disease, immunocompromise, aspiration risk	Insidious onset of low-grade fever, dyspnea, sputum production
Streptococcus pneumoniae	Diabetes, sickle cell disease, splenectomy, malignancy, alcoholism, cardiovascular disease, immunocompromise, elderly, children <2 years	Abrupt onset of single shaking chill, pleuritic chest pain, bloody or rust-colored sputum

possible etiologic organism. For example, lobar consolidation is typical of *Streptococcus pneumoniae* or *Klebsiella*. *Staphylococcus aureus*, *Pseudomonas*, and *Haemophilus influenzae* typically cause multilobar disease. Patchy infiltrates are consistent with *Legionella*, *Mycoplasma*, and chlamydial infection. Aspiration pneumonias usually result in infiltrates in dependent areas of the lungs (posterior segment of upper lobe or superior segment of lower lobe). Cavitary lesions, pleural effusions, and pneumatoceles may also be seen with bacterial pneumonias. Immunocompromised patients are especially likely to have atypical radiographic findings (eg, more diffuse or multilobar infiltrates).

Treatment

The initial management of patients with pneumonia includes assessment of the ABCs (airway, breathing, and circulation) and, if needed, cardiopulmonary stabilization, which may require supplemental oxygen or intubation for patients with severe respiratory distress or respiratory failure.

Antibiotics should be initiated promptly in order to decrease mortality and improve patient outcome. Antibiotics are usually chosen based on the most likely pathogens as determined by assessment of risk factors, clinical presentation (including severity of symptoms and presence of sepsis), and radiographic findings. Healthy patients without any use of antimicrobials in the past 3 months with presumed CAP are best treated with a **macrolide (azithromycin)**. Patients with comorbid diseases, antimicrobial use in the past 3 months, or high risk of macrolide-resistant *Streptococcus pneumoniae* should receive a respiratory **fluoroquinolone (levofloxacin) or a beta-lactam (cefpodoxime) plus a macrolide** as a reasonable alternative. Patients whose conditions require admission to the ICU should receive antibiotics that cover a broader range of organisms. A beta-lactam (ceftazidime) plus either azithromycin or a fluoroquinolone may be used. If *Pseudomonas* or community-acquired methicillin-resistant *Staphylococcus aureus* (MRSA) infection is suspected, additional antimicrobial coverage (vancomycin) is required. If concerned for aspiration pneumonia, consider adding anaerobic coverage, such as clindamycin.

Patients with concern for HAP or HCAP are at a risk for multidrug-resistant pathogens and should receive a three-drug combination therapy: (1) antipseudomonal cephalosporin (cefepime or ceftazidime), antipseudomonal carbapenem (imipenem or meropenem), or piperacillin-tazobactam; (2) antipseudomonal fluoroquinolone (ciprofloxacin or levofloxacin); and (3) anti-MRSA coverage (linezolid or vancomycin).

Disposition

Factors to be considered include the patient's age and comorbidities, physical examination and diagnostic findings, ability to tolerate oral medications, social situation, and ability to obtain close follow-up. Two commonly used clinical prediction rules are **CURB-65 and the Pneumonia Severity Index (PSI)**. The CURB-65 severity score uses mental state, BUN, BP, and age, in which each parameter gets 1 point, and a score of 0-1 = outpatient management; 2 = careful outpatient supervision vs in-patient; 3-5 = inpatient management:

- Confusion
- BUN > 19 mg/dL
- Respiratory Rate > 30/min
- Systolic **BP** < 90 or diastolic BP < 60
- Age > **65**

The PSI uses similar parameters and also incorporates coexisting conditions, HR, and temperature.

Obviously, any patient with unstable vital signs, respiratory distress, hypoxia, severe infection, or intractable vomiting requires a hospital stay.

CASE CORRELATION

- See also Case 1 (Airway Management/Respiratory Failure), Case 13 (Asthma), and Case 14 (Pulmonary Embolism).

COMPREHENSION QUESTIONS

15.1 A 55-year-old man with a history of alcoholism complains of a month of subjective fevers and a productive cough with greenish sputum tinged with blood. Examination reveals poor dentition with halitosis, coarse breath sounds, and clubbing of his fingers. On chest x-ray, there is a 2-cm cavitary lesion with an air-fluid level in the right lower lobe. Which of the following is the most appropriate treatment?

A. Isolate the patient and initiate antituberculosis treatment

B. Admit and start intravenous clindamycin

D. Schedule an outpatient bronchoscopy

E. Discharge with oral amoxicillin-clavulanate

15.2 A 25-year-old woman with no past medical history presents with fever and productive cough. Her vital signs include temperature 38.8°C (101.9°F), heart rate 115 beats per minute, respirations 20 breaths per minute, blood pressure 115/89 mm Hg, and pulse oximetry 97% on room air. On examination, rhonchi are present in the right lung field. Chest x-ray shows a right middle lobe infiltrate. Which of the following should her treatment include?

A. Admission for intravenous ceftriaxone and vancomycin

B. Admission for intravenous ceftriaxone and azithromycin

C. Outpatient treatment with oral azithromycin

D. Outpatient treatment with oral amoxicillin

15.3 A 65-year-old smoker with past medical history of chronic obstructive pulmonary disease and diabetes presents with productive cough, chills, and pleuritic chest pain. His vital signs include a temperature of 38.9°C (102.1°F), heart rate of 110 beats per minute, blood pressure of 140/89 mm Hg, respiratory rate of 24 breaths per minute, and pulse oximetry of 92% on room air. On examination, he has a barrel chest with diffuse wheezes bilaterally. His chest x-ray reveals a left-lower-lobe infiltrate and pleural effusion. Which of the following is the best treatment?

A. Outpatient treatment with azithromycin

B. Outpatient treatment with levofloxacin

C. Inpatient treatment with ceftriaxone, azithromycin, and vancomycin

D. Inpatient treatment with ceftriaxone and azithromycin

15.4 An 89-year-old was brought by ambulance from a nursing home for fever and cough. His vital signs are as follows: temperature 39.9°C (103.9°F), heart rate 120 beats per minute, blood pressure 89/69 mm Hg, respiratory rate 36 breaths per minute, and pulse oximetry 88% on a nonrebreather face mask. He is clammy and lethargic. He has coarse breath sounds bilaterally although decreased on the left. Which of the following is the most appropriate initial intervention?

A. Administer intravenous antibiotics and IV fluids

B. Draw blood cultures

C. Intubation

D. Obtain a chest x-ray

ANSWERS

15.1 **B.** The history of alcoholism, presence of periodontal disease, duration of illness, and radiographic findings suggest aspiration pneumonia. The differential diagnosis for a cavitary lesion includes anaerobes, *Staphylococcus aureus*, *Klebsiella*, *Pseudomonas*, tuberculosis, and fungal infections. Clindamycin provides the appropriate antimicrobial coverage for a presumed anaerobic infection.

15.2 **C.** This is a healthy individual with CAP who can be treated as an outpatient with an oral macrolide. She has no risk factors for drug-resistant *Streptococcus pneumonia*.

15.3 **D.** This patient is a candidate for inpatient treatment due to his comorbidities and abnormal vital signs. However, he does not appear to require ICU admission based on his clinical picture. Thus, ceftriaxone and azithromycin are the best options of those listed.

15.4 **C.** Although these are all appropriate interventions, this patient has hypoxic respiratory failure requiring intubation. This patient will need a definite airway and ventilatory support, early antibiotics and IV fluid resuscitation, appropriate cardiovascular support, and ICU admission.

CLINICAL PEARLS

▶ Historical information may help narrow the list of likely pathogens based on clinical symptomatology and risk factors for specific infections.

▶ Patients at the extremes of age and those who are immunocompromised may present atypically (clinically as well as radiographically).

▶ The chest x-ray is the most important diagnostic study in patients with suspected pneumonia.

▶ Empiric antibiotics are chosen based on the most likely pathogens (as determined by assessment of risk factors, clinical presentation, and radiographic findings).

▶ Factors to be considered when determining need for admission include the patient's age and comorbidities, physical examination and diagnostic findings, ability to tolerate oral medications, social situation, and ability to obtain close follow-up.

REFERENCES

American Thoracic Society, Infectious Diseases Society of America. Guidelines for the management of adults with hospital-acquired, ventilator-associated, and healthcare-associated pneumonia. *Am J Respir Crit Care Med*. 2005;171:399-416.

File TM. Community-acquired pneumonia. *Lancet*. 2003;362:1991-2001.

Fine MJ, Auble TE, Yealy DM, et al. A prediction rule to identify low-risk patients with community-acquired pneumonia. *N Engl J Med*. 1997;336:243-250.

Mandell LA, Wunderink RG, Anzueto A, et al. Infectious Diseases Society of America/American Thoracic Society consensus guidelines on the management of community-acquired pneumonia in adults. *Clin Infect Dis*. 2007;44:S27-72.

Marx JA, Hockberger RS, Walls RM, eds. *Rosen's Emergency Medicine: Concepts and Clinical Practice*. 8th ed. Philadelphia, PA: Saunders; 2014.

Metlay JP, Kapoor WN, Fine MJ. Does this patient have community-acquired pneumonia? Diagnosing pneumonia by history and physical examination. *JAMA*. 1997;278:1440-1445.

You are working in the emergency department (ED) of a 15-bed rural hospital without CT scan capabilities, and a 25-year-old, previously healthy woman presents for evaluation of abdominal pain. The patient describes her pain as having been present for the past 3 days. The pain is described as constant, exacerbated by movements, and associated with subjective fevers and chills. She denies any recent changes in bowel habits, urinary symptoms, or menses. Her last menstrual period was 6 days ago. The physical examination reveals temperature of 38.4°C (101.1°F), pulse rate of 110 beats per minute, blood pressure of 112/70 mm Hg, and respiratory rate of 18 breaths per minute. Her skin is nonicteric. Cardiopulmonary examination is unremarkable. The abdomen is mildly distended and tender in both right and left lower quadrants. Involuntary guarding and localized rebound tenderness are noted in the right lower quadrant. The pelvic examination reveals no cervical discharge; cervical motion tenderness and right adnexal tenderness are present. The rectal examination reveals no masses or tenderness. Laboratory studies reveal white blood cell (WBC) count of 14,000 cells/mm^3, a normal hemoglobin, and a normal hematocrit. The urinalysis reveals 3-5 WBC/high-power field (HPF), few bacteria, and trace ketones.

▶ What are the most likely diagnoses?
▶ How can you confirm the diagnosis?

ANSWERS TO CASE 16:

Acute Abdominal Pain

Summary: A 25-year-old, previously healthy woman presents with a 3-day history of lower abdominal pain and subjective fever. Her examination indicates the presence of fever and lower abdominal tenderness (right > left). The rectal examination is unremarkable. Her laboratory studies indicate leukocytosis.

- **Most likely diagnoses:** Likely diagnoses include complicated acute appendicitis, pelvic inflammatory disease (PID), ovarian torsion, or other pelvic pathology.

- **Confirmatory studies:** Begin with pregnancy test and pelvic ultrasonography to evaluate for possible ovarian and pelvic pathology. If these suggest pelvic source of pathology, then strong consideration should be given to perform exploratory laparoscopy or laparotomy.

ANALYSIS

Objectives

1. Learn the relationships between symptoms, findings, and pathophysiology of the various types of disease processes capable of producing acute abdominal pain.

2. Learn to develop reasonable diagnostic and treatment strategies based on clinical diagnosis, resource availability, and patient characteristics.

3. Learn the diagnosis and severity stratification for acute pancreatitis (AP).

Considerations

This is a healthy young woman who presents with acute pain in the lower abdomen. Based on patient age and location of pain, acute appendicitis and gynecological pathology are the most likely sources of pathology, and additional history and diagnostic studies may help to differentiate these possibilities.

Pertinent gynecological history should include history of sexual contacts, menstrual pattern, previous gynecological problems, and the probability of pregnancy. A pregnancy test should be obtained early during the evaluation process to verify the presence or absence of pregnancy, and if the history and physical examination suggest the source of pathology to have originated from the pelvic organs, a pelvic ultrasound should be obtained.

In the event that the patient is pregnant, an ultrasound should be performed to verify intrauterine gestational sac and estimate the gestational age. If an intrauterine gestational sac is not visualized by ultrasound, the possibility of ectopic pregnancy should be considered, and an immediate referral should be made for a gynecologic evaluation and possible operative intervention. However, if the pregnancy test is negative and pelvic pathology is strongly suspected, the initial priority would be to identify potential life-threatening and fertility-reducing processes, including tubo-ovarian abscesses, PIDs, and ovarian torsion. **Pelvic ultrasonography** would be very valuable as the initial study to identify or rule out these processes. In the event that the pelvic ultrasound does not identify any pelvic pathology, a computed tomography (CT) scan of the abdomen and pelvis may be useful. The management approach for patient with abdominal pain varies depending on resource and expertise availability. For this patient at a 15-bed facility without CT capability, the general surgeon should be consulted early on regarding the potential need for transfer to another facility or further evaluation by laparoscopy or laparotomy.

APPROACH TO:
Acute Abdominal Pain

DEFINITIONS

ACUTE ABDOMEN: "Acute abdomen" describes the recent onset of abdominal pain. Patients with acute abdomen require urgent evaluation and not necessarily urgent operations.

FOREGUT: Foregut extends from oropharynx to mid-duodenum, including liver, biliary tract, pancreas, and spleen.

HINDGUT: Hindgut extends from distal transverse colon to rectum.

MIDGUT: Midgut extends from distal duodenum to mid-transverse colon.

REFERRED PAIN: This pain usually arises from a deep structure to a remote deep or superficial structure. The pattern of referred pain is based on the existence of shared central pathways between the afferent neurons of cutaneous dermatomes and intra-abdominal structures. Frequently, referred pain is associated with skin hyperalgesia and increased muscle tone. (Classic example of referred pain occurs with irritation of the left hemidiaphragm from ruptured spleen that causes referred pain to the left shoulder because of shared innervation by the same cervical nerves.)

SOMATIC PAIN: This pain arises from the irritation of the parietal peritoneum. This type of pain is mediated mainly by spinal nerve fibers supplying the abdominal wall and is perceived as sharp, constant, and generally localized to one of four quadrants. **Somatic pain may arise as a result of changes in pH and temperature (infection and inflammation) or pressure increase (surgical incision).**

VISCERAL PAIN: This pain is generally characterized as dull, cramping, deep, or aching. Normal embryological development of abdominal viscera results in symmetrical bilateral autonomic innervations leading to visceral pain being perceived in the midline location. Visceral stimulation can be produced by stretching and torsion, chemical stimulation, ischemia, or inflammation. Visceral pain from gastrointestinal (GI) tract structures correlate with pain location based on their embryonic origins. Foregut pain is perceived in the epigastrium, midgut pain is perceived in the periumbilical region, and hindgut pain is perceived in the hypogastrium.

CLINICAL APPROACH

Abdominal pain is a common chief complaint of patients seen in the ED, comprising approximately 5% to 8% of total visits. Overall, 18% to 25% of patients with abdominal pain evaluated in the ED have serious conditions requiring acute hospital care. In a recent series, the distribution of common diagnoses of adult ED patients with abdominal pain were listed as the following: 18% admitted, 25% undifferentiated abdominal pain (UDAP), 12% female pelvic, 12% urinary tract, and 9.3% surgical GI. **Approximately 10% of patients required urgent surgery, and most patients with UDAP were young women with epigastric symptoms who did not progress to develop significant medical problems.**

Understanding of disease pathophysiology, epidemiology, clinical presentation, and limitations of laboratory and imaging studies are important during evaluation of patients with abdominal pain in the ED. Abdominal pain can be initially categorized as "surgical" or "nonsurgical;" alternatively, pain may be approached from an organ-system approach. Overall, the surgical causes are encountered more commonly than nonsurgical causes when considering all patients presenting with acute abdominal pain.

Surgical causes (or causes that may require surgical corrections) may be categorized by mechanism into (1) **hemorrhagic,** (2) **infectious,** (3) **perforating,** (4) **obstructive,** (5) **ischemic,** and (6) **inflammatory.** Hemorrhagic conditions causing abdominal pain include traumatic injuries to solid and hollow viscera, ruptured ectopic pregnancy, tumor rupture/hemorrhage (eg, hepatic adenomas and hepatocellular carcinomas), and leaking or ruptured aneurysms. Infectious conditions may include appendicitis, cholecystitis, diverticulitis, infectious colitis, cholangitis, pyelonephritis, cystitis, primary peritonitis, and PID. Perforations causing abdominal pain can occur from peptic ulcers, diverticulitis, esophageal perforations, and traumatic hollow viscus injury. Obstructive processes leading to abdominal pain can occur from small intestinal obstruction, large bowel obstruction, ureteral obstruction, and biliary obstruction (see Figure 16–1 for radiograph). Ischemic causes are subcategorized as microvascular or macrovascular. Macrovascular ischemic events can occur from mechanical causes, including torsion (intestines and ovaries are most common) and vascular obstruction from thrombosis, embolism, and non-occlusive low-flow states. These can include small bowel and colonic ischemia. Microvascular ischemic events are uncommon and can occur from causes such as cocaine intoxication. Inflammatory conditions causing abdominal pain may include acute pancreatitis (AP) and Crohn disease; the mechanism of pain production associated with AP is not clearly known but is likely related to the local release of inflammatory mediators. Although not all patients with abdominal pain produced by the above listed conditions need surgical interventions, the potential for surgical or other forms of invasive interventions are high in these patients; therefore, early surgical consultation is advisable.

Nonsurgical causes of acute abdominal pain are less common and occur most frequently in patients with history of prior endocrine, metabolic, hematologic, infectious, or substance abuse history. The endocrine and metabolic causes of abdominal pain may include diabetic ketoacidosis, Addisonian crisis, and uremia. Hematologic causes of abdominal pain include sickle cell crisis and acute leukemia.

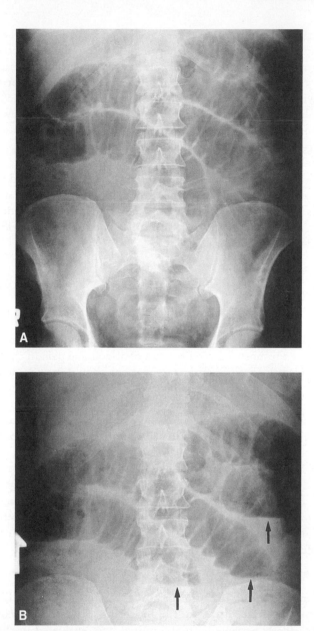

Figure 16–1. Abdominal radiographs in the supine (A) and upright (B) positions show a dilated small bowel with air-fluid levels. Source: Reproduced, with permission, from Zinner MJ, Schwarz SI, Ellis H, et al. *Maingot's Abdominal Operations*. 10th ed. New York, NY: McGraw-Hill Education; 1997:24.

Systemic infectious causes of abdominal pain can include acute meningitis, TB peritonitis, acute hepatitis, and varicella zoster infections. Because the differences between surgical and nonsurgical causes of abdominal pain are often subtle, it is advisable to consult a surgical colleague for all patients with acute abdominal pain. In addition, because of the potential for complications development in some of the patients with initially nonsurgical causes of abdominal pain, surgical consultations and follow-up are essential for the management of these complex patients.

Patient evaluations should be directed toward identifying potentially serious medical conditions. Analgesia, including narcotics, should not be withheld in patients with pain. In the event that a diagnosis is not identified following a thorough evaluation, it may be appropriate to discharge the patient with the diagnosis of "abdominal pain of uncertain etiology." Usually, **individuals still under the effect of analgesia without a diagnosis should not be discharged.** For patients whose abdominal pain etiologies are not clearly determined, it is important to provide them with the reassurance that the pain most likely will improve and resolve; however, because of the broad overlap in the early manifestation of serious disease, the patient needs to be instructed to seek early follow-up if symptoms do not resolve. Furthermore, the use of narcotic pain medications should be withheld in individuals without clear diagnosis or follow-up.

Abdominal Pain in Women

Women make up approximately 75% of all patients evaluated in the ED with abdominal pain. Women of childbearing age represent a complex patient population from the diagnostic standpoint because of a broader differential for pain. Acute appendicitis, biliary tract disease, urinary tract infection, and gynecological problems are the most common sources of abdominal pain in childbearing-age women. The history obtained from each patient should include details of menstrual history, sexual practices, gynecological and obstetrical history, and surgical history. For most individuals, the initial history and physical examination can help to direct the workup toward an organ system or body region. Laboratory evaluations, including CBC with differential, serum amylase, urinalysis, pregnancy test, and liver functions test, may provide additional information to help rule in or rule out certain diagnoses. When indicated, imaging such as ultrasonography and CT scans can be helpful in assessing for biliary tract and pelvic pathology and for acute appendicitis. **Because over-reliance on laboratory and/or imaging can contribute to misdiagnoses, laboratory and imaging results should always be interpreted within the proper clinical context; clinical judgment should be exercised regarding the acquisition of consultation and/or observation.**

Abdominal Pain in Elderly Patients

Elderly patients (age >65) account for approximately 15% of all ED visits, and about one-third of these visits result in inpatient admissions. In comparison to young adults, **elderly patients** with abdominal pain evaluated in the ED generally **have increased prevalence of serious diseases** causing abdominal pain, where the frequency of illnesses requiring surgical intervention has been estimated to be as high as 30%. Furthermore, the mortality rate associated with abdominal pain is increased in this population as a consequence of the increase in catastrophic illnesses (including mesenteric ischemia, leaking or ruptured aneurysm, and myocardial infarction). **Common diagnoses among elderly patients** include **biliary tract disease** (23%), **diverticular disease** (12%), **bowel obstruction** (11%), and undetermined (11%).

Due to various reasons that include atypical clinical presentations and difficulty with communications, **abdominal pain in the elderly is associated with high frequency of inaccurate diagnosis (up to 60%).** Inability to accurately diagnose the cause of abdominal pain contributes to delayed treatment and increased mortality, as elderly patients whose abdominal pain was not accurately diagnosed in the ED have been shown to have a twofold increase in mortality when compared to elderly patients whose causes of abdominal pain were accurately diagnosed.

For most elderly patients, the evaluation should be broadened to help identify cardiac, pulmonary, vascular, neoplastic, and neurologic causes of abdominal pain. Often symptoms in this population are attributable to an underlying medical comorbidity. It is important to bear in mind that medications taken by many elderly patients may contribute to abdominal problems as well as alter clinical presentations (eg, beta-blockers may blunt pulse rate response to stress). When indicated, ancillary testing should be applied to assist in establishing the diagnosis; however, it is important to remember that **the diagnostic accuracy of any test is dependent on the pretest probability, specificity, sensitivity, and disease prevalence of the test population.** Because abdominal pain in the elderly population is more frequently associated with serious pathology, appropriate consultations should be sought out and a liberal policy regarding inpatient or ED observation should be applied when causes cannot be clearly identified.

Patients with Acute Pancreatitis

Acute pancreatitis (AP) is an acute inflammatory condition of the pancreas that can affect adults of all ages, and in its severe forms, AP can affect all organ systems in the body. Patients are said to have severe AP when the process is associated with organ dysfunction, APACHE II scores ≥ 8, Ranson scores ≥ 3, or presence of local complications based on contrast-enhanced CT scans (eg, pancreas necrosis, pseudocysts, or peripancreatic fluid collections). Severe AP is reported in 15% to 20% of patients with AP. Mortality rates associated with mild AP are approximately 5%, whereas severe AP is associated with mortality rates up to 25%. The diagnosis of pancreatitis should be suspected when patients present with persistent abdominal or back pain associated with elevated levels of serum lipase and/or amylase. In the ED setting, the etiology of AP can be assessed by clinical history (these should include inquiries regarding gallstones, alcohol use, medications, infections, metabolic and autoimmune disorders, family history, and history of trauma) and laboratory studies that include liver function tests, calcium, and triglyceride levels. In approximately 80% of patients with AP, the cause can be determined based on the clinical history and initial clinical evaluation. Identifying cause of AP is generally not critical during the initial management of patients in the emergency center but could have implications in the prevention of future disease recurrences. Severity stratification for patients is helpful during the initial evaluation, as it may help direct the triage of patients to intensive care units or specialty care facilities.

Early management of patients is directed toward the **recognition and prevention of organ dysfunction in those patients with severe AP.** Prompt repletion of intravascular volume is essential in the prevention of renal dysfunction. When patients do not respond appropriately to their initial fluid management, central venous pressure monitoring, pulse oximetry monitoring, and urine output monitoring should be considered to help direct these efforts and avoid fluid overloading patients.

Disease recurrences are common among patients with AP, especially when the cause is alcohol, metabolically induced, or produced by anatomic abnormalities such as pancreas divisum and periampullary duodenal diverticulum. It is important to identify patients with AP that is gallstone-related because most recurrences in these patients can be prevented by cholecystectomies.

CT scan of the abdomen is not necessary for the diagnosis or confirmation of AP. CT scans in the emergency center setting may be indicated to help confirm the diagnosis of AP when the clinical picture and/or biochemical values are not sufficient for the confirmation of diagnosis. In addition, CT scan may help identify patients with significant pancreas necrosis, which often correlates with disease severity and regional pancreatic complications (Table 16–1). CT scan with intravenous contrast performed in patients with depleted intravascular volume and severe AP could contribute to acute kidney injuries and further injuries to the pancreas; therefore, these studies should be withheld until the patients' volume depletions have been corrected.

Patients with severe pancreatitis determined by the presence of end-organ dysfunction, APACHE II ≥8, Ranson score ≥3, or CT demonstrating pancreas necrosis may benefit from close monitoring and admissions to intensive care units. Over the past several years, there has been a continued trend toward the nonoperative or delayed-operative (>14 days) management of patients with severe AP. Critically ill patients with AP would still benefit from early consultation by a surgical specialist because other intra-abdominal processes that would require surgical interventions could mimic AP or develop as the result of severe AP.

Patients with Chronic or Recurrent Abdominal Pain

Patients with chronic or recurrent abdominal pain represent one of the most difficult diagnostic and management challenges for emergency medicine physicians.

Table 16–1 • CT SEVERITY INDEX (CTSI) FOR ACUTE PANCREATITIS	
CT Findings	Point
Pancreatic inflammation	
None	0
Focal diffuse enlargement of the pancreas	1
Pancreatic inflammation associated with inflammatory changes in the peripancreatic fat	2
Single, fluid collection, or phlegmon	3
Two or more fluid collections or presence of gas in the peripancreatic region	4
Pancreatic necrosis	
No necrosis	0
≤30% necrosis	2
30%-50% necrosis	4
>50% necrosis	6
Total score (Inflammation score + necrosis score)	0-10

Scores of 0-3 = mild acute pancreatitis; 4-6 = moderate acute pancreatitis; 7-10 = severe pancreatitis.

The dilemma facing ED physicians during encounters with these patients include establishing the accurate diagnosis, determining appropriate use of diagnostic studies, determining the appropriateness of analgesic medications, and follow-up.

Similar to the approach taken toward patients with acute abdominal pain, the **evaluation of chronic abdominal pain should begin with a thorough history.** Events and activities that trigger or alleviate the symptoms may be helpful in identifying the organ systems of pain origin. Furthermore, detailed description of the patterns and location of pain are helpful for categorization of pain as visceral pain, somatic pain, or referred pain; based on these determinations, organ system and anatomical sources of abdominal pain also may be delineated.

The physical examinations in these patients should be focused to help sort out the differential diagnosis formulated on the basis of history rather than a search for pathology. Unfortunately, the physical examination findings are sometimes difficult to interpret because of psychologic and personality changes, especially if the pain has been chronic, recurrent, and severe.

Unfortunately, no specific laboratory or imaging studies are completely sensitive or specific for the diagnosis of abdominal pain. As a general rule, diagnostic studies should be selected only if results of the studies will lead to specific additional evaluations or treatment. The CBC might be helpful in identifying leukocytosis, which may indicate an inflammatory or infectious condition, and the presence of anemia might help to verify the presence of ischemic colitis, GI tract malignancy, or inflammatory bowel disease. Abnormalities within the liver function panel may help identify choledocholithiasis, stenosing papillitis, and periampullary malignancy. Serum amylase elevation is generally seen in the setting of chronic or acute pancreatitis. Elevation in erythrocyte sedimentation rate may suggest the presence of autoimmune processes or collagen vascular disorders.

Frequently, even after the completion of extensive, appropriate evaluations, the patient's condition may remain unrecognized. If possible, the results of the evaluation and diagnostic studies should be discussed with the patient's primary care physician so that the patient may be provided with additional testing and follow-up. For those patients without primary care physicians, evaluation and consultation by an appropriate primary care physician or specialist should be obtained prior to discharge from the ED.

CASE CORRELATION

- See also Case 17 (GI Bleeding), Case 19 (Intestinal Obstruction), Case 20 (Acute Diarrhea), and Case 21 (Nephrolithiasis).

COMPREHENSION QUESTIONS

16.1 A 30-year-old woman presents with epigastric pain that developed following dinner. The patient describes having similar pain prior to the current
episode, but previous episodes were less severe. The patient was diagnosed
as having gastroesophageal reflux disease by her primary care physician and
prescribed a proton pump inhibitor, which has been ineffective in resolving
her pain. The current pain episode has been severe and persistent for 3 hours.
The patient has a temperature of 38°C (100.4°F), heart rate of 100 beats per
minute, respiratory rate of 20 breaths per minute, and blood pressure of
130/90 mm Hg. The abdominal examination reveals no abdominal tenderness.
The administration of 30 mL of antacids and 4 mg of morphine sulfate resulted
in some relief of pain. Which of the following is the most appropriate next step?

A. Obtain CBC, amylase, liver function tests, and ultrasound of the gallbladder. Discuss with surgical consultants regarding admission to the hospital.

B. Follow-up with her primary care physician in 2 weeks.

C. Admit the patient to the hospital for upper GI endoscopy.

D. Prescribe antacids and discharge the patient from the ED, with follow-
up by her primary care physician.

E. Obtain an ultrasound of the gallbladder, prescribe oral antibiotics, analgesics, and arrange for an outpatient follow-up with her primary care
physician.

16.2 Which of the following features best characterizes somatic pain?

A. Midline location

B. Sharp, persistent, and well-localized pain in the left lower quadrant

C. Intermittent pain

D. Pain improved with body movement

E. Poorly localized

16.3 For which of the following patients is CT of the abdomen contraindicated?

A. A 60-year-old man with persistent left lower quadrant pain, fever, and a
tender mass

B. A 45-year-old alcoholic man with diffuse abdominal pain, WBC
18,000 cells/mm^3, and serum amylase of 2000

C. A nonpregnant 18-year-old woman with suprapubic and right
lower quadrant pain, fever, right lower quadrant mass, and WBC of
15,000 cells/mm^3

D. A 70-year-old man with abdominal pain and distention, a 10-cm pulsatile mass in the epigastrium, and blood pressure of 70/50 mm Hg

E. A 24-year-old man with a new finding of painful, irreducible umbilical
hernia who presents with 12-hour history of abdominal distention and
vomiting

ANSWERS

16.1 **A.** This patient has recurrent epigastric pain that was formerly attributed to gastroesophageal reflux disease. However, the fact that her symptoms have been poorly controlled with proton pump inhibitors in the past suggests that the diagnosis is probably inaccurate. Her recurrent symptoms are likely caused by biliary tract disease, and her current presentation is highly suspicious for complicated biliary tract disease, such as acute cholecystitis. Choice A represents testing for the evaluation of biliary tract disease, which is appropriate in this setting. Because of her fever, the outpatient management approach described in choice E is inappropriate.

16.2 **B.** Somatic pain is generally associated with irritation of the parietal peritoneum, resulting in localized, persistent, and sharp pain. This type of pain is aggravated by movement and can produce spasm in the overlying abdominal wall musculature, which is manifested as involuntary guarding.

16.3 **D.** The patient in "D" is hemodynamically unstable and possesses signs and symptoms suggestive of ruptured abdominal aneurysm. A CT scan would likely delay his care and is contraindicated in this situation. The patient described in choice A likely has diverticulitis, where CT may be appropriate for severity staging. The patient described in choice B likely has AP, where CT is helpful for the stratification of disease severity. The patient described in choice C may have complicated appendicitis or some other complicated GI or gynecological process, where CT can be useful for differentiation. The patient described in choice E has an incarcerated umbilical hernia with signs and symptoms of intestinal obstruction related to this finding. Surgical intervention is indicated based on his presentation alone.

CLINICAL PEARLS

▶ Most patients with the diagnosis of "undifferentiated abdominal pain" determined after thorough ED evaluation will have spontaneous resolution of pain.

▶ Abdominal pain can be initially categorized as "surgical" or "nonsurgical;" alternatively, pain may be approached from an organ-system approach.

▶ Elderly patients with acute AP are more likely to have pathology. Common diagnoses include biliary tract disease, diverticular disease, and bowel obstruction.

▶ Narcotic medications will affect the characteristics and intensity of all abdominal pain, regardless of etiology.

▶ Up to one-third of elderly patients with abdominal pain evaluated in the ED have conditions that may require surgical intervention.

REFERENCES

Delrue LJ, De Waele JJ, Duyck PO. Acute pancreatitis: radiologic scores in predicting severity and outcome. *Abdom Imaging.* 2009;35:349-361.

Gravante G, Garcea G, Ong SL, et al. Prediction of mortality in acute pancreatitis: a systematic review of the published evidence. *Pancreatology.* 2009;9:601-614.

McNamara R, Dean AJ. Approach to acute abdominal pain. *Emerg Med Clin N Am.* 2011;29:159-173.

Pezzilli R, Zerbi A, Di Carlo V, et al. Practice guidelines for acute pancreatitis. *Pancreatology.* 2010;10:523-535.

Privette Jr TW, Carlisle MC, Palma JK. Emergencies of the liver, gallbladder, and pancreas. *Emerg Med Clin N Am.* 2011;29:293-317.

Spangler R, Pham TV, Khoujah D, Martinez JP. Abdominal emergencies in the geriatric patient. *Int J Emerg Med.* 2014;7:43-51.

A 43-year-old man is brought in on an EMS (emergency medical services) stretcher after a syncopal episode. After obtaining a palpated pressure of 80 mm Hg systolic and heart rate of 120 beats per minute, EMS placed an 18-gauge IV and initiated normal saline (NS) infusion en route to the hospital. The patient relates a history of a 3 to 4 days of dark, tarry stools (about 3-4 times per day). Today he passed out when rising from a seated position. He is currently complaining of mild epigastric pain and lightheadedness. He denies any hematemesis, hematochezia, chest pain, shortness of breath, and any similar past episodes. He admits to tobacco use and drinking 1-2 beers each day and is not regularly under the care of a physician.

On examination, his vital signs are temperature 36.6°C (97.9°F), blood pressure 92/45 mm Hg (after 900-mL IV fluid prior to arrival), heart rate 113 beats per minute, and respiratory rate 24 breaths per minute. The patient is pale with dried, dark stool on the perineum. He has mild tenderness to palpation in the epigastrium but no rebound or guarding. He does not have spider angioma, gynecomastia, palmar erythema, or ascites. The rectal examination reveals grossly melenic stool.

▶ What is the most likely diagnosis?
▶ What is the best therapy?

ANSWERS TO CASE 17:

Gastrointestinal Bleeding

Summary: This 43-year-old man presents tachycardic and hypotensive after several episodes of melena.

- **Most likely diagnosis:** Upper gastrointestinal (GI) bleed with hemorrhagic shock.

- **Best therapy:** Stabilization of the ABCs (airway, breathing, and circulation), including IV access and volume resuscitation. Consider the use of blood products and proton pump inhibitors. Endoscopy is indicated for early diagnosis and treatment.

ANALYSIS

Objectives

1. Learn the differences in presentations and outcomes between upper and lower GI bleeding.

2. Understand the priorities, evaluations, and management of patients with GI hemorrhage.

Considerations

Based on his heart rate and hypotension at rest, this 43-year-old man is in class III hemorrhagic shock (see Case 2). These findings correlate with up to 1500-2000 mL of acute blood loss. Prior to establishing the source of the hemorrhage, the most important priority is to stabilize the patient by addressing the ABCs, including placing two large-bore intravenous lines, giving boluses of NS, and monitoring the blood pressure, heart rate, pulse oximetry, and urine output. Laboratory evaluations should include complete blood count (CBC), electrolytes, renal and liver function tests, and coagulation studies, in addition to the typing and cross matching of blood. The initial priorities are to determine whether there has been significant blood loss, maintain hemodynamic stability, and determine if the bleeding is active.

After stabilization, a focused history should be taken to determine the probable etiology of the gastrointestinal bleeding. Chronic non-steroidal anti-inflammatory drug (NSAID) or aspirin use may indicate gastritis. His history and physical examination do not reveal obvious causes or signs of portal hypertension. Although the history of tar-colored stools suggests an upper GI bleeding source and directs the initial evaluation to this source, the possibility of bleeding distal to the ligament of Treitz (lower GI bleeding) cannot be excluded at this time. An initial room-temperature water lavage via a nasogastric (NG) tube may identify gross blood or "coffee-ground" fluid, which may help to establish the diagnosis of upper GI bleeding, determine if the bleeding is active, and determine the rate of hemorrhage, though this is not required for the diagnosis of an upper GI bleed. **Upper endoscopy**

is likely to be the most valuable diagnostic and treatment modality of choice for this patient. Differentiation of GI bleeding patients as possessing potential **upper GI bleeding sources versus lower GI bleeding sources** is important early on, as patients with **upper GI bleeding have significantly greater potential for rapid and large volume** hemorrhage in comparison to those with lower GI bleeding sources. Similarly, the differentiation of patients with **upper GI bleeding into those with variceal bleeding and those with non-variceal bleeding is helpful to begin empirical pharmacologic therapy with octreotide in those patients with suspected bleeding from a variceal source.**

APPROACH TO:
GI Bleeding

CLINICAL APPROACH

GI bleeding is classified as upper or lower based on whether it arises proximal or distal to the ligament of Treitz, the junction between the duodenum and the remainder of the small bowel. Common causes of upper GI bleeding include peptic ulcer disease, esophageal or gastric varices, Mallory-Weiss tear, esophagitis, and gastritis (Figure 17–1). The most common etiologies of **lower GI bleeding are upper GI bleeding, hemorrhoids, diverticulosis, angiodysplasia, malignancy, inflammatory bowel disease, and infectious conditions** (Figure 17–2). In children,

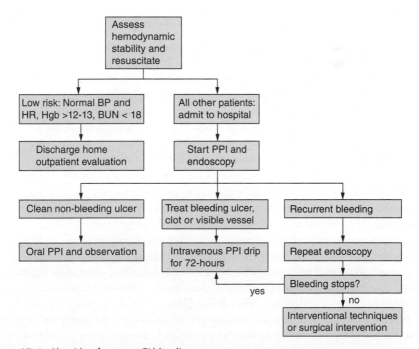

Figure 17–1. Algorithm for upper GI bleeding.

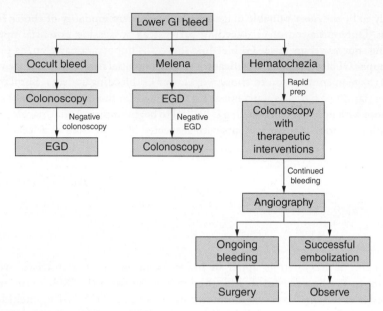

Figure 17–2. Algorithm for lower GI bleeding.

Meckel diverticulum, polyps, volvulus, and intussusception are the common causes of GI bleeding.

GI bleeding is also classified as either overt or occult. Overt bleeding is clinically obvious bleeding that presents as hematemesis, coffee-ground emesis, melena, or hematochezia, and occult GI bleeding is when a patient presents with either clinical anemia and/or microcytic anemia from chronic GI tract blood loss. From the standpoint of emergency medical care, overt GI bleeding needs to be addressed on an urgent basis to resuscitate and control the bleeding source, whereas occult GI bleeding may require treatment of symptomatic anemia and referral to a gastroenterology and/or surgical specialist to identify and treat the chronic bleeding source.

When taking a history, the clinician should focus on the nature, duration, and amount of bleeding. Classically, patients with an upper GI bleed present with hematemesis and melena, while hematochezia suggests a lower GI source. However, this is not always the case, depending on the speed and amount of bleeding. It is important to ask about syncope, weakness, chest pain, dyspnea, and confusion because these symptoms suggest significant blood loss. In addition, risk factor assessment may help determine the cause of the bleeding (Table 17–1).

Signs for evidence of hypovolemic shock (tachypnea, tachycardia, and hypotension) should be sought. Cool, pale, or diaphoretic skin suggests hypovolemia, and pale conjunctiva, nail beds, or mucous membranes suggest anemia. If stigmata of chronic liver disease (jaundice, caput medusae, spider angiomata, palmar erythema, and gynecomastia) are present, variceal bleeding should be considered as a potential bleeding possibility. The abdominal examination should focus on searching for peritoneal signs such as guarding and rebound, though most patients with GI bleeding do not exhibit abdominal pain.

Table 17–1 • GI BLEEDING SOURCES AND CLINICAL FEATURES/RISK FACTORS	
Etiology	Risk Factors
Esophageal and/or gastric varices	Alcoholism, cirrhosis
Peptic ulcer disease	*Helicobacter pylori* infection, NSAID use, alcohol use, tobacco use, heredity
Gastritis	NSAID use, alcohol use, steroids, burns, major trauma, head injury
Mallory-Weiss tear	Recent vomiting or retching, alcohol use, esophagitis
Aortoenteric fistula	History of prior abdominal aortic reconstruction
Diverticulosis	High-fat diet, older age
Colon cancer	Weight loss, change in bowel habits
Angiodysplasia	Older age, cardiovascular comorbidities

Bedside testing includes a rectal examination to check for hemorrhoids, anal fissures, and occult blood in the stool. Historically, it has been recommended that all patients have a nasogastric tube with room temperature NS or water lavage. If blood is present (bright red or "coffee ground"), an upper GI source is more likely. This is now considered an optional maneuver in the evaluation of GI bleeding. One advantage of NGT placement is the ability to rapidly prepare the colon for endoscopy.

After IV access is obtained, blood should be sent for CBC, electrolytes, blood urea nitrogen (BUN)/creatinine, coagulation studies, and type and screen or cross-match. In patients with chest pain, dysrhythmia, or risk factors for coronary artery disease, an electrocardiogram (ECG) should be obtained.

Treatment

Treatment begins with stabilizing the ABCs. Intubation may be necessary to protect the patient's airway and to prevent aspiration. **IV access (large-bore peripherals or central) is a high priority.** Volume resuscitation should begin with crystalloid solution using vital signs and urine output to guide the volume infused. For patients who are hemodynamically unstable after crystalloid infusion, have ongoing blood loss, or whose hemoglobin is less than 7 g/dL, transfusion of packed red blood cells (PRBCs) should be considered. A recent randomized controlled clinical trial comparing liberal versus restrictive transfusion thresholds found better clinical outcomes with a restrictive transfusion threshold of 7 g/dL hemoglobin, instead of a targeted hemoglobin of 9 g/dL. Prior to this trial, patients with GI bleeding were typically transfused to a hemoglobin level of 10 mg/dL in order to provide a buffer in the setting of ongoing bleeding. This liberal transfusion strategy was shown to be ineffective at improving outcomes in this study. **Reversal of anticoagulation agents** may be indicated in patients with coagulopathies caused by anticoagulation therapy. As a general rule, **a proton pump inhibitor should be given to patients with upper GI bleeding to decrease rebleeding rates.** Surgery is indicated for massive or refractory bleeding.

In patients with variceal bleeding, a somatostatin analog such as octreotide or vasopressin can be helpful. However, vasopressin has fallen out of favor because of the side effects and the risk of end-organ ischemia. Prophylactic antibiotics directed at bowel flora should be given to cirrhotic patients to decrease infection rates.

In patients with massive variceal bleeding, balloon tamponade with a **Sengstaken-Blakemore tube may be useful for the temporary control of bleeding while arrangements for definitive therapy are made.**

Various modalities exist to identify the source of bleeding. In upper GI bleeding patients, endoscopy is the study of choice because the procedure can also be therapeutic through use of lasers, electrocoagulation, sclerosant injections, clip placements, and band ligations. For lower GI bleeds, anoscopy, sigmoidoscopy, or colonoscopy are preferred for the localization of bleeding sources. Tagged red blood cell (RBC) scans are an alternative in stable patients. When lower GI bleeding is massive or continuous, angiography can be useful to localize the bleeding, and for some cases angiography-directed embolization can be applied to stop the bleeding.

In general, patients with lower GI bleeding rarely exhibit hemodynamic instability unless the process has gone on unrecognized for some time. Most lower GI bleeding episodes are self-limited. The treatments for lower GI bleeding are therefore less urgent than treatments for upper GI bleeding, and the majority of patients with lower GI bleeding can be managed outside of an ICU environment following their management in the emergency department. The number one priority following the initial management of lower GI bleeding patients is localization of the bleeding site so that endoscopic therapy, interventional radiology techniques, or surgical therapy can be implemented in the unusual event that the bleeding does not stop.

CASE CORRELATION

- See also Case 2 (Hemorrhagic Shock), Case 16 (Acute Abdominal Pain), Case 18 (Swallowed Foreign Body), and Case 19 (Intestinal Obstruction).

COMPREHENSION QUESTIONS

17.1 Which of the following conditions is the strongest risk factor for peptic ulcer disease?

A. Age greater than 50 years

B. Estrogen replacement therapy

C. Acetaminophen use

D. *Chlamydia trachomatis*

E. *Helicobacter pylori* infection

17.2 A 43-year-old man complains of an acute onset of vomiting bright red blood. He denies alcohol use and history of peptic ulcer disease. He complains of dizziness, appears anxious, and his blood pressure is 120/70 mm Hg and heart rate is 90 beats per minute. Which of the following is the best next step in managing his condition?

    A. Morphine sulfate

    B. Endoscopic examination

    C. Chest radiograph

    D. Intravenous fluid resuscitation

    E. Orotracheal intubation

17.3 In the patient described in Question 17.2, which of the following modalities is best to identify the source of bleeding?

    A. Tagged RBC scan

    B. Endoscopy

    C. Angiography

    D. Laparotomy

    E. Serial hemoglobin determination

17.4 A 58-year-old woman is brought into the ED complaining of bright red bleeding per rectum that was of acute onset. She denies abdominal pain. She is hemodynamically stable. Which of the following is the most likely etiology of her condition?

    A. Varices

    B. Gastritis

    C. Diverticulosis

    D. Mallory-Weiss tear

    E. Peptic ulcer disease

ANSWERS

17.1 **E.** Risk factors for peptic ulcer disease include *H. pylori* infection, NSAID use, alcohol use, heredity, and tobacco use.

17.2 **D.** Stabilization of the patient is always the first priority. The ABCs come first; assuming that his airway and breathing are stable, then circulation is next. Fluid administration very likely will be helpful, as the patient's dizziness and anxiety are signs of hypovolemic shock.

17.3 **B.** Endoscopy is the preferred modality to identify the source of bleeding in upper GI bleeding. Tagged red cell studies are more commonly used for the evaluation of lower GI bleeding.

17.4 **C.** This patient's clinical presentation is suggestive of lower GI bleeding. Common causes of lower GI bleeding are diverticulosis, upper GI bleeding, hemorrhoids, angiodysplasia, malignancy, inflammatory bowel disease, and infectious conditions. Bleeding with diverticulosis is described as painless and abrupt, "as though a water faucet was suddenly turned on." The other choices are common causes of upper GI bleeding.

CLINICAL PEARLS

▶ Although most GI bleeds resolve spontaneously, each case is potentially life threatening. The main priorities are to determine whether there has been significant blood loss and to maintain ABCs, including hemodynamic stability.

▶ In upper GI bleeds, endoscopy is the study of choice because it can also be therapeutic.

▶ Anoscopy, sigmoidoscopy, or colonoscopy is preferred in lower GI bleeds.

▶ In general, all patients with GI bleeding are admitted. If they are hemodynamically unstable or actively bleeding, they should be admitted to an ICU setting.

REFERENCES

Hwang JH, Shergill AK, Acosta RD, et al. Role of endoscopy in the management of variceal hemorrhage. *Gastrointest Endosc*, 2014;80(2):221-227.

Laine L, Jensen DM. Management of patients with ulcer bleeding. *Am J Gastroenterol*. 2012;107: 345-360.

ASGE Standards of Practice Committee, Pasha SF, Shergill A, et al. Role of endoscopy in the patient with lower GI bleeding. *Gastrointest Endosc*. 2014;79(6):875-885.

Villanueva C, Colomo A, Bosch A, et al. Transfusion strategies for acute upper gastrointestinal bleeding. *NEJM*. 2013;368(1):11-21.

A 2-year-old boy is brought to the emergency department (ED) because of an episode of "choking." The patient was playing with marbles when his mother left the room for a few minutes. She ran back in when she heard the patient gagging and coughing. She denies any recent fever, cough, or other upper respiratory infectious symptoms. When asked, she denies her son turning blue, having difficulty breathing or vomiting. The patient was a term baby without any significant past medical history. He is not taking any medications, and his immunizations are all up-to-date. He attends day care and has no recent sick contacts.

On examination, his temperature is 37.7°C (99.9°F), blood pressure is 93/55 mm Hg, heart rate is 105 beats per minute, respiratory rate is 24 breaths per minute, and the O$_2$ saturation is 98% on room air. The patient is playful and alert. His examination Is unremarkable except for intermittent gagging. He has no intercostal retractions or accessory muscle use.

▶ What are the potential complications in this patient?
▶ What is the most appropriate next step?

ANSWERS TO CASE 18:

Swallowed Foreign Body

Summary: This is a 2-year-old boy with probable ingestion of a foreign body (marble).

- **Potential complications:** Esophageal stricture, perforation, mediastinitis or peritonitis, paraesophageal abscess, vocal cord paralysis, and aortotracheo-esophageal fistula.

- **Most appropriate next step:** Because the child is stable, x-ray to localize the foreign body.

ANALYSIS

Objectives

1. Recognize the clinical scenario, signs, and symptoms of swallowed foreign bodies.

2. Learn the diagnostic and therapeutic approach to the various types of swallowed foreign bodies.

Considerations

Patients with swallowed foreign bodies may be asymptomatic or may present in extremis. Although most objects will pass through the gastrointestinal (GI) tract without problems, it is important to recognize which patients require observation and which will need intervention (Table 18–1).

APPROACH TO:

Swallowed Foreign Body

CLINICAL APPROACH

Although **children 18-48 months account for nearly 80% of cases,** edentulous adults, psychiatric patients, and prisoners also commonly swallow foreign objects. Children most commonly ingest things they can pick up and place in their mouths, such as coins, buttons, toys, and crayons. **Adults are more likely to have trouble swallowing meat and bones.** Although objects can be located anywhere throughout the alimentary tract, there are several areas where they lodge more frequently. In the pediatric patient, most obstructions occur in the proximal esophagus at one of five areas: the cricopharyngeal narrowing (most common), thoracic inlet, aortic arch, tracheal bifurcation, and hiatal narrowing. In contrast, most adult patients have distal esophageal obstructions caused by a structural or motor abnormality (eg, stricture, malignancy, scleroderma, and achalasia).

Table 18–1 • SPECIAL TYPES OF SWALLOWED FOREIGN BODIES		
Foreign Body	Comments	Treatment
Food impaction	Avoid proteolytic enzymes because of risk of esophageal perforation. Avoid gas-forming agents if perforation suspected. Barium swallow after treatment to confirm clearance of the impaction and to rule out esophageal pathology.	Expectant management if handling secretions and impacted <12 hours. Otherwise, endoscopy preferred. Alternatives: Intravenous glucagon, sublingual nifedipine, sublingual nitroglycerin, oral gas-forming agents.
Coin	Often asymptomatic. X-ray to confirm location (esophageal coins lie with flat side showing on anteroposterior x-ray).	Endoscopy preferred if at the level of the cricopharyngeus muscle. Alternative: Foley catheter removal under fluoroscopy if lodged <24 hours, bougienage (pushing object into stomach). Expectant management may be considered if impacted <24 hours.
Button battery	High risk of mucosal burns and esophageal perforation if lodged in esophagus. X-ray to confirm location.	Surgical consult for endoscopy if in esophagus and has not passed through the pylorus or patient symptomatic. Expectant management if past the esophagus and no symptoms. Repeat radiographs until battery cleared.
Sharp or pointed objects	X-ray to confirm location.	If foreign body proximal to or in duodenum, endoscopic removal recommended given risk of intestinal perforation. If symptomatic, impacted, or foreign body past duodenum, surgical consult for endoscopy or laparotomy. Otherwise, expectant management with serial radiographs.
Body packing	Ingestion of packets of drugs (most commonly cocaine or heroin). Rupture of packet may be fatal (especially with cocaine). May cause symptoms because of drug effect or GI obstruction. Avoid endoscopy because of risk of rupture.	If packet intact, may observe and use whole bowel irrigation with polyethylene glycol to hasten passage of packets through GI tract. Otherwise, surgery to remove packets.

Source: Data from Tintinalli J, Judith E, Stapczynski J S. Tintinalli's Emergency Medicine: A Comprehensive Study Guide. New York, NY: McGraw-Hill; 2011.

Most adult patients will be able to relate a history of ingesting a foreign object or of feeling food becoming lodged. They may complain of anxiety, foreign body sensation, chest or epigastric pain, retching, vomiting, wheezing, stridor, or difficulty swallowing. In children, the history may be less clear. Parents may have seen the child with an object in his or her mouth and suspect ingestion. Children can present with vomiting, gagging, choking, refusal to eat, or neck or chest pain. Increased salivation, drooling, or an inability to swallow suggests a complete obstruction.

Table 18–2 • SWALLOWED VS ASPIRATED FOREIGN BODIES		
	Swallowed Foreign Body	**Aspirated Foreign Body**
Most Common Objects	Children: Coins, toys, crayons Adults: Meat, bones	Children: Grapes, nuts, hot dogs, candy Adults: Nonfood items more common than in children
Most Common Location	Children: Cricopharyngeal narrowing Adults: Distal esophagus	Children: Bronchial tree Adults: Proximal airway
Clinical Presentation	Anxiety, pain (neck, retrosternal, and epigastric), foreign body sensation, choking, vomiting, dysphagia, inability to swallow, and drooling Air hunger and dyspnea generally less common	Choking, coughing, hoarse voice, dyspnea, stridor, wheezing, respiratory distress (retractions, accessory muscle use, hypoxia, and cyanosis). May present in delayed fashion with infectious complications (eg, recurrent pneumonia)
Treatment	Depends on symptomatology, location, type of foreign body May include expectant management or removal of foreign body	Removal of foreign body

Patients with airway foreign bodies tend to present with more respiratory symptoms (Table 18–2).

The physical examination should focus on identifying patients with **airway compromise, inability to tolerate fluids, or active bleeding.** It should include a careful evaluation of the oropharynx, neck, chest, and abdomen. Findings such as fever, subcutaneous air, or peritoneal signs suggest perforation. In patients with a suspected oropharyngeal foreign body, direct or indirect laryngoscopy can be useful. Plain x-rays may help locate radiopaque foreign bodies throughout the GI tract and be used to follow their progression (if repeated every 2-4 hours). Many foreign bodies are not radiopaque, including chicken and fish bones.

If plain films do not reveal the object, an esophagogram, computed tomography (CT), or endoscopy are other options. **If perforation is suspected, the esophagogram should be performed with a water-soluble contrast agent.** If aspiration is a concern, barium is the preferred contrast agent; however, barium can obscure the visual field if endoscopy is subsequently performed. CT can be useful to identify the location and orientation of swallowed foreign bodies as well as the presence of any complications, such as perforations or fistulae. Endoscopy is usually the study of choice because the object may be removed once it is visualized.

Eighty to ninety percent of patients with normal GI anatomy will pass swallowed foreign bodies without complications. Thus most patients are treated expectantly at first. If symptomatic, in-hospital observation should be considered for serial examinations. **In general, once a foreign object passes the pylorus, it will continue through the GI tract without incident.** However, if it cannot pass the esophagus or pylorus, it must be removed, with endoscopy usually being the method of choice. Surgery may be necessary if there is evidence of obstruction or perforation, if the object is too big to pass safely, or if the object contains toxins.

There are several special considerations when dealing with certain types of swallowed foreign bodies, such as esophageal button batteries, which generally need to be removed because of their toxic effects on mucosa (see Table 18–1).

> ## CASE CORRELATION
>
> - See also Case 16 (Acute Abdominal Pain) and Case 19 (Intestinal Obstruction).

COMPREHENSION QUESTIONS

18.1 Which of the following gastric foreign bodies requires emergent removal in an asymptomatic patient?

    A. Button battery

    B. Capsule full of heroin

    C. Condom full of cocaine

    D. Needle less than 6 cm in length

18.2 A 21-year-old woman accidentally swallowed a penny. At which of the following locations is the coin most likely to be lodged?

    A. Aortic arch

    B. Cricopharyngeal narrowing

    C. Lower esophageal sphincter

    D. Thoracic inlet

18.3 A 3-year-old girl accidentally swallowed a button battery from her mother's camera. She does not appear to be in respiratory distress. She has normal vital signs and is afebrile. Plain x-ray shows the battery in the esophagus. Which of the following is the best management for this patient?

    A. Avoidance of citrus drinks

    B. Avoidance of magnets

    C. Endoscopy

    D. Expectant management

18.4 An 8-year-old girl presents to the ED having swallowed a coin. The abdominal radiograph reveals that the coin is in the stomach. Thirty-six hours later, it is still in the stomach. Which of the following is the best next step?

    A. Endoscopy

    B. Laparotomy

    C. Lithotripsy

    D. Observation

    E. Rigid bronchoscopy

ANSWERS

18.1 **D.** Sharp objects in the stomach and duodenum warrant emergent endoscopic or surgical retrieval. Once the object makes it past those areas, expectant management can be taken with follow-up imaging within 48 hours.

18.2 **C.** In adults, a swallowed object will most commonly lodge in the esophagus at the lower esophageal sphincter. In children, the most common location is the proximal esophagus at the cricopharyngeal narrowing.

18.3 **C.** Immediate endoscopy is required. Button battery ingestion is a true emergency if lodged in the esophagus, with the potential for mucosal burns within 4 hours and esophageal perforation within 6 hours of ingestion. A button battery in the esophagus must be removed as soon as possible.

18.4 **A.** In general, if the foreign body has not moved past the pylorus after 24 hours, it should be removed. The preferred method of swallowed foreign body removal is endoscopy (except in body packers due to the risk of packet rupture).

CLINICAL PEARLS

▶ Children account for the vast majority of cases of swallowed foreign bodies.

▶ In the pediatric patient, objects most commonly lodge in the proximal esophagus, whereas most adult patients have distal esophageal obstructions.

▶ Findings such as fever, subcutaneous air, or peritoneal signs suggest perforation and necessitate an emergent surgical consult.

▶ Button batteries in the esophagus as well as sharp, pointed objects in the stomach must be removed as soon as possible. In general, the preferred method of swallowed foreign body removal is endoscopy (except in body packers because of the risk of packet rupture).

REFERENCES

Aghababian R. *Essentials of Emergency Medicine*. 2nd ed. Sudbury, Mass: Jones and Bartlett Publishers; 2011.

Anderson KL, Dean AJ. Foreign Bodies in the gastrointestinal tract and anorectal emergencies. *Emerg Med Clin N Am*. 2011;29(2):369-400.

Harrigan R, Ufberg JW, Tripp ML. *Emergency Medicine Review: Preparing for the Boards*. St. Louis, MO: Saunders/Elsevier; 2010.

Marx JA, Hockberger RS, Walls RM, eds. *Rosen's Emergency Medicine: Concepts and Clinical Practice*. 8th ed. Philadelphia, PA: Saunders; 2014.

Tintinalli JE, Stapczynski JS, Ma OJ, et al., eds. *Emergency Medicine: A Comprehensive Study Guide*. 9th ed. New York, NY: McGraw-Hill; 2015.

Tseng, H, Hanna TN, Shuaib W, Aized M, Khosa F, Linnau KF. Imaging foreign bodies: ingested, aspirated, and inserted. *Ann Emerg Med*. 2015;66(6):570-582.

A 55-year-old man presents to the emergency department (ED) complaining of abdominal pain. The patient relates that he has been having intermittent pain throughout the abdomen for the past 12 hours, and since the onset of pain, he has vomited twice. His past medical history is significant for hypertension and colon cancer, for which he underwent laparoscopic right colectomy 8 months ago. The patient indicates that he has not had any recent abdominal complaints. His last bowel movement was 1 day ago, and he denies any weight loss and hematochezia. On physical examination, the patient is afebrile. The pulse rate is 98 beats per minute, blood pressure is 132/84 mm Hg, and respiratory rate is 22 breaths per minute. His cardiopulmonary examination is unremarkable. His abdomen is obese and mildly distended, with well-healed surgical scars. No tenderness, guarding, or hernias are noted. His bowel sounds are diminished, with occasional high-pitched sounds. The rectal examination reveals normal tone, empty rectal vault, and hemoccult-negative stool.

▶ What is the most likely cause of this patient's problems?
▶ What are the next steps in this patient's evaluation?

ANSWERS TO CASE 19:
Intestinal Obstruction

Summary: A 55-year-old man with history of laparoscopic surgery 8 months previously for the resection of right colon carcinoma presents with intermittent abdominal pain and vomiting. The physical examination reveals no abdominal wall or groin hernias, no tenderness, and high-pitched bowel sounds.

- **Most likely diagnosis:** Bowel obstruction. It is unclear whether the intestinal obstruction is involving the large or small bowel or whether it is complete or partial obstruction.

- **Next steps in evaluation:** Diagnostic radiography, which can be either plain x-rays or a computed tomography (CT).

ANALYSIS

Objectives

1. Learn to recognize the clinical presentations of intestinal obstruction (small bowel and colon).

2. Learn the common causes of bowel obstructions.

3. Learn the approach in the selection of imaging modalities for the evaluation of patients with possible bowel obstruction.

4. Learn to recognize clinical and radiographic signs of complicated obstruction and the urgency associated with its management.

Considerations

In this patient scenario, the differential diagnosis for obstruction includes intestinal ileus, adhesions, ischemia, and obstruction from recurrence of metastatic colon carcinoma. For this individual, the probability of ileus is unlikely because he has a history of crampy abdominal pain and findings of high-pitched bowel sounds, which are clinical features compatible with mechanical obstruction and not functional obstruction. **The first imaging study to consider can be an abdominal series or CT scan.** The radiographic studies will help to distinguish partial obstruction from high grade, complete obstruction. The abdominal series may delineate the level of obstruction. **The presence of stool or air in the rectal vault may suggest a partial obstruction,** whereas the presence of air and fluid levels in the small intestine, with the absence of stool and air throughout the colon, indicate a high-grade small-bowel obstruction. His past history of colon cancer points to the possibility that recurrent cancer may be the cause of his bowel obstruction; thus, a computed tomography (CT) scan of the abdomen may be helpful in identifying any obstructing tumor masses. In addition, CT scan can help identify a transition point in the GI tract where the luminal diameter of the bowel changes, thus differentiating a mechanical obstruction from a functional obstruction.

APPROACH TO:
Bowel Obstruction

DEFINITIONS

CLOSED-LOOP OBSTRUCTION: Blockage occurs both proximal and distal to the dilated segment, preventing decompression. Examples include an isolated loop of small bowel caught in a tight hernia defect, a twisting of the bowel on itself causing a volvulus, or a complete large-bowel obstruction in a patient with a competent ileocecal valve. These obstructions are unlikely to resolve with nonoperative therapy.

COMPLICATIONS OF BOWEL OBSTRUCTION: Ischemia, necrosis, or perforation as a result of obstruction.

CT SCAN OF THE ABDOMEN: This modality is increasingly used in the evaluation of patients with bowel obstruction. CT can help to differentiate functional obstruction from mechanical obstruction. It is also useful in the evaluation of patients with previous abdominal malignancy to help determine if the obstruction is related to tumor recurrence. In addition, there are a number of CT characteristics that will identify high-grade, complicated obstructions or decreased intestinal perfusion and will differentiate these from uncomplicated obstructions. CT scans can also identify mesentery swirling, which is a finding that is highly suggestive of intestinal volvulus and a condition that might benefit from early surgical consultation and intervention. Disadvantages of CT in comparison to plain abdominal radiographs include intravenous contrast exposure that has the potential of causing acute kidney injury in a patient who is hypovolemic and excessive exposure to ionizing radiation that could have significant late carcinogenic effects.

FUNCTIONAL OR NEUROGENIC OBSTRUCTION: Luminal contents cannot pass because of bowel motility disturbances preventing peristalsis. Etiologies include neurogenic dysfunction, medication-related or metabolic problems, bowel wall infiltrative processes such as collagen vascular diseases, and extraluminal infiltrative processes such as peritonitis or malignancy. Surgery generally does not improve the above conditions; however, complications related to the above conditions may require operative intervention.

MECHANICAL OBSTRUCTION: Luminal contents cannot pass through the gastrointestinal (GI) tract because of a mechanical obstruction. The treatment can be operative or nonoperative depending on the cause, severity, and duration of the obstructive process.

OPEN-LOOP OBSTRUCTION: Intestinal blockage is distal, allowing proximal bowel decompression of obstruction via nasogastric (NG) suction or emesis.

SIMPLE (UNCOMPLICATED) BOWEL OBSTRUCTION: Partial or complete obstruction of the bowel lumen without compromise to the intestinal blood flow.

UPPER GI–SMALL-BOWEL FOLLOW THROUGH: This is contrast radiography done following the administration of oral contrast. The study accurately localizes obstruction site and caliber in the small bowel. The administration of contrast can lead to worsening of obstruction and aspiration. Patients need to be closely monitored during and after this procedure for potential complications. This study is rarely indicated in the ED setting.

CLINICAL APPROACH

The causes of bowel obstruction in young children (<5 years of age) are quite different than those found in the adult population. The following discussion is limited to adult patients. **Adhesions** represent the most common cause of **small-bowel obstruction,** whereas **colorectal carcinoma** is the most common cause of **large-bowel obstruction in developed countries.** Table 19–1 lists the distribution and clinical features associated with obstructive causes.

Pathophysiology

With mechanical obstruction, **air and fluid accumulate in the bowel lumen.** The net result is an **increase in the intestinal intraluminal pressure,** which inhibits fluid absorption and stimulates the influx of water and electrolytes into the lumen. Eighty percent of air found inside the bowel lumen is swallowed air (see Figure 16–1). Because of this, NG tube decompression may be useful in preventing progression of bowel distention. Initially following the onset of mechanical obstruction, there is an increase in peristaltic activity. However, as the obstructive process progresses (usually >24 hours), coordinated peristaltic activity diminishes along with the contractile function of obstructed bowel, giving rise to dilated and atonic bowel proximal to the point of obstruction. With this progression, the patient may

Table 19–1 • SMALL- VS LARGE-BOWEL OBSTRUCTION	
Small-Bowel Obstruction	**Large-Bowel Obstruction**
Causes • Adhesions (70%-75%) • Malignancy (8%-10%) • Hernia (8%-10%) • Volvulus (3%) • Inflammatory bowel disease (1%) • Intussusception, gallstone ileus, radiation enteritis, intra-abdominal abscess, bezoar (all <1%)	**Causes** • Carcinoma (65%) • Volvulus (15%) • Diverticular disease (10%) • Hernias, peritoneal carcinomatosis, fecal impaction, ischemic colitis, foreign body, inflammatory bowel disease (total 10%)
Symptoms • Vomiting (more common with proximal obstruction) • Cramping pain (common, early) • Distention (variable, with greater distension seen with distal obstruction)	**Symptoms** • Distention (common and usually significant) • Postprandial cramps and bloating (very common) • Vomiting (unusual) • Bowel habit changes (common)

actually appear to improve clinically with less frequent and less intense crampy abdominal pain. The effects of mechanical obstruction on intestinal blood flow include an initial increase in blood flow. **With unrelieved obstruction, blood flow diminishes, leading to a breakdown of mucosal barriers and an increased susceptibility to bacterial invasion and ischemia.**

Clinical Presentation

The **common clinical manifestations of bowel obstruction are pain, emesis, constipation,** obstipation, distention, tenderness, visible peristalsis, and/or shock. The presence or absence of these signs and symptoms are dependent on the severity of the obstruction. Pain associated with bowel obstruction is generally severe at the onset and is characterized as intermittent and poorly localized. With the progression of small-bowel obstruction, spastic pain decreases in intensity and frequency. However, continuous pain may develop as the result of ischemia or peritonitis. Patients with **large-bowel obstruction usually have pain with postprandial cramp-like discomfort,** and some patients with chronic large-bowel obstruction may describe their symptoms as indigestion. Continuous pain may also develop with the progression of marked distention, ischemia, or perforation.

Emesis is a symptom found commonly in patients with intestinal obstruction. In general, patients with proximal obstruction of the small bowel report the most dramatic episodes, whereas patients with distal obstructions may not experience as much emesis. The quality of the material vomited may help indicate the level of obstruction, as obstruction in the distal small bowel may produce feculent vomitus. Contrary to common beliefs, **obstruction of the large bowel often is not associated with vomiting** because the presence of a competent ileocecal valve (found in 50%-60% of individuals) frequently contributes to a closed-loop obstruction.

Absence of bowel movements and flatus are suggestive of a high-grade or complete obstruction. With the stimulation of peristalsis at the initiation of an obstructive episode, it is not unusual for a patient to describe having bowel movements. The presence of a recent bowel movement does not rule out the diagnosis of a bowel obstruction. The classic description of decreased stool caliber is infrequently reported by patients with large-bowel obstruction and when reported, this finding is not specific for colonic obstruction. On the other hand, diarrhea is frequently reported by patients with progressive large-bowel obstruction. Presumably, with high-grade narrowing of the bowel lumen, passages of the solid and semisolid contents are blocked; therefore, the stools become more liquid in character. Distention to some degree is generally observed in most patients with intestinal obstruction; however, this finding may be absent in patients with obstruction of the proximal small bowel. Therefore, the absence of distention does not eliminate the possibility of intestinal obstruction.

Patients with uncomplicated obstruction usually have mild, ill-defined, nonlocalized abdominal tenderness. The tenderness results from distention of the bowel wall, leading to the aggravation of visceral pain. In the case of open-loop obstruction, decompression by emesis or NG tube frequently produces improvement or resolution of abdominal tenderness. **Localized tenderness is a finding that**

Table 19–2 • CT FINDINGS ASSOCIATED WITH INTESTINAL CONDITIONS	
CT Finding	Clinical Implications Associated with Finding
Dilated small bowel (>2.5 cm) with transition to normal-sized bowel	Mechanical small bowel obstruction (SBO)
>50% diameter difference between proximal dilated small bowel and distal small bowel	High-grade SBO
Small-bowel feces	Moderate- to high-grade obstruction
Intraperitoneal free fluid	This finding in the setting of SBO suggests high-grade SBO
Thickened small bowel wall	High-grade obstruction
Target sign	Intussusception
Swirl sign*	Internal hernia or volvulus
Reduced bowel wall enhancement	Ischemic bowel wall
Pneumatosis intestinalis	Ischemic bowel wall/necrosis

*Swirl sign: small bowel wrapping around superior mesenteric artery in a "C shape" or "U shape."

is infrequently encountered in patients with uncomplicated bowel obstruction. However, it **is suggestive of complications involving an isolated bowel segment.** The presence of this finding should raise the suspicion for a closed-loop obstruction, bowel necrosis, or perforation; consequently, patients with localized tenderness should be approached with more urgency, as these patients may need early operative treatments or early CT evaluation to help delineate the cause and severity of the process (Table 19–2).

MANAGEMENT OF SMALL-BOWEL OBSTRUCTION

When identified early, patients with uncomplicated small-bowel obstruction should be managed by NPO status, intravenous hydration, and NG tube decompression. This therapy is directed at correcting the fluid and electrolyte deficits and reversing the cycle of inflammatory and metabolic events associated with increased intestinal luminal pressures. Many patients with early, partial small-bowel obstruction can be successfully managed without further problems. Patients with suspected small-bowel obstruction should undergo CT imaging, which may help differentiate uncomplicated small-bowel obstructions from complicated obstructions and help identify patients at risk of developing complicated obstructions.

Typically, **patients who present late in the course of obstruction are less likely to resolve with nonoperative management.** Furthermore, in these patients with prolonged obstruction, the probability of **bowel ischemia and necrosis** is increased. The development of complicated small-bowel obstruction is associated with increased morbidity and mortality; therefore, every effort should be made to identify and initiate early treatment in these patients. No clinical, laboratory, and radiographic criteria will reliably predict and identify patients with small-bowel obstruction who will go on to develop bowel necrosis. **The presence of fever, tachycardia, persistent** abdominal pain, abdominal tenderness, leukocytosis, and high-grade obstruction are associated with the increased likelihood of bowel necrosis. These findings should prompt early referral to a surgeon, and patients with these findings are more likely to benefit from early surgical interventions.

The nonoperative approach does not address the source of the small-bowel obstruction. Therefore, prolonged nonoperative therapy would be considered inappropriate for patients with surgically correctable causes, such as abdominal wall and groin hernias and obstructing neoplasms. Similarly, patients with no previous abdominal operations and no defined causes for intra-abdominal adhesions should undergo resuscitation and prompt evaluation to identify a possibly treatable source of obstruction (eg, Crohn disease, tumors, volvulus, and internal hernias).

MANAGEMENT OF LARGE-BOWEL OBSTRUCTION

Patients with **large-bowel obstruction are often older and more severely dehydrated** and should be managed with **nasogastric suction, intravenous fluid hydration, and close monitoring for their responses to fluid** resuscitation. Patients with inappropriate response to fluid resuscitation may require admission to an intensive care unit, where invasive monitoring may be used to guide the resuscitation efforts; alternatively, poor response to initial fluid resuscitation could indicate complications such as perforations and/or bowel necrosis, in which case early surgical interventions may be needed.

The major diagnostic dilemma in patients with suspected large-bowel obstruction is differentiating mechanical obstruction from functional obstruction (dysmotility). In most patients, a CT scan will help make the differentiation. When mechanical and functional obstruction cannot be differentiated by CT imaging, a contrast enema without bowel preparation may be obtained.

Colorectal carcinoma is by far the most common cause of mechanical large-bowel obstruction. The site of obstruction of colon carcinoma correlates to the luminal diameter of the large bowel, rather than with the frequency of distribution of carcinoma. The generally reported frequency of distribution of obstructing colorectal carcinoma is **splenic flexure (40%), hepatic flexure (25%), descending and sigmoid colon (25%), transverse colon (10%), and ascending colon and cecum (10%).** Less commonly, sigmoid volvulus and diverticular disease may cause large-bowel obstruction; in these settings the plain radiographs generally will identify the sigmoid volvulus. When identified, the volvulus may be evaluated and resolved by proctosigmoidoscopy performed without bowel preparation. Because nearly all patients with large-bowel obstruction will require operative treatment, surgical consultations should be obtained early in these patients.

One of the most devastating complications associated with large-bowel obstruction is colonic perforation, which generally occurs in the cecum or right colon. **The risk for developing colonic perforation is increased among patients with a severely dilated colon (>10 cm cecal diameter).** These patients may or may not present with frank peritonitis; however, most patients will have severe volume contraction as a consequence of the ongoing inflammatory changes. The diagnosis of colonic perforation should be entertained when patients fail to improve with aggressive fluid management.

> **CASE CORRELATION**
>
> - See also Case 16 (Acute Abdominal Pain), Case 17 (Gastrointestinal Bleeding), and Case 18 (Swallowed Foreign Body).

COMPREHENSION QUESTIONS

19.1 A 44-year-old woman with a past history of appendicitis that was treated by appendectomy 2 years ago presents with abdominal pain of 4-day duration. Her temperature is 38.5°C (101.3°F), pulse rate is 120 beats per minute, and blood pressure is 100/84 mm Hg. Her abdomen is distended and diffusely tender, with guarding. An occasional, high-pitched bowel sound is present. A kidneys, ureters, bladder (KUB) x-ray reveals a markedly dilated small bowel without air or stool in the colon. Which of the following is the most appropriate course of management?

A. Place IV, NG tube, and Foley catheter, initiate broad-spectrum antibiotics, and obtain CT of abdomen.

B. Place IV, NG tube, and Foley catheter, initiate broad-spectrum antibiotics, and prepare patient for operation.

C. Place IV, NG tube, and Foley catheter, initiate broad-spectrum antibiotics, and attempt nonoperative treatment.

D. Place IV, NG tube, and Foley catheter, initiate broad-spectrum antibiotics, obtain CT scan of abdomen, and prepare patient for an operation.

E. Place IV, NG tube, and Foley catheter. Admit the patient to the ICU for monitoring.

19.2 Which of the following is the most likely cause of small-bowel obstruction in a 25-year-old woman with no previous abdominal operations?

A. Adhesions

B. Hernia

C. Crohn disease

D. Adenocarcinoma of the small bowel

E. Endometriosis

19.3 A third-year medical student has been given an assignment to assess the relative value of methods to differentiate between functional intestinal obstruction and mechanical obstruction. The patient scenario is that of a 90-year-old woman with Alzheimer disease, urinary tract infection, and abdominal distention. Which of the following statements is most accurate for this clinical learning issue?

A. The history and physical examination is most important to differentiate between the two disorders.

B. The history and physical examination, while often unhelpful, is better than imaging tests in differentiating between the two disorders.

C. The history and physical examination is typically unhelpful in differentiating between the two disorders.

D. Imaging tests are rarely helpful and may exacerbate the condition and worsen the prognosis.

E. CT scan is helpful in differentiating between the two pathological conditions in this patient.

ANSWERS

19.1 **B.** This patient presents with signs and symptoms of high-grade small-bowel obstruction. The physical examination is highly suspicious for presence of intra-abdominal complications associated with the obstruction; therefore, CT scan is unlikely to contribute further in the diagnosis, and nonoperative therapy is inappropriate for a patient who is already exhibiting signs and symptoms of complicated small-bowel obstruction.

19.2 **B.** Statistically speaking, a hernia would be the most likely cause of small-bowel obstruction in a patient without previous abdominal operations or other causes of adhesions.

19.3 **E.** History and physical examination is often inadequate in differentiating mechanical large-bowel obstruction from functional large-bowel obstruction; this would be especially true in a patient with Alzheimer disease due to being a poor historian, and because the dementia is a possible cause for functional large-bowel obstruction. CT scan of the abdomen, barium enema and/or 4-view radiographs of the abdomen are some of the imaging tests used in this setting.

CLINICAL PEARLS

▶ Persistent pain in a patient with small-bowel obstruction is usually suggestive of bowel ischemia or impending bowel necrosis.

▶ Localized tenderness in a patient with small-bowel obstruction may indicate an isolated segment of closed-loop obstruction, localized ischemic injury, or localized perforation.

▶ Because the symptoms and physical findings associated with large-bowel obstruction are nonspecific, they can be easily overlooked by both the patient and the physician.

▶ Adhesions represent the most common cause of small-bowel obstruction, whereas colorectal carcinoma is the most common cause of large-bowel obstruction.

REFERENCES

Bornstein JE, Berger DL. Large bowel obstruction. In: Cameron JL, Cameron AM, eds. *Current Surgical Therapy*. 11th ed. Philadelphia, PA: Mosby Elsevier; 2014:177-181.

Kodadek LM, Makary MA. Small bowel obstruction. In: Cameron JL, Cameron AM, eds. *Current Surgical Therapy*. 11th ed. Philadelphia, PA: Mosby Elsevier; 2014:109-113.

Tavakkolizadeh A, Whang EE, Ashley SW, Zinner MJ. Small intestine. In: Brunicardi FC, Andersen DK, Billiar TR, Dunn DL, Hunter JG, Mathews JB, Pollock RE, eds. *Schwartz's Principle of Surgery*. 9th ed. New York, NY: McGraw-Hill; 2011:979-1012.

A 19-year-old woman is brought into the emergency department (ED) complaining of abdominal pain and diarrhea of 3-day duration. She has also been nauseous and has not been able to drink much liquid. Five days ago she returned from a camping trip in New Mexico but did not drink from natural streams. She denies fever but states that she has had some chills. Her stools have been watery, brown, and profuse. The patient denies health problems. On examination, the patient is thin and pale. Her mucous membranes are dry. Her temperature is 37.2°C (99°F), heart rate is 110 beats per minute, and blood pressure is 90/60 mm Hg. The skin has no lesions. Her heart and lung examinations are unremarkable except tachycardia. The abdominal examination reveals hyperactive bowel sounds and no masses. There is diffuse mild tenderness but no guarding or rebound. Rectal examination demonstrates no tenderness or masses and is hemoccult negative. The complete blood count reveals a leukocyte count of 16,000 cells/mm^3. The pregnancy test is negative.

▶ What is the most likely diagnosis?
▶ What is the next diagnostic step?
▶ What is the next step in therapy?

ANSWERS TO CASE 20:
Acute Diarrhea

Summary: A 19-year-old healthy woman presents to the ED with a 3-day history of abdominal pain, nausea, and non-bloody, watery, profuse diarrhea. Five days ago, she was on a camping trip in New Mexico but did not drink from natural streams. Her mucous membranes are dry. Her temperature is 37.2°C (99°F), heart rate is 110 beats per minute, and blood pressure is 90/60 mm Hg. The abdominal examination reveals hyperactive bowel sounds, no masses, and diffuse mild tenderness without peritoneal signs. Rectal examination is occult blood negative. The leukocyte count is 16,000 cells/µL. The pregnancy test is negative.

- **Most likely diagnosis:** Acute volume depletion and possible electrolyte abnormalities secondary to acute diarrhea.

- **Next diagnostic step:** Test stool for fecal leukocytes.

- **Next step in therapy:** Intravenous fluid hydration.

ANALYSIS

Objectives

1. Know a diagnostic approach to acute diarrhea, including the role of fecal leukocytes and assessment for occult blood in the stools.

2. Understand that volume replacement and correction of electrolyte abnormalities are the first priorities in treatment of patients with diarrhea.

3. Be familiar with a rational workup for acute diarrhea, and know the common etiologies of diarrhea, including *Escherichia coli*, *Shigella*, *Salmonella*, *Giardia*, and amebiasis.

Considerations

This 19-year-old woman developed severe diarrhea and nausea following a camping trip. Her most immediate problem is volume depletion as evidenced by her dry mucous membranes, tachycardia, and hypotension. The **first priority** should be **acute replacement of intravascular volume; intravenous normal saline** would be an appropriate choice. The patient's serum electrolytes should be assessed, and abnormalities, such as hypokalemia, should be corrected. After volume repletion, the next priority is to determine the etiology of the diarrhea. **Up to 90% of acute diarrhea is infectious in etiology.** This patient does not have a history consistent with inflammatory bowel disease (IBD) or prior abdominal surgeries. She had been camping in New Mexico recently, which predisposes her to several pathogens: *E coli*, *Campylobacter*, *Shigella*, *Salmonella*, and *Giardia*. She does not have grossly bloody stools, which would usually mandate an evaluation and suggests invasive bacterial infections, such as hemorrhagic or enteroinvasive *E. coli* species, *Yersinia* species, *Shigella*, and *Entamoeba histolytica*. Additionally, the stool for occult blood is negative. Fecal leukocyte is an inexpensive and good test to differentiate between the various types of infectious diarrhea. If fecal leukocytes are present in the stool, the ED physician may have a higher suspicion for *Salmonella, Shigella, Campylobacter, Clostridium difficile, Yersinia,* enterohemorrhagic and enteroinvasive *E. coli,* and *E. histolytica.* Stool cultures are helpful. However, ova and parasite evaluation is generally unhelpful unless the history strongly points toward a parasitic source, or when the diarrhea is prolonged. Most diarrheas are self-limited and do not need extensive evaluations. Table 20–1 summarizes the danger signs. Because of the severity of this patient's symptoms, empiric antibiotic therapy, such as with ciprofloxacin, might be indicated.

APPROACH TO:
Acute Diarrhea

DEFINITIONS

ACUTE DIARRHEA: Diarrhea present for less than 2-week duration.

CHRONIC DIARRHEA: Diarrhea present for greater than 4-week duration.

DIARRHEA: Passage of abnormally liquid or poorly formed stool in increased frequency.

SUBACUTE (PERSISTENT) DIARRHEA: Diarrhea present for 2- to 4-week duration.

CLINICAL APPROACH

Etiologies

Approximately 90% of the acute diarrhea cases are caused by infectious etiologies, and the remainder is caused by medications, ischemia, or toxins. Infectious etiologies often depend on the patient population. For instance, **travelers to Mexico or Asia are likely to contract enterotoxigenic *E. coli* as a causative agent.** Those traveling to Russia and campers and backpackers are susceptible to infections by *Giardia* and *Campylobacter,* and *Shigella* and *Salmonella* are also common causative agents.

Consumption of foods is frequently the culprit. *Salmonella* or *Shigella* can be found in **undercooked chicken, enterohemorrhagic *E. coli* in undercooked hamburger,** and ***Staphylococcus aureus* or *Salmonella* in mayonnaise.** Raw seafood may harbor *Vibrio, Salmonella,* or hepatitis A, B, or C. Sometimes the timing of the diarrhea following food ingestion is helpful to pinpoint the infectious organism.

For example, illness within **6 hours of eating a salad** containing mayonnaise suggests *S. aureus,* **symptoms 8-12 hours post-ingestion suggest *Clostridium perfringens*, and symptoms 12-14 hours post-ingestion suggest *E. coli*** (see Table 20–1).

Day-care settings are particularly common locales for *Shigella, Giardia,* and rotavirus transmission. Patients in nursing homes and who were recently in the hospital may develop *C. difficile* colitis from antibiotic use. In addition,

Table 20–1 • ETIOLOGIES OF DIARRHEA

Etiologic Agent	Incubation Time	Diarrhea	Emesis	Abdominal Pain	Fever	Comments
S. aureus, C. perfringens	4-12 hours	Watery, profuse	Pronounced	Mild	Absent	Preformed toxin, may be in foods
Vibrio cholerae, enterotoxigenic E. coli	8-72 hours	Watery, profuse	Moderate	Mild	Absent	Enterotoxin produced
E. Coli, Giardia	2-7 days	Variable, watery	Mild	Moderate	Variable	Enteroadherent or enteropathogenic
Hemorrhagic E. coli, C. difficile	1-3 days	Variable, often bloody	Mild	Severe	Mild	Cytotoxin producing, causing cell necrosis and inflammation
Salmonella, Campylobacter, Shigella, enteroinvasive E. coli, E. histolytica	1-4 days	Often bloody	Mild	Severe	Moderate to high	Invasive organisms leading to inflammation, abdominal pain, and fever

Source: Data from Ahlquist DA, Camilleri M. Diarrhea and constipation. In: Braunwald E, Faucis AS, Kaspar DL, et al, eds. Harrison's Principles of Internal Medicine. 15th ed. New York, NY: McGraw Hill; 2001.

immune-compromised patients with prior history of C. *difficile* infections may remain colonized and develop recurrent clinical infections despite appropriate treatment.

Clinical Presentation

Most patients with acute diarrhea have self-limited processes and do not require much workup. Exceptions to this rule include **patients with profuse diarrhea, dehydration, fevers exceeding 38.5°C (101.3°F), grossly bloody diarrhea, elderly patients, patients with severe abdominal pain, symptom duration exceeding 48 hours without improvement, and occurrence in an immunocompromised host.** Mortalities related to diarrheal illnesses are generally due to the inadequate recognition and treatment of dehydration, electrolyte disturbances, and acidosis.

The history should be meticulous to identify prior history of GI complaints and exposure history, including medications, foods, travel history, and contact with individuals with similar symptoms. A history of recent viral illness may provide clues to help identify the infectious etiology. Occupational history may also help identify infectious sources. The clinician should determine what the patient can tolerate orally; in other words, if the patient is both vomiting and having profuse diarrhea, severe dehydration is likely. The quantity and character of the stools may be helpful to determine etiology, as well as direct therapy.

The physical examination should focus on the vital signs, clinical impression of the patient's hydration status, indicators of sepsis, mental status, and the abdominal examination. The patient's hydration status is determined by observing whether the mucous membranes are moist or dry, skin has good turgor or is tenting, the presence or absence of jugular venous distention, and capillary refill.

The principal laboratory test involves the stool for microscopic and microbiological examination. Stool culture results generally require several days to become finalized and are not useful in the ED setting; however, these results may be helpful for follow-up evaluations and for patients who do not improve with initial management. Ova and parasite evaluation is generally unhelpful except in selected circumstances of very high suspicion. Stool for **C. *difficile* toxin** may yield the etiology in patients who develop symptoms after healthcare contact or **antibiotic use,** and in most instances, the enzyme immunoassay results may be available in as little as 2 hours. Although pseudomembranous colitis was classically associated with clindamycin usage, fluoroquinolones are reported recently as the most common antibiotics contributing to the condition. C. *difficile* infections are also being increasingly reported in patients with IBD, where the symptoms may be difficult to differentiate from an exacerbation of IBD. A complete blood count, electrolytes, and renal function tests are sometimes indicated to help determine illness severity.

Traveler's diarrhea most often presents as watery diarrhea occurring a few days after traveling to Mexico, South America, Africa, South Asia, or other endemic regions. This type of diarrhea is most often caused by enterotoxigenic E. *coli*, which can produce diarrhea from the generation of toxin leading to cholera-like symptoms; infections by enteroinvasive strains of E. *coli* causing a shigella-like illness that is manifested by bloody mucous-producing diarrhea; and chronic infections related to E. *coli* overgrowth. Fluid and electrolyte replacements are the mainstay of treatment for traveler's diarrhea. A number of agents are helpful in reducing stool frequency, and these agents include bismuth subsalicylate and loperamide.

Antibiotic therapy may be indicated when symptoms do not resolve with supportive care and stool-reducing agents. For travelers returning from the non-coastal regions of Mexico, double-strength trimethoprim-sulfamethoxazole (Bactrim) twice a day is recommended. Alternatively, ciprofloxacin (750 mg), levofloxacin (500 mg), norfloxacin (800 mg), or azithromycin (1000 mg) can be prescribed. For immune compromised patients and elderly patients with comorbidities traveling to high-risk regions, prophylaxis with trimethoprim-sulfamethoxazole or a fluoroquinolone should be prescribed.

If the etiology is still unclear and the patient is not improving while off oral intake, hospital admission and consultation with a gastroenterologist may be indicated. Radiological studies or endoscopy may be needed to determine the cause. Diseases such as IBD or ischemic bowel disease must be considered.

Treatment

Fluid and electrolyte replacement are fundamental to the treatment of acute diarrhea. For mildly dehydrated individuals who can tolerate oral fluids, **sports drinks,** such as Gatorade orally, are often all that is needed. In developing countries, the oral rehydration solution (ORS) introduced by the World Health Organization (WHO) has been shown to be well tolerated by patients and well received by care givers. For those with more serious volume deficits, or elderly patients or infants, hospitalization and intravenous hydration may be necessary. **Bismuth subsalicylate** may be used to alleviate the gastrointestinal symptoms but should not be used in an immune-compromised individual because of the risk of bismuth encephalopathy. Many physicians choose to treat patients with moderately ill or severely ill appearance empirically with ciprofloxacin 500 mg twice daily for 5 days. Antimicrobial treatment may not alter the course of the disease.

Traveler's Prophylaxis

The best method in preventing traveler's diarrhea, which is principally caused by enterotoxigenic E. coli, is avoidance of food and water in areas of high risk. Travelers should be advised to drink only bottled water and avoid eating foods from street vendors or unhygienic locations. "Boil it, cook it, peel it, or forget it" remains sound advice for individuals traveling to Latin America, the Caribbean, Africa, and South Asia. The CDC endorses **bismuth subsalicylate, two 262-mg tablets chewed well four times a day** (with meals and at bedtime) but does not advocate the use of antimicrobial agents because a false sense of security or antibiotic resistance may result. Nevertheless, many practitioners prescribe **ciprofloxacin 500 mg once a day. Medical prophylaxis (either bismuth subsalicylate or antibiotic) should not be used for longer than 3 weeks.**

CASE CORRELATION

- See also Case 16 (Acute Abdominal Pain), Case 17 (Gastrointestinal Bleeding), and Case 19 (Intestinal Obstruction).

COMPREHENSION QUESTIONS

Match the following etiologies (A to F) to the clinical situations in Questions 20.1 to 20.4:

  A. *E. coli*

  B. *Giardia* lamblia

  C. Rotavirus

  D. *S. aureus*

  E. *Vibrio* species

  F. *Cryptosporidium*

20.1 During the winter, a 24-year-old woman who works at a day care develops profuse watery diarrhea.

20.2 A 22-year-old college student takes a trip during spring break to Cozumel and develops diarrhea.

20.3 Several workers develop watery diarrhea and significant emesis within 4 hours after eating food at a potluck dinner.

20.4 A 45-year-old man eats raw oysters and 2 days later develops abdominal cramping, fever of 38.3°C (101°F), and watery diarrhea.

ANSWERS

20.1 **C.** Rotavirus usually causes a watery diarrhea and is especially common in the winter. It is the most common cause of diarrhea in infants and children worldwide. The vaccine has decreased the incidence in the United States significantly, but rotavirus is still a common infection. This patient who works at a day care would be susceptible to exposure.

20.2 **A.** Enterotoxic *E. coli* is the most common etiology for diarrhea in travelers visiting Mexico. This is followed by *Campylobacter jejuni*, *Shigella* spp, and *Salmonella* spp.

20.3 **D.** *S. aureus* usually causes prominent vomiting and diarrhea within a few hours of food ingestion as a consequence of the toxin produced.

20.4 **E.** Raw seafood may harbor *Vibrio* spp; thus, the history of eating raw oysters makes *Vibrio*-related infection likely.

CLINICAL PEARLS

▶ The vast majority of acute diarrhea is caused by an infectious etiology.

▶ Most acute diarrheas are self-limited.

▶ One should be cautious when assessing acute diarrhea in immunosuppressed, very young, or elderly patients.

▶ Significant dehydration, grossly bloody diarrhea, high fever, and nonresponse after 48 hours are warning signs of possible complicated diarrhea.

▶ In general, acute uncomplicated diarrhea can be treated with oral electrolyte-fluid solution with or without empiric ciprofloxacin.

REFERENCES

Engels PT, Tremblay. Jaundice, diarrhea, obstruction, and pseudoobstruction. In: Hall JB, Schmidt GA, Kress JP, eds. *Principle of Critical Care*. 4th ed. New York, NY: McGraw Hill Education; 2015: 998-1008.

Hill DR, Beeching NJ. Travelers' diarrhea. *Curr Opin Infect Dis.* 2010;23:481-487.

Pigott DC. Foodborne illness. *Emerg Med Clin N Am.* 2008;26:475-497.

White MB, Rajagopalan S, Yoshikawa TT. Infectious diarrhea: norovirus and clostridium difficile in older adults. *Clin Geriatr Med.* 2016;32:509-522.

A 30-year-old white man presents to the emergency department (ED) complaining of sudden onset of abdominal bloating and back pain. The patient states he was sleeping comfortably but then developed a sudden onset of severe, constant pain that radiates from his back to his abdomen and down toward his scrotum and caused him to be awakened. He is unable to find a comfortable position and feels best when he is able to get up to move around. He admits to having had occasional hematuria but denies ever having this type of pain in the past. He has no other significant medical problems. On physical examination the patient is diaphoretic and in moderate distress. His blood pressure is 128/76 mm Hg, heart rate is 106 beats per minute, temperature is 37.4°C (99.4°F), and respiratory rate is 28 breaths per minute. His cardiovascular examination reveals tachycardia without murmurs. Lung examination is clear to auscultation. Abdominal examination demonstrates normoactive bowel sounds, no abdominal distension, and significant costovertebral angle tenderness. A midstream voided urine specimen demonstrates gross hematuria.

▶ What is the most likely diagnosis?
▶ How would you confirm the diagnosis?
▶ What is the next step in treatment?

ANSWERS TO CASE 21:

Nephrolithiasis

Summary: A 30-year-old healthy man complains of the acute onset of severe back pain and a history of gross hematuria. He appears to be in moderate distress and has not previously experienced these symptoms.

- **Most likely diagnosis:** Nephrolithiasis.

- **Confirmation of the diagnosis:** Perform a urinalysis, complete blood count (CBC), serum chemistries, kidneys, ureters, bladder (KUB) radiograph, and intravenous pyelogram (IVP) or computed tomography (CT) scan of the abdomen.

- **Next step in treatment:** Start IV fluids and provide sufficient pain management for the patient before sending him for the appropriate imaging study. Strain all urine once the diagnosis of nephrolithiasis is suspected and perform stone analysis on any stone passed.

ANALYSIS

Objectives

1. Recognize the history and typical presentation of a patient with nephrolithiasis.

2. Learn to order the appropriate laboratory and radiographic studies to diagnose nephrolithiasis.

3. Learn to treat and manage nephrolithiasis in an acute care setting.

Considerations

This patient has a very typical presentation for nephrolithiasis: male (three times more common in men than in women) and the history of the sudden onset of pain that radiates from his back toward his abdomen. The ED physician must remain vigilant and rule out other acute abdominal etiologies that may be associated with a similar clinical presentation (Table 21–1 lists the differential diagnosis). Patients with nephrolithiasis often have difficulty finding a comfortable position. This is in contrast to patients with an acute abdomen, who often feel better when they

Table 21–1 • DIFFERENTIAL DIAGNOSIS OF NEPHROLITHIASIS	
Appendicitis	Biliary stones
Ectopic pregnancy	Ovarian torsion
Salpingitis	Peptic ulcer disease
Diverticulitis	Abdominal aortic aneurysm
Bowel obstruction	Gastroenteritis
Renal artery embolism	

remain supine without moving or with their knees bent toward their chest. The pain associated with nephrolithiasis can be described as constant, colicky, or waxing and waning. A history of dark-brown-tinged urine may represent old blood in the urine (ie, from a stone high in the calyx), while a complaint of bright red blood in the urine may be more consistent with a lower urinary tract stone. A family history of nephrolithiasis or a personal history of stones within the urinary tract may make the diagnosis easier. On physical examination, the patients are usually normotensive and afebrile, but tachycardic. The presence of fever would suggest urinary tract infection such as pyelonephritis or some other disease process (appendicitis). The increase in heart rate in this patient is most likely caused by his pain. Furthermore, costovertebral angle tenderness and hematuria on urinalysis are highly suggestive of a urinary tract process.

APPROACH TO:
Nephrolithiasis

DEFINITIONS

CALCIUM OXALATE: The most common type of renal stone; it is radiodense.

EXTRACORPOREAL SHOCK WAVE LITHOTRIPSY (ESWL): Fluoroscopically focused shockwaves which result in disintegration of the stone into fragments that are usually small enough to pass in the urine.

NEPHROLITHIASIS: A condition in which stone formation has occurred within the urinary tract system.

STONE COMPOSITION ANALYSIS: This is helpful in conjunction with metabolic workup to determine the underlying cause for stone formation when the history and physical examination does not identify risk factors for stone formation.

CLINICAL APPROACH

Epidemiology

Urinary calculus disease is a common condition that **affects up to 10% of the US population.** Nephrolithiasis is caused by urinary supersaturation; therefore, increases in urinary ion excretion and/or decrease in urinary volume are common factors that contribute to the process. The incidence of stone formation depends on a multitude of extrinsic and intrinsic risk factors, including socioeconomic status, diet, occupation, climate, medications, sex, and age (Table 21–2). **Nephrolithiasis is more common in men** than in women (3:1) and has its peak incidence between the ages of 30 and 50 years. Individuals exposed to high temperature either by geographic location or through occupational exposures are at increased risk of dehydration, which contributes to the risk of stone formation. Individuals with excessive sun exposure have increased calcium absorption due to the increased production of vitamin D, and they therefore experience an increased risk of urinary

Table 21–2 • RISK FACTORS	
Metabolic factors	**Environmental factors**
• Hypercalciuria	• Hot, dry, increased sunlight
• Hyperuricosuria	**Drugs**
• Hypocitraturia	• Loop diuretics
• Hyperoxaluria	• Antacids
Primary hyperparathyroidism	• Acetazolamide
• Renal tubular acidosis	• Glucocorticoids
Age	• Theophylline
• 30-50 years	• Allopurinol
Sex	• Probenecid
• Male 3:1	• Triamterene
Diet	• Acyclovir
• Increased intake of calcium,	• Indinavir
• protein and oxalate	• Vitamins D and C
Socioeconomic status	

calculus formation. Medications can also predispose individuals to stone formation (see Table 21–2).

Calcium-based (calcium oxalate and/or calcium phosphate) stones are the most common types of stones and account for more than 75% of urinary stones. Other types of stones include magnesium ammonium phosphate, uric, and cystine stones. Uric acid stones tend to occur in patients with low urine pH (<6.0) and with hyperuricosuria. Cystine stones occur in the setting of cystinuria, which is a relatively common autosomal-recessive condition causing defects in the gastrointestinal and renal transport of cystine, ornithine, arginine, and lysine. **Magnesium ammonium phosphate (struvite) stones are more common in women and are usually associated with urinary infections with urease-producing organisms (*Proteus, Pseudomonas,* and *Klebsiella*).**

Clinical Presentation

The vast majority of patients with renal stones will present to the ED complaining of **acute onset of colicky or non-colicky renal pain.** Non-colicky pain is most likely caused by an upper urinary tract stone, whereas colicky pain is more likely caused by the stretching from the stone in the ureter. In addition, the presenting symptoms may include tachycardia, tachypnea, and hypertension, which are produced in response to pain. **Fever, pyuria, and severe costovertebral angle tenderness usually indicate a medical emergency because pyelonephritis caused by obstruction often leads to sepsis and rapid clinical deterioration.** Persistent nausea and vomiting due to stimulation of the celiac ganglion may require the patient to be hospitalized.

A dipstick and microscopic examination of the voided midstream urine is very helpful, but the **amount of hematuria does not correlate with the degree of obstruction.** Although microscopic hematuria is present in 90% of cases of nephrolithiasis, a complete ureteral obstruction may present without hematuria. A careful analysis of urine sediment for crystals by an experienced individual should be performed promptly. In addition to the microscopic evaluation, a culture and sensitivity should be performed.

A KUB radiograph is sometimes helpful in identifying a urinary tract stone, as 90% of stones are radiopaque. Traditionally, the IVP has been the gold standard

Table 21–3 • RISK FACTORS FOR NEPHROTOXICITY WITH CONTRAST DYE	
Age >60 years	Debilitated condition
Dehydration	Known cardiovascular disease, especially
Hypotension	on a diuretic
Multiple myeloma	Asthma
Hyperuricemia	Renal insufficiency
History of intravenous contrast within	Diabetes mellitus
72 hours	

in evaluating a renal stone because it gives information about degree of obstruction as well as renal function. In many institutions, **newer-generation helical CT imaging without contrast is the preferred imaging method of choice for the evaluation of acute renal colic;** its sensitivity and specificity are greater than that of IVP, but it does not assess the degree of excretion compromised in the affected kidney. CT imaging also has the advantage of assessing the appendix, aorta, and diverticulitis. Regardless of the test, the clinician should interpret the clinical picture in conjunction with the imaging results. Before an IVP, the patient should be questioned about allergy to contrast dye or shellfish, the possibility of pregnancy, and preexisting renal disease. Pregnant women and children generally should have ultrasound imaging first to avoid the radiation exposure. Table 21–3 lists the risk factors of nephrotoxicity associated with contrast dye.

Management

The critical issues surrounding nephrolithiasis are pain control, determination of the degree of obstruction, and identification of infection. Adequate analgesia is critical in treating a patient with nephrolithiasis, and analgesic administration should not be delayed pending test results. Depending on the severity of the pain, intravenous opiates, acetaminophen with codeine, meperidine, nonsteroidal anti-inflammatory drugs (NSAIDs), or morphine may be necessary. **NSAIDs should be used with caution in patients with renal insufficiency, in older patients, and in those with diabetes mellitus.** Evaluation of the patient's volume status will determine how much and what kind of intravenous fluids are necessary. Excessive fluid administration to dislodge a stone is not therapeutic and should not be attempted. Because definitive therapy is guided by the type of stones that are being formed, recovery of any passed stones and straining all urine is important to guide long-term management.

Conservative management, including analgesics, hydration, and antibiotics if urinary tract infection is suspected, may be all the patient needs. Most small stones (<6 mm) in diameter will produce symptoms but will typically pass without the need for interventions. **Indications for urgent urologic consultation are inadequate oral pain control, persistent nausea and vomiting, associated pyelonephritis, large stone (>7 mm), solitary kidney, or complete obstruction.** If the patient is being managed expectantly, the patient should be instructed to increase fluid intake and strain the urine until the stone is passed. Medical therapy, including calcium channel blocker or α-blocker, is being increasingly applied to facilitate stone passage and has been shown to be associated with a 65% increase in the likelihood of stone passage. Surgery is indicated in patients with stones larger than 8 mm, persistent pain, or failure to pass the stone despite conservative management. Stones located in the lower urinary tract system may be removed using a ureteroscope; upper urinary tract stones can be treated by ESWL.

CASE CORRELATION

- See also Case 16 (Acute Abdominal Pain), Case 17 (Gastrointestinal Bleeding), and Case 24 (Acute Pyelonephritis).

COMPREHENSION QUESTIONS

21.1 After passing a kidney stone, a 38-year-old woman is told by her primary care physician that she had passed a magnesium ammonium phosphate stone. She is most likely to have had a urinary infection caused by which of the following organisms?

  A. *Proteus*

  B. *Escherichia coli*

  C. *Enterococcus* species

  D. Group B *Streptococcus*

  E. *Staphylococcus aureus*

21.2 A 55-year-old man presents to the ED complaining of right flank pain for the past 2 weeks. He has noted some gross hematuria and has been unable to eat anything secondary to nausea and vomiting. Which of the following is an indication for hospitalization?

  A. Gross hematuria

  B. Right flank pain

  C. Nausea and vomiting despite antiemetics

  D. Age greater than 50 years

  E. Presence of a 6-mm stone

21.3 A 39-year-old man complains of the sudden onset of severe left flank pain after running a marathon. He describes the pain as constant with radiation to his left groin area. A urinalysis shows microscopic hematuria and the presence of cystine crystals. Where is the stone most likely to be located?

  A. Renal pelvis

  B. Proximal ureter

  C. Distal ureter

  D. Ureterovesicular junction

  E. Bladder

21.4 A 33-year-old woman is pregnant at 12 weeks' gestation and presents with right flank pain and gross hematuria. She is afebrile. Which of the following imaging tests is most appropriate for this patient?

   A. Ultrasonography
   B. KUB
   C. IVP
   D. Retrograde pyelography
   E. Helical CT without contrast

ANSWERS

21.1 **A.** This woman has a magnesium ammonium phosphate stone, which are common in women and are associated with urease-producing organisms. *Proteus, Pseudomonas*, and *Klebsiella* are all urease-producing organisms.

21.2 **C.** Hospitalization is required if the patient is unable to tolerate anything by mouth. Gross hematuria and flank pain are expected with nephrolithiasis. Appropriate analgesics should be prescribed for patients if they will not be hospitalized. Stones 6 mm or less will generally pass spontaneously without interventions.

21.3 **A.** Constant pain is most likely to be due stone located in the kidney. Colicky pain is most likely to be due to a stone located in the ureter and is related to the stretching caused by the stone and inflammatory processes in the lumen of the ureter. Most stones in the renal pelvis or bladder are asymptomatic, but if symptoms are present, it is usually constant.

21.4 **A.** Because the patient is pregnant during the first trimester, the initial imaging test should be sonography to avoid the radiation-related teratogenic/ mutagenic effects on the fetus.

CLINICAL PEARLS

▶ The acute presentation of nephrolithiasis resembles other pathologies; the correct studies and appropriate interpretation of laboratory data will help to establish the diagnosis.

▶ Any patient with severe nausea, vomiting, fever, or signs of infection should be hospitalized.

▶ Adequate pain control for patients with suspected nephrolithiasis is a priority even before all test results return.

▶ All urine should be strained to confirm the diagnosis and for the stone composition to be discerned.

▶ The absence of pain does not mean follow-up is unnecessary. Identifying the etiology of stone formation is important to prevent recurrence.

REFERENCES

Qaseem A, Dallas P, Forciea TD, the American College of Physicians Guidelines Committee. Dietary and pharmacologic management to prevent recurrent nephrolithiasis in adults: a clinical practice guideline from the American College of Physicians. *Ann Intern Med.* 2014;161:659-667.

Shah S, Calle JC. Dietary and medical management of recurrent nephrolithiasis. *Cleve Clin J Med.* 2016;83:463-471.

A 17-year-old adolescent male arrives at the emergency department (ED) after he developed an acute onset of severe right testicular pain about 4 hours ago while at soccer practice. The patient does not recall any recent trauma to the area and denies any fever, dysuria, or penile discharge. Although he has nausea, he does not have any abdominal pain or vomiting.

On examination, his temperature is 99.5°F, blood pressure is 138/84 mm Hg, heart rate is 104 beats per minute, and respiratory rate is 22 breaths per minute. He is in acute distress due to pain. His abdomen is benign. On visual inspection, he has right scrotal erythema and swelling, although there are no penile lesions or discharge. Because his scrotum is so diffusely tender, it is difficult to examine it more closely. However, there is no testicular rise when his inner thigh is stroked. His urinalysis shows 3-5 white blood cells (WBCs)/high power field (hpf).

▶ What is the most likely diagnosis?
▶ What is the next diagnostic step?

ANSWERS TO CASE 22:

Scrotal Pain

Summary: This is a 17-year-old adolescent male who presents with acute onset right testicular pain without any preceding trauma.

- **Most likely diagnosis:** Testicular torsion.

- **Next diagnostic step:** Urological consultation. Manual detorsion can be attempted while awaiting the consultant.

ANALYSIS

Objectives

1. Learn the differential diagnosis for acute scrotal pain.

2. Recognize the clinical signs and symptoms associated with testicular torsion.

3. Understand the diagnostic and therapeutic approach to suspected testicular torsion.

Considerations

The differential diagnosis of acute testicular pain includes testicular torsion, epididymitis, orchitis, torsion of the testicular appendages, hernia, hydrocele, and testicular tumor (Table 22–1). Because of the risk of ischemia and infarction of the testes, testicular torsion is the priority condition that must be promptly recognized and treated. This patient is 17-years-old without a history of trauma. Adolescents during puberty are especially at risk for testicular torsion because of high hormonal stimulation. This patient's history of acute onset, especially associated with vigorous physical activity, is classic. The involved testis is firm, tender, and located higher in the scrotum on examination. The cremasteric reflex is absent, again consistent with testicular torsion. When the clinical presentation is unclear, Doppler flow studies of the intratesticular blood flow may be helpful. This patient, however, has a classic history and examination, and time is of the essence.

APPROACH TO:

Scrotal Pain

CLINICAL APPROACH

When any patient presents with scrotal pain, **testicular torsion must be considered.** Prompt diagnosis and intervention is vital because delay can lead to ischemia, loss of the testicle, and impaired fertility. In general, the best salvage time of the testis is attained **within 4-6 hours after the onset of pain,** but clinical parameters are often unreliable. Patients with testicular torsion often have a congenital "bell clapper"

Table 22–1 • DIFFERENTIAL DIAGNOSES FOR ACUTE SCROTAL PAIN

Diagnosis	Comments	Clinical Findings	Treatment
Epididymitis	Young boys: may be due to sterile reflux or coliform bacteria. <35-40 years old: usually due to *Chlamydia trachomatis* or *Neisseria gonorrhoeae*. >35-40 years old: usually due to *E. coli* and *Klebsiella*. More gradual onset. May be associated with fever and urinary symptoms	Tenderness, erythema, warmth of scrotum (may be isolated to epididymis/posterolateral testis initially). ± urethral discharge. Pain improves with scrotal elevation (Prehn sign). Doppler US: increased testicular blood flow, enlarged hypoechoic epididymis	Antibiotics, analgesia, bed rest with scrotal elevation, scrotal support, ice packs
Fournier gangrene	Polymicrobial infection causing necrotizing fasciitis of perineal, genital, or perianal regions. Risk factors: diabetes, immunocompromise, chronic alcoholism. 40% mortality	Systemically ill. Scrotal pain (initially pain out of proportion to examination), perineal erythema and swelling. Induration, ecchymosis, crepitus as later findings. US: diffuse swelling and thickening of scrotum	Fluid resuscitation, intravenous antibiotics, surgical debridement. Consider hyperbaric oxygen therapy
Hydrocele	Gradual onset	Scrotal swelling and transillumination. US: fluid-filled cavity	Urology follow-up
Inguinal hernia	Variable presentation depending on age and type of hernia	Inguinal and scrotal swelling and pain. ± Signs of intestinal obstruction if incarcerated or strangulated	Surgery
Orchitis	Most commonly viral etiology (eg, mumps). Bacterial orchitis usually associated with epididymitis. Gradual onset	Testicular tenderness and swelling. ± Systemic symptoms with bacterial orchitis or parotitis with mumps orchitis	Antibiotics if bacterial etiology. Otherwise symptomatic care (analgesia, bed rest, scrotal support, and ice packs)
Testicular tumor	Most common malignancy in young men. Seminomas most common. Gradually progressive	Often painless swelling although pain may occur with hemorrhage into tumor. Testicular mass, firmness, swelling. US: intratesticular mass	Urgent urologic referral. Radical orchiectomy, radiation therapy, and chemotherapy may be needed
Appendageal torsion	Twisting of one of four vestigial structures of the testes (most commonly the appendix testes). Most common in boys 7-14 years old. Nausea and vomiting less common than with testicular torsion	Acute scrotal pain (although less severe than with testicular torsion), tender nodule (near head of testis or epididymis), "blue dot sign." Doppler US: normal or increased testicular blood flow	Analgesia, bed rest, scrotal support. Usually resolves within 3-10 days. Consider surgical excision if severe or refractory

Abbreviations: US = ultrasound.

deformity, which allows the epididymis and testicle to hang freely and rotate in the scrotum. When torsion occurs, the spermatic cord becomes twisted, cutting off the blood supply to the testicle. Although torsion can occur at any age, it is most common in children less than 1 year old and around puberty.

When obtaining the history, the clinician should focus on the onset and duration of pain, alleviating and aggravating factors, and any associated symptoms, such as nausea and vomiting, fever, urethral discharge, or dysuria. He/she should also remember that some patients may complain of abdominal rather than scrotal pain. In addition, it is important to inquire about any previous similar episodes or any recent trauma. A typical patient with **testicular torsion** presents with the **sudden onset of severe pain in the lower abdomen, inguinal area, or scrotum.** Associated nausea and vomiting are common. The pain is often preceded by strenuous physical activity or trauma, though episodes can occur during sleep. Pain that persists for more than 1 hour after scrotal trauma is not normal and merits further investigation. Past episodes that resolved spontaneously are not uncommon.

On examination, the clinician should pay close attention to any abdominal findings, such as scrotal swelling, skin changes, penile discharge or rash, inguinal lymphadenopathy or hernia, and testicular tenderness or a palpable mass. Classically, a **torsed testicle is diffusely tender and swollen with an abnormal (horizontal) lie.** There is usually a loss of the cremasteric reflex on the affected side; however, no historical or examination findings can definitively distinguish testicular torsion from other disease processes. In addition, infants and children may lack the typical examination findings.

Testicular torsion is largely a clinical diagnosis, and no diagnostic test should delay urological evaluation. If the diagnosis is uncertain, **ultrasound (US) with color Doppler imaging is recommended.** US not only helps in confirming the diagnosis by providing valuable information on vascular perfusion of the testis, but sonographic findings also allow other diagnoses to be made in patients presenting who do not have torsion. It is important to note that patients with partial torsion or spontaneous detorsion may have blood flow detectable on US. Many times, leukocytes are found in the urine of men with testicular torsion. This finding should not distract the clinician from the diagnosis.

TREATMENT

Definitive treatment involves an emergent attempt at manual detorsion or surgical intervention if the former is unsuccessful. Because most torsions occur in a lateral to medial direction, the testis should initially be turned in a medial to lateral direction like "opening a book." Successful detorsion results in significant pain relief. If the pain does not improve or worsens, the maneuver should be tried in the opposite direction. Intravenous analgesics are necessary prior to beginning the procedure. Although pain may be significantly relieved with manual detorsion, surgery is the definitive treatment and may be scheduled electively after manual detorsion. The differential diagnosis for acute scrotal pain includes several benign and emergent conditions (Table 22–1).

CASE CORRELATION

- See also Case 21 (Nephrolithiasis) and Case 16 (Acute Abdominal Pain).

COMPREHENSION QUESTIONS

22.1 A 22-year-old baseball player comes to the ED complaining of 10 hours of severe right testicular pain. He denies a history of trauma. On examination, his right testis is diffusely tender and indurated, and the pain does not change with patient position. He has a cremasteric reflex on the right side. Which of the following is the best next step?

A. Continued observation

B. Oral antibiotics

C. Bed rest, ice to scrotum, and elevation of the scrotum

D. Emergent testicular ultrasound with color Doppler

22.2 A 32-year-old jogger is brought into the emergency room with the acute onset of severe left testicular pain. A diagnosis of testicular torsion is made, and manual detorsion is successfully accomplished. Which of the following is the most appropriate advice to this patient?

A. Likely no further therapy is needed

B. Surgical exploration may be needed if another episode of torsion occurs

C. Surgical correction will be needed but does not necessarily need to be done urgently

D. Surgical exploration still needs to be performed and should occur within 24 hours

Match the probable diagnoses (A-F) to the clinical scenarios in Questions 22.3 to 22.6:

A. Torsion of the appendix testis

B. Testicular torsion

C. Epididymitis

D. Orchitis

E. Testicular tumor

F. Acute prostatitis

22.3 A 24-year-old man complains of severe left scrotal pain increasing over 24 hours. Urinalysis shows 25 WBC/hpf, and Doppler flow shows increased intratesticular flow.

22.4 A 58-year-old man complains of urgency, dysuria, lower back pain, and pain with ejaculation.

22.5 A 14-year-old adolescent complains of 2 days of testicular pain. On examination, there appears to be a tender nodule of the testis. Transillumination reveals a small blue spot at the affected area.

22.6 A 28-year-old man complains of heaviness in his scrotum. On examination, there is a firm, non-tender mass involving his right testis.

ANSWERS

22.1 **D.** The clinical history is consistent with testicular torsion. The presence of a cremasteric reflex does not rule out the disease. Emergent testicular ultrasound is the next best step when the history and physical examination is concerning for testicular torsion.

22.2 **C.** Detorsion of the torsed testis converts an emergent condition into one that is amenable to elective correction. Manual detorsion is not definitive therapy.

22.3 **C.** The Doppler ultrasound finding consistent with epididymitis is increased or preserved blood flow. Also, epididymitis usually has a more gradual onset of pain. Fifty percent of patients with epididymitis have pyuria or bacteriuria.

22.4 **F.** Acute prostatitis usually occurs in older patients. Urinary urgency, hesitancy, frequency, and perineal pain with ejaculation are common symptoms. The most common causative organism is *Escherichia coli*. Appropriate antibiotic choices include fluoroquinolones (ciprofloxacin, ofloxacin, and norfloxacin) as well as trimethoprim-sulfamethoxazole.

22.5 **A.** Torsion of a testicular appendage classically presents as a tender testicular nodule, and upon transillumination, a "blue dot" may be seen. Color Doppler blood flow is increased or normal.

22.6 **E.** Testicular carcinoma classically presents as a painless scrotal mass.

CLINICAL PEARLS

▶ Testicular torsion should always be considered in the differential diagnoses of acute scrotal or abdominal pain.

▶ No single historical or examination finding can definitively distinguish testicular torsion from other processes.

▶ Time is testicle. If testicular torsion is suspected, prompt urological consultation is mandatory.

▶ Definitive treatment of testicular torsion is surgery. Manual detorsion may be attempted as a temporizing measure.

REFERENCES

Lewis AG, Bukowski TP, Jarvis PD, Wacksman J, Sheldon CA. Evaluation of acute scrotum in the emergency department. *J Pediatr Surg.* 1995;30:277-282.

Marx JA, Hockberger RS, Walls RM, eds. *Rosen's Emergency Medicine: Concepts and Clinical Practice.* 8th ed. Philadelphia, PA: Saunders; 2014.

Mufti RA, Ogedegbe AK, Lafferty K. The use of Doppler ultrasound in the clinical management of acute testicular pain. *Br J Urol.* 1995;76:625-627.

Paushter D, Lin E. Testicular Torsion Imaging Medscape. Aug 12, 2015.

Rabinowitz R. The importance of the cremasteric reflex in acute scrotal swelling in children. *J Urol.* 1984;132:89-90.

Ringdahl E. Testicular torsion. *Am Fam Physician.* 2006;74(10):1739-1743.

Tintinalli JE, Stapczynski JS, Ma OJ, et al., eds. *Emergency Medicine: A Comprehensive Study Guide.* 8th ed. New York, NY: McGraw-Hill; 2016.

A 54-year-old man is brought to the emergency department with complaints of generalized weakness, nausea, and nonspecific feelings of illness. The symptoms have progressed insidiously over 2-3 days. His past medical history is remarkable for long-standing diabetes and poorly controlled hypertension (HTN). He is currently taking many medications that include oral hypoglycemics, a diuretic, and an angiotensin-converting enzyme inhibitor (ACEI). On physical examination, the patient appears lethargic and ill. His temperature is 36.0°C (96.8°F), pulse rate is 70 beats per minute, blood pressure is 154/105 mm Hg, and respiratory rate is 22 breaths per minute. Head and neck examination shows normal conjunctiva and mucous membranes. There is moderate jugular venous distention, and the lungs have minor bibasilar rales. The cardiac examination reveals normal rate, no murmurs or rubs, and a positive S_4. The abdomen is soft and nontender, with hypoactive bowel sounds and no organomegaly. Rectal examination is normal. Skin is cool and dry. Extremities demonstrate pitting edema to the knees bilaterally. On neurologic examination the patient moans and weakly localizes pain. He is oriented to person and place but cannot provide any further history. The initial rhythm strip is shown in Figure 23–1.

► What is the most likely diagnosis?
► What is the next step?

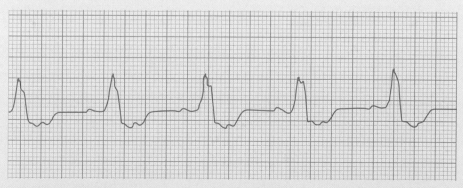

Figure 23–1. ECG rhythm strip.

ANSWERS TO CASE 23:

Hyperkalemia Due to Renal Failure

Summary: A 54-year-old man with HTN and diabetes mellitus (DM) complains of weakness, nausea, and a general sense of illness. Symptoms have progressed slowly over 3 days. His medications include hypoglycemics, a diuretic, and an ACEI. On examination he appears ill. He is moderately hypertensive and tachypneic but afebrile. Examination reveals moderate jugular venous distention, some minor bibasilar rales, and lower extremity edema. He is awake and oriented to person and place but is not able to give further history. The ECG confirms a wide complex rhythm (Figure 23–2).

- **Most likely diagnosis:** Hyperkalemia.

- **Next step:** Management of the ABCs (airway, breathing, and circulation), including immediate vascular access and continuous cardiac monitoring, rapid stepwise administration of medication to reverse the effect of excess potassium (calcium), shift potassium into cells (insulin, sympathomimetics, and possibly sodium bicarbonate), and remove potassium from the body (sodium polystyrene sulfonate or diuretics). Arrange for emergency dialysis, and admit to the hospital.

ANALYSIS

Objectives

1. Recognize the clinical settings, signs and symptoms, and complications of hyperkalemia.

2. Understand the diagnostic and therapeutic approach to suspected hyperkalemia.

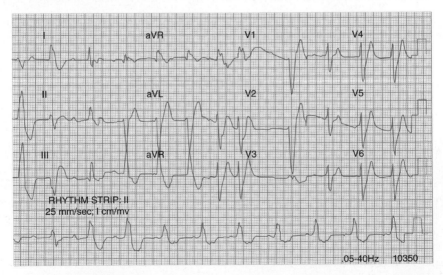

Figure 23–2. 12 Lead ECG.

Considerations

This patient has developed end-stage renal failure (also referred to as chronic kidney disease [CKD], stage 5), due to his longstanding HTN and diabetes. His damaged kidneys have very little capacity to excrete potassium. ACE inhibitor therapy contributes to his potassium retention. Acidosis and blunted insulin response both lead to potassium shifts into the extracellular space. His cardiac cell membranes are destabilized by the high-potassium level, and he is at high risk of death by arrhythmia. His weakness and general sense of illness, while non-specific and compatible with many illnesses, are very typical of untreated renal failure. Weakness can also be a prominent feature of severe hyperkalemia. It is important to suspect this condition from the history and ECG because labora-tory test results may be delayed and the patient could die before those test results become available.

Suppose you perform laboratory studies on this patient. In this case, the leu-kocyte count is 9000 cells/L, and the patient is mildly anemic with hemoglobin 10.5 g/dL and hematocrit 32%. Electrolytes show sodium of 134 mEq/L, potas-sium of 7.8 mEq/L, chloride of 101 mEq/L, and bicarbonate of 18 mEq/L. BUN is 114 mg/dL and creatinine is 10.5. The serum glucose is 180 mg/dL (10 mmol/L). The serum lipase, bilirubin, AST, ALT, and alkaline phosphatase are within normal limits. A 12-lead ECG confirms the wide-complex rhythm shown previously. His CXR shows mild cardiomegaly and pulmonary vascular congestion.

This clinical presentation is fairly representative of hyperkalemia in renal failure. Hyperkalemia is a common complication of advanced CKD, though it can occur in many other clinical conditions. Symptoms of hyperkalemia may be nonspecific or even nonexistent and are most often dominated by whatever ill-ness has predisposed the patient to elevated potassium. Morbidity and mortal-ity may result from delayed or inadequate treatment since severe hyperkalemia may rapidly progress to arrhythmia and cardiac arrest. Early suspicion, prompt recognition of associated ECG changes, and prompt resuscitation with effec-tive agents are essential. Once resuscitated, the patient will require emergent hemodialysis.

APPROACH TO:
Suspected Hyperkalemia

CLINICAL APPROACH

Hyperkalemia is a severe metabolic emergency. A delay in treatment may lead to death. Up to **one-quarter of patients with end-stage CKD will have at least one epi-sode of life-threatening hyperkalemia.** Hyperkalemia can occur from many other conditions, including medication side effects and medication errors, ingestion of potassium-containing supplements, crush injuries and burns, and redistribution resulting from acidotic states such as diabetic ketoacidosis. Many cases of hyperka-lemia are discovered as an incidental laboratory finding. Clinical findings associated with hyperkalemia are summarized in Table 23–1.

Table 23–1 • SYMPTOMS OF RENAL FAILURE AND HYPERKALEMIA		
	Hyperkalemia	Chronic Renal Failure
Fatigue	+	++
Weakness	++	+
Paresthesias	+	+
Paralysis	+	
Palpitations	+	
Anorexia, nausea, vomiting	+	+
Edema		+

Potassium Homeostasis

The body has a very large intracellular store of potassium, with the serum potassium representing only about 2% of the total body store of approximately 3500 mEq. The average diet contains about 100 mEq of potassium per day, and most is excreted in the urine, with a smaller amount excreted in the stool. Long-term balance is regulated in large part by the aldosterone system. **Renal excretion can be markedly affected by any impairment of kidney function and by a wide variety of medications.** Two common and potent inhibitors of renal potassium excretion are the **ACEIs and the potassium-sparing diuretics.** In the normal state, serum K level is tightly regulated to maintain appropriate gradients across cell membranes. Those gradients (most K intracellular, most Na extracellular) are in turn responsible for the electrical charge that makes action potentials possible. Potassium is actively transported into cells in exchange for sodium by Na-K-ATPase. Na-K-ATPase is a target of digitalis glycosides, so hyperkalemia is a prominent feature of severe digoxin poisoning. Potassium uptake into cells is stimulated by insulin and beta-adrenergic drugs. In states of increased hydrogen ion concentration (acidosis), potassium may shift out of cells. Also, potassium follows osmotic gradients, so hyperosmolar states (such as DKA and mannitol or dextrose infusions) may cause increased serum potassium.

Classification of Hyperkalemia

From a laboratory perspective, the normal range for serum potassium is 3.5-5.0 mEq/L. Levels from 5.1 to 5.5 mEq/L are generally not significant elevations. The range from 5.5 to 6.0 mEq/L is mild hyperkalemia, and significant ECG changes would be unusual. **Levels of 7.0 mEq/L or greater constitute severe hyperkalemia;** prompt aggressive treatment is almost always warranted, even if ECG changes are not severe. Although pseudohyperkalemia can result from hemolysis of the blood specimen prior to measurement, most clinical laboratories are attuned to this problem and will note hemolysis when it is detected.

ECG Changes of Hyperkalemia

One of the earliest ECG changes of hyperkalemia is a **"peaked" appearance to the T wave.** Unfortunately, there is no widely accepted scientific definition of a peaked T wave, though some authors have suggested imagining the T wave as a seat. If it is too pointed to sit upon comfortably, then it is likely peaked. Other changes of hyperkalemia include widening of the QRS, prolongation of the PR interval, QT prolongation, ST changes (which may mimic myocardial infarction), wide P waves or the disappearance of P waves. Severe hyperkalemia generally causes a very wide QRS, which may progress to a sine-wave pattern and asystole. A variety of blocks and dysrhythmias may also be seen.

Many textbooks describe a classic progression of ECG changes and attempt to correlate those changes with usual levels of potassium. It is vitally important to understand that this correlation is poor. **Patients may have severe hyperkalemia with minimal ECG changes or prominent ECG changes with mild hyperkalemia.** It is well described that patients with mild ECG changes may suddenly progress to severe changes, and a stepwise progression cannot be counted upon. Despite these caveats, the ECG remains the best available guide to the initial therapy of hyperkalemia.

Therapy

Intravenous calcium is first-line, lifesaving treatment. Calcium stabilizes cardiac cell membranes and can counteract hyperkalemia within seconds to minutes. Unfortunately, the effect is not sustained and fades within 10-20 minutes, so additional agents are required. Because of the short-lived effect and potential downsides of hypercalcemia, this author reserves calcium for patients who demonstrate ECG changes suggestive of hyperkalemia. Calcium should be given to all dialysis patients who are in cardiac arrest, as hyperkalemia is very frequently a contributing cause of the arrest. Historically, it was believed that calcium was contraindicated in potential digoxin toxicity because the heart might undergo a tetanic contraction from which the patient could not be resuscitated. This historical concern has not been supported by current science (see Table 23–2).

Calcium injection is available in two forms: calcium chloride and calcium gluconate. Calcium chloride contains approximately three times as much elemental calcium per unit volume and is considerably more caustic to soft tissue. Thus, general practice is to use calcium chloride for patients in cardiac arrest or near-arrest situations and calcium gluconate for patients with less severe ECG changes or who require prolonged infusion.

Table 23–2 • MEDICATIONS USED IN TREATMENT OF HYPERKALEMIA			
Medication	**Available Forms**	**Dose**	**Duration of Action**
Calcium	Calcium chloride 10% (14 mEq/10 mL) Calcium gluconate (4.65 mEq/10 mL)	10-20 mL slow IV 20-30 mL slow IV	Minutes
Sodium bicarbonate	44.6 mEq/50 mL	50-150 mL	Minutes-hour
Insulin	Regular	5-10 units IV	1-2 hours
Dextrose	50% dextrose in water	25-50 g	1-2 hours
Albuterol	5 mg/mL concentrate	10-20 mg nebulized	1-3 hours
SPSS (Kayexelate)	15 g/60 mL suspension	15-60 g q6h	Hours–days
Patiromer (Valtessa)	Powder for suspension	8.4-25.2 g daily	Days

Sodium bicarbonate given intravenously is a traditional second-line agent for hyperkalemia. It is thought to shift potassium into cells by reversing acidosis. It also raises extracellular sodium levels, which may have beneficial effects on membrane potentials. Considerable research has called into question the benefit of sodium bicarbonate. In animal studies using induced acidosis, no consistent K-lowering effect could be demonstrated. However, this may not be an adequate model of CKD patients, and even some nephrologists who have questioned the efficacy of bicarbonate continue to recommend it.

Insulin therapy is a mainstay in the acute management of hyperkalemia. Five to ten units of regular insulin given IV can reliably lower serum potassium approximately 0.5 mEq/L for 1-2 hours. Of course, this therapy can cause hypoglycemia, so the insulin is usually given with 25 g or 50 g of 50% dextrose. Some have advocated giving just the D50, expecting the patient's own insulin response to lower the potassium. However, many patients who experience hyperkalemia will be diabetic and may have impaired or absent insulin release. Furthermore, it has been shown in animal studies that large osmolar loads (such as a bolus of dextrose) may transiently *increase* serum potassium.

Albuterol, administered as an aerosol in doses of 10-20 mg, reliably lowers the serum potassium by an average of 0.5 mEq/L for 1-3 hours. The effect is additive with the effect of insulin. **Albuterol also reduces the incidence and severity of rebound hypoglycemia often seen after glucose and insulin therapy.** Albuterol has the advantage of requiring no IV access and therefore can be started quickly. Side effects of tremor and tachycardia may limit its use in some patients, especially those with severe cardiovascular disease. Note that this is a substantially higher dose than is typically used for the initial treatment of asthma.

Sodium polystyrene sulfonate (SPSS) (Kayexalate and others) is an ion-exchange resin that is usually administered orally. It can also be given rectally as an enema, but this is generally less effective and carries some risk of colon injury. SPSS exchanges sodium for potassium across the gut, so patients who are severely volume overloaded may not tolerate this therapy. Onset of action takes several hours. This medication is contraindicated in cases of ileus or suspected bowel obstruction or perforation. It is more effective for maintenance therapy than for acute management. Other binding agents such as patiromer (Veltassa) and sodium zirconium cyclosilicate show promise for maintenance therapy but do not yet have an established role in emergency management of hyperkalemia.

If the patient is not completely anuric, **diuresis** is a remarkably effective way to excrete large quantities of potassium. This will not be effective for the end-stage kidney disease patient who has been on dialysis for years, but it is appropriate for many patients with acute hyperkalemia due to dehydration, rhabdomyolysis, or medication effects. Once intravascular volume is restored with crystalloid, loop diuretics such as furosemide can be given to promote potassium excretion.

Dialysis is the ultimate treatment of choice for all kidney disease patients with significant hyperkalemia. However, it is time consuming and not always immediately available. Reliable vascular access and reasonably stable vital signs are prerequisites for hemodialysis, while the less-common peritoneal dialysis requires a peritoneal catheter.

> **CASE CORRELATION**
>
> - See also Case 5 (Diabetic Ketoacidosis), Case 21 (Nephrolithiasis), and Case 24 (Acute Pyelonephritis).

COMPREHENSION QUESTIONS

23.1 A 55-year-old man collapses pulseless and with a wide bizarre-looking rhythm. A dialysis fistula is present in the right arm. In addition to standard ACLS therapies, which of the following is most appropriate for this patient?

A. 25 g of 50% dextrose, IV push.

B. Sodium bicarbonate, 50-mL IV push.

C. Begin immediate hemodialysis.

D. Calcium chloride, 20-mL slow intravenous push.

23.2 A 45-year-old man is brought into the emergency center due to significant dehydration and weakness. His potassium level is noted to be 7.2 mEq/L. Which of the following statements is most accurate regarding his potassium level?

A. Hyperkalemia can usually be diagnosed by symptoms alone.

B. An ECG showing peaked T waves means the patient is stable and treatment can safely wait until laboratory results are obtained.

C. Hyperkalemia can mimic a myocardial infarction on the ECG.

D. Hyperkalemia is synonymous with kidney disease.

23.3 Which of the following statements is incorrect regarding treatment of hyperkalemia in patients with some renal function?

A. Administration of normal saline may hasten the excretion of potassium.

B. Administration of furosemide can hasten the excretion of potassium.

C. The combination of saline with a diuretic is often indicated because hyperkalemic patients are frequently dehydrated.

D. Patients with some preserved renal function do not need dialysis, even for severe hyperkalemia.

23.4 A patient with severe renal disease is found to have hyperkalemia with tall, peaked T waves on ECG. Vascular access cannot be readily obtained, but vital signs are stable. Which of the following would be appropriate temporizing measures?

A. Inhaled albuterol 2.5 mg in 3 mL saline

B. Oral sodium bicarbonate with rectal sodium polystyrene sulfonate

C. Inhaled albuterol 20 mg with oral sodium polystyrene sulfonate, 30 g

D. Oral dextrose 25 g

ANSWERS

23.1 **D.** Calcium is the only agent with rapid and reliable enough onset to potentially help this patient. Bicarbonate might be appropriate, but its onset is slower than calcium and its effect is more disputed. Dialysis requires a hemodynamically stable patient. If the patient is resuscitated, dextrose and insulin will be important in the ongoing management of hyperkalemia.

23.2 **C.** The ST-segment and T-wave changes of hyperkalemia may mimic the ECG appearance of myocardial infarction. The nonspecific symptoms typical of hyperkalemia are also often seen in patients with MI, particularly elderly patients. Peaked T waves indicate that the heart is significantly affected by hyperkalemia and the patient should not be considered stable. Many conditions and medications may cause hyperkalemia, not just renal failure.

23.3 **D.** Dialysis is the definitive therapy for hyperkalemia. Patients who have residual kidney function can sometimes be managed without resorting to dialysis, but it should always be available for those who fail to respond quickly. Severe dehydration is fairly common in the scenario of the elderly patient "found down" for an unknown period. Such dehydration may promote potassium retention by the kidneys, as well as potassium shifts from acidosis and ischemia of vital organs.

23.4 **C.** High-dose inhaled albuterol (10-20 mg) can reliably lower serum potassium with reasonable safety. SPSS can remove potassium through the GI tract, but its effect is slow. Rectal administration is falling out of favor due to risk of colon injury. Oral dextrose and oral bicarbonate have no role in emergency management. Standard 2.5 mg doses of albuterol have too slight an effect on potassium levels.

CLINICAL PEARLS

▶ In a patient with known or suspected renal failure, ECG changes consistent with hyperkalemia should be treated immediately as a life-threatening emergency. Do not await laboratory confirmation.

▶ The ECG findings of hyperkalemia can progress very rapidly and do not reliably pass through all the stages of the "typical" textbook presentation.

▶ Intravenous calcium is the antidote of choice for life-threatening arrhythmias related to hyperkalemia, but its effect is brief and additional agents must be used.

▶ Symptoms of renal failure and hyperkalemia are usually nonspecific, so risk factors must be used to suspect the diagnosis.

▶ Dialysis is the definitive therapy for hyperkalemia, though patients who have residual kidney function can sometimes be managed without resorting to dialysis.

REFERENCES

Evans KJ, Greenberg A. Hyperkalemia: a review. *J Intensive Care Med.* 2005;20(5):272-290.

Kamel KS, Wei C. Controversial issues in the treatment of hyperkalaemia. *Nephrol Dial Transplant.* 2003;18:2215-2218.

Levine M, Nikkanen H, Pallin DJ. The effects of intravenous calcium in patients with digoxin toxicity. *J Emerg Med.* 2011;40(1):41-46.

Mahoney BA, Smith WA, Lo DS, Tsoi K, Tonelli M, Clase CM. Emergency interventions for hyperkalaemia. *Cochrane Database Syst Rev.* 2005;(2):CD003235.

Sood MM, Sood AR, Richardson R. Emergency management and commonly encountered outpatient scenarios in patients with hyperkalemia. *Mayo Clin Proc.* 2007;82(12):1553-1561.

Sterns RH, Grieff M, Bernstein PL. Treatment of hyperkalemia: something old, something new. *Kidney Int.* 2016;89(3):546-54. doi: 10.1016/j.kint.2015.11.018. Epub 2016 Feb 2.

Watson M, Abbott KC, Yuan CM. Damned if you do, damned if you don't: potassium binding resins in hyperkalemia. *Clin J Am Soc Nephrol.* 2010;5(10):1723-1726.

A 24-year-old woman presents to the emergency department (ED) with complaints of flank pain and fever for the last 1-2 days. She describes feeling pain with urination over the previous week. She is currently feeling febrile and nauseated but has not vomited. The pain in her right flank is a dull, constant, nonradiating ache that she rates as 5/10 for pain. She took 600 mg of ibuprofen last night to help her sleep, but this morning the pain persisted, so she came into the ED for evaluation. She reports that she is sexually active and that her last menstrual period was 1 week ago. She denies any vaginal discharge or abdominal pain. Her vital signs include a temperature of 38.3°C (101°F), heart rate of 112 beats per minute, respiratory rate of 15 breaths per minute, and blood pressure of 119/68 mm Hg. Her examination is significant for tenderness to palpation on her right costovertebral angle (CVA).

▶ What is the most likely diagnosis?
▶ What is the best treatment?

ANSWERS TO CASE 24:

Acute Pyelonephritis

Summary: This otherwise healthy young woman presents with dysuria, flank pain, fever, and nausea. She is febrile, tachycardic, and has CVA tenderness.

- **Most likely diagnosis:** Urinary tract infection (UTI) complicated by pyelonephritis. This should be confirmed with a urinalysis.

- **Treatment:** Antibiotics, hydration, analgesia, antipyretics, and exclusion of other pathology.

ANALYSIS

Objectives

1. Recognize the clinical signs and symptoms of UTIs.

2. Understand the diagnosis and treatment of UTIs.

3. Understand the spectrum of UTIs and their variable treatment.

Considerations

Urinary tract infections are a spectrum of diseases that can affect any part of the urinary system. They are second only to respiratory tract infections as problems encountered by emergency physicians. Individuals who present to the ED with genitourinary complaints often warrant a rapid but thorough history and physical examination. This patient presentation (ie, dysuria, flank pain, nausea, and fever) is consistent with **acute pyelonephritis,** an **infection of the renal parenchyma.** Generally, the clinical features of acute pyelonephritis **include fever, chills, dysuria, and flank and CVA pain.** Patients may feel **nauseated** and **vomit.** The initial workup includes assessing the patient stability and immediately addressing any life threats. As the workup proceeds, the patient should receive an antipyretic (eg, acetaminophen) and intravenous fluids for hydration.

The differential diagnosis for patients with urinary complaints is broad and includes cystitis, pyelonephritis, urethritis, and vaginitis. In addition, patients who exhibit signs of systemic involvement (eg, fever) should be evaluated for other pathologies, including ectopic pregnancy, perforated viscous, infected kidney stone, appendicitis, pancreatitis, colitis, and pneumonia. A good history and physical examination will help the physician narrow down these possibilities.

Laboratory studies are helpful in confirming the diagnosis. A urinalysis typically reveals leukocytes, red blood cells, and bacteria. A **urine culture is essential to guide antibiotic therapy.** Blood cultures should be obtained if the patient has a fever. A complete blood count, electrolytes, and renal function studies are also recommended. Patients with suspected pyelonephritis typically do not require imaging studies. However, patients who clinically exhibit pyelonephritis but whose urinalysis is negative, as well as patients with a suspected urinary obstruction, should undergo imaging. In the ED, this is usually an ultrasound or contrast-enhanced CT scan. **Supportive care** consists of **IV hydration, analgesia, antipyretics, and antiemetics.** In uncomplicated acute pyelonephritis, patients can receive a **10- to 14-day course of oral antibiotics** (eg, fluoroquinolone) and be discharged home. In more **severe cases,** patients should be **admitted to the hospital** and receive **intravenous antibiotics.**

APPROACH TO:
Urinary Tract Infections

DEFINITIONS

DYSURIA: Painful urination.

CYSTITIS: Inflammation of the urinary bladder that generally results in dysuria, urinary frequency, urgency, and suprapubic pain.

ACUTE PYELONEPHRITIS: Inflammation of the kidney secondary to a UTI of the renal parenchyma and collecting system. It typically presents as the clinical syndrome of fever, chills, and flank pain.

BACTERIURIA: Presence of bacteria in the urine.

HEMATURIA: Blood in the urine, which may be micro- or macroscopic.

PYURIA: Pus in the urine.

UNCOMPLICATED UTI: An infection of a structurally and functionally normal urinary tract that is generally eradicated by a 3- to 5-day course of antibiotics.

COMPLICATED UTI: An infection in patients with underlying immunological, structural, or neurological disease that diminishes the efficacy of standard antimicrobial therapy.

URETHRITIS: Inflammation of the urethra.

CLINICAL APPROACH

UTIs are a common diagnosis in the ED. They can range from simple cystitis to pyelonephritis resulting in sepsis and shock. Urinary tract infections affect women more commonly than men. However, in children, boys are affected more commonly until 1 year of age. Urinary tract infections in children warrant further sonographic evaluation of the urinary tract to rule out congenital anomalies. The lifetime prevalence of UTIs is estimated to be 14,000 per 100,000 men and 53,000 per 100,000 women.

UTIs can be divided into **lower tract (urethra and bladder) and upper tract (ureters and kidneys)** infections. The symptoms of lower infections are localized and are commonly crampy suprapubic pain, dysuria, foul-smelling or dark-colored urine, hematuria, urinary frequency, and urgency. Patients with upper-tract infections usually appear more ill and are more likely to have abnormal vital signs and systemic symptoms (eg, fever, chills, nausea, and vomiting). It is important to distinguish lower- from upper-tract infections since the treatments differ vastly, as will be discussed later.

Commonly, the infecting organism gains access to the urinary tract by direct entry from the urethra. The human body has many defenses against UTIs, including frequent urinary flow, urine urea concentration and acidification, and urethral epithelial lining. The normal periurethral flora includes the bacteria *lactobacillus* that provides a symbiotic protective mechanism. The perirectal area and the vagina are both potential sites of bacterial colonization and are in much closer proximity to the urethral meatus in women. The female urethra is also much shorter than in males and brings the urethral meatus in closer proximity to the bladder, thus increasing the risk of infection by external organisms. A UTI in a man is usually the result of benign prostatic hypertrophy, kidney stones that become infected, urethral instrumentation (surgery or catheterization), or immunocompromised states.

Care should be taken to exclude other etiologies in patients who present with urinary complaints. Cervicitis, vulvovaginitis, and pelvic inflammatory diseases are important conditions to exclude in women and are more likely to present with discharge, lack of bacteria on urinalysis, and lack of urinary frequency and urgency. In considering these diagnoses, the patient should undergo a pelvic examination. Sampling with DNA probes for gonococcus and *Chlamydia* should be obtained, a wet mount slide examination performed, and treatment for these conditions considered. Pregnancy should also be considered and tested for in all women of reproductive age with any urinary symptoms. In men, urethritis and prostatitis should be excluded before the diagnosis of cystitis or pyelonephritis is confirmed.

UTIs are typically caused by a single bacterial species. **Eighty percent of infections are caused by *Escherichia coli*, a gram-negative rod.** *Staphylococcus saprophyticus* is the second most common cause of UTI and is common in young women. Other organisms include *Proteus*, *Klebsiella*, *Enterococci*, and *Pseudomonas*. The identification of an exact organism is rarely indicated in the ED. The "gold standard" of quantitative culture takes several days but will significantly assist in treatment if the patient is being admitted to the hospital or failed outpatient therapy.

Major risk factors for women aged 16-35 years include sexual intercourse, pregnancy, bladder catheterization, and diaphragm usage. Later in life, additional risk factors include gynecologic surgery and bladder prolapse. In both sexes, conditions resulting in urinary stasis increase with age, as does the incidence of UTIs. Benign prostatic hypertrophy is a major risk factor in older men.

Laboratory Studies

The **mainstay in the diagnosis of a UTI is urinalysis and culture.** Collection of sterile urine is critical because a contaminated specimen can result in a false-positive urinalysis. Suprapubic aspiration and catheterization provide the best samples; however, both are invasive and uncomfortable to the patient. Clean catch urine sample, obtained by the patient collecting urine in midstream, is standard and provides an

Table 24–1 • URINALYSIS SENSITIVITY AND SPECIFICITY		
Diagnostic Test	Sensitivity (%)	Specificity (%)
Leukocyte esterase	83 (67-94)	78 (64-92)
Nitrite	53 (15-82)	98 (90-100)
LE or N	93 (90-100)	72 (58-91)
WBCs	73 (32-100)	81 (45-98)

Abbreviations: LE = leukocyte esterase; N = nitrite; WBCs = white blood cells.

adequate sample if done properly. In children, "bag" urine collection, by placing a bag over the perineum, should be avoided due to the high rates of contamination. Condom catheterization collection of urine is not acceptable for urinalysis due to the contact of the male glans to the collection vessel. Typically, contaminated urine will exhibit cellular elements (eg, epithelial cells) and should not be used to determine the presence of a UTI.

Urinalysis can include urine dipstick testing, urine microscopy, and urine culture with sensitivities. Table 24–1 lists the sensitivity and specificity of different components of the urinalysis.

Urine dipstick Urine dipsticks test urine for infection by measuring two specific entities: leukocyte esterase, a compound released by white blood cell breakdown in the urinary tract, and nitrite, a compound produced by the reduction of dietary nitrates by some gram-negative bacteria (eg, *E. coli*).

Urine microscopy It examines the urine for white blood cells, bacteria, and other visible structures. Classically, the criteria for diagnosis of UTI on microscopy include the presence of more than five leukocytes or red blood cells per high-powered field or 2+ bacteria. Microscopic criteria are highly debated, and the presence of WBCs, RBCs, and bacteria should be used in conjunction with clinical presentation to confirm the diagnosis of a UTI.

Urine culture Diagnosis and treatment of a UTI based on the urinalysis (UA) result is presumptive, as the true diagnosis requires a culture with greater than (10×5)/mL colony count. ED urine cultures should be sent on high-risk populations, including infants and children. Cultures are also obtained in the elderly, adult men, pregnant women, individuals with comorbid illness, or those who failed initial antimicrobial therapy. Gram staining of the urine can also be helpful but is not routinely indicated.

Imaging

The majority of patients with urinary complaints do not require imaging in the ED. However, it is indicated in certain clinical settings. Patients who exhibit clinical signs or symptoms of a urinary infection but have a negative urinalysis, those with a suspected urogenital obstruction, and those with complicated UTIs often require imaging studies. In addition, first episodes of UTIs in girls younger than 4 years and in men should undergo an imaging study.

Imaging of the urinary tract consists of ultrasound, computed tomography (CT) scans, intravenous pyelography (IVP), and radionucleotide scans. Ultrasound testing is an acceptable initial study in the ED because it is quick, noninvasive, and can detect many abnormalities, including perinephric abscess, hydroureter, urinary tract stone, pyelonephritis, and congenital anomalies. CT scans are more sensitive at detecting these abnormalities but expose the patient to higher levels of radiation and often require the administration of IV contrast. IVP and radionucleotide scans are generally not performed during ED evaluation and are reserved for inpatient or outpatient workups.

Treatment

The correct choice of antibiotic can be difficult for the emergency physician. There are many factors that affect this decision, including patient drug allergies, bacterial susceptibility, community versus hospital flora, local antibiotic resistance rates, the presence of medical comorbidities, as well as the patient ability to pay for the prescription. Table 24–2 lists the most commonly used antibiotics for the treatment of UTIs.

Patients with **uncomplicated cystitis** are treated as outpatients. Antibiotic choices must be effective against *E. coli* and include trimethoprim-sulfamethoxazole (TMP-SMX), amoxicillin/clavulanate, nitrofurantoin, ciprofloxacin, and levofloxacin. Typically, patients are treated for 3-5 days. Longer therapy generally offers no benefit. However, in patients with suspected subclinical upper-tract infection, communities with high resistance rates, extremes of age, and comorbidities, a longer course (ie, 7-10 days) is recommended. For symptomatic relief, physicians often prescribe phenazopyridine, a drug that concentrates in the urine and often relieves the pain and irritation of urination. The drug causes a distinct color change in the urine, typically to a dark orange to reddish color. Phenazopyridine is contraindicated in patients with glucose-6-phosphate dehydrogenase deficiency because it can lead to drug-induced hemolysis of red blood cells.

Uncomplicated pyelonephritis can be treated in the outpatient setting, provided the patient can tolerate oral medications, has mild symptoms, gets good follow-up,

Table 24–2 • UTI TYPES AND TREATMENT CHOICES		
Infection Type	Dosing Regimen	Considerations
Lower uncomplicated	TMP-SMX DS 1 tab bid for 3-5 days Ciprofloxacin 250 mg bid for 3-5 days Nitrofurantoin sustained-release 100 mg bid for 3-5 days Amoxicillin/clavulanate 875/125 mg bid for 3-5 days	No culture indicated[a] Tailor to community susceptibilities
Upper uncomplicated or complicated lower	Ciprofloxacin 500 mg bid for 7-14 days Nitrofurantoin sustained-release 100 mg bid for 7-14 days Amoxicillin/clavulanate 875/125 mg bid for 7-14 days	Cultures recommended Admit if severe

[a]*Due to increasing resistance patterns, urine culture should be considered.*

Table 24–3 • ADMISSION CRITERIA FOR PYELONEPHRITIS
Sepsis/shock (consider intensive care setting)
Inability to tolerate oral antibiotics
Obstruction of the urogenital (UG) tract
Pregnant
Extremes of age
Failed outpatient management
Immunocompromised host
Inadequate follow-up/poor social setting

and is not pregnant. TMP-SMX, amoxicillin/clavulanate, or a fluoroquinolone antibiotic should be prescribed for 10-14 days. All pregnant patients with pyelonephritis require admission (see Table 24–3).

Complicated pyelonephritis requires admission and IV antibiotics. The antibiotic choices are TMP-SMX, ceftriaxone, gentamycin (with or without ampicillin), and fluoroquinolones. In more severe cases where urosepsis or a resistant organism is suspected, cefepime, ampicillin plus tobramycin, or piperacillin-tazobactam may be indicated.

All children and men who are discharged with the diagnosis of UTI require urological follow-up to assess for underlying anatomical abnormalities. Adults with complicated UTIs also need follow-up and evaluation of the genitourinary system.

Pregnant patients require special attention. Simple, asymptomatic bacteriuria **necessitates treatment** due to the **increased risk of preterm labor, perinatal mortality, and maternal pyelonephritis.** It is important that the bacteriuria is eliminated despite the patient being clinically asymptomatic. First-line agents include penicillins (eg, amoxicillin and ampicillin) and cephalosporins. Fluoroquinolones and tetracyclines are contraindicated, as they are known teratogens. Admission should be considered in patients in their third trimester, patients with suspected pyelonephritis, and those who cannot tolerate fluids by mouth.

Some patients require chronic placement of **indwelling catheters,** which serve as a nidus for infection. Treatment of asymptomatic bacteriuria in these patients is not indicated because frequent antibiotic administration results in increased microorganism resistance. Generally, removal of the catheter results in elimination of bacteria. Symptomatic patients who cannot be without the catheter should be treated with antibiotics, have the catheter replaced, and be considered for admission to the hospital due to the high risk for systemic infection.

CASE CORRELATION

- See also Case 16 (Acute Abdominal Pain), Case 21 (Nephrolithiasis), and Case 31 (Lower Back Pain).

COMPREHENSION QUESTIONS

24.1 A 64-year-old woman is brought to the ED by her family for mental status changes. She has multiple sclerosis and self-catheterizes for urine. The family reports that over the past several days she has not been feeling well. They state that the patient vomited that day and was behaving bizarrely. Her vital signs are blood pressure of 83/38 mm Hg, heart rate of 135 beats per minute, respirations of 26 breaths per minute, and rectal temperature of 38.8°C (101.9°F). After a history and physical examination, which of the following is the most appropriate next step in management?

A. Obtain a urinalysis and culture

B. Start broad-spectrum antibiotics

C. Perform a lumbar puncture

D. Establish IV access and place the patient on a cardiac monitor

E. Discharge the patient after close follow-up is arranged

24.2 A 34-year-old woman complains of mild crampy suprapubic abdominal pain, dysuria, and urinary frequency for the last 3 days. She has no fever. Her blood pressure is 125/70 mm Hg, heart rate is 88 beats per minute, respiratory rate is 16 breaths per minute, and temperature is 36.8°C (98.3°F). She has no significant past medical history and is able to drink oral fluids with difficulty. She has a clean-catch urinalysis that reveals 2+ leukocyte esterase, 1+ nitrite, 1+ blood, and 2+ bacteria. Her beta-hCG is negative. Which of the following organisms is most likely responsible for her presentation?

A. *Klebsiella* spp

B. *E. coli*

C. *Pseudomonas aeruginosa*

D. *Proteus mirabilis*

E. *Enterobacter* spp

24.3 A 24-year-old woman presents to the ED for painful urination over the last 2 days that is associated with urinary urgency. She states that she is pregnant and the fetus is at 12-weeks' gestational age as measured by ultrasound. On examination, she is well appearing and sitting comfortably in bed. Her blood pressure is 115/70 mm Hg, heart rate is 81 beats per minute, respiratory rate is 16 breaths per minute, and temperature is 37.2°C (98.9°F). A urinalysis reveals 5 WBC/mm^3, 1+ leukocyte esterase, and 1+ bacteria. The urine is negative for nitrite and blood. As you return to the patient bed to tell her the results, she states that her pain has resolved, she is urinating without difficulty, and she wants to go home. Which of the following is the most appropriate course of management?

A. Admit the patient for intravenous antibiotics.

B. Discharge the patient with a prescription for antibiotics and tell her to fill the prescription only if the culture results are positive.

C. Ask the patient to undergo another examination to evaluate for gonorrhea and *Chlamydia*.

D. Administer a dose of ciprofloxacin in the ED and have the patient call the hospital to find out her culture results.

E. Prescribe the patient nitrofurantoin for 5-7 days and have her follow-up with her obstetrician.

24.4 A 65-year-old man with hypertension and benign prostatic hyperplasia (BPH) presents to the ED with urinary retention and a UTI on a catheterized urine analysis. He was evaluated by the urologist and is being discharged home with an in-dwelling Foley catheter and follow-up in the urology clinic in 1 week. Which of the following is the most appropriate antibiotic for this patient?

A. TMP-SMX bid for 3 days

B. Nitrofurantoin 100 mg for 14 days

C. Amoxicillin 100 mg tid for 14 days

D. Ciprofloxacin 500 mg bid for 14 days

E. Levofloxacin 250 mg qd for 3 days

24.5 Which of the following patients with pyelonephritis can be safely discharged home with close follow-up?

A. A 23-year-old woman in her second trimester of pregnancy

B. A 13-year-old woman who cannot tolerate her diet despite antiemetics

C. An 88-year-old man with urinary retention and dehydration

D. A 67-year-old woman with 3+ bacteria, a sulfa allergy, and a history of lupus

E. A 44-year-old woman with a kidney stone and hydroureter on CT scan

ANSWERS

24.1 **D.** This woman may indeed have a UTI; however, her vital signs are unstable. The mainstay of treatment in emergency medicine is to first address the patient airway, breathing, and circulation (ABCs). This patient is hypotensive (BP 83/38 mm Hg). The first step in her management is placing an IV line and administering fluids. She should also be placed on a cardiac monitor to monitor her blood pressure, heart rate, and rhythm. Once her ABCs are addressed, laboratory studies should be obtained, including a urinalysis and culture. She should also receive broad-spectrum antibiotics and an antipyretic. This patient may need a lumbar puncture, but not until her ABCs are addressed. This patient requires admission to the hospital.

24.2 **B.** *E. coli* is the infecting organism in more than 80% of all UTIs. All of the other choices cause UTIs but are less common. *S. saprophyticus* is a common organism in young, sexually active women. In hospitalized or nursing home patients, *Pseudomonas* spp and *Staphylococcus* spp are frequent pathogens. Lactobacilli are normal urethral flora and are not considered a causative organism. Complicated UTIs are more likely to be caused by other organisms.

24.3 **E.** The patient is pregnant and has evidence of a UTI on the urinalysis. Pregnant patients are at high risk for preterm labor and perinatal mortality if a urinary infection goes untreated. Therefore, this patient should receive a 5-7 days course of nitrofurantoin or a penicillin-based antibiotic and follow-up with her obstetrician. The patient does not need to be admitted to the hospital for intravenous antibiotics. This would likely be the case if she were diagnosed with pyelonephritis. The patient should not wait for culture results and delay receiving her antibiotics. It is important to eradicate the bacteriuria as quickly as possible. This patient does not report the symptoms of gonorrhea or *Chlamydia* (eg, vaginal discharge) at this time and does not require further evaluation for these conditions. Fluoroquinolones (eg, ciprofloxacin) are contraindicated in pregnant patients due to the risk of fetal abnormalities (eg, tendon maldevelopment).

24.4 **D.** Men with UTIs automatically fit into the "complicated" variety of UTIs. Therefore, the most appropriate therapy is ciprofloxacin for 14 days. With the exception of amoxicillin as monotherapy, all of the above choices are appropriate for treatment of certain types of UTIs. Complicated UTIs mandate 14 days of therapy with an appropriate antibiotic. The emergency physician should also consider sending urine cultures on this patient and provide good follow-up. Patients with benign prostatic hypertrophy or other lower urinary tract obstructions may be discharged with a Foley catheter if they have good follow-up, understand how to manage their catheter, and have no significant medical comorbidities.

24.5 **D.** Despite a chronic medical condition, this patient may be safely discharged home. Because this patient has a sulfa allergy, TMP-SMX should not be administered. Other treatment options include quinolones, amoxicillin/clavulanate, and nitrofurantoin. All of the other patients should be admitted for treatment. All pregnant patients with pyelonephritis require admission. The 13-year-old and 88-year-old are not tolerating their diet and require intravenous hydration. The 44-year-old has a urinary obstruction with a UTI, which makes it a complicated UTI. These patients are at high risk for developing sepsis. For most admitted patients, urine cultures should be sent to guide antibiotic therapy.

CLINICAL PEARLS

▶ All UTIs in men are considered complicated.

▶ The definitive diagnosis of a UTI is made on urine culture from a noncontaminated urine sample.

▶ Care should be taken to exclude other etiologies, such as cervicitis, vulvovaginitis, and pelvic inflammatory disease in female patients who present with urinary complaints.

▶ All pregnant patients with bacteriuria require antibiotic treatment to prevent complications.

▶ Patients with a UTI and an obstructed kidney stone are at high risk for morbidity and require urgent urologic consultation.

▶ Antibiotic therapy should be tailored to the type of UTI, the community resistance rates, and the patient's ability to tolerate the medications.

REFERENCES

Askew K. Urinary tract infections and hematuria. In: Tintinalli JE, Stapczynski JS, Cline DM, Ma OJ, Cydulka RK, Meckler GD, eds. *Tintinalli's Emergency Medicine: A Comprehensive Study Guide.* 8th ed. New York, NY: McGraw-Hill; 2015.

Ban KM, Easter JS. Selected urologic problems. In: Marx JA, Hockberger RS, Walls RM, eds. *Rosen's Emergency Medicine: Concepts and Clinical Practice.* 8th ed. Philadelphia, PA: Mosby Elsevier; 2013.

Dielubanza EJ, Schaeffer AJ. Urinary tract infections in women. *Med Clin N Am.* 2011;95:27-41.

Lane DR, Takhar SS. Diagnosis and management of urinary tract infection and pyelonephritis. *Emerg Med Clin N Am.* 2011;29:539-552.

Nicolle LE. Uncomplicated urinary tract infection in adults including uncomplicated pyelonephritis. *Urol Clin N Am.* 2008;35:1-12.

Schrock JW, Reznikova S, Weller S. The effect of an observation unit on the rate of ED admission and discharge for pyelonephritis. *Am J Emerg Med.* 2010;26:682-688.

A 76-year-old nursing home patient is transferred to the emergency department (ED) for reported altered mental status (AMS). He is confused and unable to provide any relevant information about his condition. According to EMS, he has been in the nursing home since he fractured his tibia 4 weeks ago. He has a past medical history of hypertension, diabetes mellitus, and chronic obstructive pulmonary disease (COPD).

His vital signs are BP 150/90 mm Hg, HR 110 beats per minute, RR 20 breaths per minute, T 36.7°C, and oxygen saturation of 92% on 4 L by nasal cannula. On physical examination, the patient appears sleepy but is arousable to verbal stimuli. He is having difficulty following directions and appears confused. His pupils are 4 mm, equal and reactive. His mucous membranes appear dry. He is tachycardic, and his lung sounds are clear and equal bilaterally. His abdomen is soft and nontender. There is a cast on his left lower extremity. The capillary refill in his toes is less than 2 seconds. He has strong femoral pulses. He has poor skin turgor and there is tenting. His motor and sensory examinations are normal.

Laboratory results include a WBC 12 cells/mm³ and hemoglobin 10 mg/dL. His sodium is 110 mEq/L, potassium 4.1 mEq/L, BUN 52 mg/dL, creatinine 1.0 mg/dL, magnesium 1.7 mEq/L, and glucose 125 mg/dL. His urine drug screen is positive for opiates and benzodiazepines. His urinalysis is negative for infection.

▶ What is the most likely diagnosis?
▶ What is the best management?

ANSWERS TO CASE 25:

Altered Mental Status

Summary: This is a 76-year-old man from a nursing home with a history of hypertension, diabetes mellitus, and COPD. He presents to the ED with AMS. He has limited mobility due to a cast on his left lower leg secondary to a tibia fracture. His examination reveals dehydration, and lab tests are consistent with significant hyponatremia and prerenal azotemia.

- **Most likely diagnosis:** Electrolyte abnormality (hyponatremia and uremia) secondary to deconditioning and dehydration.

- **Next step in management:** Intravenous fluid hydration (0.9% normal saline) and consideration of hypertonic saline.

ANALYSIS

Objectives

- Recognize the diversity in presentation of patients with AMS and understand the diagnostic approach.

- Know the appropriate workup for patients and initial management of patients with AMS.

Considerations

This is a 76-year-old man who presents to the ED from a nursing home. The presentation of AMS in a nursing home patient should elicit concerns for underlying **infection** (eg, pneumonia, meningitis, and UTI), **electrolyte and metabolic abnormalities** (eg, hypoglycemia, hyperglycemia, hyponatremia, and uremia), **endocrine abnormalities** (eg, hypothyroidism and adrenal crisis), **intracranial pathology** (eg, CVA and subdural hemorrhage), **polypharmacy** (eg, benzodiazepines, sedatives, opiates, and anticholinergics), **delirium,** and **hypoxia.** It is important to keep in mind other common causes of AMS, such as **intoxication** and **withdrawal syndromes.**

Once the patient's airway, breathing, and circulation (ABCs) are addressed, the first step in management is to **obtain a capillary blood glucose to rule out hypoglycemia.** The patient appears dehydrated; therefore, an electrolyte panel should be sent to the lab immediately and intravenous fluids (0.9% normal saline) started for resuscitation.

APPROACH TO:

Altered Mental Status

DEFINITIONS

DELIRIUM: Global disturbance in consciousness and cognition, with an inability to relate to the environment and process sensory input that is not better explained by preexisting or evolving dementia.

DEMENTIA: Progressive, irreversible decline in mental function affecting judgment, memory, reasoning, and comprehension.

AGITATION: Excessive restlessness.

OBTUNDED: Level of diminished arousal or awareness, frequently from extraneous causes (eg, infection, intoxication, and metabolic states).

STUPOR: Level of decreased responsiveness in which an individual requires aggressive or unpleasant stimulation.

COMA: Severe alteration of consciousness from which one cannot be aroused.

CLINICAL APPROACH

AMS and confusion are estimated to occur in 2% of all ED patients, 10% of all hospitalized patients, and 50% of elderly hospitalized patients. The phrase "altered mental status" generally refers to a change from an individual's "normal" mental state. This may reflect a change in behavior, speech, comprehension level, judgment, mood, or level of consciousness. Changes in mental status should be thought of in three classes: organic, functional (or psychiatric), and mixed disorders. Organic causes have a pathological basis primarily with a systemic or metabolic root; however, structural lesions in the central nervous system or vasculature must also be considered. Functional or psychiatric diseases do not have a clearly defined physiologic foundation.

The reticular activating system (RAS) is physiologically responsible for our level of arousal. Signals from the RAS run through the pons in the brainstem, through the thalami, and then project to both cerebral hemispheres. Any disruption in this pathway will lead to a decreased level of arousal. Examples of this include chemical depression via endogenous or exogenous agents or via structural abnormalities, such as decreased blood flow causing cerebral ischemia.

The evaluation of a patient with AMS can be a diagnostic challenge, and a **complete history** and **physical examination** (Table 25–1) is imperative to the workup. Because the patient often cannot provide a reliable history, it is important **to obtain information from all available sources** (eg, family, friends, bystanders, and nursing home staff). EMS may be able to provide clues by describing the scene from where they transported the patient (eg, an empty pill vial on scene). Family may be able to describe recent illnesses or concerns and the patient's baseline mental status, and they may be able to confirm when the patient was last seen normal.

Assessing the patient's ABCs and quickly recognizing and managing reversible causes of AMS (eg, hypoglycemia and hypoxia) are critical steps in early management. The severity of illness must be quickly assessed, and any life-threatening issues must be rapidly addressed (Table 25–2). Once the ABCs are addressed and stabilized, a systemic approach guided by the history and physical examination should be used to develop a differential diagnosis and treatment plan. The mental state examination screening tool or Quick Confusion Scale (QCS) can be used to gauge mental status. These instruments are 4-7 questions that can be used in reassessment to monitor change in mental status.

Special consideration must be given to the **pediatric and geriatric** populations. Seizures with prolonged postictal states, head injuries, and accidental ingestions are common causes for AMS in the pediatric population. In the geriatric population, a change in mental status may occur concomitant with existing dementia. In elderly patients who are confused and forgetful, understanding the differences between dementia and delirium is critical (Table 25–3). Electrolyte abnormalities

Table 25–1 • PHYSICAL EXAMINATION FINDINGS SUGGESTING MEDICAL CONCERNS FOR ALTERED MENTAL STATUS	
Blood pressure	**Neurologic (motor/sensory) findings**
• *Significant hypertension* Hypertensive encephalopathy, increased intracranial pressure, thyrotoxicosis, intracranial hemorrhage, eclampsia, toxicologic (eg, sympathomimetic, serotonin syndrome) • *Significant hypotension* Septic shock, cardiogenic shock, neurogenic shock, medication reaction, myocardial infarction	• *Focal motor or sensory deficit* Stroke, space-occupying lesion, hypoglycemia, Todd's paralysis (postictal), Wernicke encephalopathy • *Asterixis* Hepatic failure, uremia, other metabolic derangements • *Rigidity* Neuroleptic malignant syndrome • *New pupil asymmetry or fixed pupils* Stroke, space-occupying lesions • *Bilaterally pinpoint pupils* Toxicologic etiology (eg, opioids, clonidine, organophosphates), pontine stroke • *Bilaterally dilated pupils* Toxicologic etiology (eg, sympathomimetic, anticholinergic, hallucinogens) • *Breath odor* Acetone—ketoacidosis, toxic ingestion; Fetor hepaticus—hepatic encephalopathy; ethanol—ethanol or other volatile intoxication
Pulse	**Funduscopic examination**
• *Bradycardia* Toxicologic (eg, beta-blockers, calcium channel blockers), increased intracranial pressure, hypothyroidism • *Tachycardia* Toxicologic (eg, tricyclic antidepressants, sympathomimetic, anticholinergic), sepsis, thyrotoxicosis, decreased cardiac output, withdrawal syndromes, hypoxia, hypoglycemia	• *Papilledema or retinal hemorrhage* Space-occupying lesion, hypertensive encephalopathy, subarachnoid hemorrhage
Respiration	**Neck**
• *Hypoventilation* Toxicologic (eg, opioids, barbiturates, benzodiazepines), stroke, increased intracranial pressure, COPD, CO_2 retention • *Hyperventilation* Thyrotoxicosis, ASA overdose, acidosis, sepsis, CHF, COPD	• *Nuchal rigidity or other meningeal signs with or without fever* CNS infection, subarachnoid hemorrhage

Continued

Table 25–1 • PHYSICAL EXAMINATION FINDINGS SUGGESTING MEDICAL CONCERNS FOR ALTERED MENTAL STATUS *Continued*	
Temperature • *Fever/hyperpyrexia* CNS infection, urinary tract infection, skin infection, sepsis, toxicologic (eg, anticholinergic, salicylate, sympathomimetic, neuroleptic malignant syndrome, serotonin syndrome, withdrawal), stroke, heat stroke, thyrotoxicosis • *Hypothermia* Sepsis, toxicologic (eg, alcohol, barbiturates), hypothyroidism, hypoglycemia	**Abdominal** • *Ascites/hepatomegaly* Hepatic encephalopathy, spontaneous bacterial peritonitis, HIV, hepatitis
General appearance • *Signs of head trauma or occult hematoma* Intracranial hemorrhage (consider occult signs like hemotympanum, retinal hemorrhage, CSF rhinorrhea)	**Skin** • *Needle marks* Parenteral substance abuse, CNS infection • *Petechiae/purpura* Intracranial hemorrhage, Rocky Mountain spotted fever, CNS infection (*Neisseria meningitidis*), sepsis

Source: Data from Karas S. Behavioral emergencies: differentiating medical from psychiatric disease. Emerg Med Prac. 2002;4(3):7-8.

and dehydration are common causes in addition to hypoglycemia, hyperglycemia, and thyroid hormone abnormalities. The elderly are more prone to subdural hematoma due to age-related cerebral atrophy, which increases the vulnerability of the bridging veins to tearing. Polypharmacy and unintentional overdoses also commonly cause an alteration in mental status in the elderly.

Many mnemonics are used to aid in the clinical workup for AMS. One popular mnemonic is **AEIOU TIPS** (Table 25–4).

Glasgow Coma Scale

The Glasgow Coma Scale (Table 25–5) was created as an assessment tool to quantify the degree of depression in the level of consciousness in patients with head trauma. Its original purpose was to track the progress of a patient's neurologic status. Its use has widened to include patients with undifferentiated changes in mental status. The scale utilizes assessments of eye opening, motor function, and verbal function to provide a rapid indication on any alteration of consciousness. A higher score corresponds to a higher level of consciousness.

Management

Stabilization of Life Threats Always start by addressing the ABCs, and treat any immediate threats to life. Opening the airway and providing a jaw thrust and supplemental oxygen are the first steps in treating hypoxia. Patients without a secure airway may require intubation. Patients with ineffective breathing can be supported with bag-valve-mask ventilation. If the underlying cause of apnea or hypoventilation

Table 25–2 • CRITICAL AND EMERGENT DIAGNOSES OF CONFUSION
Critical
• Hypoxia/diffuse cerebral ischemia
○ Respiratory failure, CHF, MI
• Systemic
○ Hypoglycemia
• CNS infections
• Hypertensive encephalopathy
• Increased intracranial pressure
Emergent
• Hypoxia/diffuse cerebral ischemia
○ Severe anemia
• Systemic disease
○ Electrolyte/fluid disturbances
○ Endocrine disease (thyroid/adrenal)
○ Hepatic failure
○ Nutrition/Wernicke's encephalopathy
○ Sepsis/infection
• Intoxication and withdrawal
○ CNS sedatives
○ Ethanol
○ Medication side effects (eg, serotonin and anticholinergic syndrome)
• CNS disease
○ Trauma
○ Infections
○ Stroke
○ Subarachnoid hemorrhage
○ Epilepsy/seizures
▪ Postictal state
▪ Nonconvulsive status epilepticus
▪ Complex partial status epilepticus
• Neoplasm

cannot immediately be corrected (eg, naloxone administration for opiate overdose), the patient may require endotracheal intubation and mechanical ventilation.

Assess the circulation by feeling for central pulses, placing the patient on a cardiac monitor, evaluating perfusion, and checking the blood pressure. The only way to fix a hypoperfused brain is to restore circulation. Begin CPR if the patient is pulseless. If the patient has a non-perfusing rhythm (eg, ventricular fibrillation and pulseless ventricular tachycardia), prepare for defibrillation. If there is a pulse but signs of shock are present (eg, mottled skin and cool extremities), you need to assure there is adequate intravascular volume by providing intravenous fluids and possibly a blood transfusion. The patient may also need additional hemodynamic support through the administration of vasopressor medications.

Neurologic　As soon as support of the ABCs has been established, perform a global assessment of neurologic functioning. Assess the Glasgow Coma Scale (GCS) score. Check for pupil size and reactivity. Look for spontaneous movements, especially noting seizure-like activity or lack of movement on one side of the body (suggesting a stroke) or below a specific spinal cord level (suggesting a spinal cord injury).

Table 25–3 • CHARACTERISTICS OF DELIRIUM AND DEMENTIA	
Delirium	Dementia
Abrupt onset—days to weeks	Gradual onset—usually progressive
Early disorientation	Late disorientation
Moment to moment variability	Often more stable
Altered level of consciousness	Level of conscious most often normal
Short attention span	Attention span is reduced

Source: Data from Smith J, Seirafi J. Delirium and dementia. In: Rosen P, Barkin R, eds. Emergency Medicine, Concepts and Clinical Practice. *7th ed. Philadelphia, PA: Mosby; 2009: 1372.*

Any suspicion of spinal cord injury requires placement of a cervical collar and spinal immobilization. Undress the patient and roll onto one side to look for any signs of trauma, drug patches, or infection sources.

Infectious Fever, recent history of infection, or any signs of infection on physical examination need to be addressed immediately. Any patient who is altered with a fever should always raise the suspicion for sepsis. It is prudent to empirically treat (intravenous ceftriaxone and vancomycin, plus pretreat with steroids) patients with suspected meningitis while you proceed with the diagnostic workup (lumbar puncture). If the history and physical examination suggests any other sources of infection (eg, decubitus ulcer, pneumonia, and UTI), appropriate antibiotics and cultures should be started immediately. Previous indwelling lines and catheters should be removed or changed. Other causes of fever should be considered (eg, toxicologic and endocrine).

Electrolyte and Metabolic Hypoglycemia is a common cause of AMS. If you cannot quickly determine a capillary glucose, then give an amp of D50 (25 g of dextrose) empirically. In addition to unconsciousness, hypoglycemia can cause seizures and prolonged postictal states. If the patient is unconscious and intravenous

Table 25–4 • AEIOU TIPS—MNEMONIC FOR TREATABLE CAUSES OF ALTERED MENTAL STATUS	
A	Alcohol (intoxication/withdrawal)
E	Epilepsy, electrolytes, encephalopathy (hepatic, hypertensive, Wernicke), endocrine (thyroid/adrenal)
I	Insulin (hypoglycemia/hyperglycemia), intussusception
O	Opioids, oxygen (hypoxia)
U	Urea (metabolic)
T	Trauma, temperature (hypothermia, hyperthermia)
I	Infection (systemic, CNS), ingestion (drugs/toxins)
P	Psychiatric, porphyria
S	Shock, subarachnoid hemorrhage, stroke, seizure, space-occupying lesion, snake bite

Table 25–5 · GLASGOW COMA SCALE		
Eye Opening		
	Spontaneous eye opening	4
	Opens to verbal commands	3
	Opens to painful stimuli	2
	No response	1
Verbal Response		
	Oriented	5
	Disoriented	4
	Inappropriate words	3
	Incomprehensible sounds	2
	No response	1
Motor Response		
	Obeys commands	6
	Localizes to pain	5
	Withdraws to pain	4
	Abnormal flexion	3
	Abnormal extension	2
	No response	1

access is difficult, obtain intraosseous (IO) access. D50 can be infused through an IO, although if diluted to D25 the fluid may infuse faster. Alternatively, you can consider administering intramuscular glucagon, which acts as a counter-regulatory hormone to increase serum glucose levels.

Hyponatremia and hypernatremia are primarily problems of water metabolism and are frequently associated with volume overload or dehydration states. Hyponatremia can cause AMS, focal neurologic abnormalities, and seizures. This should be treated with hypertonic (3%) saline if the patient is seizing. Hypernatremia should respond to appropriate rehydration. These patients typically require admission to the intensive care unit.

Hypocalcemia and hypercalcemia can result from several metabolic abnormalities or paraneoplastic syndromes. Hypocalcemia should be treated with calcium, whereas the initial treatment for hypercalcemia is intravenous fluid hydration.

Uremia from renal failure can result in uremic encephalopathy, which can cause delirium, as well as asterixis and seizures. Emergent treatment is to correct the underlying electrolyte derangement with intravenous hydration and possibly hemodialysis.

Endocrine Dysfunction of the pancreas (see metabolic for discussion of hypoglycemia and hyperglycemia), thyroid, and adrenal glands can lead to AMS.

Both primary (dysfunction of the thyroid gland) and secondary (deficiency in thyroid stimulating hormone from the pituitary gland) can cause delirium and, in severe cases, coma. Treatment for hypothyroidism is replacement of thyroxine intravenously with T3 or T4. Once the patient's AMS has resolved, thyroid hormone replacement can continue with oral levothyroxine.

Both primary (hyperactivity of the thyroid gland) and secondary (excess production of thyroid releasing hormone or thyroid stimulating hormone from the hypothalamic pituitary axis) hyperthyroidism can result in agitation and anxiety. Thyrotoxicosis is a state of excess circulating thyroid hormone from the thyroid gland itself, ectopic tissue that is secreting thyroid hormone, or supratherapeutic exogenous thyroid hormone administration. Symptoms of thyrotoxicosis include confusion, psychosis, coma, tremor, hyperreflexia, and paralysis. Thyroid storm is an extreme, life-threatening form of thyrotoxicosis, characterized by fever, tachycardia, pulmonary edema, lethargy, vomiting, diarrhea, abdominal pain, and jaundice. Thyroid storm is managed with multiple medications administered in a specific order to avoid worsening the condition. First, decrease sympathetic hyperactivity with a beta-blocker (eg, propranolol). Second, propylthiouracil (PTU) or methimazole must be administered to block the synthesis of T4. Third, giving iodine inhibits the release of stored T4. Finally, steroids can be used to treat an underlying autoimmune process, such as Grave's disease.

Adrenal crisis is a life threatening form of adrenal insufficiency with neurological manifestations including confusion, disorientation, and lethargy. Treatment includes correcting the underlying condition, steroid replacement with hydrocortisone, and blood pressure support with IV fluids and vasopressors if necessary.

Primary CNS Seizure is a common cause for AMS. Always rule out hypoglycemia first. Benzodiazepines are the first-line therapy for seizures. Serum drug levels should be checked if the patient is on anticonvulsant medications with measurable levels or metabolites. If levels are low, then you should load subtherapeutic patients with the appropriate anticonvulsant.

An intracranial mass may present as AMS. Any previous cancer history, focal neurologic findings, headache, or papilledema should prompt a head CT scan. If there is evidence of edema or mass effect, consider administering steroids to help reduce vasogenic edema. Intravenous contrast enhances the ability of CT to identify a mass lesion, specifically brain abscess. These patients should immediately be placed on antibiotics. Obtain an emergent neurosurgical consultation for significant CT abnormalities. These patients typically require admission to the intensive care unit.

Drugs and Toxins Many overdoses can lead to AMS. Look for signs and symptoms of a toxidrome (eg, sedative/hypnotic, sympathomimetic, anticholinergic, cholinergic, or opioid). Most toxidromes can be treated with supportive measures, though specific antidotes exist for each.

Ethanol is a common ingestion for ED patients. These patients need to be thoroughly evaluated to exclude other causes of AMS (eg, stroke, hypoglycemia, Wernicke encephalopathy, intracranial hemorrhage, and toxic alcohol ingestion). Once serious causes are ruled out, these patients require supportive care until they reach clinical sobriety and can be safely discharged.

Withdrawal states can lead to AMS. Patients with ethanol and benzodiazepine withdrawal are typically hyperadrenergic, agitated, and confused. These patients require administration of benzodiazepines, supportive care, and inpatient admission.

Trauma A head CT scan should be performed immediately in patients with evidence of head trauma and AMS. It is important to rule out an intracranial injury such as acute hemorrhage, skull fracture, and evidence of increased intracranial pressure. The trauma or neurosurgical service should be contacted for any positive findings.

Disposition

The majority of patients who present to the ED with AMS will require admission for further inpatient workup unless the patient presents to the ED with an identifiable, reversible cause for his or her change in mental status (eg, heroin overdose).

CASE CORRELATION

- See also Case 26 (Syncope), Case 28 (Stroke), Case 30 (Seizure), Case 39 (Bacterial Meningitis), Case 52 (Heat-Related Illness), Case 56 (Cocaine Intoxication), and Case 58 (Ethanol Withdrawal).

COMPREHENSION QUESTIONS

25.1 A 77-year-old woman presents to the ED with her daughter. The patient is usually alert and oriented. At baseline she independently performs all of her activities of daily life (ADLs). Over the past week, she has been eating and drinking less and tells her daughter that she is not hungry. Yesterday she had an episode of urinary incontinence. This morning, she woke up confused, was unable to follow commands, and kept asking where her husband was (he has been deceased for over 5 years). Her HR is 132 beats per minute, and her temperature is 39°C. She appears dehydrated. What is the most likely cause of her AMS?

   A. Alzheimer's dementia

   B. Alcohol intoxication

   C. Polypharmacy

   D. Urinary tract infection

25.2 A 45-year-old man presents to the ED with AMS. He runs his own business and has been struggling financially since undergoing three surgeries on his right shoulder. He has visited multiple doctors to help control his pain. EMS was called to his office after an employee found him on the floor with a bottle of vodka and a prescription medication bottle. Which of the following is the most appropriate next step?

   A. Administer naloxone

   B. Administer thiamine

   C. Obtain a capillary blood glucose

   D. Assess the patient's ABCs

25.3 A 68-year-old woman presents to the ED with AMS. While visiting with friends, she began slurring her speech and became confused. She then developed jerking movements of her extremities and became unresponsive. When EMS arrived, she was conscious and her BP was 160/90 mm Hg. She was not talking or following commands. She was transported to the ED without incident. After addressing her ABCs, what is the most appropriate next step in the management of this patient?

A. Administer lorazepam

B. Check a capillary glucose

C. Obtain a head CT scan

D. Administer labetalol

ANSWERS

25.1 **D.** Infection is a common cause of AMS, especially in the elderly population. The history and physical examination suggests a urinary tract infection with concomitant dehydration as the cause of her AMS. Alzheimer's does not develop rapidly, but rather gradually over time. The history and physical examination is not suggestive of alcohol abuse or polypharmacy.

25.2 **D.** An assessment of the ABCs always takes priority in a patient with AMS. The patient's airway, breathing, and circulation should be assessed, and any concerns should be addressed before moving forward with diagnostic and therapeutic interventions. This patient may require naloxone if the examination is consistent with an opiate overdose (eg, pinpoint pupils, respiratory depression, and hypotension), although ABC assessment is the first priority. The patient is at risk for hypoglycemia, and a capillary blood glucose should also be obtained once the ABCs have been addressed. If the patient requires dextrose administration, thiamine administration should also be considered; glucose infusion in a thiamine deficient patient can lead to Wernicke encephalopathy.

25.3 **B.** Hypoglycemia can mimic stroke symptoms and can lead to seizures. A quick capillary glucose should be obtained in all patients with stroke or seizure symptoms. The history obtained from friends in this case is critical to making a diagnosis. She likely had a seizure and may be in a postictal state. However, the history of slurred speech and confusion raise suspicion for stroke. She should undergo a CT scan once she is stable, but this should come after capillary glucose testing. Her blood pressure does not require immediate treatment. Therefore, labetalol treatment is unnecessary. She is no longer displaying seizure activity. Therefore, treatment with lorazepam is unnecessary.

CLINICAL PEARLS

▶ Be sure to utilize all possible resources (family, bystanders, EMS, nursing home providers, medical alert bracelets, and previous medical records) to find important clues that may help determine the underlying cause of AMS.

▶ The differential diagnosis of AMS is broad (AEIOU TIPS). A detailed history and physical examination can help guide the differential diagnosis and diagnostic workup.

▶ An assessment of the ABCs should take priority to a detailed history and physical examination in critically ill patients.

▶ A capillary glucose should be checked in all patients with AMS.

▶ Be careful not to classify a confused elderly patient as demented without first ruling out organic causes of their confusion.

REFERENCES

Cooke JL. Depressed consciousness and coma. In: Rosen P, Barkin R, eds. *Emergency Medicine, Concepts and Clinical Practice.* 7th ed. Philadelphia, PA: Mosby; 2009.

Han J, Wilber S. Altered mental status in older patients in the emergency department. *Clin Geriatr Med.* 2013;29(1):101-136.

Huff JS. Altered mental status and coma. In: Tintinalli JE, et al., eds. *Emergency Medicine: A Comprehensive Study Guide.* 8th ed. New York, NY: McGraw-Hill; 2016.

Huff JS. Confusion. In: Rosen P, Barkin R, eds. *Emergency Medicine, Concepts and Clinical Practice.* 7th ed. Philadelphia, PA: Mosby; 2009.

Nassisi D, Okuda Y. ED management of delirium and agitation. *Emerg Med Prac.* 2007;9(1):1-20.

Odiari E, Sekhon N, Han J, David E. Stabilizing and managing patients with altered mental status and delirium. *Emerg Med Clin North Am.* 2015;33(4):753-764.

Smith J, Seirafi J. Delirium and dementia. In: Rosen P, Barkin R, eds. *Emergency Medicine, Concepts and Clinical Practice.* 7th ed. Philadelphia, PA: Mosby; 2009.

Young J, Rund D. Psychiatric considerations in patients with decreased levels of consciousness. *Emerg Med Clin North Am.* 2010;28(3):595-609.

A 64-year-old man is brought into the emergency department (ED) by his family after fainting at home. He was standing, dusting a bookshelf, when he fell backward onto the couch. He was noted to be pale and clammy during the incident, and recovered spontaneously in approximately 30 seconds. He does remember the moments just prior to and after the incident. He felt lightheaded and had palpitations just prior to falling but does not describe any shortness of breath, chest pain, headache, nausea, diplopia, or loss of bowel or bladder control. His history includes a myocardial infarction 2 years prior. The patient has been taking his regular medicines as directed, which include aspirin, a beta-blocker, and a cholesterol-lowering agent. His primary medical doctor has not recently started any new medicines or changed his doses. On presentation to the ED, the patient's vitals are: blood pressure of 143/93 mm Hg, heart rate of 75 beats per minute, respiratory rate of 18 breaths per minute, temperature of 37.1°C (98.8°F), and oxygen saturation of 97% on room air. His examination is significant for a cardiac gallop. No carotid bruits, neurological abnormalities, rectal bleeding, or orthostatic changes are noted. A 12-lead electrocardiogram (ECG) demonstrates a normal sinus rhythm at 75 beats per minute, with normal intervals and Q waves in leads II, III, aVF, not significantly changed from a prior study 6 months earlier. The patient now states he feels fine and would like to go home.

► What is the most likely diagnosis?
► What is your next step?

ANSWERS TO CASE 26:

Syncope

Summary: This is a 64-year-old man with a medical history that includes a myocardial infarction who presents with an episode of syncope. The patient's ECG shows inferior Q waves but no acute changes at the time of presentation.

- **Most likely diagnosis:** Syncope, most likely caused by a cardiac dysrhythmia with spontaneous resolution.

- **Next step:** Management of ABCs (airway, breathing, circulation), intravenous access, and initiation of continuous cardiac monitoring.

ANALYSIS

Objectives

1. Recognize worrisome historical and physical features of syncope.

2. Understand the emergency physician's (EP's) role in evaluation of patients with syncope and the role of selective diagnostic testing.

3. Learn to recognize which patients need to be admitted to the hospital.

Considerations

Syncope has many etiologies that are often difficult to identify with certainty in the ED. The goal of the EP is to identify and treat any life threats. If there is no critical immediate treatment needed, the goal is then to risk-stratify patients for the likelihood of an adverse outcome. The patient in this case is at high risk for a cardiac etiology of his syncope. This patient should immediately be placed on a cardiac monitor and receive an intravenous line. The physician should treat any abnormal findings. If the patient appears dehydrated, he should receive intravenous fluids. If a dysrhythmia exists (eg, ventricular tachycardia), it should be immediately addressed with either cardioversion or defibrillation. If the patient appears stable, the workup should proceed with the patient maintained on the cardiac monitor. The decision to admit or discharge the patient depends on many factors. However, if there is suspicion that there is a cardiac etiology for syncope, this patient should be admitted to a monitored hospital bed.

APPROACH TO:

Syncope

DEFINITIONS

SYNCOPE: A transient loss of consciousness with a corresponding loss of postural tone, with a spontaneous and full recovery.

PRESYNCOPE: A sensation that one is about to lose consciousness, usually with nonspecific symptoms consistent with a prodrome of syncope, such as lightheadedness, weakness, dizziness, blurred vision, or nausea.

VASOVAGAL SYNCOPE: A form of neurocardiogenic syncope, which occurs in the setting of increased peripheral sympathetic activity and venous pooling.

CLINICAL APPROACH

Syncope is an extremely common presenting symptom in the ED, accounting for approximately 5% of all ED visits in this country. Between 1% and 6% of hospitalized patients are admitted for an evaluation of syncope. The list of potential etiologies of syncope is extensive; causes include cardiac, reflex-mediated, orthostatic (eg, postural hypotension caused by volume depletion, sepsis-related peripheral vasodilation, or medications), psychiatric, hormonal, neurologic, and idiopathic. Unnecessary or inappropriate ancillary testing can consume thousands of dollars per patient and increase ED length of stay. With a carefully taken history and physical examination, clinicians can better risk stratify patients and determine who needs to be admitted to the hospital for further evaluation and who can be safely discharged for outpatient workup.

Etiologies

Cardiac syncope refers to the loss of postural tone secondary to a sudden and dramatic fall in cardiac output. **Bradydysrhythmias, tachydysrhythmias,** heart block, and mechanisms that **disrupt outflow or preload** are the functional physiologic abnormalities that cause these sudden changes in blood flow and ultimately inadequate perfusion of the brain. Patients with various forms of organic heart disease (eg, aortic stenosis, hypertrophic cardiomyopathy, and arrhythmogenic right ventricular dysplasia), and those with coronary artery disease, congestive heart failure, ventricular hypertrophy, and myocarditis are at highest risk. Causes of bradydysrhythmias include sinus node disease, second/third-degree heart block, and pacemaker malfunction. **Tachydysrhythmias** include ventricular tachycardia, ventricular fibrillation, torsades de pointes, and supraventricular tachycardia of both nodal and atrial origin, some of which may be associated with conditions such as Wolfe-Parkinson-White syndrome, Brugada syndrome, or long QT syndrome. When syncope is precipitated by a tachydysrhythmia, patients may complain of palpitations. Mechanical etiologies, such as pericardial tamponade and aortic dissection, should be considered in causes of cardiac syncope since both entities will result in a significant fall in functional cardiac output. Massive pulmonary embolism must also be considered, as it can lead to syncope caused by right ventricular outflow obstruction which, in turn, leads to a fall in left-sided filling pressure. Right-sided ventricular strain and dilatation can also lead to dysrhythmia.

Reflex-mediated syncope, also known as situational syncope, includes **vasovagal, cough, micturition, defecation, emesis, swallow, Valsalva, and emotionally** (eg, fear, surprise, and disgust) related syncope. Loss of consciousness and motor tone is caused by stimulation of the **vagal reflex,** resulting in transient bradycardia and hypotension. Warmth, nausea, lightheadedness, and the impending sense that often precedes loss of consciousness are common complaints of those affected by vagal syncope. Carotid sinus disease or stimulation of overly sensitive baroreceptors in the neck (a tight collar) are other causes of sudden reflex-related syncope. These patients will often note a specific activity that is temporally related to their syncopal episodes (turning the head in a certain direction). A recent examination of the Framingham cohort found that patients who were clearly identified to have syncope of vasovagal etiology were not at any increased risk of cardiovascular morbidity or mortality. Unfortunately, making a firm diagnosis of vasovagal syncope in the setting of the ED is difficult, and it should be a diagnosis of exclusion.

Orthostasis is another common cause of syncope. It is defined by a drop in systolic blood pressure of 20 mm Hg or more, drop in diastolic blood pressure of 10 mm Hg or more, or increase in heart rate of 20 points or more. Diaphoresis, lightheadedness, and graying of vision may suggest orthostatic syncope, and recurrence of these symptoms on standing is more significant than the actual numeric change in blood pressure. However, orthostasis may be present in up to 40% of patients older than the age of 70 who are asymptomatic. Orthostatic hypotension can be related to volume depletion, sepsis-related peripheral vascular dilation, medications, and autonomic instability, which can develop in a number of chronic illnesses such as diabetes, Parkinson's disease, multiple sclerosis, and other neuromuscular disorders. Volume depletion secondary to sudden blood loss needs to be considered in all patients with syncope. Patients of all ages can develop a sudden gastrointestinal (GI) bleed, and the initial blood flow can be occult because it is confined to the lower GI tract. Elderly patients can lose massive amounts of blood from a leaking or ruptured abdominal aortic aneurysm, with abdominal or flank pain as common associated complaints; however, syncope alone can also be the presenting complaint. In the female patient of childbearing age, normal intrauterine or ruptured ectopic pregnancy may present with syncope. The former may cause orthostasis as a result of the normal cardiovascular changes associated with pregnancy, and the latter as the only manifestation of life-threatening hemorrhage.

Hypotension leading to syncope is not necessarily related to volume loss. Patients, particularly the elderly, may present with syncope as the first overt manifestation of sepsis. Hypotension in these patients is caused by relative lack of intravascular volume secondary to decreased vascular tone as part of the inflammatory response. Patients with a history of hypertension may have what appears to be a "normal" blood pressure when they are actually in a state of relative hypotension.

Medication, especially polypharmacy, a common problem in the elderly, is another important cause of syncope. **Antihypertensives, antidepressants, antianginals, analgesics, central nervous system depressants**, medications that can **prolong the QT interval** (eg, erythromycin, clarithromycin, haloperidol, amiodarone, droperidol, and others), **insulin, oral hypoglycemics, and recreational polypharmacy** are common culprits. Geriatric patients with complicated medical histories are particularly at risk, although a detailed ingestion history should be obtained from all patients presenting with syncope. One should look closely for recent additions or changes to a medication regimen, including over-the-counter medications.

Neurologic causes of **syncope** are **rare,** unless seizure is included in the differential diagnosis; seizure and syncope should be differentiated and thought of as discrete diagnoses. Seizure can usually be quickly identified by the history of witnessed seizure activity, especially if accompanied by a history of seizures in the past. It is also suggested by physical examination findings (eg, tongue biting and loss of bowel/bladder control), especially the observation of a postictal state, which commonly resolves over a period from several minutes to many hours. Sometimes, it is not straightforward. **Brief tonic-clonic activity can result from** transient brain stem hypoxia, which leads to loss of consciousness; these situations can appear as epilepsy. However, the duration of confusion or lethargy following the episode is short lived. The sudden onset of a severe headache associated with loss of consciousness suggests a subarachnoid hemorrhage as the cause of syncope. Other neurological causes of syncope include migraines, subclavian steal, and transient ischemic attack or stroke of the vertebrobasilar distribution.

Sometimes patients with **psychiatric disease** will present with the complaint of sudden loss of consciousness. The history of these patients may include several prior episodes of syncope. Typically, these incidents will present with **minimal physical trauma** and none of the signs or symptoms that are commonly associated with cardiac syncope. Anxiety, with or without hyperventilation, conversion disorder, somatization, panic attacks, and breath-holding spells are all manifestations of psychiatric illness that can cause syncope. However, psychiatric and emotional etiologies of syncope are considered a diagnosis of exclusion. This diagnosis should be considered only after appropriate laboratory or ancillary testing has ruled out more serious etiologies. Furthermore, it must be recognized that many of the most commonly prescribed **neuroleptics** cause **QT prolongation,** which in turn can lead to ventricular dysrhythmia.

Diagnosis

Much to the frustration of patients and providers, the **underlying cause of the syncopal presentation is not elucidated in approximately half of patients who present to the ED with syncope.** Unfortunately, patients in this category represent a mixed population in which it is estimated that anywhere between 45% and 80% may have had a cardiac cause. Most of the young and otherwise healthy patients will be discharged home without a clearly defined cause for their loss of consciousness. Many of the elderly patients will be admitted for additional testing and observation. Of all the diagnostic tools available to physicians in the evaluation of syncope, a thorough history, physical examination, and ECG are the only level A recommendations from the American College of Emergency Physicians (ACEP). The information gathered from the history and physical examination alone will identify the potential cause of syncope in 45% of cases.

The goal of the initial evaluation is not only to find out exactly what happened to the patient, but also to ensure no injuries occurred as a result of the syncopal event. It is critical to ascertain a step-by-step history of the event. This includes getting a detailed account from any bystanders or family members, which can be valuable in making the correct diagnosis. The **history and complete physical examination,** combined with the **ECG,** form the preliminary workup of patients with syncope. Orthostatic vital signs should be obtained if orthostasis is likely.

This approach is often suggestive of a diagnosis in cases of vasovagal, situational, orthostatic, polypharmacy, and some cardiac-related syncope. Although vasovagal and situational syncope may be strongly suspected based upon the history, a true diagnosis of vasovagal syncope requires additional testing not available in the ED. While vasovagal/situational syncope does occur in elderly patients, it is a diagnosis that cannot be safely relied upon in the ED unless the history is completely indicative (ie, syncope at the sight of blood) and there are no physical or diagnostic test findings that raise concern for more ominous causes. Conversely, young, healthy patients with histories consistent with vasovagal syncope may be approached with less diagnostic testing. Younger patients should be questioned regarding a family history of early cardiac or sudden death. Rare, certain genetic conditions such as Brugada syndrome, hypertrophic cardiomyopathy, and long QT syndrome may present with syncope.

Laboratory Tests

Although laboratory testing rarely elucidates the cause of the syncope, it can be helpful in a **limited number of situations and should be guided by the history and physical examination.** Inexpensive laboratory tests include a complete blood count (CBC) for anemia, glucometer for hypoglycemia, and a basic metabolic panel for electrolyte derangements and evidence of dehydration. Toxicology screening for drug-related syncope is rarely helpful for the immediate evaluation and stabilization of the patient. Furthermore, assumption of a toxicologic cause should not deter the physician from performing a complete evaluation. A urinalysis is an inexpensive and useful screening test that can provide information about glucose, infection, the patient's state of hydration, and the presence or absence of ketones. **A urine pregnancy test should always be obtained in women of childbearing age** because previously unknown pregnancy and ectopic pregnancy can present with syncope.

Management

Patients with history or examination findings suggestive of a particular pathology should undergo further testing that may include continuous **cardiac monitoring, echocardiography, Doppler vascular studies,** or contrast **computed tomography (CT) imaging.** Point-of-care ultrasound is increasingly helpful in the initial ED workup for evaluation of cardiac tamponade, acute valvulopathies, aortic aneurysms/dissections, and right heart strain suggestive of pulmonary embolism. Those patients with unexplained syncope and high-risk clinical features (eg, advanced age, abnormal ECG, previous cardiac history, and exertional syncope) require admission for further investigation such as cardiac stress testing, tilt-table testing, cardiac enzymes, cardiac catheterization, electrophysiologic studies, and extended continuous cardiac monitoring.

While diagnosis and treatment are the goals in the evaluation of syncope, the decision tree for EM physicians is more focused than that of the specialist or outpatient physician (Figure 26–1). Unstable patients presenting after a syncopal

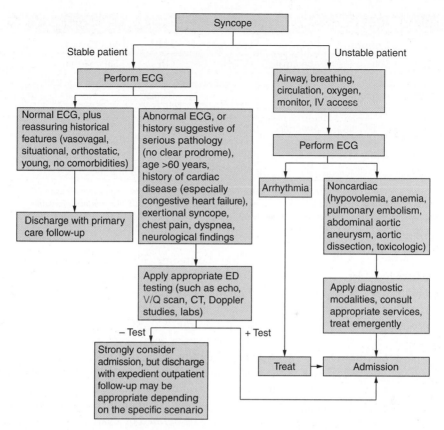

Figure 26–1. Algorithm of syncope evaluation.

episode, including those with persistent hypotension, life-threatening dysrhythmias, active blood loss, acute coronary syndromes, hemodynamically significant pulmonary emboli, and cardiac tamponade must be managed emergently. **The "ABCs"** approach to the unstable patient applies in this scenario as in all presentations with unstable vital signs. History and physical examination in the context of syncope should guide diagnostic thinking but should not be a substitute for emergent management considerations.

Disposition

For the patient who presents after syncope but is hemodynamically normal at the time of presentation, the decision to admit versus discharge from the ED with outpatient follow-up is dependent on other clinical features suggesting that the patient is at high risk for a short-term adverse outcome.

Several studies have tried to aid the EM physician in identifying high-risk patients by using clinical decision rules (Table 26–1). The **San Francisco Syncope Rule,** the **OESIL** (Osservatorio Epidemiologico sulla Sincope nel Lazio), and the **ROSE** (Risk Stratification of Syncope in the Emergency Department) are decision rules that attempt to provide clinicians with patient characteristics associated

Table 26–1 • SYNCOPE RULES						
	Symptoms	ECG	Laboratory	PMH	Vital Signs	Age
SFSR	SOB	Abnormal ECG	HCT<30	CHF	SBP <90 mm Hg	
OESIL	No prodrome	Abnormal ECG		Cardiac disease		>65 y
ROSE	Chest pain associated with syncope	Abnormal ECG	HB <9 (+) Fecal occult Blood BNP ≥300		O₂ SAT ≤94% Bradycardia (HR ≤ 50 bpm)	

Abbreviations: CHF = Congestive heart failure; OESIL = Osservatorio Epidemiologico sulla Sincope nel Lazio; PMH = Past medical history; ROSE = Risk stratification of syncope in the emergency department; SOB = Shortness of breath. Based on data from SFSR: San Francisco Syncope Rules.

with an increased likelihood for an adverse outcome. The San Francisco Syncope rule uses five criteria—history of CHF, abnormal ECG, hematocrit <30, shortness of breath, and/or systolic BP of <90 mm Hg at triage—to predict who requires hospitalization. The OESIL score is based upon abnormal ECG, history of cardiac disease, age >65, and syncope without prodrome. The **ROSE** predictors are: presence of associated chest pain, BNP >300, positive fecal occult blood, hemoglobin <9, oxygen saturation <94% on room air, bradycardia <50, and Q waves present on ECG. The ROSE rule is the first to incorporate a biochemical marker, BNP, into the criteria and claims a sensitivity and negative predictive value of 87.2% and 98.5%, respectively. **An abnormal ECG is the only common thread in all three rule sets** (Figure 26–2), although "abnormal" may be defined in a variety of ways. If the biochemical marker BNP in the ROSE criteria is considered a surrogate for a history of CHF, this reinforces that known cardiac disease is a factor associated with high-risk patients. **Regardless of which rule set one considers, it should be recognized that decision tools and algorithms should never be used as a substitute for a full evaluation and individualized clinical judgment of all aspects of the patient's presentation.** Many of these decision rules are still undergoing evaluation in an effort to gain validation. In fact, a recent analysis comparing the efficacy of risk stratification using the San Francisco and OESIL rule sets versus clinical judgment on short-term prognosis found that both rule sets had relatively low sensitivities. Furthermore, both rule sets would need to be employed to identify all patients who subsequently died; the best results were obtained if the clinician used a combination of clinical knowledge with either rule set.

The **ACEP clinical policy guidelines** emphasize risk stratification of patients presenting with syncope in a similar fashion to those presenting with chest pain. It is generally accepted that historical or physical examination findings consistent with heart failure, structural or coronary heart disease, as well as an abnormal ECG are linked with high risk of poor outcomes. Advancing age is coupled with a continuum of growing cardiovascular risk and should also be a consideration. It also bears mentioning that in the high-risk groups, however they are defined, presyncopal events should be evaluated and managed as syncope, as the etiologies are the same

COMPARATIVE DIAGRAM OF THREE SYNCOPE RISK RULES

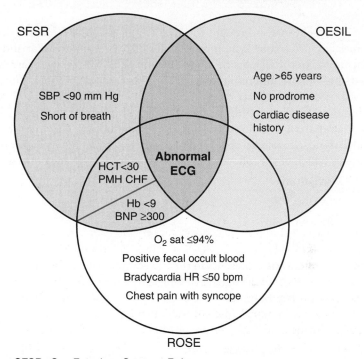

SFSR

OESIL

SBP <90 mm Hg

Short of breath

Age >65 years

No prodrome

Cardiac disease history

HCT<30
PMH CHF

Abnormal ECG

Hb <9
BNP ≥300

O_2 sat ≤94%

Positive fecal occult blood

Bradycardia HR ≤50 bpm

Chest pain with syncope

ROSE

SFSR: San Francisco Syncope Rules
OESIL: Ossevatorio Epidemiologico sulla Sincope nel Lazio
ROSE: Risk Stratification of Syncope in the Emergency Department

Figure 26–2. Predictor variables of risk rules. Each of the three syncope risk rules aim to identify those patients at risk for sudden death or morbidity. Each uses a slightly different strategy. The best clinician will understand the rationale, utility, and limitations of each.

and are distinguished only by the degree of hypoperfusion of the brain. The younger patient with no comorbidities, reassuring first-time symptoms, and a normal ECG can usually be discharged from the ED. Referral to a primary medical doctor should be made for coordination of any outpatient studies that may be warranted in the evaluation of recurring syncope. Patients with specific job-related concerns, such as heavy machine operators, pilots, or physicians, may require more expeditious referral and notification of the appropriate State authorities. **Even benign causes of syncope, such as vasovagal syncope, can be fatal when the patient is driving.**

CASE CORRELATION

- See also Case 2 (Hemorrhagic Shock), Case 6 (Anaphylaxis), Case 9 (Atrial Fibrillation), Case 10 (Regular Rate Tachycardia), Case 28 (Stroke), Case 30 (Seizure Induced by Traumatic Brain Injury), Case 36 (Ectopic Pregnancy), and Case 52 (Heat-Related Illness).

COMPREHENSION QUESTIONS

26.1 A 37-year-old man is brought into the ED because he fainted at work. He denies any prodromal symptoms. Family history is negative for sudden cardiac death. In the ED, his BP lying down is 125/75 mm Hg, heart rate is 75 beats per minute, and respiratory rate is 14 breaths per minute. The patient's blood pressure and heart rate standing are 120/75 mm Hg and 77 beats per minute, respectively. His ECG shows a sinus rhythm with a rate of 72. Physical examination does not reveal any abnormal findings. Currently, he is lucid and has no neurologic abnormalities. After a complete evaluation of this patient, which of the following is the most common etiology of syncope?

A. Dysrhythmia

B. Orthostasis

C. Idiopathic

D. Situational

26.2 A 35-year-old woman presents to the ED complaining of feeling lightheadedness. She noticed some vaginal bleeding earlier in the day. Her blood pressure is 85/53 mm Hg, heart rate is 130 beats per minute, and respiratory rate is 18 breaths per minute. Which of the following is the most appropriate next step in management?

A. Obtain a urine pregnancy test.

B. Obtain a serum quantitative beta human chorionic gonadotropin (β-hCG).

C. Obtain immediate IV access and begin fluid resuscitation.

D. Obtain stat OB/GYN consult.

26.3 A 21-year-old man is brought to the ED after collapsing to the ground while playing basketball. He is alert and oriented, denies chest pain, difficulty breathing, or any other physical complaints. There was no trauma. He denies any past medical problems. Physical examination is unremarkable. Which of the following elements on his ECG is concerning for a life-threatening cause of syncope?

A. Heart rate of 55

B. P-wave inversion in lead aVR

C. Sinus arrhythmia

D. QTc of 495 msec

26.4 A 72-year-old man is brought to the ED by paramedics after fainting at the supermarket. His syncopal episode was witnessed by shoppers who stated the patient collapsed, hitting his head. The patient is currently alert and oriented and denies any persistent symptoms. His past medical history is significant for carotid stenosis, for which he takes aspirin and clopidogrel. What is most appropriate next step in the management of this patient?

A. Head CT scan

B. Order a carotid duplex ultrasound

C. Obtain an ECG

D. Chest radiograph

ANSWERS

26.1 **C.** Idiopathic. Approximately 50% of all patients with a presenting complaint of syncope will not have a definitive cause. Cardiac causes of syncope (eg, dysrhythmia) are the most worrisome because patients are at increased risk for sudden cardiac death. Situational syncope is a common cause of syncope. It is a result of an abnormal autonomic reflex response to a physical stimulus. Some triggers of this response include coughing, swallowing, defecation, and micturition. The patient does not have evidence for orthostatic hypotension as demonstrated by his vital signs.

26.2 **C.** Obtain IV access and begin fluid resuscitation. Investigating the possibility of pregnancy, specifically ectopic pregnancy, is critical. However, initial stabilization of the patient takes precedence. Hypotension must be treated emergently with fluids. Obtaining a consult early in the patient's course is important. Definitive management will be in the operating room.

26.3 **D.** The upper level of normal for the corrected QT interval is approximately 440 msec for men and 460 msec for women. A finding of a prolonged QT interval should prompt a more thorough investigation into this patient's medications, family history, and potential electrolyte imbalances. Prolonged QT syndrome is associated with sudden death, especially in young athletes. Mild bradycardia alone in a young, healthy patient who has fully recovered from an episode of syncope is of little concern. P-wave inversion in lead aVR is a normal finding. Sinus arrhythmia is a normal variation in the RR interval with respiration.

26.4 **C.** Obtain an ECG. This patient has a high probability for a cardiac cause of his syncope. Initial management includes placing the patient on a cardiac monitor and obtaining an ECG to monitor for dysrhythmias. A head CT scan should be performed after an ECG is obtained. A carotid duplex ultrasound and chest radiograph may aid in the workup for syncope, but it is most important to first rule out a dysrhythmia.

CLINICAL PEARLS

▶ The primary goal of the EP in the evaluation of patients with syncope is to be able to identify those who are at high risk for morbidity and mortality.

▶ The causes of syncope are varied, and a successful diagnosis hinges on diligent history collection and appropriate use of diagnostic tools.

▶ Even the most experienced clinician will be unable to determine the cause of syncope in up to 50% of patients.

▶ Reassuring clinical signs in syncope are youth, a normal ECG, absence of comorbidities, and reassuring historical features.

▶ Unstable patients should be treated emergently and stabilized, first addressing the ABCs.

REFERENCES

American College of Emergency Physicians. Clinical policy: critical issues in the evaluation and management of patients presenting with syncope. *Ann Emerge Med*. 2007;49:431-444.

Carlson MD. Syncope. In: *Harrison's Principles of Internal Medicine*. 19th ed. New York, NY: McGraw-Hill; 2015.

Colivicchi F, Ammirati F, Melina D, et al. Development and prospective validation of a risk stratification system for patients with syncope in the emergency department: the OESIL risk score. *Eur Heart J*. 2003;24:811-819.

De Lorenzo RA. Syncope. In: *Rosen's Emergency Medicine: Concepts and Clinical Practice*. 6th ed. St Louis, MO: Mosby; 2005.

Dipaola FCG, Perego F, Borella M, et al. San Francisco Syncope Rule, Osservatorio Epidemiologico sulla Sincope nel Lazio risk score, and clinical judgment in the assessment of short-term outcome of syncope. *Am J Emerg Med*. 2010;28:432-439.

Dovgalyuk J, Holstege C, Mattu A, Brady WJ. The electrocardiogram in the patient with syncope. *Am J Emerg Med*. 2007;25(6):688-701.

Huff JS, Decker WW, Quinn JV, et al.; American College of Emergency Physicians. Clinical policy: critical issues in the evaluation and management of adult patients presenting to the ED with syncope. *Ann Emerg Med*. 2007;49:431-434.

Kessler C, Tristano JM, DeLorenzo R. The emergency department approach to syncope: evidence-based guidelines and prediction rules. *Emerg Med Clin N Am*. 2010;28:487-500.

Linzer M, Yang EH, Estes NA, et al. Diagnosing syncope part 1: value of history, physical examination, and electrocardiography. *Ann Intern Med*. 1997;126(12):989-996.

Linzer M, Yang EH, Estes NA, et al. Diagnosing syncope part 2: unexplained syncope. *Ann Intern Med*. 1997;127(1):76-84.

Quinn, J. Syncope. *Tintinalli's Emergency Medicine: A Comprehensive Study Guide*. 8th ed. McGraw-Hill; 2015.

Quinn JV, Stiell IG, McDermott DA, et al. Derivation of the San Francisco syncope rule to predict patients with short-term serious outcomes. *Ann Emerg Med*. 2004;43:224-232.

Reed MJ, Newby DE, Coull AJ, et al. The ROSE (Risk Stratification of Syncope in the Emergency Department) Study. *J Am Coll Cardiol*. 2010;55 (8):713-721.

Schipper JL, WN Kapoor. Cardiac arrhythmias: diagnostic evaluation and management of patients with syncope. *Med Clin North Am*. 2001;85(2):423-456.

Serrano LA, Hess EP, Bellolio MF, et al. Accuracy and quality of clinical decision rules for syncope in the emergency department: a systematic review and meta-analysis. *Ann Emerg Med*. 2010;56(4):362-373.

Soteriades ES, Evans JC, Larson MG, et al. Incidence and prognosis of syncope. *New Engl J Med*. 2002;347:878-885.

Sun BC, Emond JA, Camargo CA Jr. Direct medical costs of syncope-related hospitalizations in the United States. *Am J Cardiol*. 2005;95(5):668-671.

A 27-year-old woman reports that her mouth has been drooping in the right corner since yesterday. As a result, it is difficult for her to drink water without drooling. She cannot close her right eye completely, and her right eye is red and irritated. She denies having headaches, visual disturbances, nausea, or vomiting. She does not have any history of trauma. Her past medical history is unremarkable. She is not taking any medications. On physical examination, the right corner of her mouth droops, and the right nasolabial fold is absent. The right lower eyelid is sagging, and the patient cannot completely close her right eye. On attempts to close the right eye, the eye rolls upward. The patient also cannot wrinkle her forehead. The other cranial nerves seem to be normal, and the neurologic examination reveals no deficits other than as stated.

▶ What is your diagnosis?
▶ How will you manage this condition?

ANSWERS TO CASE 27:

Bell Palsy (Idiopathic Facial Paralysis)

Summary: A 27-year-old woman has acute onset of right facial weakness and right eye irritation. She denies trauma and has no other cranial nerve or neurological problems.

- **Most Likely Diagnosis:** Facial nerve palsy, most likely idiopathic (Bell palsy).

- **Management of condition:** Protection of the eye and a course of prednisone.

ANALYSIS

Objectives

1. Differentiate an upper motor neuron process from a lower motor neuron process, and review the differential diagnoses for each.

2. Understand the clinical presentation of Bell palsy.

3. Learn the management of Bell palsy.

Considerations

This 27-year-old woman is affected by the abrupt onset of right facial weakness. Notably, her upper facial muscles are affected, which is consistent with a peripheral neuropathy. She has none of the findings suggestive of a more complicated process (Table 27–1). Her symptoms are likely caused by paralysis of the seventh cranial nerve, which is mainly a motor nerve supplying all the ipsilateral muscles of facial expression. The drooping of the right corner of the mouth represents paralysis of the orbicularis oris muscle. Tearing of the right eye (epiphora) occurs because paralysis of the orbicularis oculi muscle prevents closure of the eyelids and causes the lacrimal duct opening to sag away from the conjunctiva. The inability to wrinkle the forehead is a result of paralysis of the frontalis muscle. Affected individuals will often have the Bell phenomenon (the eye on the paralyzed side rolls upward) upon attempted closure of the eyelids.

Table 27–1 • RED FLAGS FOR SUSPECTED FACIAL NERVE PALSY
Cranial nerve involvement other than VII
Bilateral facial weakness
Weakness, numbness of arms or legs
Unaffected upper facial muscles (forehead)
Headache, visual deficits, nausea or vomiting
History of travel through woods, tick bite
Recurrent unilateral facial paralysis
Slow progression of symptoms
Ulceration or blisters near ear

APPROACH TO:
Facial Paralysis

Approach to Bell Palsy

The seventh cranial nerve exits the cranium through the stylomastoid foramen and supplies all the muscles concerned with facial expression. It also has a small sensory component which conveys taste sensation from the anterior two-thirds of the tongue and cutaneous impulses from the anterior wall of the external auditory meatus. A complete interruption of the facial nerve at the stylomastoid foramen paralyzes all the muscles of the face on the affected side. Taste sensation is intact because the lesion is beyond the site where the chorda tympani has separated from the main trunk of the facial nerve. If the nerve to the stapedius muscle is involved, there is often hyperacusis. If the geniculate ganglion or the motor root proximal to it is involved, lacrimation and salivation may be reduced.

Although the most common cause of facial paralysis is Bell palsy, this is a diagnosis of exclusion. In other words, the emergency department (ED) physician should be careful of presuming a facial palsy is Bell palsy without considering other possible etiologies. Other causes of nuclear or peripheral facial nerve palsy include Lyme disease, tumors of the temporal bone (carotid body, cholesteatoma, and dermoid), Ramsey Hunt syndrome (herpes zoster of the geniculate ganglion), and acoustic neuromas. Malignant otitis externa, stroke, Guillain-Barré disease, polio, sarcoid, and human immunodeficiency virus (HIV) infection are other processes that must be considered.

All forms of peripheral facial nerve palsy must be distinguished from the supra-nuclear type. In the latter, the frontalis and orbicularis oculi muscles are spared because the innervation of the upper facial muscles is bilateral and that of the lower facial muscles is mainly contralateral. In other words, **if the patient has drooping of the mouth but is able to wrinkle his or her forehead normally, an intracranial process should be suspected.** With supranuclear lesions, there may also be a dissociation of emotional and voluntary facial movements. Because Bell palsy is a diagnosis of exclusion, a very careful history and physical examination are critical to detect any other neurological abnormalities.

The onset of Bell palsy is abrupt, and symptoms can progress from weakness to complete paralysis over a week. Over half of the patients with Bell palsy will recall a preceding viral prodrome. Associated symptoms may include pain behind the ear, ipsilateral loss of taste sensation, decreased or overflow tearing, and hyperacusis. The patient may complain of heaviness and numbness on the affected side of the face; however, no sensory loss is demonstrable. Eighty percent of patients recover within weeks to a few months. The presence of incomplete paralysis in the first week is the most favorable prognostic sign. If the presentation is atypical or there is no improvement at 6 months, laboratory studies, imaging studies (eg, computed tomography and magnetic resonance imaging [MRI]), or motor-nerve conduction studies should be considered.

Treatment

The patient should use an **eye patch while sleeping** to protect the eye and prevent corneal drying and abrasions. While awake, he or she should apply artificial tears to the affected eye every hour. Massaging of the weakened muscles may improve muscle tone and aid in recovery.

Medical therapy should be started as soon as possible but can be considered for up to 1 week after the onset of symptoms. Although treatment regimens are controversial, most experts recommend the use of corticosteroids. **Corticosteroids are hypothesized to decrease facial nerve edema.** Thus, prednisone 1 mg/kg/day can be given orally for 7-10 days (with or without a taper). Because some studies implicated herpes simplex virus as a causative agent of Bell palsy, antivirals have been routinely incorporated into the treatment regimen. However, further studies have shown conflicting results regarding the efficacy of antiviral therapy combined with steroids. If physicians choose to prescribe antiviral agents, valacyclovir and famciclovir are favored due to their less frequent dosing and greater bioavailability. These agents do cost substantially more than acyclovir, which requires more frequent dosing. If medical therapy is unsuccessful, patients may benefit from surgical decompression of the facial nerve.

CASE CORRELATION

- See also Case 25 (Altered Mental Status), Case 28 (Stroke), Case 29 (Headache), and Case 39 (Bacterial Meningitis).

COMPREHENSION QUESTIONS

27.1 A 32-year-old woman complains of facial weakness for several weeks that has gradually worsened. The upper face and lower face are both affected. She does not have weakness of the arms or legs. Which of the following would suggest a diagnosis other than Bell palsy?

   A. Absence of symptoms in arms

   B. Absence of symptoms in legs

   C. Gradual onset over several weeks

   D. Upper facial weakness

27.2 A 55-year-old woman complains of weakness of her right facial muscles along with numbness of her right cheek region. Which of the following is the next step?

   A. Obtain MRI of the brain

   B. Obtain a rapid plasma reagin (RPR) serology

   C. Perform a lumbar puncture

   D. Recommend eye protection and observation

Match the following mechanisms (A to E) to the clinical scenarios presented in Questions 27.3 to 27.5:

A. Pressure on the cerebellopontine nucleus

B. Edema of the nerve at the stylomastoid foramen

C. Immunoglobulins against the acetylcholine receptor

D. Multifocal myelin destruction in the central nervous system

E. Autoimmune attack on myelinated motor nerves, particularly of the lower extremities

27.3 A 22-year-old woman is on the ventilator because of inability to breathe. This condition began 3 weeks ago when she had weakness of both legs following a bout of gastroenteritis. Her deep tendon reflexes are absent.

27.4 A 32-year-old woman has a 5-year history of progressive weakness during the day. She cannot look upward for long periods of time because of fatigue.

27.5 A 35-year-old man had eye weakness 2 years ago with full resolution. Now he has difficulty with his right handgrip. His deep tendon reflexes are normal to increased.

ANSWERS

27.1 **C.** The onset of Bell palsy is abrupt, with maximum weakness occurring within 1 week. Facial nerve palsy due to tumors of the temporal bone is insidious, and the symptoms gradually progress.

27.2 **A.** The numbness over the cheek is concerning and inconsistent with Bell palsy. For this reason, an MRI of the brain should be performed. The facial nerve supplies all the muscles of the face. Injury to this nerve produces paralysis of the facial muscles. Drooping of the corner of the mouth is one of the findings. The tongue is supplied by the hypoglossal nerve. Middle ear lesions producing facial palsy will cause loss of taste over the anterior two-thirds of the tongue, but alteration of taste sensation does not occur. The sensory component of the facial nerve is limited to the anterior wall of the external auditory meatus. Further evaluation with MRI may be warranted.

27.3 **E.** This presentation of ascending paralysis is classic for Guillain-Barré syndrome, in which the deep tendon reflexes are typically absent.

27.4 **C.** Myasthenia gravis is characterized by progressive weakness throughout the day, particularly involving the eye muscles. These symptoms are due to immunoglobulin G antibodies against the acetylcholine receptors.

27.5 **D.** Multiple sclerosis typically affects young individuals with waxing and waning weakness and full recovery between exacerbations. The mechanism is multifocal destruction of the myelin in the central nervous system.

CLINICAL PEARLS

▶ Bell palsy is an idiopathic seventh cranial nerve peripheral neuropathy, leading to both upper and lower facial weakness.

▶ The diagnosis of Bell palsy is one of exclusion. A careful history and physical examination can usually exclude other diagnoses such as stroke, Guillain-Barré, or acoustic neuroma.

▶ The most important assessment in a patient who presents with possible Bell palsy is to rule out serious disorders such as intracranial tumors and strokes.

▶ Protection of the eye to prevent corneal drying and abrasions is accomplished with an eye patch during sleep and lubricants to the affected eye.

▶ The prognosis of Bell palsy is usually favorable, but persistent weakness, the appearance of other neurologic deficits, or blisters that appear on the ear are indications for referral.

REFERENCES

Axelsson S, Lindberg S, Stjernquist-Desatnik A. Outcome of treatment with valacyclovir and predni-sone in patients with Bell's palsy. *Ann Otol Rhinol Laryngol.* 2003;112:197-201.

Baringer JR. Herpes simplex virus and Bell's palsy. *Ann Intern Med.* 1996;124:63-65.

Benatar M, Edlow J. The spectrum of cranial neuropathy in patients with Bell's palsy. *Arch Intern Med.* 2004;164:23-83.

Brodal A. The cranial nerves. *Neurological Anatomy in Relation to Clinical Medicine.* 3rd ed. New York, NY: Oxford; 1980:448-577.

Engstrom M, Berg T, Stjernquist-Desatnik A, et al. Prednisolone and valaciclovir in Bell's palsy: a ran-domised, double-blind, placebo-controlled, multicentre trial. *Lancet Neurol.* 2008;7:993-1000.

Fahimi J, Navi BB, Kamel H. Potential misdiagnoses of Bell's palsy in the emergency department. *Ann Emerg Med.* 2014:63(4)428-434.

Gilden DH, Tyler KL. Bell's palsy—is glucocorticoid treatment enough? *N Engl J Med.* 2007;357:1653-1655.

Hato N, Yamada H, Kohno H, et al. Valacyclovir and prednisolone treatment for Bell's palsy: a multi-center, randomized, placebo-controlled study. *Otol Neurotol.* 2007;28:408-413.

Hauser WA, Karnes WE, Annis J, Kurland LT. Incidence and prognosis of Bell's palsy in the population of Rochester, Minnesota. *Mayo Clin Proc.* 1971;46:258-264.

Karnes WE. Diseases of the seventh cranial nerve. In: Dyck PJ, Thomas PK, Lambert EH, et al., eds. *Peripheral Neuropathy.* 2nd ed. Philadelphia, PA: WB Saunders; 1984: 1266-1299.

Marx JA, Hockberger RS, Walls RM, eds. *Rosen's Emergency Medicine: Concepts and Clinical Practice.* 8th ed. Philadelphia, PA: Saunders; 2014.

Sullivan FM, Swan IR, Donnan PT, et al. Early treatment with prednisolone or acyclovir in Bell's palsy. *N Engl J Med.* 2007;357(16):1598-1607.

Worster A, Keim SM, Sahsi R, Pancioli AM; Best Evidence in Emergency Medicine (BEEM) Group. Do either corticosteroids or antiviral agents reduce the risk of long-term facial paresis in patients with new-onset Bell's palsy? *J Emerg Med.* 2010;38(4):518-523. Epub 2009 Oct 21.

A 59-year-old man with a history of hypertension presents to the emergency department (ED) with right-sided paralysis and aphasia. The patient's wife states he was in his normal state of health until 1 hour ago, when she heard a thud in the bathroom and walked in to find him collapsed on the floor. She immediately called emergency medical services, which transported the patient to your ED. En route, his fingerstick blood sugar was 108 mg/dL. On arrival in the ED, the patient is placed on monitors and an IV is established. His temperature is 36.8°C (98.2°F), blood pressure is 169/93 mm Hg, heart rate is 86 beats per minute, and respiratory rate is 20 breaths per minute. The patient has a noticeable left-gaze preference and is verbally unresponsive, although he will follow simple commands such as raising his left thumb. He has a normal neurologic examination on the left, but on the right he has a facial droop, no motor activity, decreased deep tendon reflexes (DTRs), and no sensation to light-touch.

▶ What is the most likely diagnosis?
▶ What is the most appropriate next step?
▶ What is the best therapy?

ANSWERS TO CASE:

Stroke

Summary: This is a 59-year-old man with acute onset of aphasia and right-sided paralysis 60 minutes prior to arrival in the ED.

- **Most likely diagnosis:** Stroke.
- **Most appropriate next step:** CT scan of the head.
- **Best therapy:** Thrombolytics.

ANALYSIS

Objectives

1. Recognize the clinical findings of an acute stroke.
2. Understand the diagnostic and therapeutic approach to suspected stroke patients.
3. Be familiar with the National Institutes of Health (NIH) Stroke Scoring system.

Considerations

This 59-year-old man presents with an acute onset of focal neurologic deficits, which are typical for a cerebrovascular accident (CVA). Management priorities include: ABCs (airway, breathing, and circulation), stabilization of vitals, and a careful history and physical to distinguish CVA from other etiologies which may present similarly, such as hypoglycemia. Non-contrast CT is used to quickly determine whether the CVA is ischemic or hemorrhagic. If the event is ischemic, the patient may be a candidate for thrombolytic administration. The goal is to complete an evaluation and, if the patient is eligible, initiate treatment within 60 minutes of the patient's arrival to the ED. **We must be cognizant that "Time is Brain Tissue."**

APPROACH TO:

Suspected Stroke

DEFINITIONS

STROKE: The rapid development of the loss of brain function due to a disturbance in the blood vessels supplying the brain. It is also referred to as a CVA.

TRANSIENT ISCHEMIC ATTACK (TIA): Occurs when the blood supply to a particular area of the brain is interrupted. It is often referred to as a "mini stroke," and the symptoms typically last minutes to hours, but resolve within 24 hours.

THROMBOLYTICS: Medications that act to degrade clots and are used in the treatment of myocardial infarctions, pulmonary embolisms, and strokes.

NATIONAL INSTITUTES OF HEALTH STROKE SCALE: A bedside assessment tool that provides a reproducible, quantitative measurement of the stroke-related neurologic deficit.

CLINICAL APPROACH

Introduction

Stroke is a serious and common disorder that affects over 795,000 persons in the United States each year. It remains the **fourth leading cause of death in the United States and the number one cause for disability.** Twenty percent of affected persons will die within 1 year. Many surviving victims are left with neurologic deficits and may be unable to care for themselves. Symptoms vary widely depending on the type of infarct, the location, and the amount of brain involved (Tables 28–1 and 28–2). Strokes are classified as either ischemic or hemorrhagic. Eighty percent of strokes are ischemic due to the blockage of a blood vessel secondary to thrombosis or embolism. They are generally seen in patients older than the age of 50 and present with the sudden onset of focal neurologic deficits. Hemorrhagic strokes are typically seen in younger patients and are due to intraparenchymal or subarachnoid cerebral vessel bleeding.

Evaluation

The history and physical examination remains the cornerstone of evaluating stroke patients. The **symptoms may include weakness, numbness, or discoordination of the limbs or face, cranial nerve palsies, dysarthria, or cognitive impairments such as aphasia or neglect.** It is critical to find out the exact onset of stroke symptoms, as thrombolytics can only be given within a 4.5-hour window from the

Table 28–1 • ISCHEMIC STROKE SYNDROMES	
Syndrome	Symptoms
Transient ischemic attack (TIA)	Neurological deficit resolving within 24 hours; highly correlated with future thrombotic stroke
Dominant hemisphere	Contralateral numbness and weakness, contralateral visual field cut, gaze preference, dysarthria, aphasia
Nondominant hemisphere	Contralateral numbness and weakness, visual field cut, contralateral neglect, dysarthria
Anterior cerebral artery	Contralateral weakness (leg > arm); mild sensory deficits; dyspraxia
Middle cerebral artery	Contralateral numbness and weakness (face, arm > leg); aphasia (if dominant hemisphere)
Posterior cerebral artery	Lack of visual recognition; altered mental status with impaired memory; cortical blindness
Vertebrobasilar syndrome	Dizziness, vertigo; diplopia; dysphagia; ataxia; ipsilateral cranial nerve palsies; contralateral weakness (crossed deficits)
Basilar artery occlusion	Quadriplegia; coma; locked-in syndrome (paralysis except upward gaze)
Lacunar infarct	Pure motor or sensory deficit

Table 28–2 • HEMORRHAGIC STROKE SYNDROMES	
Syndrome	Symptoms
Intracerebral hemorrhage	May be clinically indistinguishable from infarction; contralateral numbness and weakness; aphasia, neglect (depending on hemisphere); headache, vomiting, lethargy, marked hypertension more common
Cerebellar hemorrhage	Sudden onset of dizziness, vomiting, truncal instability, gaze palsies, stupor

onset of symptoms in ischemic strokes. If the patient awoke with symptoms or is unable to communicate, the physician must determine when the patient was last awake and "normal." Strokes are more common in the elderly (75% occur in patients older than 75 years), males, and African Americans. Other risk factors for stroke include a history of TIA or previous stroke, hypertension, atherosclerosis, cardiac disease (eg, atrial fibrillation, myocardial infarction, and valvular disease), diabetes, carotid stenosis, dyslipidemia, hypercoagulable states, tobacco, and alcohol use. It is possible, although challenging, to clinically infer the location of the anatomic insult to the clinical presentation by correlating symptoms with circulatory region (Figure 28–1). For instance, aphasia usually corresponds to a left hemispheric stroke; neglect generally indicates a right hemispheric stroke; crossed signs (eg, right-sided facial droop with left-sided extremity weakness) typically indicate brainstem involvement.

The evaluation should include the use of the NIH Stroke Scale (NIHSS) (Table 28–3), a standardized system that measures the level of impairment caused

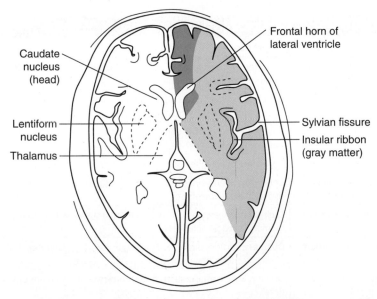

Figure 28–1. Anatomy of brain and blood flow. (*Modified, with permission, from Schwartz DT. Emergency Radiology: Case Studies. New York, NY: McGraw-Hill Education, 2008: 505.*)

Table 28–3 • NATIONAL INSTITUTES OF HEALTH STROKE SCALE

Category	Patient Response	Score
Level of consciousness questions (know month and age?)	Answers both questions correctly Answers one correctly Answers none correctly	0 1 2
Level of consciousness commands (patient instructed to open and close eyes and then to grip and release nonparetic hand)	Obeys both correctly Obeys one correctly Obeys none correctly	0 1 2
Best gaze (horizontal gaze tested)	Normal gaze Partial gaze palsy Forced deviation or total gaze paresis	0 1 2
Best visual (visual fields tested by confrontation)	No visual loss Partial hemianopsia Complete hemianopsia Bilateral hemianopsia (blind including cortical blindness)	0 1 2 3
Facial palsy (patient instructed to show teeth or raise eye brows or close eyes)	Normal symmetric movement Minor paralysis Partial paralysis Complete paralysis of one or both sides	0 1 2 3
Best motor arm Right _____ Left _____	No drift Drift <10 seconds Falls <10 seconds No effort against gravity No movement	0 1 2 3 4
Best motor leg Right _____ Left _____	No drift Drift <10 seconds Falls <10 seconds No effort against gravity No movement	0 1 2 3 4
Limb ataxia (finger-nose-finger and heel-toe bilaterally)	Absent Ataxia in one limb Ataxia in two limbs	0 1 2
Sensory (sensation or grimace to pinprick)	No sensory loss Mild sensory loss Severe sensory loss	0 1 2
Best language (describe picture, name items on sheet)	No aphasia, normal Mild to moderate aphasia Severe aphasia Mute, global aphasia	0 1 2 3
Dysarthria (read or repeat words from a sheet)	Normal Mild to moderate Severe	0 1 2
Extinction and Inattention	No abnormality Visual, tactile, spatial, or personal inattention or extinction to bilateral simultaneous stimulation Profound hemi-attention or hemi-attention to more than one modality	0 1 2

Source: Reproduced from the National Institutes of Health, 2000.

by stroke. It measures several aspects of brain function such as consciousness, vision, sensation, movement, speech, and language. A score above 20 to the maximal score of 42 represents a severe stroke. Current guidelines allow strokes with scores above 4 to be treated with tissue-type plasminogen activator (tPA).

Many hospitals have a "Stroke Team" or a "Code Stroke" protocol that facilitates the prompt diagnosis and treatment of stroke patients, as the treatment of stroke is highly time sensitive. The National Institute of Neurological Disorders and Stroke (NINDS) has established door-to-treatment time frames in responding to acute stroke. These include a **physician evaluation within 10 minutes of arrival, specialist/neurologist notification within 15 minutes, CT of head within 25 minutes and CT interpretation within 45 minutes.** For ischemic strokes, the guideline for the administration of rtPA (recombinant tissue-type plasminogen activator) in eligible patients is within 60 minutes of arrival to the facility, within the "golden hour" of stroke care (Table 28–4).

Diagnostic Studies: Most of the diagnostic studies in acute stroke patients are used to exclude other etiologies of neurologic impairments and identify possible contraindications to tPA administration. Oxygen saturation is needed to exclude hypoxia as etiology of neurologic impairments. Because cardiac abnormalities are common among stroke patients, an ECG should be obtained. The most common

Table 28–4 • CRITERIA FOR INTRAVENOUS THROMBOLYSIS[a] IN ISCHEMIC STROKE
INCLUSIONS
• Age 18 years or older
• Clinical criteria of ischemic stroke
• Time of onset well established, <3 hours
EXCLUSIONS
• Minor stroke symptoms
• Rapidly improving neurological signs
• Prior intracranial hemorrhage or intracranial neoplasm
• Arteriovenous malformation or aneurysm
• Blood glucose <50 mg/dL or >400 mg/dL
• Seizure at onset of stroke
• Gastrointestinal or genitourinary bleeding within preceding 21 days
• Arterial puncture at a noncompressible site or lumbar puncture within 1 week
• Recent myocardial infarction
• Major surgery within preceding 14 days
• Sustained pretreatment severe hypertension (systolic blood pressure >185 mm Hg, diastolic blood pressure >110 mm Hg)
• Previous stroke within past 90 days
• Previous head injury within past 90 days
• Current use of oral anticoagulant or prothrombin time >15 seconds or INR >1.7
• Use of heparin within preceding 48 hours or prolonged partial thromboplastin time
• Platelet count <100,000/mm³

[a]Recombinant tissue plasminogen activator (rtPA) should be used with caution in individuals with severe stroke symptoms, NIHSS >22.
Source: Data from Adams HP, Brott TG, Furlon AJ, et al. Guidelines for thrombolytic therapy for acute stroke. Circulation. 1996;94:1167.

dysrhythmia is atrial fibrillation. Although further cardiovascular studies will ultimately be performed, they should be done as an inpatient so that the acute care of the patient is not delayed. Another critical bedside test that should be performed is a capillary blood glucose (CBG). Severe hypoglycemia and occasionally hyperglycemia can mimic acute stroke, and these conditions can be rapidly ruled out with a normal glucose level. Other blood tests usually include a complete blood count including platelets (platelets should also be above 100,000 per mm^3 to administer thrombolytics), coagulation studies, and cardiac markers. Coagulation studies are important on patients with anticoagulation who are supratherapeutic and at higher risk for an intracerebral bleed.

Patients with suspected strokes should undergo diagnostic imaging, **commonly a non-contrast head CT scan.** Because of the difficulty in clinically differentiating a hemorrhagic from an ischemic stroke, the CT is vital for ruling out an intracerebral bleed, which is an absolute contraindication to thrombolytic therapy and often requires neurosurgery consultation. An early CT finding in ischemic stroke is loss of the gray-white differentiation due to increased water concentration in ischemic tissues, leading to a loss of distinction among the basal ganglia nuclei, gyri swelling, and sulcal effacement. Another early CT finding is increased density within the occluded vessel, which represents the thrombus. Other imaging modalities, such as contrast-enhanced CT and MRI, may equal CT's efficiency in detecting intracerebral hemorrhage. MRI is superior to CT for the demonstration of subacute and chronic hemorrhage, and gradient-echo MR can also detect other vascular lesions such as malformations and amyloid angiopathy. However, the time required to obtain these studies may delay the time-sensitive administration of tPA.

Differential Diagnoses

The differential for stroke is broad and may include: neurologic entities such as seizure/Todd's paralysis; complicated migraine headaches; nonconvulsive status epilepticus; flares of demyelinating disorders such as multiple sclerosis, and spinal cord lesions. Toxic/metabolic abnormalities such as hypo- and hyperglycemia, hypo- or hypernatremia, drug overdose, and botulism are possibilities. It is also important to consider infectious etiologies, such as systemic infection, Bell palsy, meningitis/encephalitis, Rocky Mountain spotted fever, and brain abscess. Cardiac or vascular causes should also be ruled out, including hypertensive encephalopathy, carotid/aortic/vertebral artery dissection, subarachnoid hemorrhage, or cerebral vasculitis. Other etiologies such as tumor, sickle cell cerebral crisis, vitamin deficiencies, depression or psychosis, and heat stroke are some of the other considerations.

Treatment

Stroke patients are managed as critically ill patients. Management imperatives include: assessment and stabilization of the ABCs, formal evaluation for possible thrombolytic administration, and addressing comorbid conditions such as hypertension. Alteplase (intravenous rtPA) may help restore tissue perfusion in ischemic stroke and is the only FDA-approved thrombolytic for stroke. The NIH/NINDS study in 1995 found that **alteplase improved functional outcomes at 3 months compared to placebo if given within 3 hours of symptom onset.** In May 2009, the American Heart Association/American Stroke Association (AHA/ASA) guidelines for the administration of rtPA following acute stroke were revised to expand the window of treatment from 3 to 4.5 hours to provide more patients with an opportunity to receive benefit from this effective therapy.

Recent studies have suggested that there may be a longer therapeutic window for the administration of thrombolytics. However, earlier administration is always better since "time is brain;" nervous tissue is lost as the stroke progresses. rtPA is usually administered 0.9 mg/kg with a maximum dose of 90 mg, with 10% of the dose administered as an IV bolus and the remainder infused over 60 minutes. Furthermore, neither heparin nor aspirin is used during the initial 24 hours. However, thrombolytics should not be withheld from a patient who has recently taken aspirin. Additionally, endovascular therapies such as intra-arterial and mechanical thrombolysis are being used for a subset of patients with acute ischemic stroke. Consideration or the use of mechanical thrombolysis should not prevent or delay administration of rtPA (see Table 28–4).

Elevated blood pressures are generally left untreated to maintain cerebral perfusion pressure. However, **systolic blood pressures >220 mm Hg and diastolic blood pressures >120 mm Hg are best treated** with easily titratable agents, such as IV labetalol and nitrates. The blood pressure should not be lowered more than 25% of the presenting mean arterial blood pressure. The treated blood pressure should be **below 185/110 mm Hg for rtPA administration.** Treatment of hemorrhagic stroke is different and includes blood pressure control with antihypertensives such as nimodipine, possibly reversing any anticoagulation with cryoprecipitate or platelets, and consultation with a hematologist and neurosurgeon.

CASE CORRELATION

- See also Case 26 (Syncope), Case 27 (Bell Palsy [Idiopathic Facial Paralysis]), and Case 30 (Seizure).

COMPREHENSION QUESTIONS

28.1 A 58-year-old man experienced a neurologic deficit and is diagnosed as having a stroke. Which of the following is the most likely etiology?

A. Ischemic

B. Hemorrhagic

C. Drug-induced

D. Trauma-induced

E. Metabolic-related

28.2 An 80-year-old man is being evaluated for possible thrombolytic therapy after presenting with 2 hours of right arm weakness and aphasia. Which of the following is a contraindication for thrombolytic therapy?

A. Bilateral cerebral infarct

B. Hemorrhagic stroke

C. Hypertension-related stroke

D. Age of 80 years

28.3 An otherwise healthy 65-year-old woman is taken to the ED with probable stroke. Which of the following are the most urgent diagnostic studies?

A. Coagulation studies

B. ECG and cardiac enzymes

C. Bedside blood glucose and CT scan of the head

D. MRI of the head with and without contrast

28.4 A 67-year-old woman is seen in the emergency room with left arm weakness and right facial droop. Her blood pressure is 180/105 mm Hg. Which of the following is the best management for the hypertension?

A. Lower the blood pressure to less than 160/80 mm Hg by giving a small dose of labetalol.

B. Lower the blood pressure to less than 120/80 mm Hg.

C. No intervention for her blood pressure, but continue to monitor.

D. Lower the blood pressure to below 160/80 mm Hg if she is eligible for tPA.

ANSWERS

28.1 **A.** Ischemia is the most common etiology of stroke (due to thrombosis, embolism, or hypoperfusion) and is responsible for up to 80% of strokes.

28.2 **B.** Indications for tPA administration include an ischemic stroke with a clearly defined time of onset, measurable neurologic deficit, and a baseline CT with no evidence of intracranial hemorrhage. Contraindications for tPA therapy vary and include, but are not limited to: seizure at the time of stroke, history of intracranial hemorrhage, persistent blood pressure greater than 185/110 mm Hg despite antihypertensive therapy, recent surgery or GI bleed, recent MI, pregnancy, elevated aPTT or INR due to heparin or warfarin use, or platelet count less than 100,000.

28.3 **C.** Bedside blood glucose and CT scan of the head are the most urgent diagnostic studies in evaluating possible stroke patients. Coagulation studies, a complete blood count or platelet count should not delay tPA administration unless the patient is taking anticoagulation or has suspected thrombocytopenia. Non-contrast head CT is generally the initial imaging study, not MRI, to exclude hemorrhage or tumor as a cause of neurologic deficits. Though MRI provides more information, its cost, limited availability, restricted patient access, and other contraindications such as patient claustrophobia or metal implants limit its use.

28.4 **C.** Emergency administration of antihypertensive agents should be withheld in acute stroke to maintain cerebral perfusion pressure, unless the blood pressure is greater than 220/120 mm Hg. In patients who are eligible for tPA, the goal BP is less than 185/110 mm Hg. If patients have concurrent conditions (eg, aortic dissection, hypertensive encephalopathy, acute renal failure, or congestive heart failure) that require acute lowering of blood pressure, a reasonable goal is to lower their mean arterial pressure 15% to 25% within the first 24 hours.

CLINICAL PEARLS

▶ Strokes may present in a variety of ways, and the differential diagnosis of stroke is broad.

▶ Clinicians must take a careful history, including the time of onset of symptoms.

▶ The NIHSS measures the impairment due to stroke.

▶ A bedside glucose measurement and a CT scan of the head are the most urgent diagnostic studies in suspected stroke.

▶ Treatment is aimed at stabilizing the ABCs, evaluating for possible thrombolytic administration, and addressing comorbid conditions such as hypertension.

▶ Thrombolytic therapy should be initiated in patient with an ischemic stroke as soon as possible since "time is brain."

▶ Some of the major contraindications to thrombolytic therapy include hemorrhagic stroke, severe hypo- or hyperglycemia, uncontrolled severe hypertension, or significant bleeding conditions.

REFERENCES

Adams HP Jr, del Zoppo G, Alberts MJ, et al. Guidelines for the early management of adults with ischemic stroke: a guideline from the American Heart Association; American Stroke Association Stroke Council; Clinical Cardiology Council; Cardiovascular Radiology and Intervention Council, and the Atherosclerotic Peripheral Vascular Disease and Quality of Care Outcomes in Research Interdisciplinary Working Groups. *Stroke.* 2007;38:1655-1711.

Asimos AW. Code stroke: a state-of-the-art strategy for rapid assessment and treatment. *Emerg Med Prac.* 1999;1(2):1-24.

Del Zoppo GJ, Saver JL, Jauch EC, Adams HP Jr. Expansion of the time window for treatment of acute ischemic stroke with intravenous tissue plasminogen activator: a science advisory from the American Heart Association/American Stroke Association. *Stroke.* 2009;40(8):2945-2948.

Diedler J, Ahmed N, Sykora M, et al. Safety of intravenous thrombolysis for acute ischemic stroke in patients receiving antiplatelet therapy at stroke onset. *Stroke.* 2010;41(2):288-294.

Hacke W, Kaste M, Bluhmki E, et al. Thrombolysis with alteplase 3 to 4.5 hours after acute ischemic stroke. *N Engl J Med.* 2008;359(13):1317-1329.

Huang P, Khor GT, Chen CH, et al. Eligibility and rate of treatment for recombinant tissue plasminogen activator in acute ischemic stroke using different criteria. *Acad Emerg Med.* 2011;18(3):273-278.

Latchaw R, Alberts M, Lev M. Recommendations for imaging of acute ischemic stroke: a scientific statement from the American Heart Association. *Stroke.* 2009;40;3646-3678.

Lewandowski C, Barsan W. Treatment of acute ischemic stroke. Ann Emerg Med. 2001;37(2):202-216.

The National Institute of Neurological Disorders and Stroke rt-PA Stroke Study G. Generalized efficacyor tPA for acute stroke. *Stroke.* 1997;28:2119-2125.

The National Institute of Neurological Disorders and Stroke rt-PA Stroke Study G. Tissue plasminogen activator for acute ischemic stroke. *N Engl J Med.* 1995;333(24):1581-1587.

Tintinalli JE, Kelen GD, Stapczynski JS, eds. *Emergency Medicine.* 8th ed. New York, NY: McGraw-Hill; 2015: 1430-1439.

U.S. Centers for Disease Control and Prevention and the Heart Disease and Stroke Statistics—2007 Update, published by the American Heart Association. Available at: http://www.strokecenter.org/patients/stats.htm. Accessed April, 2011.

A 50-year-old woman presents with a severe headache of abrupt onset of 10 hours' duration. The pain is diffuse, throbbing, and worsened when she went outside into the sunlight. She denies any recent fever, neck pain, numbness, weakness, vomiting, and any change in vision. She was concerned because she has never had a headache as strong as this before. Her past medical and family histories are unremarkable. She does not take any medications, does not smoke, and only drinks alcohol socially.

On examination, her temperature is 36.9°C (98.4°F), blood pressure is 136/72 mm Hg, heart rate is 88 beats per minute, and respiratory rate is 16 breaths per minute. She is not in any acute distress but appears to be mildly uncomfortable. Her pupils are equal and reactive bilaterally. There is no evidence of papilledema on fundoscopic examination. Movement of her neck causes her some increased discomfort. Her neurological examination is normal, including cranial nerves, strength, light touch sensation, deep-tendon reflexes, and finger-to-nose. The computed tomography (CT) scan of her head is normal.

▶ What is the most likely diagnosis?
▶ What is the next diagnostic step?

ANSWERS TO CASE 29:

Headache

Summary: This is a 50-year-old woman with acute onset of "the worst headache of her life."

- **Most likely diagnosis:** Subarachnoid hemorrhage.
- **Next diagnostic step:** CT scan of the head followed by lumbar puncture.

ANALYSIS

Objectives

1. Learn to differentiate emergent, urgent, and non-urgent causes of headache.

2. Understand the treatment of various types of headache.

Considerations

This 50-year-old woman has an acute onset of severe headache, described as the "worst headache of her life." The acute onset and severity of her symptoms are concerning for subarachnoid hemorrhage (SAH). Headache is a very common chief complaint in the emergency department (ED). When evaluating patients with headaches, the clinician's goals are to identify those with serious or life-threatening conditions and to alleviate pain. The physical examination should screen for non-neurological causes of headache, including palpation of the sinuses (looking for tenderness consistent with sinusitis) and palpation of the temporal arteries (for tenderness or reduced pulsations suggestive of temporal arteritis). A thorough eye examination is important and should consist of assessment of the pupils, visual acuity, and fundoscopy. A detailed neurological examination should also be performed. This patient's CT scan of the head is unremarkable, which does not definitively rule out SAH. A CT scan is often performed to rule out an intracranial mass before performing lumbar puncture (LP). Erythrocytes in the cerebrospinal fluid (CSF) or a xanthochromic CSF are considered diagnostic for SAH. However, xanthochromia may take up to 12 hours to appear. Therefore, a negative LP in the face of clinical suspicion for SAH may necessitate repeat LP or other neuroimaging such as CT angiogram, magnetic resonance imaging (MRI), or conventional angiography.

APPROACH TO:

Headache

CLINICAL APPROACH

Headaches can be caused by many intracranial and extracranial processes and can be subdivided into **emergent versus non-emergent causes.** Emergent headaches have an etiology that mandates immediate identification and treatment (Table 29–1).

Table 29–1 • CRITICAL AND EMERGENT CAUSES OF HEADACHE
Anemia
Anoxia
Brain abscess
Carbon monoxide poisoning
Glaucoma
Hypertensive encephalopathy
Meningitis/encephalitis
Mountain sickness
Shunt failure
Subarachnoid/other intracranial hemorrhage
Temporal arteritis
Tumor/cerebral mass

In contrast, non-emergent causes are benign and do not present any immediate threat to life. This category includes primary headache syndromes and post-LP headaches. Although only a minority of patients with headache have a potentially life-threatening etiology, identification of these patients is paramount.

When evaluating patients with headaches, the history should focus on the nature of the pain (location, severity, character, and onset), any associated symptoms, and aggravating or alleviating factors. Past medical history (including history of head trauma and medications) and family history are important to identify risk factors for serious disease. A history of prior headaches and any previous diagnostic studies can also be helpful. Potentially ominous historical findings include sudden onset, pain described as the "worst headache of my life," headaches that are dramatically different from past episodes, immunocompromised patients, and new onset after age 50 or with exertion.

A complete physical examination with a **detailed neurological evaluation** can also help to separate emergent from non-emergent causes. Abnormal vital signs can be a sign of life-threatening conditions. Other warning signs include **altered mental status, abnormal fundi, meningeal signs, focal neurological deficits, and a rash suspicious for meningococcemia.** Some types of headache have classic historical or examination findings that will aid in narrowing the differential (Table 29–2).

Because there is no routine workup of headaches, testing should be based on clinical suspicion of serious illness (Table 29–3). Diagnostic imaging of the head should be considered for patients with sudden-onset severe headaches, immunocompromised patients with a new headache, and headaches with new abnormal findings (eg, focal deficit and altered mental status). Management includes stabilizing any life-threatening conditions, controlling pain, and addressing any underlying disease or specific etiologies.

SUBARACHNOID HEMORRHAGE

Most cases of SAH occur in patients 40-60 years old. The presentation can be very subtle with a normal neurological examination, little or no nuchal rigidity, normal level of consciousness, and normal vital signs. Nevertheless, the mortality

Table 29–2 • CLASSIC HISTORICAL AND EXAMINATION FINDINGS

Etiology	History	Examination
Brain tumor	Headache with nausea and vomiting, gradual onset, worse in morning, most commonly metastatic	Papilledema, cognitive difficulties, focal neurological deficits
Cluster	Severe, unilateral periorbital pain with lacrimation, rhinorrhea; worse at night; attacks "clustered" in short time period; more common in men	Ipsilateral conjunctival injection, ptosis, miosis
Hypertensive encephalopathy	Diffuse, throbbing headache; worse in morning	Diastolic blood pressure >120-130 mm Hg, altered mental status, papilledema
Idiopathic intracranial hypertension (pseudotumor cerebri)	Headache with visual complaints, classically young obese females of childbearing age	Papilledema, visual field defects
Meningitis	Febrile illness	Fever, meningismus, altered mental status; Kernig and Brudzinski signs
Migraine	Unilateral, throbbing headache with nausea, vomiting, photophobia, phonophobia; may be accompanied by visual, motor, or sensory disturbances; more common in women	
Post lumbar puncture	Bilateral, throbbing headache; worse upon standing, better when lying down	
Subarachnoid hemorrhage	"Thunderclap" onset, "worst headache of life," nausea, vomiting	Retinal or subhyaloid hemorrhages, meningismus, third or sixth nerve palsy
Temporal arteritis	Pain over temporal artery; visual problems, jaw claudication; fever, malaise, weight loss; joint pains; worse at night; more common in women >50 years old	Tenderness or induration of temporal artery, decreased or absent pulse in temporal artery, optic nerve edema
Tension type	Dull, "band-like" headache	Pericranial muscle tenderness

associated with SAH approaches 50%. Thus, the ED physician must maintain a high index of suspicion in a patient with acute onset of severe headache. CT scan is the most common initial imaging study and is most sensitive when performed within 6-12 hours of symptom onset (up to 98% sensitivity). Although CTs have high sensitivity, no imaging procedure can definitively rule out SAH. Thus, many authorities advocate performing an LP on patients suspected of having SAH, even with a normal CT scan. **The LP revealing xanthochromic CSF is considered the gold standard of diagnosis.** Because xanthochromia may take up to 12 hours to develop,

Table 29–3 • DIAGNOSTIC TESTS AND TREATMENT		
Etiology	Diagnostic Tests	Treatment
Brain tumor	CT; consider CT with contrast or MRI	Neurosurgical consultation. If increased intracranial pressure, consider intubation and mild hyperventilation, osmotic agents, steroids
Cluster		High-flow oxygen, sumatriptan, DHE; consider intranasal lidocaine
Hypertensive encephalopathy	CT; rule out other end-organ damage	Control blood pressure (eg, nicardipine and labetalol)
Idiopathic intracranial hypertension	CT to rule out other causes of increased intracranial pressure; LP with opening pressure	Serial LPs, acetazolamide; surgical intervention may be required
Meningitis	CT may be needed prior to LP; LP	Intravenous antibiotics (without delay); consider steroids
Migraine		Acetaminophen, NSAIDs, antiemetics (eg, metoclopramide and prochlorperazine), serotonin agonists (sumatriptan), ergot alkaloids (DHE); narcotics if refractory pain; consider steroids
Post-lumbar puncture		Hydration, bed rest, NSAIDs, narcotics, caffeine; consider epidural blood patch for severe, prolonged symptoms
Subarachnoid hemor-rhage	CT, LP if CT negative; MRI or angiography may be required	Neurosurgical consult, control blood pressure, analgesia, nimodipine, antiemetics, antiseizure medications
Temporal arteritis	Erythrocyte sedimentation rate; consider temporal artery biopsy (may be done as outpatient)	Steroids
Tension type		Aspirin, acetaminophen, NSAIDs, stress reduction

Abbreviations: CT = computed tomography; MRI = magnetic resonance imaging; DHE = dihydroergotamine; LP = lumbar puncture; NSAIDs = nonsteroidal anti-inflammatory drugs.

persistently bloody CSF is also worrisome for SAH. Neurosurgical evaluation is important once the diagnosis of SAH is established. Further imaging is usually obtained to assess for lesions requiring surgical intervention, such as berry aneurysms. Prognosis generally correlates with initial neurological status.

CEREBRAL CAUSES

Viral or bacterial meningitis can cause severe headache. LP is the definitive method of assessing for these infections. Immunocompromised states such as human immunodeficiency virus (HIV) infection may cause subtle or atypical symptoms (eg, lack of fever or meningismus). Pre-LP CT does not necessarily need to be performed for an immunocompetent patient with a non-focal neurological examination, normal level of consciousness, and absence of papilledema. Stroke or transient ischemic attack (TIA) may present as headache, but usually there is a history of or continued neurological deficit. The classic presentation of a brain tumor (headache associated with nausea or vomiting, sleep disturbances) is uncommon. A persistent atypical headache (such as new onset after age 50 years, severe pain, or associated with subtle cognitive or neurological function) should be investigated, usually with CT.

TEMPORAL ARTERITIS

Temporal arteritis (TA) almost always occurs in patients older than age 50 years and is more common in women. It is caused by systemic arteritis and presents as a severe, throbbing headache located over the frontotemporal region. Often, the temporal artery has a diminished pulse or is tender to palpation. Patients are diagnosed with TA if they fulfill three of the following criteria: **age older than 50 years, new-onset localized headache, decreased pulse or tenderness over the temporal artery, an erythrocyte sedimentation rate exceeding 50 mm/h, and/or an abnormal temporal artery biopsy.** As permanent vision loss is a potential complication, immediate treatment should include prednisone 40-60 mg/day and urgent referral.

PRIMARY HEADACHE SYNDROMES

Migraine headaches are common and usually begin during the teenage years. Women are more often affected, and a family history is often positive. The most common presentation is migraine without aura, which is usually slow in onset, unilateral, and throbbing. Photophobia, phonophobia, nausea, and vomiting frequently accompany the pain. Patients with migraines with aura have a similar type of headache that is preceded by reversible visual phenomena, paresthesias, motor deficits, or language difficulties. Treatment includes intravenous hydration if the patient is dehydrated and placing the patient in a dark, quiet room. Pharmacological options include nonsteroidal anti-inflammatory agents (eg, ketorolac), dihydroergotamine (a nonspecific serotonin agonist), sumatriptan (a selective serotonin agonist), dopamine antagonists (eg, metoclopramide, chlorpromazine, or prochlorperazine), steroids (eg, dexamethasone or methylprednisolone), or valproate. In general, opiates are used for patients with refractory pain.

Tension headaches are extremely common. They are usually characterized by bilateral, non-pulsating, "band-like" pain around the forehead that radiates to the occiput and are commonly associated with nausea and vomiting. Treatment includes acetaminophen, non-steroidal anti-inflammatory drugs (NSAIDs), muscle relaxants, and stress-reduction techniques.

Cluster headaches are rarer than other types of primary headache syndromes. They occur more commonly in **men** and usually start after 20 years of age. Patients typically present with unilateral, severe, orbital, or temporal pain, often associated with ipsilateral lacrimation, nasal congestion, rhinorrhea, miosis, and/or ptosis. The headaches tend to occur in "clusters" for several weeks and then remit for months or years. High-flow oxygen is usually effective. Sumatriptan can also help relieve symptoms.

CASE CORRELATION

- See also Case 12 (Hypertensive Encephalopathy), Case 25 (Altered Mental Status), Case 26 (Syncope), Case 28 (Stroke), Case 30 (Seizure Induced by Traumatic Brain Injury), and Case 39 (Bacterial Meningitis).

COMPREHENSION QUESTIONS

29.1 Several patients have been brought into the ED with a chief complaint of headache. Which of the following patients should be seen first (ie, which is most likely to have a potentially life-threatening condition)?

   A. A 52-year-old man with headache of 8-hours' duration and blood pressure of 210/120 mm Hg.

   B. A 24-year-old woman with a severe, squeezing headache involving the front of her head that radiates to her neck.

   C. A 32-year-old woman who underwent an outpatient bilateral tubal ligation under spinal anesthesia and now complains of a severe bilateral headache, especially with sitting up.

   D. A 35-year-old woman with a severe headache and a prior diagnosis of pseudotumor cerebri.

29.2 A 22-year-old man complains of a severe headache of 45 minutes' duration that is described as unilateral, periorbital and associated with ipsilateral nasal congestion. Which of the following is the best treatment?

   A. High-flow oxygen

   B. Propranolol

   C. Ergotamine

   D. Prednisone

29.3 A 34-year-old woman is brought into the ED for "the worst headache of her life." She has some lethargy, photophobia, and nuchal rigidity. An LP is performed after examining her eye grounds. Which of the following findings in cerebrospinal fluid is most concerning for SAH?

   A. Red blood cells

   B. White blood cells

   C. Elevated opening pressure

   D. Xanthochromia

ANSWERS

29.1 **A.** The first patient is most likely to have a potentially life-threatening condition (hypertensive crisis). If untreated, stroke, MI or acute kidney failure may ensue.

29.2 **A. High-flow oxygen is an effective treatment for cluster headaches.** Cluster headaches are more common in men, are usually periorbital, and are associated with ipsilateral conjunctival injection, lacrimation, nasal congestion, rhinorrhea, miosis, ptosis, or facial sweating.

29.3 **D.** Xanthochromia in cerebrospinal fluid is most concerning for SAH. Because it results from hemoglobin metabolism, xanthochromia may take up to 12 hours to develop.

CLINICAL PEARLS

▶ Potentially ominous historical findings include sudden onset, "the worst headache of life," headaches dramatically different from past episodes, immunocompromised states, new onset after age 50 years, and onset with exertion.

▶ Diagnostic testing must be based on clinical suspicion. For example, if there is a concern for a subarachnoid hemorrhage, a CT scan of the head and LP (if CT is negative) are warranted.

▶ In general, management includes stabilizing any life-threatening conditions, controlling pain, and addressing any underlying disease or specific etiologies.

REFERENCES

American College of Emergency Physicians. Clinical policy: critical issues in the evaluation and management of adult patients presenting to the emergency department with acute headache. *Ann Emerg Med.* 2008;52:407-436.

Godwin SA, Villa J. Acute headache in the ED: evidence-based evaluation and treatment options. *Emerg Med Pract.* 2001;3(6):1-32.

Goldstein JN, Camargo CA Jr, Pelletier AJ, et al. Headache in United States emergency departments: demographics, work-up and frequency of pathological diagnoses. *Cephalalgia.* 2006;26:684-690.

Hamilton GC, Sanders AB, Strange GR, Trott AT, eds. *Emergency Medicine: An Approach to Clinical Problem-Solving.* Philadelphia, PA: WB Saunders; 2003:535-551.

Kotapally M, Josephson SA Common neurologic emergencies for non-neurologists: when minutes count. *Cleve Clin J Med.* 2016;83(2):116-126.

Marx JA, Hockberger RS, Walls RM, eds. *Rosen's Emergency Medicine: Concepts and Clinical Practice.* 8th ed. Philadelphia, PA: Saunders; 2014.

Mick NW, Peters JR, Silvers SM. *Blueprints in Emergency Medicine.* Malden, MA: Blackwell Publishing; 2002:139-142.

Tintinalli JE, Stapczynski JS, Ma OJ, et al., eds. *Emergency Medicine: A Comprehensive Study Guide.* 8th ed. New York, NY: McGraw-Hill; 2016.

A 37-year-old insulin-dependent diabetic (IDDM) man is brought into the emergency department (ED) by ambulance after a motor vehicle accident. Per EMS, he was the restrained driver of a vehicle that lost control and collided into the center divider at highway speeds. Witnesses reported that the severely damaged vehicle rolled over multiple times but that the air bag did not deploy. Vital signs taken in the field showed a blood pressure of 110/85 mm Hg, heart rate 140 beats per minute, respiration rate 24 breaths per minute, and oxygen saturation 98% on 15 L of oxygen via nonrebreather mask. Paramedics report that during transport to the ED, the patient seized with tonic-clonic movements of all four extremities. He was given lorazepam 2-mg IV push with almost immediate resolution of the seizure. In the ED, he is no longer seizing but has a depressed level of consciousness with a Glasgow coma scale (GCS) of 8. HIs airway is patent, breath sounds are equal bilaterally, and pulses are bounding throughout. His blood glucose is 75 mg/dL. It is noted that his right pupil is 5 mm and nonreactive, and his left pupil is 3 mm and reactive. His tone is normal in all four extremities. His reflexes are 2+ throughout. His toes are downgoing bilaterally. His cardiovascular, respiratory, and abdominal examinations are unremarkable. He is not wearing a medic-alert bracelet. His CT scan of the head reveals a large right-frontal intraparenchymal hemorrhage.

▶ What is the most likely diagnosis?
▶ What is your next step?

ANSWERS TO CASE 30:

Seizure Induced by Traumatic Brain Injury

Summary: A 37-year-old man was a restrained driver in motor vehicle accident. He has no known history of seizures but did seize en route to the ED; he is found to have right-sided blown pupil and a GCS of 8.

- **Most likely diagnosis:** Seizure likely secondary to acute intraparenchymal bleed from a traumatic brain injury.

- **Next step:** Aggressive management of ABCs (airway, breathing, and circulation) with rapid sequence intubation to protect the airway, management of intracranial pressure (ICP), and anticonvulsant treatment to prevent reoccurrence of seizures.

ANALYSIS

Objectives

1. Develop a methodological approach to the assessment of the patient who presents to the ED with first-time seizure and status epilepticus.

2. Understand the diagnostic and therapeutic approach to patients presenting with first-time seizure and status epilepticus.

Considerations

This 37-year-old man with IDDM presents with a seizure after being involved in a motor vehicle accident. It is important to consider the order of events in traumas such as this, especially when the history is limited. One must question whether a medical event preceded the crash; did the patient have a seizure while driving secondary to hypoglycemia, does he have a past medical history of epilepsy and is subtherapeutic on his anticonvulsant medications, or did he become distracted or confused for some other reason? Despite the confirmed head injury, the provider must cast a broad net to make sure no additional injuries are missed.

APPROACH TO:

Seizure Disorders

DEFINITIONS

SEIZURE: A **seizure** is any event involving an abnormal, excessive, and synchronous firing of neurons characterized by changes in sensory perception or motor activity. **Provoked seizures** occur in the presence of precipitating factors such as hypoglycemia, electrolyte imbalance, fever, head injury, alcohol withdrawal, and exposure to drugs/toxins.

EPILEPSY: The term **epilepsy** is applied when two or more unprovoked seizures occur more than 24 hours apart. A seizure is a neurologic event, and epilepsy is a disease involving recurrent unprovoked seizures.

STATUS EPILEPTICUS: Status epilepticus (SE) is now defined as continuous seizure activity lasting greater than 5 minutes, or two or more sequential seizures without return to normal mental baseline. Historical definitions used a 30-minute time limit, a period after which irreversible neuronal damage occurs.

CLINICAL APPROACH

Classifications

Seizures can be divided into two major classifications based on their origin. *Neurogenic* seizures represent the majority of seizures seen in the ED and result from excessive discharge of cortical neurons. *Psychogenic*, or nonepileptic seizures (NES) are increasingly common and may be extremely difficult to distinguish from true seizures. Unlike neurogenic seizures, these *pseudoseizures* are not the result of abnormal cortical discharge and are often associated with major stress or emotional trauma. *Unclassified* seizures are difficult to fit into a single class and are considered when there is inadequate data.

Neurogenic seizures are either *generalized seizures,* involving abnormal neuronal activity in both hemispheres of the brain and accompanied by a loss of consciousness, or *partial (focal) seizures,* involving neuronal discharge in a localized area of one cerebral hemisphere. *Partial seizures* are subclassified into simple (consciousness is maintained) and complex (impaired level of consciousness). They can be further characterized based on the pattern of motor activity, such as tonic (rigid trunk and extremities), clonic (symmetrical rhythmic jerking of the trunk and extremities), tonic clonic (tonic phase followed by clonic phase), atonic (sudden loss of postural tone), and myoclonic (brief, shock-like muscular contractions).

SE is present when patients have more than 5 minutes of continuous seizure activity or experience two or more sequential seizures without full recovery of consciousness in between. SE is the initial presentation of a seizure disorder in approximately one-third of cases. The most common cause of SE is discontinuation of anticonvulsant medications. The catecholamine surge that accompanies SE can cause tachycardia, hypertension, hypotension, cardiac arrhythmias, respiratory failure, hyperglycemia, acidosis, and rhabdomyolysis. *Nonconvulsive SE* must be ruled out by EEG in any patient who does not regain consciousness after 30 minutes from the cessation of a single generalized seizure, and it should be considered in any patient with unexplained confusion or coma.

Etiology

It is important to consider the etiology of a patient's seizure, as it may influence the clinical approach. Primary, unprovoked seizures in a patient with a known history of epilepsy are usually managed pharmacologically with the goal of restoring normal neuronal function. However, seizures can also present as secondary manifestations of other primary diseases.

Common etiologies of secondary seizures include head trauma, intracranial masses or hemorrhages, post cerebral vascular accident and scar tissue formation, infections such as meningitis or encephalitis, metabolic disturbances (ie, glucose or electrolyte abnormalities), and drugs or toxins. Additional common conditions that may present as seizures include hypertensive encephalopathy and anoxic-ischemic injury secondary to cardiac arrest or severe hypoxemia. Eclampsia must also be considered in pregnant women and up to 4 weeks postpartum as a potential etiology of seizures.

Diagnosis

History: History is essential in the evaluation of a seizure patient, especially in a first-time seizure. It is important to ask the patient and/or witnesses about the circumstances leading up to the seizure, including a description of the ictal movements and the postictal period. Any symptoms associated with the seizure should also be addressed to help direct workup and management. For example, a headache prior to the seizure is concerning for intracranial hemorrhage, while a fever and/or lethargy in a patient who presents with a seizure is worrisome for infectious causes. Patients with a known seizure disorder should be questioned about the type and frequency of their seizures as well as medication compliance. Past medical history, medications, and social history including drug use, alcohol use, and HIV risk factors are also important to consider.

Examination: Patients presenting to the ED with seizure require a thorough physical examination. A detailed neurologic examination is the key component of the evaluation. Focal neurologic deficits may represent a well described transient postictal neurologic condition referred to as Todd's paralysis that can last up to 48 hours. The head and neck examination should include the tongue to look for lacerations, the head and face for evidence of trauma, and the neck for tenderness and rigidity. Cardiopulmonary examination should include auscultation for heart murmurs or an irregular rhythm suggesting an embolic or syncopal event. Although rare, extremity fractures or dislocations may be missed and should be ruled out by a thorough musculoskeletal examination.

Diagnostic Workup: Appropriate laboratory studies in patients with first-time seizures include glucose, serum electrolytes such as sodium, calcium, and magnesium, assessment of renal function, and drug and/or toxicology screen. Women of childbearing age also require a pregnancy test, although seizures secondary to eclampsia would be rare before the late second or early third trimester.

Neuroimaging studies should be performed when a clear etiology to the seizure is not identified or when an acute intracranial process is suspected. American College of Emergency Physicians (ACEP) guidelines recommend a head CT be performed in patients with a history of recent head trauma, persistent altered mental status/headache, fever, malignancy, immunocompromised status, anticoagulation, or in patients who have a new focal deficit, are over 40, or have a partial-onset seizure.

A **lumbar puncture** is an essential part of the workup if clinical presentation is suggestive of an infectious process. Use of EEG is uncommon and often unavailable in the ED evaluation of first-time seizure, but it is necessary when nonconvulsive SE is suspected.

MANAGEMENT

Initial stabilization of the patient requires (a) **ABCs,** (b) bedside **glucose** analysis, (c) **pulse oximetry,** (d) **cardiac monitoring,** and (d) **anticonvulsant** therapy if seizure activity continues at the time of evaluation.

Aggressive airway protection is critical, as seizure patients have decreased gag reflexes and are at risk for aspiration. Positioning the patient on their side with frequent suctioning, if necessary, will lower the risk for aspiration. Patients who continue to seize despite therapy or those unable to protect their airway with conservative measures require intubation.

Pharmacologic Therapy

Parenteral **benzodiazepines** are first-line therapy for active seizures (including SE) and are effective in terminating seizures in 75% to 90% of patients. They suppress seizure activity by directly enhancing GABA (gamma-aminobutyric acid)-related neuronal inhibition. Intravenous **lorazepam** is generally preferred (0.1 mg/kg IV maximum dose 4 mg) up to two doses. **Lorazepam** and **diazepam** (0.2 mg/kg IV maximum dose 10 mg) are equally effective at terminating the initial seizure, while lorazepam is superior for preventing recurrence of the seizure. Options for patients without intravenous access include IM **midazolam** (**10 mg for >40 kg, 5 mg for 13-40 kg**) or rectal **diazepam** (0.5 mg/kg maximum dose 20 mg).

If a benzodiazepine does not terminate seizure activity after two rounds, second-line agents for abortive therapy include **phenytoin/fosphenytoin, valproic acid, and levetiracetam. There is no evidence to suggest which second-line agent is superior.** Phenytoin does not directly suppress electrical activity at the seizure focus but rather slows recovery of voltage-activated sodium channels and thus suppresses neuronal recruitment. Thus, concurrent benzodiazepine administration is necessary when treating active seizures. The IV loading dose of phenytoin is 20 mg/kg but must be given at a rate no greater than 50 mg/min to avoid **hypotension** and potentially fatal **cardiac dysrhythmias** associated with its propylene glycol diluent. Cerebellar findings, such as nystagmus and ataxia, are the most common neurological side effects associated with phenytoin. While parenteral loading is most common, oral loading with a maximum of 400 mg PO every 2 hours is appropriate in stable patients who report medication noncompliance or are found to have a subtherapeutic phenytoin level. **Fosphenytoin** is **water soluble** and is preferred to phenytoin in actively seizing patients due to its safety profile.

Parenteral **valproic acid** has shown some recent promise as an abortive seizure therapy and is considered an alternative in cases where benzodiazepine or phenytoin use is limited by hypotension or hypersensitivity. Although it is similar to phenytoin in mechanism of action, it is generally well tolerated with mild side effects. Recommended loading dose for valproic acid is 20-40 mg/kg (maximum dose 3 gm) at a rate of 3-6 mg/kg/min, though more rapid bolus infusions have been safely administered. **Levetiracetam** is a relatively new anti-epileptic drug (AED) with a mechanism of action that is atypical compared to other AEDs. Recently updated 2016 clinical guidelines from the American Epilepsy Society have included **levetiracetam** as a second-line agent for SE and can be loaded intravenously 20-60 mg/kg (maximum dose 4500 gm) at a rate of 2-5 mg/min.

Phenobarbital is a CNS depressant that directly suppresses cortical electrical activity and may be used as an alternative second-line agent. The onset of intravenous phenobarbital is 15-30 minutes with a long duration of action of up to 48-96 hours. Adverse effects of phenobarbital include profound **respiratory depression** and **hypotension,** limiting its use as abortive seizure therapy.

Refractory SE necessitates consideration of continuous infusions of additional abortive seizure therapeutics, including **propofol, barbiturates** (other than phenobarbital), and midazolam; refractory SE also requires intubation for airway protection. **Propofol** acts as a direct GABA agonist and global CNS depressant. While studies regarding its efficacy in SE are limited, it has been shown to provide almost immediate suppression of seizure activity after a 1-2 mg/kg bolus infusion. Barbiturates (**pentobarbital** and **thiopental**) directly enhance GABA-mediated neuronal inhibition while suppressing all other brainstem functions and thus can also induce respiratory arrest, myocardial depression, and hypotension. Inhaled **isoflurane anesthesia** suppresses electrical seizure foci and is the treatment of last resort for the patient in SE.

It may be very difficult to determine if patients who are profoundly sedated or paralyzed are still seizing. In these situations, anticonvulsant therapy should be continued and **EEG monitoring** of the patient should be arranged.

SPECIAL CASES

Drug-Induced Seizures

Therapy for drug-induced seizures is guided by general seizure management principles. There are no clear evidence-based guidelines for the management of drug-related seizures, and they usually require therapy that is specific to the etiological agent. **Cocaine is one of the most frequent causes of drug-induced seizures.** Approximately 15% of cocaine users will experience a drug-induced seizure. Seizures caused by cocaine are a result of a combination of a lowered seizure threshold and hypersympathetic state. These seizures are usually self-limited, but in cases **of SE they should be treated with high doses of benzodiazepines.**

Tricyclic antidepressants cause seizures as a consequence of their anticholinergic properties. In addition to standard seizure therapy, patients with SE secondary to tricyclic overdose should be treated with sodium bicarbonate in an effort to obtain a blood pH of approximately 7.5. Alkalinization will decrease the free form of the drug in the patient's CNS as well as mitigate the drug's sodium channel–blocking effect on the heart.

Isoniazid-induced seizures are associated with a high mortality rate and typically occur within 120 minutes of an acute overdose. Isoniazid (INH) binds pyridoxine, the active form of vitamin B_6, a cofactor for glutamic acid decarboxylase, and GABA transaminase. INH toxicity and depleted **vitamin B_6 lead to a reduction in** levels of CNS inhibitory transmitter GABA and ultimately can result in SE. Treatment of seizures secondary to isoniazid toxicity is often refractory to standard measures and **should be treated with IV pyridoxine.** The dose of pyridoxine is based upon the amount of drug ingested.

Alcohol Withdrawal Seizures

Alcohol withdrawal seizures (AWS) are a leading cause of seizures in adults. These seizures often occur as part of a constellation of early withdrawal symptoms, **typically within 6-48 hours after the last drink.** Other withdrawal symptoms often occur prior to the onset of seizures; these symptoms include sweating, anxiety, tremor, auditory/visual hallucinations, agitation, nausea/vomiting, headache, and disorientation. The more serious withdrawal syndrome of delirium tremens can be associated with seizures that may occur as long as 7 days post-alcohol cessation. The more common and classic early AWS often occur in bunches of up to 4-6 seizures. However, these almost always cluster over a fairly brief period of time, and they rarely persist past 12 hours from onset. Recent evidence recommends the use of benzodiazepines to reduce the incidence of seizures and delirium. Phenytoin does not have a role in managing either AWS or controlling recurrent alcohol-related seizures in the ED; however, it may play a role in alcoholics who have underlying seizure disorders. The data for use of other anticonvulsants like carbamazepine in alcohol withdrawal seizures are limited.

CT imaging of the head has a high diagnostic yield in patients with their first alcohol-related seizure, as these patients have a high incidence of structural intracranial lesions, such as subdural hematomas or other intracranial hemorrhages. Alcoholism is also a common cause of hypoglycemia and other metabolic abnormalities, so electrolytes should be checked. IV fluid hydration with a glucose-containing solution in addition to thiamine, magnesium, potassium, and multivitamins is also indicated.

Neurocysticercosis

Neurocysticercosis (NCC) is an infection of the brain with larvae of *Taenia solium* (pork tapeworm) and is the most common cause of adult onset seizures in the developing countries of Latin America, sub-Saharan Africa, and Southeast Asia. It is also becoming increasingly prevalent in nonendemic countries with large immigrant populations. Seizures can vary from simple partial seizures to generalized tonic clonic. Diagnosis is confirmed via neuroimaging with visualization of active or calcified cysts in the brain. Treatment is usually initiated by a neurologist and consists of an antihelminth medication, such as albendazole, combined with an antiepileptic medication.

Psychogenic Seizures

Pseudoseizures, also known as **psychogenic seizures,** are often the result of major stress or emotional trauma. These psychogenic nonepileptic seizures are often difficult to distinguish from physiologic seizures. Patients with **psychogenic seizures tend to have multiple seizure patterns,** which are usually **not followed by a postictal period.** Urinary incontinence and injury such as tongue biting has been reported in up to 20% of patients with psychogenic seizure. Unlike in physiologic seizures, noxious stimuli such as ammonia capsules may elicit responses from patients having psychogenic seizures. The observation of purposeful movement during a psychogenic seizure also is typical. Management of pseudoseizures involves reassurance and patient education, with psychiatric consultation recommended.

Patient Disposition

Disposition of patients depends on the etiology of their seizure (if known), the known seizure history, and the availability of adequate outpatient follow-up. All patients need to be provided detailed **seizure precautions,** and locally mandated reporting requirements must be noted in the patient's chart. Patients should also be warned about limiting activities when and where sudden loss of consciousness would be especially dangerous, such as operating heavy equipment, swimming alone, cooking with hot water, or even bathing. The Department of Motor Vehicles must be notified and the patients instructed not to drive until cleared by their physician.

In patients with known epilepsy who present with a single seizure, it is acceptable to send laboratory test results for anticonvulsant levels (if appropriate), give a loading dose of the appropriate anticonvulsant, and then discharge them with the appropriate follow-up. Subtherapeutic levels of antiseizure medication can be a result of medical noncompliance or increased metabolism, often caused by concurrent medication intake. Any history or physical examination findings consistent with a new seizure pattern should be addressed, as would be the case in a first-time seizure patient (Tables 30–1 and 30–2). Patients should also be thoroughly educated regarding the risks and benefits of noncompliance with antiepileptic medications.

In patients without a history of epilepsy who present with a single unprovoked seizure, a more thorough workup is indicated. If this initial workup is unremarkable, it is acceptable to discharge the patient home with follow-up neuroimaging and an appointment with a neurologist. They will not necessarily need to be discharged on new antiepileptic medications, but they will need education about restrictions and precautions in patients with seizures.

Table 30–1 • COMMON CAUSES OF REACTIVE SEIZURES
Metabolic encephalopathies: Hypomagnesemia, hyponatremia, hypocalcemia, hypoglycemia, hepatic or renal failure
Infectious encephalopathies: Central nervous system abscess, meningitis, encephalitis
Central nervous system lesions: Neoplasm, arteriovenous malformations, vasculitis, acute hydrocephalus, intracerebral hematomas, cerebrovascular accident, posttraumatic seizures, migraine/vascular headache, degenerative disease (multiple sclerosis)
Intoxications: Medications (tricyclic antidepressants, isoniazid, theophylline), recreational drugs (cocaine), alcohol and drug withdrawal, lead, strychnine, camphor, eclampsia

Table 30–2 • ACUTE SEIZURE MANAGEMENT: DRUG THERAPY			
Drug	Adult Dose	Pediatric Dose	Comments
First Line			
Lorazepam	0.1 mg/kg IV up to 4 mg/dose. May repeat x 1.	0.05-0.1 mg/kg IV	Rapid acting; longer duration of action than diazepam; prolonged CNS depression possible
Diazepam	0.2 mg/kg IV up to 10 mg/dose. May repeat x 1	0.2-0.5 mg/kg IV up to 20 mg	Rapid acting; short effective half-life
Midazolam	0.2 mg/kg IM up to 10 mg	10mg IM (>40 kg) 5mg IM (13-40 mg)	Significant amnestic effect
Second Line			
Phenytoin	20 mg/kg IV at <50 mg/min	20 mg/kg IV at 1 mg/kg/min	Hypotension and arrhythmias at high infusion rates; cardiac monitoring required
Fosphenytoin	20 mg PE/kg IV at 150 mg PE/min	15-20 mg PE/kg IV	Hypotension and arhythmias
Valproic Acid	20-40 mg/kg IV at 3-6 mg/kg/min. May repeat 20 mg/kg x 1	20 mg/kg at 1.5-3 mg/kg IV	Hyperammonia, pancreatitis, hepatotoxic thrombocytopenia
Levetiracetam	60 mg/kg IV up to 4500 mg at 2-5 mg/min	20-60 mg/kg IV	Minimal drug interactions
Phenobarbital	20 mg/kg IV at 60-100 mg/min	10-20 mg/kg IV	Long lasting; may be given as IM loading dose
Third Line			
Propofol	1-2 mg/kg IV bolus, then 20 mcg/kg/min	1 mg/kg IV bolus	Hypotension, respiratory depression, cardiac failure
Pentobarbital	5 mg/kg IV at 25 mg/min, then titrate to EEG	1-3 mg/kg	Intubation, ventilation, and pressor support required; respiratory arrest, hypotension, and myocardial de pression common
Isoflurane	Via general endotra-cheal anesthesia		Monitor with EEG

Patients without a history of seizure who do not return to baseline and remain postictal should be admitted to the hospital until they return to their baseline mental status and the underlying etiology of their seizures is determined. Patients in SE are usually admitted to the ICU for management and evaluation.

CASE CORRELATION

- See also Case 25 (Altered Mental Status), Case 26 (Syncope), Case 28 (Stroke), Case 29 (Headache), and Case 34 (Febrile Seizure).

COMPREHENSION QUESTIONS

30.1   A 34-year-old man is brought into the ED with a seizure of new onset. It is
determined that it was likely to be metabolic in etiology. Which of the following is the most likely diagnosis?

   A.   Hyperthyroidism

   B.   Hypocalcemia

   C.   Hypoglycemia

   D.   Hypomagnesemia

30.2   A 28-year-old woman is brought into the ED by paramedics because of seizure activity that has persisted for 40 minutes despite intravenous valium at
the house and en route. Which of the following is the most likely reason for
this patient's condition?

   A.   Meningitis

   B.   Noncompliance with seizure medications

   C.   Cocaine

   D.   Benzodiazepine allergy

30.3   A 21-year-old man is brought into the ED for a seizure that was witnessed. It
was described as tonic clonic and lasting for 3 minutes. Currently, the patient
appears alert, oriented, and with normal vital signs. He has no nuchal rigidity. He admits to being diagnosed with HIV disease, but otherwise he has no
medical problems. He denies head trauma and alcohol or illicit drug use. He
denies headache. Which of the following is the best next step?

   A.   Emergent CT or MRI imaging of the brain

   B.   Begin fosphenytoin for seizure disorder

   C.   Observation because this is his first seizure

   D.   Stat EEG

30.4   A 42-year-old woman with a history of epilepsy is experiencing a sudden
tonic-clonic seizure in the hospital. There is no IV access. Which of the following is the best treatment?

   A.   Oral phenytoin

   B.   Intramuscular phenobarbital

   C.   Rectal propofol

   D.   Intramuscular midazolam

ANSWERS

30.1 **C.** New-onset seizure in the ED caused by metabolic abnormalities is rare. Hypoglycemia is considered the most common metabolic cause of seizure. Symptomatic hypoglycemia occurs most commonly as a complication of insulin or oral hypoglycemic therapy in diabetics. Hyperglycemia, hypocalcemia, and hypomagnesemia are other, less-common metabolic causes of seizure.

30.2 **B.** A patient who experiences more than 5 minutes of continuous seizure activity or a series of seizures without return to full consciousness between seizures is considered to be in SE. The most common cause of SE is discontinuation of anticonvulsant medications.

30.3 **A.** Diagnostic imaging with head CT or MRI is recommended for seizure patients with suspicion of head trauma, elevated ICP, intracranial mass, persistently abnormal mental status, focal neurologic abnormality, or HIV disease.

30.4 **D.** IM midazolam is a good agent to use for a patient with seizures and no IV access. Benzodiazepines are effective agents in stopping an acute seizure.

CLINICAL PEARLS

▶ Identifying the patient within one of the following subgroups facilitates the evaluation and management of the seizure patient in the ED: (a) new-onset (first-time) seizure, (b) recurrent seizures in patients with epilepsy, (c) febrile seizures, (d) post-traumatic seizures, and (e) alcohol- and drug-related seizures.

▶ The possibility of provoked seizures should be considered in all seizure patients who present to the ED, including patients with a history of epilepsy. Failure to treat the underlying cause of reactive seizure is a major pitfall.

▶ Seizures may be confused with other nonictal states such as syncope, hyperventilation, breath-holding spells in children, migraines, transient global amnesia, cerebral vascular disease, narcolepsy, and psychogenic seizures.

▶ Prolonged altered mental status following a seizure should not be attributed to an uncomplicated postictal state.

REFERENCES

Armon K, Stephenson T, MacFaul R, et al. An evidence and consensus based guideline for the management of a child after a seizure. *Emerg Med J.* 2003;20(1):13-20.

Beghi E. Treating epilepsy across its different stages. *Ther Adv Neurol Disord.* 2010;3(2):85-92.

Epilepticus in Children and Adults: Report of the Guideline Committee of the American Epilepsy Society. *Epilepsy Currents.* 2016;16(1):48.

Glauser T, Shinnar S, Gloss D, et al. Evidence-based guideline. Treatment of convulsive status epilepticus in children and adults: Report of the guideline committee of the American Epilepsy Society. *Epilepsy Currents.* 2016;16(1):48-61.

Harden CL, Huff JS, Schwartz TH, et al. Reassessment: neuroimaging in the emergency patient presenting with seizure (an evidence-based review): report of the Therapeutics and Technology Assessment Subcommittee of the American Academy of Neurology. *Neurology.* 2007;69:1772.

Krumholz A, Wiebe S, Gronseth G, et al. Evidence-based guideline: management of an unprovoked first seizure in adults: Report of the Guideline Development Subcommittee of the American Academy of Neurology and the American Epilepsy Society. Epilepsy Currents: May/June, Vol. 15, No. 3, pp. 144-152. Available at: http://dx.doi.org/10.5698/1535-7597-15.3.144. Accessed July 1, 2016.

Krumholz A, Wiebe S, Gronseth G, et al. Evidence-based guideline: management of an unprovoked first seizure in adults. Report of the Quality Standards Subcommittee of the American Academy of Neurology and the American epilepsy Society. *Neurology.* 2015;84:1705-1713.

Martindale JL, Goldstein JN, Pallin DL. Emergency Department Seizure Epidemiology. *Emerg Med Clin N Am.* 2011;(29):15-27.

Matthaiou DK, Panos G, Adamidi ES, Falagas ME. Albendazole versus praziquantel in the treatment of neurocysticercosis: a meta-analysis of comparative trials. *PLoS Negl Trop Dis.* 2008;2(3):e194.

Prasad K, Al-Roomi K, Sequeira R, Krishnan PR. Anticonvulsant therapy for status epilepticus (Review). *The Cochrane Database of Systematic Reviews.* 2014(9):CD003723.

Trinka E, Cock H, Hesdorffer D, et al. A definition and classification of status epilepticus—Report of the ILAE Task Force on Classification of Status Epilepticus. *Epilepsia.* 2015;56(10):1515-1523.

Turnbull TL, Vanden Hoek TL, Howes DS. Utility of laboratory studies in the emergency department patient with a new-onset seizure. *Ann Emerg Med.* 1990;19(4):373-377.

A 57-year-old man presents to the emergency department (ED) with a 1-month history of worsening low back pain. The pain radiates down the back of both legs and suddenly increased yesterday. For the past 2 days, the patient has been having difficulty voiding and has had "to force the urine out." He has also noticed that the skin around his anus feels numb when he wipes with toilet tissue. He works in a warehouse but has been on light duty for the past month due to his back pain. He denies prior trauma to or surgery on his back.

▶ What is the most likely diagnosis?
▶ What is the next diagnostic step?

ANSWERS TO CASE 31:

Low Back Pain

Summary: A 57-year-old warehouse worker has a 1-month history of worsening low back pain with radiation bilaterally to his legs. The pain increased suddenly and is now associated with perianal numbness and difficulty voiding. He denies trauma or prior surgery.

- **Most likely diagnosis:** Cauda equina syndrome (CES).

- **Next diagnostic step:** STAT magnetic resonance imaging (MRI) of the lumbar and sacral spine, since this is a potential surgical emergency.

ANALYSIS

Objectives

1. Review the possible etiologies of low back pain.

2. Learn how to evaluate a patient with low back pain.

3. Identify the "red flags" associated with serious causes of low back pain.

Considerations

This 57-year-old man has a history of low back pain that has worsened significantly and is now associated with difficulty voiding and with perianal numbness. In contrast to this patient's emergency condition, most low back pain is not as urgent. Low back pain is a common complaint and can be caused by a multitude of disease processes. Although benign mechanical causes are most common, the ED physician must consider the "cannot miss" diagnoses: cauda equina syndrome, spinal fracture, spinal infection (epidural abscess or spondylitis), and malignancy. A careful history and physical examination are important to identify "red flags" that may herald the presence of serious disease (Table 31–1). Most patients with back pain do not require any diagnostic studies in the ED. However, if a serious etiology is suspected, laboratory studies and imaging may be necessary. In general, pain control is a high priority for these patients.

APPROACH TO:

Low Back Pain

CLINICAL APPROACH

Back pain is a common complaint that accounts for about 3% of ED visits. Seventy to ninety percent of adults suffer from acute low back pain during their lifetime. The differential diagnosis of low back pain is extensive. Common causes include muscle strain, ligamentous injury, osteoarthritis, disk herniation, spondylolisthesis, and

Table 31–1 • "RED FLAG" SIGNS AND SYMPTOMS OF LOW BACK PAIN
Age <18 years or >50 years
Significant trauma (or mild trauma in patients >50 years)
Chronic steroid use
Osteoporosis
History of cancer
Recent infection
Immunocompromise
History of intravenous drug use
Pain worse at night, lasting >6 weeks, or refractory to analgesics and rest
Associated systemic symptoms (fever, unexplained weight loss, malaise, night sweats, diaphoresis, nausea, and syncope)
Acute onset
Use of anticoagulants or coagulopathy
Abnormal vital signs (including unequal blood pressures or pulse deficits)
Neurologic deficits (including extremity weakness, numbness, paresthesias, loss of rectal sphincter tone, and urinary retention)

fracture. Infectious etiologies are epidural abscess, spondylitis, diskitis, and herpes zoster. Malignancies that cause low back pain may be primary or, more commonly, metastatic. Rheumatologic diseases, such as ankylosing spondylitis and Reiter syndrome, are other considerations. Back pain may also be referred from various gastrointestinal, genitourinary, gynecologic, and vascular sources (most ominously from an abdominal aortic aneurysm). Miscellaneous causes include sickle cell pain crisis and functional back pain.

The history and physical examination are important to distinguish benign causes from potentially life-threatening ones. Table 31–2 describes the typical findings for patients with the "cannot miss" causes of low back pain. Important historical questions include location, duration, and onset of pain; aggravating and alleviating factors; associated symptoms; work history; history of trauma; and past medical history (including comorbidities, medications, and family history).

The ED physician should note the patient's vital signs because any abnormalities may herald a life-threatening disease process (eg, hypotension due to sepsis or a ruptured abdominal aortic aneurysm [AAA]). **The physical examination should screen for signs of systemic disease and possible sources of referred back pain.** If possible, gait and range of motion of the back should be observed. Inspection of the back can identify bony abnormalities such as scoliosis and skin lesions that suggest infection (erythema and warmth) or trauma (swelling and ecchymosis). The back should be palpated to isolate the area of maximal tenderness. Point tenderness over the spinous processes may indicate a destructive lesion of the spine. Pain that is severe or excessive has increased suspicion of acute spinal infection or AAA. The neurologic examination should focus on identifying any focal weakness, dermatomal sensory loss, and decreased or absent deep tendon reflexes. Straight-leg raise (SLR) testing involves the examiner passively elevating the supine patient's leg (with knee extended) 30-70 degrees. If the SLR elicits radicular pain in the low back radiating down the leg to below the knee, it is indicative of sciatic nerve root

Table 31–2 • "CANNOT MISS" CAUSES OF LOW BACK PAIN				
Disease	Etiology	Clinical Presentation	Diagnostics	Treatment
Cauda equina syndrome	Central disk herniation bilateral nerve roots	Bilateral leg pain and weakness, urinary retention and overflow incontinence, decreased rectal tone, saddle anesthesia	CT, MRI (preferred imaging)	Emergent surgical decompression, +/− IV dexamethasone
Spinal fracture	Significant blunt trauma or minimal trauma in patient with osteoporosis	Midline tenderness along spine	Plain x-ray, CT	Orthopedic consultation May require admission
Spinal infection	Most commonly due to *Staphylococcus aureus*. Risk factors: intravenous drug use, elderly, immunocompromised, alcoholism, recent bacterial infection or back trauma	Back pain (even at rest/night), fever, midline cultures, tenderness along spine Focal neurologic deficits as late finding	CBC, ESR, plain x-ray, CT, myelography, MRI (preferred imaging)	Intravenous antibiotics, surgical drainage and decompression
Malignancy	Most commonly metastatic (breast, prostate, lung common). May also be primary (eg, multiple myeloma, leukemia, lymphoma)	Pain lasting >1 month, worse at night, unrelieved by rest; unexplained weight loss; mild to moderate spinal tenderness	CBC, ESR, plain x-ray, CT, MRI	May benefit from intravenous dexamethasone and radiation therapy

Abbreviations: CBC = complete blood count; CT = computed tomography; ESR = erythrocyte sedimentation rate; MRI = magnetic resonance imaging.

irritation. This test is more sensitive (up to 80%) than specific (40%). A positive crossed SLR (elevation of the unaffected leg causes radicular pain in the affected leg) is very specific (90%) but insensitive (25%). Digital rectal examination should be performed on patients with severe pain or neurologic deficits to assess sphincter tone and perianal sensation.

Most patients who present with low back pain do not require any diagnostic tests or imaging studies in the ED. The history and physical examination can help separate the majority of patients with simple, self-limited musculoskeletal back pain from the minority with more serious underlying causes. If rheumatologic causes, malignancy, or infection are concerns, a complete blood count, erythrocyte sedimentation rate, and urinalysis may be helpful. Indications for plain x-rays include age less than 18 years or older than 50 years; recent trauma; history or suspicion of malignancy; pain lasting longer than 4-6 weeks; history of fever, intravenous drug use, or immunocompromise; and progressive neurologic deficits. Further imaging by computed tomography or magnetic resonance imaging may be required if a strong suspicion of fracture, spinal infection, malignancy, or cauda equina syndrome exists.

Treatment

If a patient with low back pain is hemodynamically unstable, cardiac monitoring and resuscitation with intravenous fluids is mandated. If infection is suspected, antibiotics should be administered. Stable patients benefit from pain management. Depending on the severity of the pain, intravenous narcotics such as morphine or fentanyl may be required. Patients with simple musculoskeletal back pain can be treated with pain control (primarily acetaminophen and NSAIDs). Oral narcotics may be used for a short period of time if the pain is not adequately controlled by the aforementioned medications. Benzodiazepines may be useful adjuncts to provide some muscle relaxation and sedation, and application of local heat or ice may provide some pain relief.

Although strict bed rest was once the recommended treatment, **resumption of normal daily activities has been shown to hasten recovery and resolution of pain.** Strenuous exercise should be avoided until the acute pain has subsided. Most patients recover with conservative management within 4-6 weeks.

Admission should be considered for patients with underlying etiologies that require inpatient management, those with abnormal vital signs, those requiring intravenous narcotics for pain control, and those who cannot walk.

CASE CORRELATION

- See also Case 24 (Acute Pyelonephritis) and Case 28 (Stroke).

COMPREHENSION QUESTIONS

31.1 Which of the following describes the most common location of herniated disk of the lumbar spine region?

   A. L1-L2

   B. L2-L3

   C. L3-L4

   D. L4-L5

31.2 Which of the following is the most sensitive finding for cauda equina syndrome?

   A. Decreased anal sphincter tone

   B. Saddle anesthesia

   C. Urinary retention

   D. Weakness or numbness in the low extremities

31.3 A 27-year-old woman with a 1-week history of progressive pain radiating from the lumbar spine down the back of the leg presents to the ED. Her physical examination is normal except for complaints of back pain with movement. Which of the following is the most appropriate imaging test?

A. No imaging is necessary; attempt conservative therapy

B. Obtain plain films of the lumbar spine

C. Perform MRI

D. Perform CT

ANSWERS

31.1 **D.** The L4-L5 interspace is the most commonly affected for a herniated disk. The common symptoms are low back pain radiating down the posterior aspect of the leg. If the patient has weakness or bowel/bladder symptoms, then it is a medical emergency.

31.2 **C.** Urinary retention with overflow incontinence is the most sensitive finding for cauda equina syndrome (90%). The other answer choices indicate other findings of CES, but these are not as common.

31.3 **A.** No imaging is necessary. If the patient has no risk factors in the history and physical examination for serious disease other than sciatica, treat conservatively and do not perform any diagnostic tests in the ED.

CLINICAL PEARLS

▶ Most patients with acute low back pain have resolution of symptoms within 4-6 weeks.

▶ Pain that interferes with sleep, significant unintentional weight loss, or fever suggests an infectious or neoplastic cause of back pain.

▶ Low back pain with associated bowel and bladder dysfunction is suspicious for cauda equina syndrome.

▶ Most patients do not require diagnostic tests or imaging studies. However, further testing may be advisable if there is a concern for rheumatologic, infectious, or neoplastic processes; fracture; or cauda equina syndrome.

▶ Pain control is important in the management of patients with low back pain. Acetaminophen, NSAIDs, and narcotics are all viable options.

REFERENCES

Borczuk P. An evidence-based approach to the evaluation and treatment of low back pain in the emergency department. *Emerg Med Pract*. 2013;15(7):1-23.

Chou R, Fu R, Carrino JA, et al. Imaging strategies for low-back pain: systematic review and meta-analysis. *Lancet*. 2009;373(9662):463-472.

Della-Giustina D. Evaluation and treatment of acute back pain in the emergency department. *Emerg Med Clin North Am*. 2015;33(2):311-326.

Deyo RA, Weinstein JN. Low back pain. *N Engl J Med*. 2001;344:363-370.

Friedman BW, Chilstrom M, Bijur PE, et al. Diagnostic testing and treatment of low back pain in United States emergency departments: a national perspective. *Spine*. 2010;35(24):E1406-1411.

Frohna WJ, Della-Giustina D. Neck and back pain. *Tintinalli's Emergency Medicine: A Comprehensive Study Guide*. 7th ed. New York, NY: McGraw-Hill; 2011; Chapter 276.

Hermance TC, Boggs LR. Arthitis and back pain. In: Stone CK, Humphries RL, eds. *Current Diagnosis and Treatment: Emergency Medicine*. 6th ed. Available at: http://www.accessmedicine.com/content. aspx?aID=3100883. Accessed May 15, 2016.

Marx JA, Hockberger RS, Walls RM, eds. *Rosen's Emergency Medicine: Concepts and Clinical Practice*. 8th ed. Philadelphia, PA: Saunders; 2014.

A 10-week-old infant is brought to the emergency department (ED) by his mother for 1 day of fever. The mother tells you that her son was delivered vaginally at full term and was the product of an uncomplicated pregnancy. He has had regular well-baby checks and has been gaining weight appropriately. He has met his normal developmental milestones, and vaccinations are up-to-date. He has had no prior illnesses. This morning his mother noticed he felt warm to the touch and discovered an axillary temperature of 101°F. There are no other signs or symptoms of infection, including runny nose, cough, difficulty breathing, rash, nuchal rigidity, seizure activity, abdominal distention, vomiting, and diarrhea. She states her son has been breast-feeding less than normal but overall has had a normal number of wet diapers. She is very concerned because this is her first child and he has never had a fever before.

On examination, the child is found to have a heart rate of 180 beats per minute, a blood pressure of 90/50 mm Hg, a respiratory rate of 40 breaths per minute, an oxygen saturation of 99% on room air, and a rectal temperature of 102.7°F. He is overall well appearing and has an unremarkable physical examination. Although he cries when you perform the examination, his mother is able to console him easily.

▶ What is the most likely diagnosis?
▶ What is the next step in management?
▶ What is the best therapy?

ANSWERS TO CASE 32:

Fever Without a Source in the 1- to 3-Month-Old Infant

Summary: A previously healthy 10-week-old infant is brought in by his mother for fever. The cause of the fever is not clearly identified by the history or physical examination. His vital signs in the ED are significant for fever and tachycardia. His examination is unremarkable.

- **Most likely diagnosis:** Fever without a source (FWS).

- **Next step:** Order CBC, blood cultures, urinalysis, and urine culture. You may also order stool studies and a chest x-ray (CXR) and perform a lumbar puncture depending on the clinical presentation.

- **Best therapy:** It is up to physician discretion to decide which well-appearing infants with fever without a source should receive antibiotics. If antibiotics are given, the best drug is ceftriaxone, either IV or IM.

ANALYSIS

Objectives

1. Understand the appropriate workup for fever without a source in the well-appearing 1- to 3-month-old infant.

2. Appreciate the controversy regarding the management of fever without a source in this age group.

3. Learn the treatment options for fever without a source in a 1- to 3-month-old infant.

Considerations

This 10-week-old infant presented with fever without any other signs or symptoms of infection, including runny nose, cough, difficulty breathing, rash, nuchal rigidity, seizure activity, abdominal distention, vomiting, and diarrhea. Importantly, the emergency physician must be aware that the 1- to 3-month-old infant will not manifest the same signs of infection as an older child. For this reason, the workup of fever in this age group must remain broad, and one must have a low threshold for both further testing and treatment with antibiotics.

APPROACH TO:

Fever Without a Source in the 1- to 3-Month-Old Infant

DEFINITIONS

FEVER WITHOUT A SOURCE: Fever without a source is an acute febrile illness in which the etiology of the fever is not apparent after a careful history and physical examination. A rectal temperature greater than 38°C (100.4°F) is defined as a fever.

SERIOUS BACTERIAL ILLNESS (SBI): Illnesses including bacteremia, pneumonia, urinary tract infection, skin and soft tissue infections, bone and joint infections, enteritis, or meningitis due to a bacterial pathogen.

CLINICAL APPROACH

Determining fever in the 1- to 3-Month-Old Infant

Temperature must be measured with a rectal thermometer in order to rule out a fever, as axillary, tympanic membrane, and temporal (forehead) temperatures inadequately measure core temperature in an infant. If an infant has had a rectal temperature more than 38°C at home but is afebrile and well appearing in the ED, this infant still requires full workup for fever. If the parent only reports a tactile fever and the infant is afebrile and well appearing in the ED, no laboratory testing for fever workup is required. While a mildly elevated temperature can result from bundling of an infant, a temperature more than 38.5°C should never be attributed to bundling.

Evaluation of Fever Without a Source in the 1- to 3-Month-Old Infant

The evaluation of fever in this age group has changed dramatically in the last 30 years, as vaccines targeting *Haemophilus influenzae* type b and *Streptococcus pneumoniae* have dramatically decreased the burden of SBI in this age group. After the introduction of the Hib vaccine, the majority (90%) of infections were due to pneumococcus. The heptavalent pneumococcal conjugate vaccine further changed the landscape of SBI, decreasing the incidence of invasive pneumococcal disease by 65% to 80% in children younger than 3 years of age. Prior to the development of these vaccines, the majority of febrile infants in this age group were often hospitalized and started on empiric antibiotic therapy, as morbidity and mortality for SBI was high and early clinical identification was difficult.

Given the controversy and difficulties identifying infants with SBI, several decision rules have been developed. These are the Rochester, Boston, and Philadelphia criteria, each using a combination of factors including history, physical examination, and laboratory parameters to identify low-risk infants (see Table 32–1). Although all these criteria use slightly different testing strategies, all of the criteria support the use of CBC, blood cultures, urinalysis, and urine cultures to identify infants at low risk for SBI. Urine specimens should always be collected by catheter, if possible, given the risk of false positives and false negatives with urine collected from a bag.

The decision to use CXR or stool studies in the workup of fever in children 1-3 months old should be based on symptoms. Only those children with respiratory symptoms (tachypnea, rales, rhonchi, retractions, wheezing, coryza, grunting, stridor, nasal flaring, or cough) need CXR. In a meta-analysis that included 361 febrile infants, the absence of respiratory symptoms had a negative predictive value of 99% against pneumonia or other diagnoses made by CXR. Similarly, febrile children aged 1-3 months without GI symptoms do not routinely need stool studies as part of their workup for fever. Greater than 5 WBC/hpf in the stool specimen is considered high risk for SBI.

Routine lumbar puncture is an area of controversy among the decision rules. Several studies suggest that infants can be identified as low risk for SBI using the

Table 32–1 • CRITERIA USED FOR THE IDENTIFICATION OF LOW-RISK FEBRILE INFANTS

Rochester Criteria	Boston Criteria	Philadelphia Criteria
Infant appears well	Infant appears well	Infants >28 days old
Born at term (>37 weeks gestation)	No skeletal, soft tissue, skin or ear infections	Infant Observation Score ≤10
Has not received antibiotics	No immunizations in preceding 48 hours	No recognizable bacterial infection on examination
Was not treated for hyperbilirubinemia	No antibiotics in preceding 48 hours	WBC <15,000/mm³
Has not been previously hospitalized	Not dehydrated	Band-to-neutrophil ratio <0.2
Has no chronic or underlying illness	CSF <10 cells/mm³	UA with WBCs <10/mm³ and few bacteria
No evidence of skin, soft tissue, bone, joint or ear infection	Urinalysis <10 WBC/hpf	CSF with <8/mm³ and a negative Gram stain in non-bloody specimen
WBC 5000 to 15,000/mm³	WBC <20,000/mm³	No infiltrate on CXR
Absolute band count ≤1500/mm³	Chest radiograph without infiltrate	Stool smear negative for blood *and* few or no WBCs
UA with ≤10 WBCs/hpf		
Stool with ≤5 WBCs/hpf on smear		

Rochester criteria without performing a lumbar puncture. However, many physicians feel that the significant morbidity and mortality associated with bacterial meningitis outweigh the low incidence of the disease, and thus they argue in support of routine lumbar puncture in the workup of fever without a source. Cerebrospinal fluid (CSF) with greater than or equal to 8 WBC/mm³ or organisms on Gram stain is considered high risk for SBI.

While this case has focused on the well-appearing infant with fever without a source, it is worthwhile to note that 45% of ill-appearing infants in this age group will test positive for SBI. All ill-appearing infants less than 3 months of age should be treated with empiric antibiotics prior to results of laboratory testing and admitted to the hospital.

Treatment

In 1- to 3-month-old infants with fever not deemed low risk by any of the validated testing strategies (see Table 32–1), antibiotics and hospitalization must be considered. The empiric antibiotic of choice is ceftriaxone, which may be given IV or IM. The regular dose is 50 mg/kg; however, if meningitis is suspected, the dose should be increased to 100 mg/kg. If, based on an absence of concerning clinical findings, a lumbar puncture is not performed, then antibiotics should be withheld. Giving empiric antibiotics in this situation could mask the presentation of bacterial meningitis on follow-up examination. For ill-appearing infants in this age group, consideration should be given to augmenting empiric ceftriaxone by targeting suspected organisms (see Table 32–2). For instance, administration of vancomycin may be considered to cover for methicillin-resistant *Staphylococcus aureus* (MRSA) and ceftriaxone-resistant *Streptococcus pneumonia*; ampicillin may also be considered for the ill-appearing infant to cover for possible *Listeria monocytogenes*.

Table 32–2 • COMMON PATHOGENS IN FEBRILE INFANTS (1-3 MONTHS)		
Bacteremia	Urinary Tract Infection	Meningitis
Coagulase-negative Staphylococcus	*E. coli*	Group B Streptococcus
Staphylococcus aureus	Klebsiella sp.	*E. coli*
E. coli	Proteus sp.	*Streptococcus pneumonia*
Candida sp.	*Pseudomonas aeruginosa*	*Neisseria meningitidis*
Enterococcus sp.	Enterobacter sp.	
Klebsiella sp.		
Group B Streptococcus		

CASE CORRELATION

- See also Case 34 (Febrile Seizure) and Case 39 (Bacterial Meningitis).

COMPREHENSION QUESTIONS

32.1 An 8-week-old previously healthy infant, product of a full-term pregnancy, is brought by his older sister to the ED for a fever up to 101.2°F. The sister, who is 17 years old, states that she is the primary caretaker for her brother because the only adult at home is her mother, who is struggling with cocaine and alcohol abuse. The sister states that although her brother has not been eating well, he is taking in a normal amount of formula and has not had cough, runny nose, altered behavior, vomiting, or diarrhea. Overall, the patient is well appearing. You perform an appropriate workup for this infant with FWS and find a WBC count of 10,000/mm^3 and a UA with 2 WBCs/hpf. You also elect to do a lumbar puncture (LP), and the CSF shows 1 WBC/mm^3 and no organisms on Gram stain. What is the most appropriate disposition for this patient?

A. Discharge the patient home after giving a dose of IV ceftriaxone.

B. Discharge the patient home but do not give any antibiotics.

C. Give a dose of IV ceftriaxone and admit the patient to the hospital.

D. Order a CXR, stool WBCs and culture, and then admit the patient to the hospital.

32.2 An 11-week-old male infant is brought in by his mother for 4 days of fever (Tmax 100.8°F) associated with cough and runny nose. The child was the product of a full-term healthy pregnancy, and his vaccines are up-to-date. He is overall well appearing and has normal vital signs. A CXR demonstrates no evidence of pneumonia. A rapid respiratory syncytial virus (RSV) test comes back positive. Which of the following statements most accurately describes the risk of SBI in the RSV positive infant?

A. SBI is just as common in RSV-positive infants as in RSV-negative infants.

B. SBI is less common in RSV-positive infants than in RSV-negative infants.

C. SBI is more common in RSV-positive infants than in RSV-negative infants.

D. There is no risk of SBI in the febrile infant with a positive RSV test.

32.3 A 9-week-old, well-appearing female infant is brought in to the ED with a chief complaint of a fever up to 102°F at home. The infant has not had any vomiting or cough, and the examination is unremarkable, including a thorough skin examination. In the ED, the infant is afebrile, but the mother states she gave the infant ibuprofen 2 hours prior to arrival. A catheter urinalysis comes back positive for 20 WBCs/hpf. What is the best management for this patient?

A. Send urine cultures, give her IV antibiotics, and admit her to the pediatric service.

B. Send urine cultures, give her PO antibiotics, and discharge her home.

C. Give her an IM shot of ceftriaxone and send her home with PO antibiotics.

D. Send urine cultures, give IV or IM antibiotics, and evaluate the social situation.

32.4 A 6-week-old male infant is brought in by his parents for evaluation of fever of 39°C. The infant is ill appearing and lethargic and does not want to breast-feed. His parents also reported that his cry sounds different. The patient is given antipyretics and a bolus of 20 cc/kg IV fluids, and labs are sent. A thorough examination including skin does not reveal any source of infection. Urinalysis, CXR, and CSF are all normal, and cultures are sent. What is the best management of this patient?

A. Give him an IM shot of ceftriaxone and discharge home with close follow-up.

B. Give him IV ceftriaxone and admit to the pediatric service.

C. Give him IV ceftriaxone, vancomycin, and ampicillin and admit to the pediatric service.

D. Do not give any antibiotics at this time, and admit to the pediatric service for observation.

ANSWERS

32.1 **C.** This case demonstrates the importance of good follow-up and an adequate social situation when considering discharging the well-appearing infant with FWS. In order to discharge a well-appearing infant with FWS, one must ensure follow-up within 24 hours. There must also be adequate social support to ensure the patient can be brought back to the hospital if his condition worsens. In general, this means that the patient's family should have access to a telephone and transportation. In this case, the social situation is less than ideal, as a minor is primarily caring for the patient and the only adult in the family is incapacitated by polysubstance abuse to the point that she has not even come to the hospital with her ill infant. There is no indication for a CXR or stool studies in this patient since he has no respiratory symptoms and no diarrhea.

32.2 **B.** A positive RSV test in a 1- to 3-month-old infant with a fever decreases the risk of SBI but does not completely eliminate this risk. Most studies demonstrate that the risk of SBI in the RSV-positive population is decreased by approximately 50%. The most common SBI in the RSV-positive patient is a urinary tract infection. There are no studies at this time which have been powered enough to detect difference in rates of bacteremia and meningitis in RSV-positive and RSV-negative patients, as both bacteremia and meningitis in this age group is relatively uncommon. Thus, RSV-positive infants in this age group with fever should at least receive a urinalysis and urine culture. It remains unclear whether or not clinicians can safely forgo blood and spinal fluid testing in these same infants.

32.3 **D.** Urinary tract infection is the most common cause of SBI in infants with fever without a source, and the prevalence has not changed with the PCV7 vaccine. A positive urine is defined as greater than 10 WBCs per high power field. A negative urine dipstick or urinalysis does not exclude UTI, as pyuria is absent on initial urinalysis in up to 20% of febrile infants with pyelonephritis. Thus, a urine culture must be obtained on all patients. Additionally, catheter samples should always be obtained since bag specimens are often contaminated. Infants younger than 8 weeks of age warrant admission to the hospital. Well-appearing infants greater than 8 weeks may be discharged home if the parents are reliable and follow-up within 24 hours is possible. Infants younger than 3 months of age should be given parenteral antibiotics (ceftriaxone 50 mg/kg) with admission or discharge and may need additional parenteral doses even if discharged home.

32.4 **C.** Infants who have an abnormal cry and temperature greater than 38.5°C or are ill appearing have an increased risk of SBI. Up to 45% of ill-appearing young infants may have SBI and thus require extensive workup including blood, urine, CSF, and CXR. Ill-appearing infants in this age group should receive parenteral antibiotic therapy to cover the likely pathogens in this age group regardless of initial laboratory results (*S. pneumoniae, S. aureus, N. meningitides, H. influenza* type b) and should be admitted to the hospital. Of note, vancomycin should be administered to infants with soft tissue infection or CSF pleocytosis. In infants 29-60 days of age, ampicillin should also be given to cover *L. monocytogenes*.

CLINICAL PEARLS

▶ Infants younger than 8 weeks of age warrant admission to the hospital, while febrile, well-appearing infants greater than 8 weeks may be discharged home if the parents are reliable and follow-up within 24 hours is possible.

▶ Ill-appearing infants 1-3 months old should receive parenteral antibiotic therapy to cover the likely pathogens in this age group regardless of initial laboratory results (*S. pneumoniae, S. aureus, N. meningitides, H. influenza* type b) and should be admitted to the hospital.

▶ All three of the criteria for identifying SBI in infants support the use of CBC, blood cultures, urinalysis, and urine cultures to identify infants at low risk for SBI.

REFERENCES

Bachur RG, Harper MB. Predictive model for serious bacterial infections among infants younger than 3 months of age. *Pediatrics.* 2001;108(2):311-316.

Bramson RT, Meyer TL, Silbiger ML, et al. The futility of the chest radiograph in the febrile infant without respiratory symptoms. *Pediatrics.* 1993;92(4):524-526.

Cheng TL, Partridge JC. Effect of bundling and high environmental temperature on neonatal body temperature. *Pediatrics.* 1993;92(2):238-240.

Hoberman A, Wald ER, Reynolds EA, et al. Is urine culture necessary to rule out urinary tract infection in young febrile children? *Pediatr Infect Dis J.* 1996;15(4):304-309.

Ishimine P. The evolving approach to the young child who has fever and no obvious source. *Emerg Med Clin North Am.* 2007;25(4):1087-1115,vii.

Jaskiewicz JA, McCarthy CA, Richardson AC, et al; Febrile Infant Collaborative Study Group. Febrile infants at low risk for serious bacterial infection—an appraisal of the Rochester criteria and implications for management. *Pediatrics.* 1994;94(3):390-396.

Rudinsky SL, Carstairs KL, Reardon JM, et al. Serious bacterial infections in febrile infants in the post-pneumococcal conjugate vaccine era. *Acad Emerg Med.* 2009;16(7):585-590.

Yiannis L, Katsogridakis MD, MPH, Kristine L, Cieslak MD. Empiric antibiotics for the complex febrile child: when, why, and what to use. *Clin Pediatr Emerg Med.* 2008;9:258-263.

A 3-year-old boy presents to the emergency department (ED) with his parents complaining of a limp for 2 days. The limp began following a fall from a playground structure, and has worsened to the point that the child is no longer willing to walk. The patient was treated 2 weeks ago for acute otitis media with Augmentin. The patient had subjective fevers for 2 days with no emesis, cough, abdominal pain, recent travel, or insect bites. His blood pressure is 95/68 mm Hg, pulse is 150 beats per minute, respirations are 25 breaths per minute, and temperature is 38.0°C (100.4°F). On physical examination, he is crying, and his right hip is noted to be flexed with slight abduction and external rotation. The joint is warm to touch, and he resists passive range of motion testing. He is unwilling to bear weight. The right knee is normal, and there are no other findings on physical examination.

▶ What are your next steps?
▶ What is the most likely diagnosis?
▶ What is the best treatment for this problem?

ANSWERS TO CASE 33:

Septic Arthritis

Summary: The patient is a 3-year-old boy with right hip pain who is refusing to ambulate. The child appears to be in pain and is febrile. His examination reveals decreased passive range of motion of the right hip.

- **Next steps:** Perform an ultrasound to evaluate for a hip effusion, consider getting a plain film x-ray in a frog leg position, and do an arthrocentesis to evaluate the synovial fluid.

- **Most likely diagnosis:** A final diagnosis cannot be confirmed, but given the acuity and severity of the patient's presentation, a septic hip is the most likely diagnosis.

- **Best treatment for this problem:** Orthopedic consultation for possible surgical drainage and lavage of the joint with subsequent admission to the hospital for IV antibiotics.

ANALYSIS

Objectives

1. Recognize the clinical presentation of septic arthritis, and appreciate the similarities of its presentation to osteomyelitis or transient synovitis.

2. Learn about the diagnosis and treatment of suspected septic arthritis.

3. Be familiar with the other etiologies of limp in a child.

Considerations

Septic arthritis is an infection that can lead to rapid destruction of the articular joint cartilage. This disease can lead to long-term morbidity if not diagnosed early. Joints of the lower extremity are affected in more than 90% of the cases, with the hip being the most common joint affected. It is most often seen in children less than 3 years old, and there is a male-to-female ratio of 2:1. Approximately 3% of children who present to the ED for limp will have septic arthritis. Causative bacterial organisms vary with age group, but *Staphylococcus aureus* is the most common organism, followed by Group A Streptococcus (*S. pyogenes*) and *Streptococcus pneumoniae*. *Kingella kingae* has recently become a common pathogen in children younger than 3, and *Neisseria gonorrhoeae* should be considered in neonates and sexually active adolescents. Empiric antibiotic coverage should include an anti-staphylococcal agent with gram-negative coverage added when age appropriate. Definitive treatment is by immediate surgical drainage and washout in addition to antibiotics. Presentation may be extremely subtle and unrevealing, and it varies significantly by age. In general, children with septic arthritis will have a history of fever, malaise and/ or anorexia within the week prior to presentation. Neonates and infants with septic arthritis may present with irritability, poor feeding, and pseudoparalysis of the affected limb. Recent antibiotic use may complicate the diagnosis and subsequent treatment. On physical examination the child will likely appear ill, and the position of maximum comfort will be with the hip flexed, abducted, and externally rotated. Passive range of motion examination will be resisted and painful. Appropriate initial laboratory studies include complete blood count (CBC), blood cultures, erythrocyte sedimentation rate (ESR), and C-reactive protein (CRP). Plain radiographs are keys to rule out several alternative diagnoses, and bedside ED ultrasound may identify a hip effusion. The definitive diagnosis of septic arthritis is made by examination of synovial fluid obtained by arthrocentesis.

APPROACH TO:
Child with a Limp

DEFINITIONS

LIMP: A limp is an uneven, jerky, or laborious gait, usually caused by pain, weakness, or deformity.

LEGG-CALVE-PERTHES DISEASE (LCP): Avascular necrosis of the femoral head leading to a childhood limp.

CLINICAL APPROACH

The differential diagnosis of the pediatric limp is broad, and the emergency physician must use a systemic approach to identify or exclude the conditions that require emergent treatment. The likely causes of limping can often be narrowed through careful history taking and physical examination. Laboratory tests, imaging, and diagnostic testing can then be applied to confirm clinical suspicions.

History

History taking is challenging in a young child who may be unable to communicate verbally or has difficulty localizing the site of the pain. Parents may attribute the limp to a recent event such as a fall. Obtaining the following information will help aid in the formulation of an appropriate differential diagnosis:

1. Age (age specific diagnoses)

2. Onset of pain (acute versus chronic)

3. Duration of pain (intermittent, constant, or worse at particular times of day)

4. Location of pain (bone, joint, soft tissue, neurologic, or intra-abdominal)

5. Preceding events (history of trauma, recent viral illness, or antibiotic use)

6. Constitutional symptoms (fever, malaise, or weight loss)

There is overlap among age groups, but knowing which diseases are common in each age group is a good place to start when making a list of potential diagnoses (Table 33–1).

Table 33–1 • COMMON CAUSES OF LIMP BY AGE

Age (y)	Infectious	Trauma	Inflammatory	Developmental	Neoplasia
Toddler (1-3)	Septic arthritis	Toddler fracture	Transient synovitis	Developmental dysplasia of the hip	Leukemia
	Osteomyelitis	Child abuse	Juvenile rheumatoid arthritis	Clubfoot	
Juvenile (4-10)	Septic arthritis	Fracture	Transient synovitis	Developmental dysplasia of the hip	Ewing sarcoma
	Osteomyelitis	Legg-Calve-Perthes disease	Juvenile rheumatoid arthritis		Osteoid osteoma
Adolescent (11-17)	Septic or gonococcal arthritis	Fracture	Juvenile rheumatoid arthritis	Osteochondritis dissecans	Osteosarcoma
	Osteomyelitis	Slipped capital femoral epiphysis	Osgood-Schlatter		Ewing sarcoma
					Osteoid osteoma

Entities that cause limping that are acute in onset are more likely to be due to trauma or infection. Chronic limping is suggestive of systemic illness, LCP disease (avascular necrosis), or slipped capital femoral epiphysis (SCFE). Pain that is worse at night is more typical of a malignancy, and morning stiffness is commonly associated with juvenile rheumatoid arthritis. The location of the pain may be typical of a musculoskeletal etiology, but referred pain and alternative diagnoses such as appendicitis, testicular or ovarian torsion, and psoas abscess should be entertained. A history of trauma can suggest fracture or contusion, while a recent illness or constitutional symptoms may direct the physician to consider osteomyelitis, septic arthritis, or transient synovitis.

Physical Examination

The gait should be observed if the child is ambulatory. The child should be fully undressed, vital signs reviewed, and the general appearance of "sick or not sick" considered. The extremities should be inspected for skin erythema, rash, tenderness, deformity, muscle atrophy and abnormal range of motion. The log roll test is particularly useful in evaluating hip rotation. To perform the log roll test, the leg is straightened, and the foot is manipulated medially (internal rotation of the hip) and laterally (external rotation of the hip). Pain with this maneuver suggests inflammation, infection, or trauma that is localized to the hip. The presence or absence of a fever has not been found to be helpful in making a definitive diagnosis. In a series of 95 children with septic arthritis, most had a low-grade fever, but one-third were afebrile at presentation. Absence of fever should not sway the clinician from this diagnosis. The presence of fever does not help separate several potential diagnoses, including transient synovitis, osteomyelitis, septic arthritis, and psoas abscess. Lastly, if there are any inconsistencies between the history and physical examination, the possibility of non-accidental trauma, or child abuse, must be explored.

Laboratory Studies

Laboratory studies are not routinely indicated in a child who has normal vital signs, appears well, and has a history consistent with an immediately preceding trauma. However, a CBC, ESR, CRP, and blood cultures are useful if entities such as osteomyelitis, neoplasm, septic arthritis, and transient synovitis remain on the differential. Synovial fluid analysis, which includes cell count, Gram stain, and culture and sensitivity testing, may be required to distinguish between septic arthritis and transient synovitis. A synovial fluid white blood cell count of greater than 50,000 cells/L with a predominance (>90%) of polymorphonuclear (PMN) leukocytes suggests septic arthritis. However, that number is not very sensitive or specific and should be considered in context with all other factors. The Gram stain may rapidly identify the organism, and the culture and sensitivity results will allow the antibiotic regimen to be narrowed. Finally, neonates and adolescents with a suspected septic arthritis should be tested for gonorrhea.

Imaging Studies

In contrast to laboratory studies, most children with a limp require radiographic evaluation. Plain films must be ordered with a minimum of two views and the joints above and below the area of concern should be included. If possible, weight-bearing

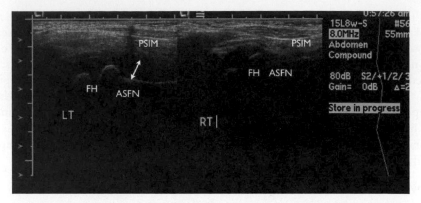

Figure 33–1. Ultrasound demonstrating a left hip effusion. The right hip is normal. The echogenic linear focus, which courses along the left femoral neck, is felt to represent periosteal new bone. An effusion is diagnosed when the distance between the anterior surface of the femoral neck and the posterior surface of the iliopsoas muscle is greater than 5 mm or when there is a greater than 2 mm difference from the contralateral hip. *Abbreviations: ASFN = anterior surface femoral head; FH = femoral head; PSIM = posterior surface iliopsoas muscle.*

views ought to be obtained, and if the hip is involved, the contralateral hip should be filmed for comparison. Radiographs can identify fracture, late avascular necrosis, soft tissue swelling, slippage of the head on the neck of the hip, and destructive bony lesions. A bone scan uses IV technetium 99m-labeled methylene diphosphonate to identify areas of increased cellular activity and blood flow. This test can be useful to detect early LCP disease, osteomyelitis, stress fractures, and osteoid osteomas. Magnetic resonance imaging (MRI) can be helpful in detecting osteomyelitis, early avascular necrosis, and bone malignancies. Computed tomography (CT) is rarely indicated for musculoskeletal complaints; however, the test may be necessary when intra-abdominal entities, such as appendicitis, psoas abscess, or pelvic etiologies, are in the differential. Ultrasound (US) is perhaps the most useful imaging study after plain films in the evaluation of the pediatric patient with limp. Recent studies have demonstrated that the use of bedside ED ultrasound can reliably detect a joint effusion (Figure 33–1). Early detection of an effusion and ultrasound guidance of arthrocentesis can decrease the time to definitive diagnosis and treatment of septic arthritis. Additionally, the detection of bilateral hip effusions raises the clinical suspicion for rheumatologic conditions and transient synovitis.

Alternate Etiologies of Pediatric Limp

Osteomyelitis of the femur or pelvis can present as hip pain. The proximal femur is the most common site of bone infection in children and may also involve the joint, given the intracapsular location (Figure 33–2). On examination, there may be focal erythema, swelling, and warmth near the location of the metaphysis. Similar to septic arthritis, the presentation may be attenuated and altered by recent antibiotic use. Plain films may not show bony changes until 10-20 days after symptoms begin. MRI is the ideal study, with a sensitivity of 92% to 100%. The most common organisms are the same as those that cause septic arthritis, and patients with

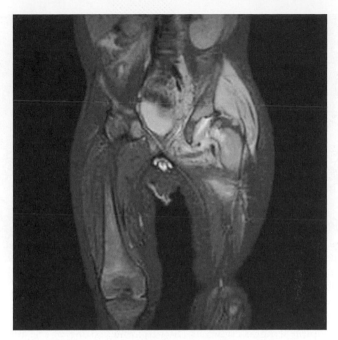

Figure 33–2. An example of osteomyelitis of the left proximal femur, ischia, and iliac bones with associated left hip septic arthritis. There is also extensive myositis surrounding the left hip. There is possible pus under pressure or necrotic changes present in the left proximal femur.

osteomyelitis require empiric antibiotic therapy and emergent orthopedic consultation for bone aspiration.

Transient synovitis is the most common cause of acute hip pain in children aged 3-10 years old. The arthralgia is caused by a temporary inflammation of the synovium, the soft tissue that lines the non-cartilaginous surfaces of the hip joint. While the etiology is not clearly understood, the disease is suspected to be secondary to an infection because up to 50% of patients report a recent upper respiratory tract infection. Fever typically is absent or, if it occurs, is low grade. Most patients will complain of unilateral hip pain, and up to 5% will have bilateral pain. There is a male-to-female predominance of slightly more than 2:1.

LCP disease (avascular necrosis of the femoral head) develops when an insufficient blood supply to the femoral head leads to necrosis. It is commonly found in boys aged 4-10 years, and though there are many theories as to its etiology, its cause is unknown. The child usually presents with a limp and may complain of hip or knee pain. On physical examination, the child will have decreased range of motion at the affected hip. X-rays may show fragmentation and then healing of the femoral head (Figure 33–3), and a bone scan will show decreased blood perfusion to the femoral head. Ten to twenty percent of patients will have bilateral disease, and the aim of treatment is to keep the femoral head within the acetabulum to allow healing to occur. A brace, cast, or splint may be required to immobilize the hip's position. Patients should be referred to an orthopedist for possible surgical management.

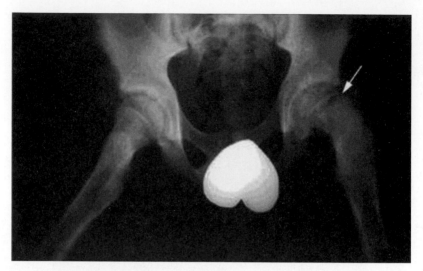

Figure 33–3. Avascular Necrosis of the Femoral Head.

Slipped capital femoral epiphysis (**SCFE**) remains one of the most common disorders affecting the hip in adolescence. SCFE is characterized by the posterior displacement of the capital femoral epiphysis from the femoral neck through the growth plate. It is most common in obese boys aged 11-15 years. Children who grow rapidly and who have hormonal imbalances such as hypothyroidism and acromegaly are also at risk. In addition to a limp, patients will complain of hip and/or knee pain. On examination, patients will have impaired internal rotation, and passive hip flexion may be associated with compensatory external rotation. Plain films of the hip or pelvis will often show displacement of the femoral head, commonly described as "fallen ice cream from the cone." Approximately 30% to 60% of patients with unilateral SCFE will eventually have SCFE of the contralateral hip. Once the diagnosis is suspected, weight-bearing should be avoided, and most patients will require surgery to reattach the femoral head to the femur.

Toddler's fracture is a nondisplaced fracture of the distal tibial shaft that occurs most commonly in a child younger than 2 years who is learning to walk. Frequently, there is no definite history of a traumatic event, and the child is brought to the office due to reluctance to bear weight on the leg. On physical examination, maximal tenderness can usually be elicited over the fracture site. On plain film, the typical findings are a nondisplaced hairline spiral fracture of the tibia and no fibular fracture. It is not uncommon for initial radiographs to be normal and the diagnosis of this fracture to be made several days after the injury when follow-up radiographs show a lucent line or periosteal reaction.

Osgood-Schlatter syndrome is caused by a reaction of the bone and cartilage of the tibial tubercle to repetitive stress (eg, jumping) and is believed to represent tiny stress fractures in the apophysis. The condition is also associated with rapid growth spurts. Physical examination reveals tenderness and swelling over the tibial tubercle. Running, jumping, and kneeling worsen the symptoms. The condition is managed with ice, anti-inflammatory medication, and a decrease in activity. Daily stretching of the quadriceps and hamstrings is also beneficial. Patients with severe pain may require immobilization using crutches or a knee immobilizer. Individual regulation of activity is usually effective; pain may recur until the tubercle matures (ie, ossifies completely).

CASE CORRELATION

- See also Case 32 (Fever in 1-3 Month Old Infants) and Case 34 (Febrile Seizure).

COMPREHENSION QUESTIONS

33.1 A 2-year-old girl presents with refusal bear weight on the left leg and a fever of 38.7°C (101.6°F) for 2 days. She has significant guarding when you attempt to assess the range of motion of her left hip. In consideration of the differential diagnosis, which of the following diagnostic tests would be most useful?

    A. Radiograph of both hips

    B. CBC

    C. Blood culture

    D. Ultrasound examination of the hip

33.2 The mother of an 8-year-old boy is told that her son's limping and knee pain is caused by LCP disease. Which of the following best explains the condition of the femoral head?

    A. Dislocation

    B. Subluxation

    C. Avascular necrosis

    D. Dysplasia

33.3 A 5-year-old girl is brought into the emergency center due to significant hip pain. There is no history of trauma or fall. She has had a recent respiratory infection. Which of the following is the most likely diagnosis?

    A. Subacute osteomyelitis

    B. Transient synovitis

    C. Developmental dysplasia of the hip

    D. Malignant degeneration of the hip

    E. SCFE

33.4 A 13-year-old overweight, adolescent boy presents to his pediatrician's office with chronic left hip pain for 2 months. He has a Trendelenburg gait and decreased range of motion of the left hip. Which of the following is the most likely diagnosis for this patient?

A. SCFE

B. Transient synovitis

C. Osgood-Schlatter

D. LCP disease

33.5 A 12-month-old male infant presents with his concerned mother after rolling off the bed in the night. X-ray reveals a femoral shaft fracture, and you note that this child has had three other visits to the ED for injury. What is your next step in the management of this patient?

A. Urgent orthopedic consultation

B. Order a skeletal survey

C. Report your concerns to the appropriate child protection services

D. All of the above

ANSWERS

33.1 **D.** Osteomyelitis, septic arthritis, and transient synovitis should be considered in the differential of this child. Osteomyelitis and septic arthritis are orthopedic emergencies and require prompt intervention. Transient synovitis is often hard to distinguish clinically from the prior two entities. To make a definite diagnosis, an ultrasound should be performed to evaluate for an effusion and guide arthrocentesis. The synovial fluid of a septic joint will have a marked neutrophilia.

33.2 **C.** LCP disease is commonly found in boys aged 4-8 years. It results in avascular necrosis of the femoral head.

33.3 **B.** Transient synovitis is the most common cause of hip pain in children aged 3-10 years. Though a benign process, it is often hard to distinguish from a septic joint or osteomyelitis. If the diagnosis is clear, the child can be safely treated with bed rest and anti-inflammatory medications.

33.4 **A.** SCFE is commonly found among overweight pubertal children. A Trendelenburg gait is described as the pelvis tilting downward on the unaffected side when a patient steps on the affected side. There is also an accompanying subtle shift of the torso. LCP is in the differential but is more common among children aged 4-8. Transient synovitis presents more acutely. Osgood-Schlatter usually presents in athletic children who have reproducible tibial tubercle tenderness.

33.5 **D.** Child abuse should be suspected, as this is likely to be a non-ambulatory child. The mechanism sounds suspicious, was not witnessed, and there may have been delay in seeking medical care. Treating the injury, alerting the appropriate authorities of your concerns, and obtaining a skeletal survey are essential for the safety of the child. A typical skeletal survey includes skull, chest, pelvis, and entire limb x-rays.

CLINICAL PEARLS

▶ Always order an ultrasound and perform arthrocentesis in a child with fever who refuses to move a joint. Transient synovitis should be a diagnosis of exclusion.

▶ Consider LCP disease in boys aged 4-8 who present with a limp, as it requires a high index of suspicion.

▶ SCFE treatment is operative, and 30% to 60% will eventually have bilateral disease. To prevent delay in diagnosis of the second slip, all patients should be followed closely by an orthopedist until the child has finished growing.

▶ Perform a thorough history (with or without the parent) and physical on children who present with fractures to evaluate for possible child abuse.

REFERENCES

Clark MC. Approach to the child with a limp. Available at: www.uptodate.com. Accessed March 19, 2016.

Frank G, Mahoney HM, Eppes SC. Musculoskeletal infections in children. *Pediatr Clin North Am.* 2005;52:1083-1106.

Kiang KM, Ogunmodede F, Juni BA, et al. Outbreak of osteomyelitis/septic arthritis caused by Kigella kingae among child care center attendees. *Pediatrics.* 2005;116:e206-213.

Kienstra AJ, Macias CG. Slipped capital femoral epiphysis. Available at: www.uptodate.com. Accessed May 9, 2012.

Kocher MS, Mandiga R, Zurakowski D, Barnewolt C, Kasser JR. Validation of a clinical prediction rule for the differentiation between septic arthritis and transient synovitis of the hip in children. *J Bone Joint Surg Am.* 2004;86A:1629-1635.

Krogstad P. Bacterial arthritis: clinical features and diagnosis in infants and children. Available at: www. uptodate.com. Accessed Feb 1, 2017.

Nelson JD. Skeletal infections in children. *Adv Pediatr Infect Dis.* 1991;6:59-78.

Nigrovic PA. Overview of hip pain in childhood. Available at: www.uptodate.com. Accessed April 16, 2012.

Shetty AK, Gedalia A. Septic arthritis in children. *Rheum Dis Clin North Am.* 1998;24:287-304.

Sonnen GM, Henry NK. Pediatric bone and joint infections: diagnosis and antimicrobial management. *Pediatr Clin North Am.* 1996;43:933-947.

Viera RL, Levy JA. Bedside ultrasonography to identify hip effusions in pediatric patients. *Ann Emerg Med.* 2010;55:284-289.

A 14-month-old child is brought in by EMS after a witnessed tonic-clonic event at home by his mother. The child was born vaginally at term after an uneventful pregnancy. His birth weight was 3700 g, and he was discharged on the second hospital day. The mother noted that the child has been well appearing, is not taking any medications, and has not traveled recently. He has been active for the past week with no apparent complaints. The mother thinks the seizure lasted about 5 minutes, but it ceased by the time EMS arrived at the home. The vital signs on the chart include a temperature of 38.4°C (101.1°F) (rectal), a heart rate of 130 beats per minute, a respiratory rate of 24 breaths per minute, and a systolic blood pressure of 100 mm Hg. On initial evaluation, the child is well appearing, well-perfused, and in no respiratory distress. His mental status is back to baseline per the mother. On further evaluation, the child has no rashes or murmurs but is noted to have a bulging erythematous tympanic membrane. No laboratory studies are ordered initially.

▶ What is the most likely diagnosis?
▶ What is the next step in management of this patient?

ANSWERS TO CASE 34:
Febrile Seizure

Summary: This is a 14-month-old child with a febrile seizure and acute otitis media (AOM). A relatively brief seizure in a febrile child in this age group who returns to baseline mental status is consistent with a diagnosis of a febrile seizure. Uncomplicated presentations require a thorough history and physical examination but rarely any additional laboratory or radiographic testing. The presence of a focal infection like otitis media is common but not essential for the diagnosis. Providing the child returns to a baseline playful state, admission to the hospital is not necessary.

- **Most likely diagnosis:** Simple febrile seizure and AOM.

- **Next step in management:** Medication to reduce the fever, such as acetaminophen, followed by a period of observation and reevaluation.

ANALYSIS

Objectives

1. Learn the specific definition of a simple febrile seizure.

2. Understand current standards for an age-based approach to the evaluation of a simple febrile seizure in the pediatric patient.

3. In cases of concurrent infection, specifically otitis media (OM), determine the need for further evaluation and/or testing in a simple febrile seizure.

Considerations

This infant has experienced a witnessed seizure at home and is noted to be febrile but well appearing, without neurologic deficits, and back at his baseline in the emergency department. As with all sick emergency department patients, the evaluation begins with assessment of airway, breathing, and circulation. After the initial assessment, the etiology of the seizure must be investigated. This subject can be complex, considering the large number of potential causes, and the clinician must address the threat of a CNS infection before less acute etiologies are considered. After the toddler has been observed in the emergency department for 1 hour, noted to be playful, active, and in no distress, and a careful physical examination is normal, the child is discharged home with his mother to follow up with his pediatrician. Parents should be instructed to return to the emergency department immediately for repeat seizure, change in behavior, vomiting, etc. The child's AOM should improve within 72 hours of antibiotic treatment, and if not, they should return to their pediatrician or the emergency department.

> # APPROACH TO:
> ## Febrile Seizures

DEFINITIONS

SIMPLE FEBRILE SEIZURE: The definition for a simple febrile seizure is very specific: age between 6 months and 60 months, generalized tonic-clonic convulsions, spontaneous cessation of convulsion within 15 minutes, return to alert mental status after convulsion, documentation of fever (>38.0°C), one convulsion within a 24-hour period, and absence of neurologic abnormality on examination.

COMPLEX FEBRILE SEIZURE: This heterogeneous group is beyond the scope of this chapter. The essential features include seizures lasting longer than 15 minutes, focal features or postictal paresis, or more than one seizure occurring in a 24-hour period. The causes, presentations, assessments, and treatments are broad and complex. A standard treatment recommendation **does not exist**, and the clinician must evaluate and treat the child with a complex febrile seizure on a case-by-case manner.

WELL-APPEARING INFANT: An infant who appears to both caretaker and healthcare practitioner to interact appropriately for age, has no increased work of breathing, has normal skin color, and no evidence of dehydration on the clinical examination.

ACUTE OTITIS MEDIA (AOM): Bacterial (suppurative) infection of middle ear associated with signs, symptoms, and visualization of middle ear effusion.

CLINICAL APPROACH

A simple febrile seizure is often a traumatic event for the caregiver. Emergency physicians are often the first clinicians to evaluate the child after the event and need to be patient and supportive of the parents. If the child does not appear toxic, distressed, or hemodynamically unstable, a period of observation is recommended. During this period (usually under 1 hour), the clinician should obtain a thorough history from the caregiver (and EMS if available) regarding the duration of the event, recent illnesses, and new medications. Additional useful history includes any possible exposures to chemicals or medications in the household and any family history of seizure disorders. A fever greater than 38.0°C should be documented, and in the presence of fever antipyretic medications can be administered (oral or rectal, based on the child's mental status).

A thorough physical examination should be performed, looking specifically for any source of infection and clinical signs that are worrisome for bacterial meningitis (petechial rash, nuchal rigidity, failure to fully engage or to return to baseline level of awareness, etc.). The child's entire body should be examined for any signs of trauma or abuse, such as old ecchymoses, scratches, or scars. The provider should observe the interaction between the child and caregiver in order to raise or lower suspicion for possible abuse.

For a child who meets the strict definition of a **simple febrile seizure**, further testing (serum electrolytes, glucose, lumbar puncture, and neuroimaging) is often not warranted. Multiple retrospective studies have demonstrated extremely low incidence of bacterial meningitis in children with a simple febrile seizure and no clinical signs of meningitis. However, for children between the ages of 6 and 12 months who are unimmunized or have an unknown immune status, the American Pediatric Association recommends a lumbar puncture to rule out meningitis. Additionally, those currently on antibiotics should also have a lumbar puncture performed since the symptoms and signs of meningitis may be masked. Infants discovered to have a concurrent infection (bacterial enteritis, urinary tract infection, or otitis media) presenting with a simple febrile seizure should be treated for the underlying illness with standard therapy.

Acute Otitis Media

The diagnosis of AOM requires a middle ear effusion and signs of middle ear inflammation. The disease exists on the same spectrum as otitis media with effusion, which lacks a bacterial infection or inflammation. Diagnosis of a middle ear effusion can be confirmed on otoscopy by finding bubbles or an air-fluid level, along with a tympanic membrane that is abnormally colored (not translucent), opaque, and/or not mobile with pneumatic pressure. Acute inflammation can be confirmed either by a history of fever and ear pain (or tugging) or by direct visualization of a bulging and red tympanic membrane.

Streptococcus pneumoniae, nontypeable *Haemophilus influenzae*, and *Moraxella catarrhalis* are thought to cause over 90% of cases of AOM; however, current vaccine patterns may alter future etiologies. Complications of AOM are rare but include hearing loss, tympanic membrane perforation, and mastoiditis. Of most concern in this case would be the rare complication of intracranial extension causing mastoiditis, meningitis, brain abscess, or central venous thrombosis. These complications must be entertained if **AOM is encountered in the setting of a seizure, especially if the child experienced a complex febrile seizure.**

Controversy exists about whether to treat AOM with antibiotics. Most professional guidelines recommend treating a child younger than the age of 2 with oral antibiotics. Children older than the age of 2 may be treated with a "watchful waiting" approach if they have mild or moderate symptoms. A prescription may be provided, but parents should be asked not to fill it unless the child fails to improve after several days. Amoxicillin remains the drug of choice.

Risk of Seizure Recurrence

One-third of children who have a simple febrile seizure will experience another by the age of 6 years old. However, children who experience a simple febrile seizure have only a small increased likelihood of developing epilepsy (approximately 1% overall risk).

Prevention and Treatment

Antibiotic and/or antipyretic therapy has not been shown to decrease the recurrence rates of simple febrile seizures. Caretakers should be made aware that even the most vigilant attempts at fever reduction after discharge may not reduce febrile seizure recurrence.

Initiation of oral antiepileptic medications (eg, valproic acid, phenobarbital, etc.) is not recommended for first-time febrile seizures. Treatment after a second seizure is controversial.

CASE CORRELATION

- See also Case 32 (Fever in 1-3 Month Old Infants) and Case 33 (Child with Limp).

COMPREHENSION QUESTIONS

34.1 A 2-year-old toddler is brought in by her family after a seizure episode today. The family states that the child was in her normal state of health when they noticed her entire body jerking rhythmically for several minutes, during which she did not respond to their voice. After 1 hour, the child remained somnolent and minimally responsive at home and was brought to the ED for evaluation. The mother states the infant was coughing and having clear nasal discharge for the past 24 hours but was otherwise well. The vital signs included a temperature of 39.0°C (102.2°F) (rectal), a heart rate of 140 beats per minute, a respiratory rate of 30 breaths per minute, and a systolic blood pressure of 80 mm Hg. On the initial evaluation (about 30 minutes after the child is brought to the emergency department), the child is somnolent and not at baseline mental status per the mother. Further evaluation finds no physical examination abnormalities other than mild clear nasal discharge. The child has a normal cardiac, lung, and skin examination. Which of the following criteria indicates this was a complex febrile seizure?

A. Age of the child involved

B. Height of the fever

C. Generalized tonic-clonic nature of the seizure

D. Lack of return to baseline mental status after convulsion

E. Preceding upper respiratory infection symptoms

34.2 A 16-month-old child is brought in by EMS after an episode of shaking visualized by the mother that lasted 3 minutes. On arrival to the ED, the child is back to baseline mental status as per the mother. The mother states the infant was coughing for the past 24 hours but was otherwise well. In the ED the child was playful and active but was noted to have a mild, nonproductive cough. The vital signs on the chart include a temperature of 39.3°C (102.7°F) (rectal), a heart rate of 150 beats per minute, a respiratory rate of 34 breaths per minute, and a systolic blood pressure of 80 mm Hg. On the initial evaluation, the child is well appearing, well perfused, and in no respiratory distress. The child has a normal cardiac and pulmonary examination and has no rashes. Discharge instructions to the parent should include:

A. Around-the-clock antipyretic therapy

B. Anticonvulsive medications to prevent development of epilepsy

C. Outpatient neurologic testing, including electroencephalography

D. Rectal diazepam if the child becomes febrile again to prevent further seizures

E. Appropriate follow-up with the toddler's pediatrician and reassurance

34.3 A 36-month-old toddler is brought in by EMS after an episode of shaking visualized by the mother that lasted 12 minutes. On arrival to the ED, the child is resting comfortable in the bed with his mother. The mother states the toddler was tugging at his left ear and coughing for the past 2 days but was otherwise well. The toddler has received all of his vaccinations and never had a seizure in the past. The vital signs on the chart include a temperature of 38.4°C (101.1°F) (rectal), a heart rate of 140 beats per minute, a respiratory rate of 22 breaths per minute, and a systolic blood pressure of 110 mm Hg. On the initial evaluation, the child is well appearing, well perfused, and in no respiratory distress. The oropharynx shows injected pharyngeal tonsils. The left tympanic membrane is erythematous and non-mobile during air insufflation. The child has a normal cardiac and pulmonary examination and has no rashes. What is the most appropriate management of the toddler?

A. Obtain laboratory testing (CBC) to determine the presence of an underlying infection

B. Neuroimaging to determine the presence of an underlying CNS infection

C. Treatment of the otitis media (OM) with conservative therapy (NSAIDs) and instructions to follow up with the child pediatrician in 24 hours

D. Lumbar puncture to determine a meningeal infection

E. Inpatient admission for ENT consultation

ANSWERS

34.1 **D.** A simple febrile seizure is characterized by strict criteria. If the child does not return to baseline mental status shortly after convulsion, even in the setting of fever, it is considered a complex febrile seizure and alternative causes must be explored.

34.2 **E.** Research has shown that a simple febrile seizure cannot be prevented by antipyretics or antiepileptics. After a first occurrence, the risk of future epilepsy is low, and no action need be taken initially as long as the symptoms fit the strict criteria for simple febrile seizure.

34.3 **C.** This patient had a simple febrile seizure, so there is a very low suspicion for a direct extension of the AOM into the intracranial space. The AOM is the cause of the fever and likely the related seizure as well. Given the patient is over 2 years old, expert recommendations endorse a watchful waiting approach to treatment.

CLINICAL PEARLS

▶ Most professional guidelines recommend treating a child younger than the age of 2 with AOM with oral antibiotics. Amoxicillin is the drug of choice. Children older than the age of 2 may be treated with a "watchful waiting" approach if they have mild or moderate symptoms.

▶ A simple febrile seizure is often a traumatic event for the caregiver. It is important to be patient and supportive of the parents.

▶ For a child who meets the strict definition of a simple febrile seizure, further testing is often not warranted. For children 6-12 months old who are unimmunized or have an unknown immune status, a lumbar puncture should be done to rule out meningitis.

REFERENCES

American Academy of Pediatrics Subcommittee on Management of Acute Otitis Media. Diagnosis and management of acute otitis media. *Pediatrics*. 2013;131(3):991-999.

Febrile seizures: clinical practice guideline for the long-term management of the child with simple febrile seizures. *Pediatrics*. 2008;121(6):1281-1286.

Fetveit A. Assessment of febrile seizures in children. *Eur J Pediatr*. 2008;167(1):17-27.

Hampers LC, Spina LA. Evaluation and management of pediatric febrile seizures in the emergency department. *Emerg Med Clin North Am*. 2011;29(1):83-93.

Neurodiagnostic evaluation of the child with a simple febrile seizure. Subcommittee on Febrile Seizure; American Academy of Pediatrics. *Pediatrics*. 2011;127(2):389-394.

An 18-year-old adolescent woman presents to the emergency department (ED) complaining of a 1-week history of abdominal pain. She tells you that she and her friends recently returned from spring break vacation in Mexico, and she has noticed a constant ache that is worse on her right side. The patient's mother is worried because her daughter has been unable to eat or drink anything for 2 days. After asking the mother to step out of the room while you examine the patient, she tells you that she has had five sexual partners, occasionally uses condom for birth control, and has never been pregnant. Her last menstrual period was 2 weeks ago and was heavier than normal. On physical examination, her blood pressure was 100/70 mm Hg, pulse 110 beats per minute, respirations 22 breaths per minute, and temperature 38.9°C (102.1°F). Her heart has a regular rate and rhythm without murmurs. Lungs are clear to auscultation bilaterally. The abdominal examination reveals a diffusely tender lower abdomen, greater on the right than left, and the patient exhibits voluntary guarding. Examination of the pelvis reveals a greenish, foul-smelling discharge with a red, friable-appearing cervix. Bimanual examination reveals an exquisitely tender cervix with fullness and pain in the right adnexal area. The wet prep of the discharge shows many white blood cells (WBCs), no clue cells, no trichomonas, and no *Candida*. A urine pregnancy test is negative.

▶ What is the most likely diagnosis?
▶ What is the next diagnostic step?
▶ What is the next step in your treatment?

ANSWERS TO CASE 35:

Acute Pelvic Inflammatory Disease

Summary: An 18-year-old nulliparous adolescent woman complains of severe abdominal pain, vaginal discharge, fever, nausea, and vomiting. She displays cervical motion tenderness and her right adnexa appear to have some fullness and tenderness on examination.

- **Most likely diagnosis:** Pelvic inflammatory disease (PID).

- **Next step:** Transvaginal ultrasound to rule out tubo-ovarian abscess, assays for gonorrhea (GC) and *Chlamydia*, complete blood count (CBC), and screen for sexually transmitted infections (STIs).

- **Next treatment step:** Admit the patient and start IV antibiotic therapy.

ANALYSIS

Objectives

1. Understand the diagnosis and workup of PID.

2. Describe the lack of clinical signs of tubo-ovarian abscess.

3. Know the criteria and treatments for both outpatient and inpatient PID.

4. Know the common differential diagnoses for lower abdominal pain and be able to consult the appropriate specialties based on the physical examination and laboratory studies.

Considerations

This nulliparous adolescent woman has lower abdominal pain, fever, abnormal vaginal discharge, adnexal tenderness/fullness, and cervical motion tenderness. Although these symptoms may occur with other diagnoses such as appendicitis, ovarian torsion, ectopic pregnancy, or inflammatory bowel disease, the clinical symptoms are most consistent with PID. **PID is defined as an ascending infection from the vagina or cervix to the upper genital tract,** such as the endometrium, fallopian tubes, or ovaries. Although the etiology may be **polymicrobial,** sexually transmitted organisms such as **Neisseria gonorrhoeae or Chlamydia trachomatis are implicated in many cases but declining in incidence.** Because the disease may mimic other common conditions, meticulous physical examination, clinical examination, and use of transvaginal ultrasound must be performed in conjunction to correctly diagnose a gynecologic disease from that of a general surgery process. This patient is admitted to the hospital due to inability to tolerate oral medication (nausea and vomiting) and also height of the temperature (37.8°C [102°F]).

APPROACH TO:
Pelvic Inflammatory Disease

DEFINITIONS

CERVICAL MOTION TENDERNESS: Also referred to as a "chandelier sign." Motion of the cervix during bimanual examination elicits extreme tenderness, so as to cause the patient to jump off the bed and hit the chandelier.

PELVIC INFLAMMATORY DISEASE (PID): An ascending infection of microorganisms from the lower genital tract to the upper genital tract that is polymicrobial and may be associated with *N. gonorrhoeae* or *C. trachomatis*. PID may also be termed salpingitis.

TUBO-OVARIAN ABSCESS (TOA): A collection of purulent material encompassing the fallopian tube and ovary comprised of predominantly anaerobic organisms. TOAs are an important complication of PID.

CLINICAL APPROACH

Pelvic inflammatory disease is an ascending infection from the lower genital tract to the upper genital tract that may be difficult to diagnose due to the variety and severity of presenting symptoms. Risk factors for the development of PID are young age, recent menstruation, multiple sexual partners, no use of barrier contraception, and lower socioeconomic status. The clinical diagnosis of PID is fairly accurate, but a broad differential diagnosis should be kept in mind in the evaluation of abdominal pain in a woman. Criteria for diagnosis include **lower abdominal tenderness, adnexal tenderness, and/or cervical motion tenderness.** Previously, all three criteria were considered necessary to make the diagnosis; however, recent studies have shown that this strategy likely misses some episodes of PID. Thus, clinical suspicion and only looking for one sign is sufficient for a possible PID diagnosis. The presence of purulent vaginal discharge, fever more than 101°F, elevated serum leukocyte count, and presence of gonorrhea or *Chlamydia* in the endocervix are supportive findings. Thus, all women who are suspected of having PID should have testing for *N. gonorrhoeae* and *C. trachomatis* as well as HIV.

The clinical presentation of tubo-ovarian abscess can be subtle. The majority of these patients have little or low-grade fever, slightly elevated white blood cell count, and may not have a palpable adnexal mass on pelvic examination. For this reason, those patients who are diagnosed with PID should have imaging of the pelvis to assess for TOA, since this diagnosis requires inpatient therapy.

Ultrasound imaging or computed tomography (CT) imaging of the abdomen and pelvis may be helpful to assess for other conditions. The differential diagnosis of acute PID includes appendicitis, ectopic pregnancy, endometriosis, ovarian torsion, hemorrhagic corpus luteum cyst, benign ovarian tumor, and inflammatory bowel disease. CT imaging is more helpful in assessing appendicitis. Finally, laparoscopy is considered the "gold standard" in establishing the diagnosis by visualizing purulent discharge from the tube, and it is generally considered when a patient has acute symptoms, sepsis, or is not improving with therapy.

The etiology of PID is polymicrobial, as many different bacteria are harbored in the vagina. Recently, it has been discovered that less than 50% of cases involve *N. gonorrhoeae* and *C. trachomatis*; other organisms, such as *Bacteroides fragilis*, *Escherichia coli*, *Peptostreptococci* sp, *Haemophilus influenzae*, and aerobic streptococci, are isolated from acute cases of PID. Thus, organisms may be classified as either sexually transmitted organisms or endogenous.

The pathogenesis of PID may include many mechanisms. First, for ascension of infection to develop from the vagina, through the cervical canal, to the endometrium of the uterus, through the fallopian tubes and to the ovaries or peritoneum, there must be a breakdown of the natural host defense system. For instance, hormonal changes unique to a woman's cycle may play a role in the ascending infection. During a normal menstrual cycle, the cervical mucus changes based on the predominate hormone, either estrogen or progesterone. At midcycle, when estrogen predominates and progesterone is low, cervical mucus is thin and may facilitate easy ascension of bacteria. However, after ovulation, when the progesterone level is high, the cervical mucous is thick and more difficult for bacteria to penetrate. For this reason, progestin-containing contraception via the oral contraceptive or depot medroxyprogesterone acetate (depo provera) decreases the incidence of PID. Menses is another time when women are at greater risk for developing PID because the cervical mucous plug is lost due to outward menstrual flow and organisms may also ascend to the upper genital tract. Retrograde menstrual flow has also been attributed to the risk of bacteria ascending from the uterus into the fallopian tubes, ovaries, or peritoneal cavity.

Treatment of PID varies widely depending on the clinical presentation of the patient. Treatment should provide broad-spectrum coverage of the suspected pathogens and should be initiated as soon as a presumptive diagnosis has been made in order to prevent long-term sequelae or complications from acute PID, such as tubal damage leading to infertility, chronic pain, or ectopic pregnancies. **Of note, postinfectious tubal infertility is the second most common reason for female infertility in the United States.**

Uncomplicated PID in a compliant patient may be treated outpatient. However, **certain criteria for hospitalization** exist for the management of complicated PID (Table 35–1). Although IV antibiotics are used to treat the symptoms of PID, laparoscopy is useful in cases with an uncertain diagnosis, suspicion of a ruptured TOA, or when a patient fails to respond to IV antibiotics. A ruptured TOA presents as

Table 35–1 • CRITERIA FOR HOSPITALIZATION
Surgical emergencies (eg, appendicitis) unable to be excluded
Pregnancy
Lack of response clinically to oral antimicrobial therapy
Patient is unable to follow or tolerate an outpatient oral regimen
Severe illness, nausea, and vomiting, or high fever
Tubo-ovarian abscess
Adolescent, nulliparous, or questionable compliance
Presence of an intrauterine device

Table 35–2 • THERAPY FOR PELVIC INFLAMMATORY DISEASE
Outpatient therapy: • Ceftriaxone 250 mg IM in a single dose *plus* doxycycline 100 mg PO bid for 14 d *with or without* metronidazole 500 mg PO bid for 14 d • Cefoxitin 2 g IM in a single dose and probenecid 1 g PO administered concurrently in a single dose *plus* doxycycline 100 mg PO bid for 14 d *with or without* metronidazole 500 mg PO bid for 14 d • Other parenteral third-generation cephalosporin (eg, ceftizoxime or cefotaxime) *plus* doxycycline 100 mg PO bid for 14 d *with or without* metronidazole 500 mg PO bid for 14 d
Inpatient therapy: • Cefotetan 2 g IV q12h or cefoxitin 2 g IV q6h and doxycycline 100 mg PO or IV q12h • Clindamycin 900 mg IV q8h and gentamycin 2 mg/kg IV loading dose followed by 1.5 mg/kg q8h

Source: Data from Centers for Disease Control and Prevention. 2010 Guidelines for treatment of sexually transmitted diseases. MMWR. 2010;59(RR-12):1.

shock and is a surgical emergency. Thus, the patient who is brought into the ED with hypotension, significant abdominal pain, and signs of infection should receive fluid resuscitation and arrangements for rapid surgical management.

Treatment is usually parenteral. Outpatient management includes **intramuscular ceftriaxone 250 mg once and oral doxycycline 100 mg twice daily for 14 days with or without metronidazole 500 mg twice daily for 14 days** (Table 35–2). Patients should ideally be seen back in 48 hours to assess for improvement. A common inpatient management is intravenous cefotetan 2 g every 12 hours and oral or IV doxycycline 100 mg every 12 hours. Improvement should occur after 24-48 hours of therapy. When a tubo-ovarian abscess is suspected, clindamycin or metronidazole is used in the place of doxycycline since anaerobic bacteria are the main concern. TOAs are an exception to the rule that "abscesses require drainage"—the majority of TOAs can be treated with antibiotic therapy and followed with imaging for resolution. Approximately one-third of TOAs will need surgical therapy.

After clinical improvement on intravenous therapy, the patient is changed to oral antibiotic therapy for 10 days. If there is no improvement after 72 hours of therapy (decreased fever, improvement in abdominal pain, reduction in uterine/adnexal tenderness), a more in-depth workup is needed. **Follow-up and treatment of a known sexual partner** is essential for decreasing the incidence of recurrence of PID. Known **complications are infertility, pelvic adhesions leading to chronic pelvic pain, risk of ectopic surgery, Fitz-Hugh-Curtis syndrome, and chronic PID.**

CASE CORRELATION

- See also Case 16 (Acute Abdominal Pain), Case 24 (Acute Pyelonephritis), Case 36 (Ectopic Pregnancy), Case 37 (Hyperemesis Gravidarum and OB Emergencies), and Case 38 (Sexual Assault).

COMPREHENSION QUESTIONS

35.1 A 22-year-old woman is noted to have lower abdominal pain associated with some dysuria and abnormal menses. Her appetite has decreased recently. The pregnancy test is negative. Which of the following findings would most likely suggest PID?

A. Endometrial biopsy showing atypical cells

B. Vaginal wet mount demonstrating clue cells

C. Cervical motion tenderness on physical examination

D. Pain on rectal examination

35.2 A 32-year-old woman is noted to have a 2-day history of low-grade fever and lower abdominal tenderness. The examination reveals cervical motion tenderness and adnexal tenderness. Which of the following is best in assessing for possible tubo-ovarian abscess?

A. Degree of temperature

B. Elevation of leukocyte count

C. Pelvic examination revealing adnexal mass

D. Ultrasound of the pelvis

E. Rebound tenderness of the abdomen

Match the following diseases (A to G) to the clinical situations in Questions 35.3 to 35.6:

A. Ectopic pregnancy

B. Appendicitis

C. Gastroesophageal reflux disease (GERD)

D. Crohn disease

E. Cholelithiasis

F. Pancreatitis

G. Ovarian torsion

35.3 A 21-year-old woman experiences crampy abdominal pain that begins near the umbilicus and moves to the lower right quadrant. The pain has progressed over days and is intermittent and crampy. The patient is afebrile and complains of some nausea.

35.4 A 41-year-old woman complains of pain in the upper abdomen, especially after eating. The pain seems to travel to her right shoulder. She has bloating at times.

35.5 A 35-year-old man complains of epigastric abdominal pain which seems to "bore straight to the back." He has nausea and vomiting.

35.6 A 22-year-old woman complains of intermittent severe abdominal pain with diarrhea. She also has some joint pain.

ANSWERS

35.1 **C.** Although cervical motional tenderness is not specific for acute salpingitis and can be seen with other acute inflammatory conditions of the lower abdomen such as diverticulitis and appendicitis, it is a classic finding of PID.

35.2 **D.** Imaging is the best way to assess for TOA. Tubo-ovarian abscess is often subtle in its presentation and may not be associated with fever or elevated WBC. Most TOAs can be treated medically with antibiotics rather than requiring surgical therapy.

35.3 **G.** The intermittent crampy abdominal pain is classic for ovarian torsion. Although this patient's pain moves from the umbilicus to the lower quadrant area, the pain has lasted longer than 24 hours and is without fever, making appendicitis less likely.

35.4 **E.** The right upper quadrant abdominal pain following meals (especially fatty meals) is very typical of cholelithiasis. The pain often radiates to the right scapula. If she had fever, cholecystitis would be suspected.

35.5 **F.** Pancreatitis usually presents with midepigastric pain that penetrates straight to the back, is constant in nature, and is associated with nausea and vomiting. Common etiologies include alcohol abuse and gall stones.

35.6 **D.** Inflammatory bowel disease (Crohn disease or ulcerative colitis) often affects individuals in their teens or twenties with abdominal pain, diarrhea (often bloody), and extraintestinal manifestations such as joint pain or eye findings.

CLINICAL PEARLS

▶ The classic triads of symptoms for diagnosing PID include lower abdominal tenderness, adnexal tenderness, and cervical motion tenderness.

▶ Laparoscopy remains the gold standard for diagnosing PID.

▶ TOAs often present in a subtle or indolent fashion and require imaging for diagnosis. TOAs require hospital antibiotic therapy, and the majority can be treated medically.

▶ Patients with a ruptured TOA present in shock. This is a surgical emergency.

▶ Long-term sequelae of PID include infertility, pelvic adhesions, chronic pelvic pain, risk of ectopic pregnancy, and Fitz-Hugh-Curtis syndrome.

▶ Disseminated gonococcal infection, although uncommon, is a serious complication of untreated gonorrhea, which is a very common infection.

▶ Persons found to have a positive gonorrhea culture should also be treated for *Chlamydia* because concomitant infection is found in as many as 40% of patients.

▶ In any person presenting with asymmetric polyarthritis, tenosynovitis, and pustular skin lesions, disseminated gonococcal infection should be considered in the differential diagnosis.

REFERENCES

Centers for Disease Control and Prevention. 2015 guidelines for treatment of sexually transmitted diseases. *MMWR*. 2015;59(RR-12):1.

Cohen CR. Pelvic inflammatory disease. In: Klausner JD, Hook III EW, eds. *Current Diagnosis & Treatment of Sexually Transmitted Diseases*. New York, NY: McGraw-Hill; 2007.

Hemsell DM. Gynecologic infection. In: Schorge J, Schaffer J, Halvorson L, Hoffman B, Bradshaw K, Cunningham F, eds. *Williams Gynecology*. 3rd ed. New York, NY: McGraw-Hill; 2015:73-76.

Sweet RL, Gibbs RS. *Infectious Diseases of the Female Genital Tract*. 5th ed. Baltimore, MD: Lippincott Williams & Wilkins; 2009.

A 26-year-old woman presents to the emergency department (ED) with a 6-hour history of worsening abdominal pain. She states the pain initially was a dull pain near her umbilicus but has since moved to her lower right side. She rates the pain as 8 on a scale of 10 and crampy in nature. The patient states that she noted some vaginal spotting this morning but denies any passage of clots or tissue. The patient ate breakfast that morning but states she has not eaten since because she feels nauseous. She denies any fever or chills or any change in her bowel habits. Upon further questioning, the patient states her last menstrual period was 2 months ago, but her periods are irregular. She also states that she was told that she had a vaginal infection a year ago but does not recall having been treated for the illness. On physical examination, her blood pressure is 120/76 mm Hg, heart rate is 105 beats per minute, and she is afebrile. In general, she is in mild distress. The abdomen reveals tenderness to palpation in her right lower quadrant that is greater than that in the left lower quadrant. The examination reveals some minimal voluntary guarding, but no rebound tenderness is appreciated. On pelvic examination, the uterus appears mildly enlarged without cervical motion tenderness. There are no masses or tenderness in the adnexal region. Her complete blood count (CBC) reveals a mildly elevated white blood cell count with a left shift. A beta–human chorionic gonadotropin (β-hCG) was 4700 mIU/mL. A transvaginal sonogram reveals an empty uterus, and no adnexal masses or free fluid is noted.

- ▶ What is the most likely diagnosis?
- ▶ What is the next step?
- ▶ What is the initial treatment?

ANSWERS TO CASE 36:

Ectopic Pregnancy

Summary: A 26-year-old woman complains of severe abdominal pain, nausea, and vaginal spotting. She has a positive pregnancy test, a quantitative β-hCG level of 4700 mIU/mL, and a transvaginal sonogram showing no intrauterine pregnancy.

- **Most likely diagnosis:** Ectopic pregnancy.

- **Next step:** Diagnostic versus operative laparoscopy.

- **Initial treatment:** Establish an IV line and stabilize the patient in preparation for surgery.

ANALYSIS

Objectives

1. Understand the diagnosis and workup of ectopic pregnancy.

2. Know the different sonographic appearances of ectopic pregnancy.

3. Know the common differential diagnoses for lower abdominal pain and be able to consult the appropriate specialties based on the physical examination.

Considerations

This patient presents to the ED with complaints of vaginal bleeding, abdominal pain, and a positive pregnancy examination. Her quantitative **hCG level is above the threshold of 1200-1500 mIU/mL**, and **no intrauterine pregnancy** is seen on **transvaginal** sonography; thus, her **risk for an ectopic pregnancy approaches 85%.** Other diagnoses should be considered, such as threatened abortion, incomplete abortion, pelvic inflammatory disease, or appendicitis. Ectopic pregnancy is defined as a pregnancy that develops after implantation of the blastocyst anywhere other than in the lining of the uterine cavity.

APPROACH TO:

Ectopic Pregnancy

DEFINITIONS

ECTOPIC PREGNANCY: Pregnancy that develops after implantation anywhere other than the lining of the uterus.

RUPTURED ECTOPIC PREGNANCY: Ectopic pregnancy that has eroded through the tissue in which it has implanted, producing hemorrhage from exposed vessels.

SALPINGECTOMY: Surgical excision and removal of the oviduct and ectopic pregnancy.

SALPINGOSTOMY: Surgical excision of the ectopic pregnancy with preservation of the tube. The tube remains opened to heal by secondary intention.

CLINICAL APPROACH

Ectopic pregnancy is defined as a pregnancy outside the lining of the uterus, most commonly occurring in the oviduct, but it may also be found in the abdomen, ovary, or cervix. The incidence of the ectopic pregnancy has increased in the United States for three reasons: (1) the increased incidence of salpingitis caused by increased infection with *Chlamydia trachomatis* or other sexually transmitted diseases, (2) improved diagnostic techniques, and (3) the increase in assisted reproductive technology pregnancies. Other risk factors include prior tubal surgery, previous ectopic pregnancy, use of exogenous progesterone, and a history of infertility agents. The most common presenting symptoms are abdominal pain, absence of menses, and irregular vaginal bleeding. Other symptoms found on physical examination may include a palpable adnexal tenderness, uterine enlargement, tachycardia, hypotension, syncope, peritoneal signs, and fever.

Approximately half of the episodes of ectopic pregnancy are linked to previous salpingitis, although these episodes may be asymptomatic. Prior infections are likely to lead to anatomic tubal pathology that prevents the normal passage of an embryo into the uterus. In the remaining incidences of ectopic pregnancy, an identifying factor cannot be determined and may be linked to a physiologic disorder. Increased levels of estrogen and progesterone interfere with tubal motility and increase the chance of ectopic pregnancy.

Approximately 97% of ectopic pregnancies occur in the oviduct, specifically in the ampullary region. The remainder of ectopic pregnancies implant in the abdomen, cervix, or ovary. Pathogenesis of ectopic pregnancy begins as the embryo invades the lumen of the tube and its peritoneal covering. As the embryo continues to grow, surrounding vessels may bleed into the peritoneal cavity, resulting in a hemoperitoneum. The stretching of the tube results in abdominal pain until necrosis ensues and results in rupture of the ectopic pregnancy.

The differential diagnosis of ectopic pregnancy includes many other gynecologic and surgical illnesses. Most common are salpingitis, threatened or incomplete abortion, ruptured corpus luteum, adnexal torsion, and appendicitis. The diagnosis of ectopic pregnancy must be considered in any woman of reproductive age with abnormal vaginal bleeding and abdominal pain.

Diagnosis of ectopic pregnancy may be aided with the use of transvaginal ultrasound. Visualization of the pelvic organs may reveal the absence of an intrauterine pregnancy, the presence of a complex adnexal mass, or the presence of an embryo in the adnexa. It is important to note that with higher resolution ultrasound, **the hCG discriminatory zone is closer to 1200-1500 mIU/mL than the traditionally quoted figure of 1500-2000 mIU/mL, in which an intrauterine pregnancy is almost always seen on transvaginal sonography.** Lack of visualization of an intrauterine gestational sac on transvaginal sonography confers up to an 85% risk of an ectopic pregnancy.

At times, sonography can visualize an ectopic pregnancy even with hCG levels lower than this threshold; the **level of hCG does not reliably correlate with the size of the ectopic pregnancy.** When hCG levels are lower than the above threshold, the ED physician should rely on the clinical impression to diagnose an ectopic pregnancy.

In a reliable and asymptomatic patient whose initial hCG level is below the threshold, a repeat hCG level can be obtained in 48 hours. The **hCG should increase by at least 66% over 48 hours;** lack of normal rise strongly implies an abnormal pregnancy, although the test does not indicate the location of the pregnancy (ectopic or miscarriage). A definitive diagnosis of ectopic pregnancy can most always be made by direct visualization of the pelvic organs using laparoscopy if the diagnosis remains uncertain.

More pregnancies are associated with in vitro fertilization (IVF), which carries a higher risk of ectopic pregnancy and multiple gestation. Notably, in women who have IVF pregnancies, a proven intrauterine pregnancy may not rule out ectopic pregnancy since these patients can have heterotopic pregnancies (concomitant intrauterine and ectopic pregnancies).

Treatment options include both medical and surgical therapy (see figure 36-1). Medical treatment consists of using intramuscular **methotrexate**, a folinic acid antagonist that interferes with deoxyribonucleic acid (DNA) synthesis, repair, and cellular replication. Actively dividing tissue, such as fetal cell growth, is susceptible to methotrexate and may be used for treatment of ectopic pregnancy under specific conditions (Figure 36–1). Methotrexate is found to be more successful if the hCG is less than 5000 mIU/mL, if the fetus is smaller than 3.5 cm, and if there is no detectable fetal cardiac activity. It is important to note that each individual patient may present with different complaints and different levels of hCG, and at times medical management involves multiple doses of methotrexate.

Potential problems associated with medical management of ectopic pregnancy include drug side effects and treatment failure. Some patients treated with methotrexate will develop acute abdominal pain due to the process of "tubal abortion." In these individuals, pelvic sonography is useful—if the vital signs are stable and the ultrasound does not show much intra-abdominal fluid, the patient may be observed in the hospital to assess for resolution of the pain. However, those patients who have hypotension or evidence of intra-abdominal bleeding should go to the operating room.

If medical therapy fails, surgical intervention is necessary. Surgical management commonly consists of laparoscopy and/or laparotomy. A few common surgical techniques used for treatment of ectopic pregnancy include salpingotomy, salpingostomy, and partial salpingectomy. These techniques can be used to treat the majority of unruptured ectopic pregnancies, whereas exploratory laparotomy may be used in cases of ruptured ectopic pregnancy.

EMERGING CONCEPTS

Because of higher resolution ultrasound and earlier diagnosis of ectopic pregnancies, there is a higher likelihood of early detection than in the past. There have been

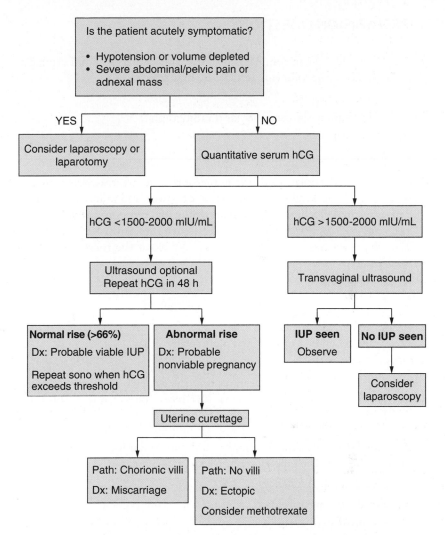

Figure 36–1. Algorithm for the management of suspected ectopic pregnancy.

some practitioners who have advocated expectant management for patients with small ectopic pregnancies, are hemodynamically stable, without symptoms, compliant with follow-up, and have appropriately declining hCG levels. Approximately 70% of candidates have successful spontaneous resolution.

CASE CORRELATION

- See also Case 2 (Hemorrhagic Shock), Case 16 (Acute Abdominal Pain), Case 35 (Acute Pelvic Inflammatory Disease), and Case 38 (Sexual Assault).

COMPREHENSION QUESTIONS

36.1 A 22-year-old woman complains of lower abdominal pain and vaginal spotting. Which of the following tests is the first priority?

A. Pelvic ultrasound

B. KUB (kidneys, ureters, bladder) radiograph

C. hCG level

D. *Chlamydia* antigen test of the cervix

36.2 A 22-year-old woman underwent methotrexate treatment for an ectopic pregnancy 1 week ago and complains of lower abdominal cramping. She denies vaginal bleeding, dizziness, or vomiting. On examination, her blood pressure is 120/80 mm Hg and her heart rate is 80 beats per minute. The abdomen reveals mild tenderness. Which of the following is the best management?

A. Observation

B. Surgical management of the ectopic pregnancy

C. Administration of folinic acid

D. Transfusion of 2 units of red blood cells

36.3 A 42-year-old woman complains of an acute onset of significant abdominal pain of 6 hours' duration. She states that she underwent in vitro fertilization and is currently 8 weeks pregnant. Her blood pressure is 90/60 mm Hg, and her heart rate is 110 beats per minute. Her quantitative hCG level is 22,800 mIU/mL. Transvaginal sonography reveals a singleton intrauterine gestation with cardiac activity and a moderate amount of free fluid in the cul de sac. Which of the following is the most likely diagnosis?

A. Heterotopic pregnancy

B. Ruptured corpus luteum

C. Cirrhosis with ascites

D. Urinary tract infection

36.4 A 33-year-old woman complains of vaginal bleeding and abdominal cramping. She passed some blood clots. Her last menstrual period was 6 weeks previously. On examination her cervical os is open to 1 cm. Her quantitative hCG level is 2000 mIU/mL. Which of the following is the most likely diagnosis?

A. Ectopic pregnancy

B. Incomplete abortion

C. Completed abortion

D. Incompetent cervix

36.5 A 28-year-old woman complains of lower abdominal cramping pain for about 3 hours and passed what was described as "liver-like" tissue, after which her pain resolved. In the ED, her blood pressure is 120/70 mm Hg and heart rate is 80 beats per minute. Her uterus is firm and the cervix is closed. The hCG level is 2000 mIU/mL. Transvaginal sonography reveals no intrauterine pregnancy. Which of the following is the next step?

A. Laparoscopy

B. Methotrexate therapy

C. Progesterone level

D. Repeat hCG level in 48 hours

ANSWERS

36.1 **C.** In general, any woman in the childbearing age group with abdominal pain or abnormal vaginal bleeding should have a pregnancy test. If pregnant, then ectopic pregnancy should be ruled out.

36.2 **A.** A large number of women who undergo methotrexate treatment of ectopic pregnancy will have some abdominal discomfort. As long as there are no signs of rupture such as hypotension, severe pain, or free fluid on ultrasound, expectant management may be practiced.

36.3 **A.** In vitro fertilization with embryo transfer produces a rate of coexisting intrauterine pregnancy and ectopic pregnancy of up to 3% (markedly higher than the spontaneous rate of 1:10,000). Thus, a woman who has undergone in vitro fertilization who presents with abdominal fluid and hypotension must be suspected as having an ectopic pregnancy, even when an intrauterine pregnancy has been visualized on sonography.

36.4 **B.** The presence of uterine cramping, vaginal bleeding, passage of tissue, and an open cervical os in a pregnant woman is consistent with an incomplete abortion. Uterine curettage would be the therapy.

36.5 **D.** This patient likely has a completed abortion with the resolution of symptoms following passage of tissue and now has a small uterus and closed cervical os. Nevertheless, there is still a possibility of ectopic pregnancy and perhaps the "tissue" passed was only a blood clot. The tissue should be sent for pathologic analysis. Also, a repeat hCG level should be performed to ensure that all tissue has passed. The hCG level should fall by about 50% in 48 hours if all tissue has passed. A plateau in the hCG level may indicate incomplete abortion or ectopic pregnancy. Dilation and curettage would generally be performed, and if chorionic villi are found, the diagnosis is miscarriage. Absence of chorionic villi establishes the diagnosis of ectopic pregnancy, which may be treated by surgery or methotrexate.

CLINICAL PEARLS

▶ In any woman of childbearing age, consider pregnancy. If the pregnancy test is positive, consider an ectopic pregnancy.

▶ Consider pregnancy even when a woman has had a tubal ligation or is using contraception.

▶ When the serum quantitative hCG level is above 1500-2000 mIU/mL and transvaginal ultrasound does not reveal an intrauterine pregnancy, the risk of ectopic pregnancy is high.

▶ Surgery, not methotrexate, is the best treatment for the patient who is hemodynamically unstable or has significant abdominal pain.

▶ Laparoscopy remains the gold standard for ectopic pregnancy.

REFERENCES

American College of Obstetricians and Gynecologists. Medical management of ectopic pregnancy. ACOG Practice Bulletin 94, June 2008, reaffirmed 2014.

Cunningham FG, Leveno KJ, Bloom SL, et al. Ectopic pregnancy. In: Cunningham FG, Leveno KJ, Bloom SL, Hauth JC, Rouse DJ, Spong CY, eds. *Williams Obstetrics*. 24th ed. New York, NY: McGraw-Hill; 2014: Chapter 10.

Hoover KW, Tao G, Kent KC. Trends in the diagnosis and treatment of ectopic pregnancy in the United States. *ACOG*. 2010;115(3):495-502.

Silva C, Sammel MD, Zhou L, et al. Human chorionic gonadotropin profile for women with ectopic pregnancy. *ACOG*. 2006;107(3):605-610.

A 25-year-old G1P0 woman at 11 weeks' gestation is noted to be lethargic by her husband. The patient was noted to have numerous episodes of nausea and vomiting over the past 1 1/2 months, which has persisted despite antiemetic therapy and adjustments in her diet. The patient was admitted to the hospital 2 weeks ago due to emesis. She was brought in by EMS when her husband arrived after work to find her unarousable. On examination, the patient is lethargic but will respond to painful stimuli and open her eyes. Her blood pressure is 92/44 mm Hg and heart rate 130 beats per minute. Her respiratory rate is 14 breaths per minute. O_2 saturation is 99% on room air. The patient's mucous membranes are dry. She otherwise has a normal examination. The fetal heart tones are 150 beats per minute. The urinalysis shows a dipstick of specific gravity 1.027 and 3+ ketones.

▶ What is the most likely diagnosis?
▶ What is your next step in management?
▶ What is the differential diagnosis?

ANSWERS TO CASE 37:

Hyperemesis Gravidarum and OB Emergencies Less Than 22 Weeks' Gestation

Summary: A 25-year-old G1P0 woman at 11 weeks' gestation has a 6-week history of persistent emesis. She is found to be lethargic and noted to be hypovolemic with blood pressure of 92/44 mm Hg and heart rate of 130 beats per minute. Her respiratory rate is 14 breaths per minute. The fetal heart tones are 150 beats per minute. The urinalysis shows a dipstick of specific gravity 1.027 and 3+ ketones.

- **Most likely diagnosis:** Hyperemesis gravidarum, severe.

- **Next step in management:** Immediate isotonic fluid replacement, and also assess for electrolyte abnormalities and correction of these problems.

- **Differential diagnosis:** Acute pancreatitis, molar pregnancy or twin pregnancy, peptic ulcer disease, hyperthyroidism, and cholelithiasis.

ANALYSIS

Objectives

1. Know the common complications in pregnant women less than 26 weeks' gestation.

2. Understand the diagnostic strategy and management of those complications.

3. Know the physiologic changes in pregnancy and their impact on common diseases in pregnancy.

Considerations

This patient described in the scenario above is significantly ill and needs aggressive fluid replacement, electrolyte replacement, and correction of metabolic abnormalities. Replacement with 2 L of normal saline quickly is warranted. Assessment of comprehensive metabolic panel, electrolytes, amylase, lipase, urinalysis for leukocytes, calcium, magnesium, and CBC with differential should be performed. She has complicated hyperemesis gravidarum and needs a diagnostic workup, such as pelvic ultrasound if not previously performed, right upper quadrant ultrasound, and thyroid function tests. The patient should be admitted to the hospital. Antiemetic therapy, fluid replacement and nothing by mouth should be initiated. The patient should be followed carefully once discharged to ensure that she does not become so volume depleted.

APPROACH TO:

Medical Complications in Pregnancies before 22 Weeks' Gestation

INTRODUCTION

There are numerous emergencies or urgencies that bring a pregnant woman to be seen in the emergency department. The gestational age of viability is changing and most recently has shifted from 26 weeks to 22-24 weeks due to the improved neonatal care and outcomes. For this chapter, the discussion will be focused on: hyperemesis gravidarum, spontaneous abortion, asthma exacerbation, hyperthyroidism/thyroid storm, preterm premature rupture of membranes, and pyelonephritis.

Hyperemesis Gravidarum

Nausea and vomiting in pregnancy is very common, affecting up to 75% of pregnant women. However, **hyperemesis gravidarum, which is defined as intractable emesis with volume depletion and/or metabolic/electrolyte alterations**, is less common, with prevalence of about 2% of pregnancies. Typically, it occurs in women in the first trimester. The emergency physician should not be lulled into complacency because nausea and vomiting is common in pregnant women. The evaluation should include addressing the degree of volume depletion and exploring the possibility of metabolic issues such as electrolyte abnormalities, renal or liver function abnormalities, and the possibility of other etiologies. A urinalysis should also be performed. Hyperemesis gravidarum is a diagnosis of exclusion.

Pregnant women are typically young and healthy and can have significant hypovolemia with compensation without appearing ill. A careful history should be taken regarding the amount of oral intake, any medications taken, and the presence of other possible causes of emesis. The differential diagnosis includes pancreatitis, gallstones, peptic ulcer disease, appendicitis, ovarian torsion, pyelonephritis, and gastroenteritis. Additionally, high hCG level, as associated with molar pregnancies or multiple gestation, is seen with hyperemesis. Thus, an **ultrasound should be performed to assess for adnexal masses and to define the type of pregnancy**, even if the patient gives a verbal history of a normal ultrasound.

Treatment depends on the severity of the patient's condition. Patients with mild volume depletion can be prescribed antiemetic medications and given IV hydration or a trial of oral fluids. Pyridoxine (vitamin B_6) has efficacy as a first-line agent. Ondansetron (Zofran), while pregnancy Class B, has become the most common parenteral and oral antiemetic used in US emergency departments due to its efficacy, and it has become the first choice in hyperemesis in the last several years. As an adjunctive agent, corticosteroids have also been used. Patients who have failed outpatient therapy or who have moderate to severe volume depletion should be hospitalized for more intensive therapy and monitoring. Rarely, patients will be so severely affected that total parenteral nutrition is required.

Spontaneous Abortion

Patients who present with vaginal bleeding during pregnancy are said to have a **threatened abortion.** In this setting, approximately 10% of cases will involve ectopic pregnancy (see Case 26), 40% will result in a spontaneous abortion, and 50% will result in a normal pregnancy carried to term. When the patient presents to the emergency department, a careful history and physical examination should be performed, including assessing for cramping, passage of tissue, risk factors for ectopic pregnancy, and hemodynamic alterations. The physical examination should be focused on assessing volume status, abdominal tenderness, pelvic examination for the state of the cervix, and the presence of adnexal masses or tenderness. **The hCG level and transvaginal ultrasound usually help to determine the type of pregnancy.** For instance, if the hCG level is above the threshold of 1500 mIU/mL and nothing is seen in the uterus indicating an intrauterine pregnancy, in the absence of history indicative of tissue passing, this is consistent with an ectopic pregnancy. Women with threatened abortion should be instructed to bring in any passed tissue for histologic analysis.

An **inevitable abortion** must be differentiated from **cervical insufficiency.** With an inevitable abortion, the uterine contractions (cramping) lead to the cervical dilation. With a cervical insufficiency, the cervix opens spontaneously without uterine contractions and, therefore, affected women present with painless cervical dilation. This disorder is treated with a surgical ligature at the level of the internal cervical os (cerclage). Hence, one of the main features used to distinguish between an insufficient cervix and an inevitable abortion is the presence or absence of uterine contractions.

The treatment of an **incomplete abortion**, characterized by the **passage of tissue and an open cervical os**, is dilatation and curettage of the uterus. The primary complications of persistently retained tissue are bleeding and infection. A completed abortion is suspected with the history of having passed tissue and cramping abdominal pain, now resolved. The cervix is closed. Serum hCG levels are still followed to confirm that no further chorionic villi are contained in the uterus.

Asthma Exacerbation

Asthma is one of the most common medical conditions complicating pregnancy, with an incidence of 4% to 9%. The clinical course of asthma in pregnancy is relatively unpredictable; however, there is evidence to suggest that worsening of asthma may be related to baseline asthma severity. Approximately one-third of pregnant asthmatics experience worsening of symptoms, while one-third improve and one-third remain the same. Exacerbations are more common in the second and third trimester and are less frequent in the last 4 weeks of pregnancy. Asthma typically follows a similar clinical course with successive pregnancies. As such, this patient would be expected to do relatively well, given that her symptoms were well controlled prior to this pregnancy and in previous pregnancies.

Asthma symptoms correlate poorly with objective measures of pulmonary function. Therefore, the next step in the evaluation of this patient is to perform an objective measure of airway obstruction. The single best measure is the **forced expiratory volume (FEV_1)**, which is the volume of gas exhaled in 1 second by a forced exhalation after a full inspiration. This value, however, can only be obtained by spirometry, thus limiting its clinical use. The **peak expiratory flow rate (PEFR)** correlates well with FEV_1 and can be measured with inexpensive, disposable portable peak flow meters. Both the FEV_1 and PEFR remain unchanged throughout pregnancy and may be used as measures of asthma control and severity.

Treatment of an acute exacerbation during pregnancy is similar to that of nonpregnant asthmatics. In other words, a rule of thumb is that **pregnant women should be treated similarly to nonpregnant asthmatics.** Patients should be taught how to recognize the signs and symptoms of early exacerbations so that they may begin treatment at home promptly. **Initial treatment consists of a short-acting inhaled beta-2-agonist** (albuterol) in up to three treatments of 2-4 puffs by MDI (metered-dose inhaler) at 20 minute intervals or in a single nebulizer treatment for up to 1 hour. A good response is characterized by PEFR greater than 80% of personal best and resolution of symptoms sustained for 4 hours. Patients may be continued on beta-2-agonists every 3-4 hours for 24-48 hours. Inhaled corticosteroids (ICS) should be initiated, or if patients are already taking ICS, the dose should be doubled. Follow-up appointments with their physicians should be made as soon as possible. Inadequate response to initial therapy (PEFR <80%) or decreased fetal activity warrants immediate medical attention.

Prevention of hypoxia is the ultimate goal for the pregnant woman who presents to the hospital during an acute asthma attack. Initial assessment should include a brief history and physical examination to assess the severity of asthma and possible trigger factors such as a respiratory infection. Patients with imminent respiratory arrest include those who are drowsy or confused, have paradoxical thoracoabdominal movement, bradycardia, pulsus paradoxus, and decreased air movement (no wheezing). Intubation and mechanical ventilation with 100% oxygen should be performed in these circumstances, and the patient should be admitted to the intensive care unit. Because of the changes in the respiratory physiology in pregnancy (ie, a respiratory alkalosis with partially metabolic compensation), different thresholds for action exist (Table 37-1). A $Paco_2$ greater than 35 mm Hg, along with a pH less than 7.35 in the presence of a falling Pao_2, is a sign of impending respiratory failure in a pregnant asthmatic. Intubation is warranted when the $Paco_2$ is 45 mm Hg or more and rising.

Premature Rupture of Membranes

Premature rupture of membranes (PROM) is defined as the ROM prior to the onset of labor. Preterm PROM (PPROM) is the ROM that occurs prior to 37 completed weeks.

Table 37-1 • ARTERIAL BLOOD GAS FINDINGS IN PREGNANCY			
Parameter	Nonpregnant	Pregnancy	Mechanism
pH	7.40	7.45	Respiratory alkalosis
Po_2	80-100 mm Hg	90-110 mm Hg	Increased minute ventilation
Pco_2	40 mm Hg	28 mm Hg	Respiratory alkalosis
HCO_3	24 mEq/L	18 mEq/L	Partial metabolic acidosis compensation

PPROM complicates approximately 3% of all pregnancies and is the underlying etiology of one-third of preterm births. Normal fetal membranes are biologically very strong in preterm pregnancies. The weakening mechanism is likely multifactorial. Studies have shown PPROM to be associated with intrinsic (intrauterine stretch/strain from polyhydramnios and multifetal pregnancies, cervical insufficiency) and extrinsic factors (ascending bacterial infections). There is evidence demonstrating an association between ascending infection from the lower genital tract and PPROM. This section will be restricted to gestational age less than 22 weeks.

PPROM is associated with significant maternal and fetal morbidity and mortality. The time from rupture of membranes to delivery is known as "latency." The latency period is inversely proportional to the gestational age at PPROM. A latency period of 1 week or less is present in 50% to 60% of PPROM patients. During this period amnionitis occurs in 13% to 60%, and abruptio placentae occurs in 4% to 12%. Multiple complications have been associated with PPROM; however, both maternal and fetal complications decrease with increasing gestational age at the time of PPROM.

The primary maternal morbidity is chorioamnionitis. Incidence varies with population and gestational age at PPROM, with reported frequency from 15% to 40%. Chorioamnionitis typically precedes fetal infection, but this is not always the case, and therefore close clinical monitoring is required. Fetal morbidity and mortality varies with gestational age and complications, particularly infection. The most common complication is respiratory distress syndrome (RDS). Other serious fetal complications include necrotizing enterocolitis, intraventricular hemorrhage, and sepsis. The three causes of neonatal death associated with PPROM are prematurity, sepsis, and pulmonary hypoplasia. Preterm infants born with sepsis have a mortality rate four times higher than those without sepsis.

Management of PPROM starts with initial evaluation and diagnosis of rupture of membranes. The primary patient complaint is experiencing a "gush" of fluid, but some patients will report persistent leakage of fluid. A patient with such a history of rupture of membranes is accurate in 90% of cases. Diagnosis is established on sterile speculum evaluation. Confirmatory findings include pooling of amniotic fluid in posterior fornix and/or leakage of fluid on Valsalva; positive nitrazine test of fluid (vaginal pH 4.5-6.0, amniotic fluid pH 7.1-7.3, nitrazine turns dark blue above 6.0-6.5); and amniotic fluid *ferning* on microscopy. Should the initial tests be ambiguous or negative in the face of continued clinical suspicion, other diagnostic modalities can be utilized. The ultrasound finding of oligohydramnios is usually confirmatory.

At the time of the initial evaluation, the patient's cervical os should be **visually** assessed for dilatation and possible prolapse of umbilical cord or fetal limb. In general, a digital examination of the cervix should be avoided since bacteria may be theoretically inoculated with an examination. Ultrasound evaluation of the gestational age, fetal weight, fetal presentation, placental location, and assessment of amniotic fluid index (AFI) are vital for treatment planning. A low AFI (<5.0 cm) and low maximum vertical fluid pocket (<2.0 cm) at the time of initial assessment is associated with shorter latency, increased RDS, and increased composite morbidity.

Management

Patients diagnosed with PPROM would benefit from an admission to the hospital in all likelihood until delivery. Once PPROM is verified, the treatment plan must balance the maternal, fetal, and neonatal risks/benefits of prolonged pregnancy or expeditious delivery and possible inclusion of medical intervention. For those gestations that are previable, observation in the hospital or careful follow-up with an obstetrician is advisable.

In the absence of clinical signs of labor, abruption, or maternal or fetal signs of infection, most patients in this gestational age will benefit from expectant management with daily assessment of the maternal and fetal well-being.

Maternal and fetal assessment

1. **Maternal:** The criteria for the diagnosis of clinical chorioamnionitis include maternal pyrexia, tachycardia, leukocytosis, uterine tenderness, malodorous vaginal discharge, and fetal tachycardia. During inpatient observation, the woman should be regularly examined for such signs of intrauterine infection. The frequency of maternal and fetal assessments (temperature, pulse, and fetal heart rate auscultation) should be between 4 and 8 hours.

2. **Fetal:** Electronic fetal heart rate tracing is useful when the gestation is considered viable, as fetal tachycardia may represent a sign of fetal infection and is frequently used in the clinical definition of chorioamnionitis in some studies. Fetal tachycardia is often the earliest sign of infection. However, checking intermittent fetal heart activity for previable gestation is preferable.

Use of steroids: A meta-analysis of 15 randomized controlled trials involving more than 1400 women with preterm rupture of the membranes demonstrated that antenatal corticosteroids reduced the risks of RDS. These are generally administered from 24 to 34 weeks' gestation to enhance fetal lung maturity in the absence of infection. The American College of Obstetricians and Gynecologists has recently recommended considering the use of corticosteroids at 23 weeks if there is a likelihood for the delivery being delayed for 1 week. More recently, ACOG has affirmed emerging studies that a single course of corticosteroids between 34 to 36 6/7 weeks may have some efficacy in reducing the severity of RDS.

Use of antibiotics: The use of antibiotics following PPROM was associated with a statistically significant reduction in chorioamnionitis. There was a significant reduction in the numbers of babies born within 48 hours and 7 days. Neonatal infection was significantly reduced in the babies whose mothers received antibiotics.

PPROM under 23 weeks: There are insufficient data to make recommendations in the setting of PPROM under 23-24 weeks, including the possibility of home, daycare, and outpatient monitoring. It would be considered reasonable to maintain the woman in hospital for at least 48 hours before a decision is made to allow her to go home. The management of these cases should be individualized, and outpatient monitoring should be restricted to certain groups of women after careful consideration of other risk factors and access to the hospital.

Hyperthyroidism

Hyperthyroidism in pregnancy is more difficult to recognize due to the hyper-dynamic physiologic changes in pregnancy. However, unintended weight loss, nervousness, palpitations, tachycardia, or tremor are clinical manifestations that warrant evaluation. The diagnosis is made based on clinical suspicion and thyroid function tests, such as thyroid-stimulating hormone (TSH) and free T4 levels. The immediate treatment includes beta-blocking agents and thioamides.

The patient who presents acutely to the emergency department should be started on beta-blockers urgently to relieve the adrenergic symptoms of tachy-cardia, tremor, anxiety, and heat sensitivity by decreasing the maternal heart rate, cardiac output, and myocardial oxygen consumption. **Longer-acting agents, such as atenolol and metoprolol 50-200 mg/day, are recommended.** Beta-blockers are contraindicated in patients with asthma and congestive heart failure and should not be used at the time of delivery due to possible neonatal bradycardia and hypoglycemia.

Thioamides inhibit thyroid hormone synthesis by reduction of iodine organifi-cation and iodotyrosine coupling. Both propylthiouracil (PTU) and methimazole have been used during pregnancy, but PTU is preferred during the first trimes-ter. After the first trimester, physicians should consider switching to methimazole because the risk of liver failure associated with PTU use becomes greater than the risk of teratogenicity. Teratogenic patterns associated with methimazole include aplasia cutis and choanal/esophageal atresia; however, these anomalies do not occur at a higher rate in women on thioamides compared to the general population.

Side effects of thioamides include transient leukopenia (10%); agranulocytosis (0.1%-0.4%); thrombocytopenia, hepatitis, and vasculitis (<1%) as well as rash, nausea, arthritis, anorexia, fever, and loss of taste or smell (5%). Agranulocytosis usually presents with a fever and sore throat. If CBC indicates agranulocytosis, the medication should be discontinued. Treatment with another thioamide carries a significant risk of cross-reaction as well.

Initiation of thioamides in a patient with a new diagnosis during pregnancy requires a dose of PTU 100-150 mg three times daily or methimazole 10-20 mg twice daily. Free T4 levels are used to monitor response to therapy in hyperthyroid patients and should be checked in 4-6 weeks. The PTU or methimazole can be adjusted in 50 mg or 10 mg increments, respectively, with a therapeutic range for free T4 of 1.2-1.8 ng/dL. The goal of treatment is to maintain the free T4 in the upper normal range using the lowest possible dose in order to protect the fetus from hypothyroidism. **The required dose of thioamide during pregnancy can increase up to 50% for patients with a history of hyperthyroidism prior to conception.** The patient's TSH should be checked at the initial prenatal visit and every trimester. Medication adjustments, testing intervals, and therapeutic goals for the free T4 are the same as for patients with new-onset disease.

The most common cause of hyperthyroidism is Graves disease, which occurs in 95% of all cases at all ages. The diagnosis of Graves disease is usually made by the presence of elevated free T4 level or free thyroid index with a suppressed TSH in the absence of a nodular goiter or thyroid mass. The differential diagnosis of hyper-thyroidism, in the order of decreasing frequency, includes subacute thyroiditis, painless (silent or postpartum) thyroiditis, toxic multinodular goiter, toxic adenoma (solitary autonomous hot nodule), iodine-induced (iodinated contrast or amiodarone), iatrogenic overreplacement of thyroid hormone, factitious thyrotoxicosis, *struma ovarii* (ovarian teratoma), and gestational trophoblastic disease. The general symptoms of hyperthyroidism include palpitations, weight loss with increased appetite, nervousness, heat intolerance, oligomenorrhea, eye irritation or edema, and frequent stools. The general signs include diffuse goiter, tachycardia, tremor, warm, moist skin, and new-onset atrial fibrillation. Diagnosis during pregnancy is even more difficult because the signs and symptoms of hyperthyroidism may overlap with the hypermetabolic symptoms of pregnancy. Discrete findings with Graves disease include a diffuse, toxic goiter (common in most young women), ophthalmopathy (periorbital edema, proptosis, and lid retraction in only 30%), dermopathy (pretibial myxedema in <1%), and acropachy (digital clubbing).

The pathogenesis of Graves disease is characterized by an autoimmune process with production of thyroid-stimulating immunoglobulins (TSIs) and TSH-binding inhibitory immunoglobulins (TBIIs) that act on the TSH receptor on the thyroid gland to mediate thyroid stimulation or inhibition, respectively. These antibodies, in effect, act as TSH agonists or antagonists, to stimulate or inhibit thyroid growth, iodine trapping, and T4/T3 synthesis. Maternal Graves disease complicates 1 out of every 500-1000 pregnancies. The frequency of poor outcomes depends on the severity of maternal thyrotoxicosis, with a risk of preterm delivery of 88%, risk of stillbirth of 50%, and risk of congestive heart failure of over 60% in untreated mothers.

Thyroid Storm

Maternal thyroid storm is a medical emergency characterized by a hypermetabolic state in a woman with uncontrolled hyperthyroidism. **Thyroid storm occurs in less than 1% of pregnancies but has a high risk of maternal heart failure.** Usually, there is an inciting event, such as infection, cesarean delivery, or labor, which leads to acute onset of fever, tachycardia, altered mental status (restlessness, nervousness, and confusion), seizures, nausea, vomiting, diarrhea, and cardiac arrhythmias. Shock, stupor, and coma can ensue without prompt intervention, which includes OB-ICU admission, supportive measures, and acute medical management. Therapy includes a standard series of drugs, each of which has a specific role in suppression of thyroid function: PTU or methimazole blocks additional synthesis of thyroid hormone, and PTU also blocks peripheral conversion of T4 to T3. Saturated solutions of potassium iodide or sodium iodide block the release of T4 and T3 from the gland. Dexamethasone decreases thyroid hormone release and peripheral conversion of T4 to T3. Propranolol inhibits the adrenergic effects of excessive thyroid hormone. Phenobarbital can reduce extreme agitation or restlessness and may increase catabolism of thyroid hormone. Fetal surveillance is performed throughout, but intervention for fetal indications should not occur until the mother is stabilized.

Pyelonephritis

A pregnant woman is at greater risk for pyelonephritis and its complications, such as sepsis and acute respiratory distress syndrome (ARDS). Most cases of

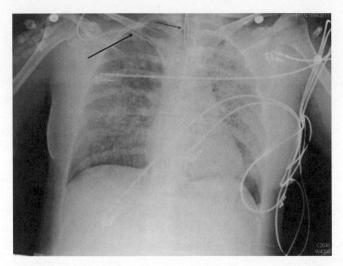

Figure 37–1. CXR showing diffuse bilateral alveolar opacities consistent with ARDS. (Reproduced, with permission, from Longo DL, Fauci AS, Kasper DL, et al. *Harrison's Principles of Internal Medicine.* 18th ed. New York, NY: McGraw-Hill Education; 2011. Figure e34-30.)

pyelonephritis in pregnancy are caused by infection with gram-negative aerobic bacteria, but an increasing number are due to group B *Streptococcus.* Approximately 7% of affected women will develop pulmonary insufficiency due to ARDS (see Figure 37–1), presumably related to release of endotoxin. For these reasons, a pregnant patient with pyelonephritis should be admitted to the hospital. The diagnosis is established with the classic triad of fever, costovertebral angle (CVA) tenderness, and pyuria.

The patient should be placed on IV hydration and antibiotics aimed at the most common etiology, *Escherichia coli*, and monitored for complications. Bacteria and/or their component toxins can produce a sepsis syndrome which, unchecked, will develop into septic shock. The cornerstone of management is early diagnosis, but often that is not easy. **A program of early goal-directed therapy has been shown to reduce mortality from septic shock.** However, not all patients with septic shock require the same treatment interventions. The woman in our case scenario, for example, requires aggressive fluid resuscitation and transfer to an intensive care unit. Per hour, 1-2 L would be appropriate. The total volume needed should be determined by monitoring central venous pressure. An arterial catheter should be placed to monitor blood pressure and obtain timely pH and blood gas measurements. If adequate fluid resuscitation does not elevate the mean arterial pressure above 65 mm Hg, then vasopressors are indicated. Adequate oxygenation should be maintained, with endotracheal intubation and mechanical ventilation, if necessary.

CASE CORRELATION

- See Case 35 (Acute Pelvic Inflammatory Disease), Case 36 (Ectopic Pregnancy), and Case 38 (Sexual Assault).

COMPREHENSION QUESTIONS

37.1 A 35-year-old woman G2P1 at 24 weeks' gestation comes into the emergency department with fever of 102°F, dysuria, and costovertebral angle tenderness. The urinalysis shows numerous bacteria and leukocytes. The patient asks whether she can be treated as an outpatient. Which of the following is the best response?

    A. Outpatient therapy with oral cephalexin is acceptable.

    B. Outpatient therapy with an initial dose of ceftriaxone IM and then oral nitrofurantoin is acceptable.

    C. Outpatient therapy is acceptable if this is the patient's first episode with these symptoms.

    D. Inpatient therapy is preferred in this patient.

37.2 The patient in Question 37.1 is treated with antibiotic therapy for 2 days and then develops acute shortness of breath and is noted to have an O_2 sat of 89% on room air. Which of the following is the most likely cause of her hypoxemia?

    A. Pulmonary embolism

    B. Pneumonia

    C. ARDS

    D. Aspiration

37.3 A 28-year-old G1P0 woman is noted to be at 7 weeks' gestation by dates. She comes into the ED with vaginal bleeding. The physical examination is otherwise unremarkable. There are no adnexal masses or tenderness, and the uterus is nontender and the cervix is closed. The hCG level is 2000 mIU/mL, and the transvaginal (TV) ultrasound shows no intrauterine gestation, no adnexal masses, and no free fluid. Which of the following is the most likely diagnosis?

    A. Ectopic pregnancy

    B. Completed abortion

    C. Incomplete abortion

    D. Molar pregnancy

37.4 A 31-year-old G3P2 woman at 19 weeks' gestation complains of jitteriness, weight loss, and palpitations. She has a history of Graves disease and had been taking PTU and propranolol until she stopped 2 weeks ago due to concern about the medications' effect on her pregnancy. The patient is noted to have a temperature of 102°F, BP of 160/100 mm Hg, and heart rate of 130 beats per minute, and she is confused and disoriented. Which of the following is the most likely diagnosis?

A. Acute β-blocker withdrawal syndrome

B. Sepsis due to PTU-induced neutropenia

C. Thyroid storm

D. Hyperparathyroidism

37.5 A 27-year-old G1P0 woman at 18 weeks' gestation complains of significant nausea and vomiting throughout her pregnancy and has not been able to keep any foods or liquids down. She has been admitted to the hospital numerous times. Her BP is 100/60 mm Hg and heart rate 110 beats per minute, and urinalysis shows negative nitrates, negative leukoesterase, and ketones 2+. Which of the following statements is most accurate about this patient?

A. The presence of ketones in the urine in consistent with significant volume depletion.

B. The patient's gestational age of 18 weeks is expected for hyperemesis gravidarum.

C. Vitamin B_1 is useful for this patient's condition.

D. The patient may be expected to have hyperkalemia.

37.6 A 31-year-old G2P1 woman is noted to be at 20 weeks' gestation. She presents to the ED with a history of leakage of fluid per vagina earlier in the day. On speculum examination, there is no fluid in the vagina. The fern and nitrazine tests are negative. Which of the following is the best next step for this patient?

A. Inform the patient that she does not have rupture of membranes.

B. Hospitalize the patient and assume that she has rupture of membranes.

C. Treat with an oral antibiotic for presumed UTI.

D. Perform an ultrasound examination.

ANSWERS

37.1 **D.** Generally, pregnant women with pyelonephritis should be admitted to the hospital because of the complications such as sepsis, preterm labor, miscarriage or ARDS. Endotoxin-induced pulmonary injury is a well-documented complication of pyelonephritis and occurs more commonly in pregnant women. Endotoxin release can also cause hypotension and shock.

37.2 **C.** A patient who develops acute shortness of breath and hypoxemia after treatment for pyelonephritis should be assumed to have endotoxin-mediated pulmonary injury, or ARDS. A chest x-ray will usually reveal patchy bilateral infiltrates in the lung fields. The treatment is supplemental oxygen and supportive therapy.

37.3 **A.** When the hCG level exceeds the threshold of 1500 mIU/mL and no gestational sac is seen on TV ultrasound, the likelihood of an ectopic pregnancy is high (in the range of 85%). These patients usually go to laparoscopy to confirm the diagnosis. When the hCG level is below the threshold, then the next step is generally to repeat the hCG level in 48 hours to assess for a normal rise (>66% rise), which would indicate a normal intrauterine pregnancy, versus an abnormal rise (<66%), which would be either an ectopic pregnancy or a miscarriage.

37.4 **C.** Thyroid storm is present with hyperthyroidism in conjunction with CNS dysfunction (seizures, confusion, and lethargy) and/or autonomic instability (fever). Thyroid storm carries a worse prognosis and usually requires immediate admission to the ICU and aggressive therapy consisting of PTU, β-blockers, and steroids. A common precursor to thyroid storm is a patient who has stopped taking medications and a stressor, such as infection or surgery.

37.5 **A.** With hyperemesis gravidarum, the presence of moderate to significant ketones is associated with significant volume depletion. The patient is typically hypokalemic. The usual gestational age for hyperemesis is the first trimester, although less commonly, women can persist later and ever rarer, throughout the pregnancy. Vitamin B_6 is a useful adjunctive treatment.

37.6 **D.** When the history suggests PROM but the speculum examination is negative, ultrasound to assess for amniotic fluid volume is helpful. If oligohydramnios is diagnosed, the patient is assumed to have ROM and should be admitted to the hospital.

CLINICAL PEARLS

► Nausea and vomiting in pregnancy are common, but hyperemesis gravidarum is less common and is associated with significant volume or metabolic derangements.

► Hyperemesis is a diagnosis of exclusion.

► The physiologic changes of pregnancy should be considered when interpreting ABGs. For instance, when the P_{CO_2} exceeds 40 mm Hg in a pregnant asthmatic, severe hypercarbia is present and intubation should be considered.

► Dyspnea and hypoxemia after treatment for pyelonephritis are usually caused by endotoxin-related pulmonary injury, ARDS.

► Hyperthyroidism is typically treated with methimazole or PTU, and a β-blocker.

► When the hCG level exceeds the threshold of 1200-1500 mIU/mL and no gestational sac is seen in the uterus on transvaginal ultrasound, then an ectopic pregnancy is highly likely.

► The history of a gush of fluid followed by constant leakage is 90% accurate for rupture of membranes.

► If there is strong clinical suspicion and the speculum examination is negative for ROM, an ultrasound assessment for amniotic fluid volume is helpful.

REFERENCES

American College of Obstetricians and Gynecologists. Diagnosis and treatment of gestational trophoblastic disease. *ACOG Practice Bulletin 53*. Washington, DC: 2004.

American College of Obstetricians and Gynecologists. Medical management of abortion. *ACOG Practice Bulletin 67*. Washington, DC: 2005.

American College of Obstetricians and Gynecologists. Premature rupture of membranes. *ACOG Practice Bulletin 160*. Washington, DC: 2016.

Andrews JI, Shamshirsaz AA, Diekema DJ. Nonmenstrual toxic shock syndrome due to methicillin-resistant *Staphylococcus aureus*. *Obstet Gynecol*. 2008;112:933-938.

Carney LA, Quinlan JD, West JM. Thyroid disease in pregnancy. *Am Fam Physician*. 2014;89(4): 273-278.

Katz VL. Spontaneous and recurrent abortion: etiology, diagnosis, treatment. In: Katz VL, Lentz GM, Lobo RA, Gersenson DM, eds. *Comprehensive Gynecology*. 6th ed. Philadelphia, PA: Mosby; 2012:335-359.

Lu MC, Hobel CJ. Antepartum care: preconception and prenatal care, genetic evaluation and teratology, and antenatal fetal assessment. In: Hacker NF, Gambone JC, eds. *Essentials of Obstetrics and Gynecology*. 6th ed. Philadelphia, PA: Saunders; 2016:76-95.

Martin SR, Foley MR. Intensive care in obstetrics: an evidence-based review. *Am J Obstet Gynecol.* 2006;195:673-689.

Neal DM, Cootauco AC, Burrow G. Thyroid disease in pregnancy. *Clin Perinatol.* 2007;34:543-557.

Parillo JE. Septic shock—vasopressin, norepinephrine, and urgency. *N Engl J Med.* 2008;358:954-956.

CASE 38

A 24-year-old G0P0 woman is brought into the emergency center by police due to a sexual assault. The preliminary information is that the woman was attacked by an unknown male assailant while she was jogging in a nearby park. She reported that she is not sexually active and uses no form of contraception. She experienced vaginal penetrated penile intercourse while being threatened with a knife. On examination, the patient appears anxious and tearful. Her blood pressure (BP) is 130/70 mm Hg, heart rate (HR) is 90 beats per minute, and she is afebrile.

▶ What are the priorities in the management of this patient?
▶ What special approach must be undertaken in the examination?
▶ What infections are most likely to be acquired?
▶ What medications (if any) should be offered?

ANSWERS TO CASE 38:
Sexual Assault

Summary: A 24-year-old nulliparous woman is brought into the emergency center by police due to a sexual assault. She is not currently sexually active and does not use contraception. She experienced vaginal penetrated penile intercourse by an unknown male assailant and was threatened with a knife. On examination, the patient appears anxious and tearful. Her vital signs are normal.

- **Priorities in management:** Treat acute and/or life-threatening medical issues, perform a careful history and physical examination, order appropriate lab and sexually transmitted infection (STI) testing, arrange for emergency contraception and STI prophylaxis, and provide psychosocial support and counseling.

- **Special approach in the examination:** Some differences to this exam include special care to gain informed consent and approach the examination with sensitivity, and collect samples appropriate for local regulation and ensuring the chain of custody for legal reasons.

- **Most common infections:** Trichomonas, Chlamydia, gonorrhea, and hepatitis B.

- **Medications offered:** Ceftriaxone intramuscular (IM), oral metronidazole, and oral azithromycin, and if not previously vaccinated, hepatitis B immune globulin (HBIG) and hepatitis B vaccine, as well as emergency contraception.

ANALYSIS

Objectives

1. Define sexual assault and the incidence and prevalence.

2. Describe the legal, emotional and social, and medical approach to the sexual assault victim.

3. Describe postexposure prophylaxis for the sexual assault victim.

4. Be aware of elder abuse and describe physical examination findings.

5. Be aware of domestic abuse, recognize the signs, and be familiar with the interventions.

Considerations

This is a case of a 24-year-old nulliparous woman brought into the emergency center by police due to a sexual assault. She reports to have been raped at knifepoint by an unknown male assailant at a nearby park. The patient appears anxious and tearful. Sexual assault is a crime of violence and can result in significant physical and emotional trauma and injury. A coordinated and multidisciplinary approach is optimal to minimize trauma and connect the patient to community resources. The examination should be victim-centered, meaning that the order of the examination may need to be modified depending on the patient's cultural or emotional needs. Informed consent is crucial and should be gained for treatment through out the process including medical care, pregnancy testing, testing and prophylaxis for STI, *human immunodeficiency virus* (HIV) prophylaxis, photographs, and permission to contact the patient for follow-up on test results. The first priority is to identify and treat any life threatening injury. As much as possible, the examination should be coordinated with evidence collection to minimize discomfort to the patient. Many emergency centers have Sexual Assault Forensic Examiners who have special training, expertise, and knowledge of how to collect evidence to meet legal requirements. Counseling should be provided in the patient's preferred language. Confidentiality is complex in these settings, and should be carefully discussed with the patient. The patient should be made aware of what information may be part of the criminal justice record (information shared with law enforcement, justice system advocates, etc.) and what evidence and lab results may become legal evidence and not privileged. Testing for STIs should be individualized. A pregnancy test should be performed. The most common infections identified after a sexual assault are trichomonas, gonorrhea, chlamydia, and hepatitis B. Thus, the patient should be encouraged to accept STI prophylaxis. A common regimen is ceftriaxone 125 mg IM, metronidazole 2 g orally, and azithromycin 1 g orally. If the patient has not been vaccinated for hepatitis B, then HBIG as well as the full hepatitis B vaccine is recommended. HIV postexposure prophylaxis should be discussed with the patient, taking into account the risk factors for exposure. Pregnancy prevention should be discussed, and emergency contraception should be offered. Finally, support of community resources, arrangements for follow-up, and referral for reporting to the legal authorities should be set up if not already done.

APPROACH TO:

Sexual Assault and Domestic Violence

DEFINITIONS

SEXUAL ASSAULT: Any sexual act, ranging from sexual coercion to contact abuse to rape including genital, oral, or anal penetration, performed by one person on another without consent.

ACQUAINTANCE RAPE: Sexual assault committed by someone known to the victim.

DATE RAPE: When the sexual assault occurs in the context of a dating relationship.

STATUTORY RAPE: Sexual intercourse with a person under an age specified by state law; in many states it is 16-18 years old.

CHILD SEXUAL ABUSE: Refers to an interaction between a child and an adult, when the child is being used for sexual stimulation of the adult.

INTIMATE PARTNER VIOLENCE: Control by one partner over another in a dating, marital, or live-in relationship. The control can include physical, sexual, emotional or economic abuse and/or threats, and isolation.

INCEST: A form of acquaintance rape in which the assailant is a family member; this includes parental figures who live in the home.

ELDERLY ABUSE: A single or repeated act, or lack of appropriate actions, which causes injury or distress to an individual 60 or more years old and occurs within a relationship where there is an assumption of trust, or when the act is directed toward an elder person due to their age or impairments. It can be physical, psychological, emotional, or sexual abuse, neglect, abandonment, or financial exploitation.

MARITAL RAPE: Forced coitus or related sexual acts within a marital relationship without consent of the partner.

SEXUAL COERCION: The use of nonphysical tactics to gain sexual contact with a nonconsenting partner. It may include intentional use of drugs or alcohol to lower inhibitions.

POSTTRAUMATIC STRESS DISORDER: A disorder developing after a traumatic event that involves re-experiencing the trauma, avoidance of activities that may be associated with the trauma, and a state of hyperarousal.

CLINICAL APPROACH

Sexual assault is a term that encompasses rape, unwanted genital touching, and sexual coercion. It is a complex problem with many medical, psychological, and legal aspects. The lifetime prevalence of sexual assault is reported as approximately 20%, but this is likely an underestimation due to reporting bias. The majority of reported assailants are known to the victim—either a current or former intimate partner, acquaintance, or family member. Fourteen percent of reported assailants are strangers. Those at increased risk for sexual assault include the physically or mentally disabled, those who are homeless, and persons who are gay, lesbian, bisexual, or transgendered. Other populations at risk are college students, alcohol and drug users, and persons under the age of 25 years.

Sexual assault can lead to physical injury in approximately half of cases, and emotional trauma, fear, and embarrassment in the majority of cases. Many victims fear that they will not be heard or believed or that details about their assault will be released to the public. They may also fear for their safety, or fear that their case will not be successfully prosecuted. Sexual assault victims may be hesitant to seek medical attention after the inciting event, so it is important for healthcare providers to understand that the patient may be guarded in verbal and nonverbal responses. Prior to examination, the patient must be instructed not to bathe, eat, drink, clean fingernails, smoke, urinate or defecate. All of these actions may alter important legal data collection.

The initial role of the healthcare provider is to rule out any life-threatening injuries as with any patient triaged through a medical facility. Although most physical injuries are reported as minor, about 1% report major injuries needing hospitalization or operative repair, and 0.1% suffer fatality. After life-threatening injuries have been ruled out, the patient must be moved to a quiet, private room for the remainder of the examination and informed consent must be obtained (Figure 38–1). A thorough history and physical examination must be taken that includes: details of the event with a description of the attacker, last menstrual period, and contraceptive use. Next, the patient should be instructed to undress on a white sheet and the clothes collected for legal purposes. A head to toe examination needs to be performed, searching for bruises, lacerations, and bite marks, including a thorough documentation of the pelvic examination. Photographs may be placed in the medical record to aid in the documentation.

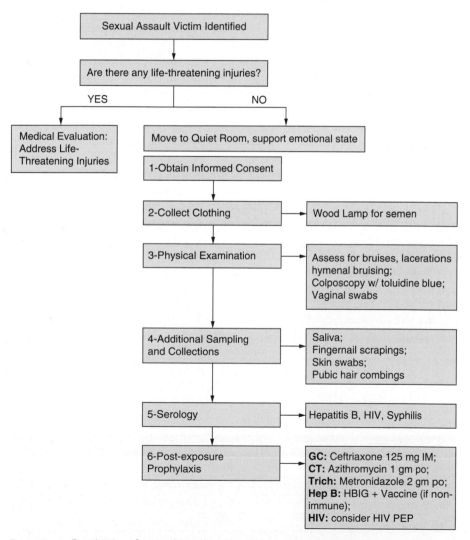

Figure 38–1. Examination of a sexual assault victim. *Abbreviations*: CT, Chlamyia; GC, gonorrhea; Hep B, hepatitis B; Trich, Trichomonas. (Reproduced, with permission, from Toy EC, Ross PJ, Baker B, et al. *Case Files®: Obstetrics and Gynecology.* 5th ed. New York, NY: McGraw-Hill Education; 2016:309. Figure 31-1.)

Vaginal swabs should be taken on speculum examination, which can be used to perform deoxyribonucleic acid (DNA) evaluation, noting the presence of motile sperm on microscopy, as well as cultures for *Neisseria gonorrhea*, *Chlamydia trachomatis*, and *Trichomonas vaginalis*. Pubic hair combings, fingernail scrapings, and skin washings need to be collected as well. A Wood's lamp can be used to assess clothing for semen. Colposcopic evaluation with toluidine blue can assess microscopic abrasions that may be missed on gross examination. **Serologic tests for hepatitis B virus, HIV, and syphilis should also be performed.** Collection of these samples and thorough documentation play a pivotal role from a legal and medical perspective, and any healthcare provider that does not feel comfortable proceeding with the necessary steps must seek assistance from experienced personnel (see Figure 38–1 for algorithm of the examination of a sexual assault victim).

The risk of pregnancy after sexual assault is estimated to be between 2% and 4%. Emergency contraceptives should be given within 72 hours of the assault but may be effective if given within 120 hours. A serum pregnancy test must be documented in the chart prior to administering any method of contraception to rule out a pre-existing pregnancy. The **most effective form of emergency contraception is the copper intrauterine device** if inserted **within 120 hours postcoital**, and patients may benefit from the long-term retention.

There are three main regimens for oral emergency contraception: progestin-only pills, combined oral contraceptives, and antiprogesterone pills (Table 38–1).

Prophylactic antibiotics for STIs are indicated for chlamydial, gonococcal, and trichomonal infections. **Administering ceftriaxone 250 mg intramuscularly in a single dose, metronidazole 2 g orally in a single dose, as well as azithromycin 1 g orally in a single dose or doxycycline 100 mg twice daily orally for 7 days are the recommended treatment for these infections (see Table 38–2).**

Post exposure prophylaxis (PEP) is also recommended for hepatitis B virus and HIV. The regimen according to the 2015 CDC guidelines includes receiving **hepatitis B immunoglobulin in addition to hepatitis B vaccine** if the assailant is hepatitis B positive and the victim unvaccinated. **HIV PEP is controversial;** however, the CDC recommends administering 28 days of zidovudine within 72 hours of assault to patients outlined in the algorithm (Figure 38–2). Additionally, Human Papilloma Virus vaccine is recommended for female victims aged 9-26 years and may be offered to the victim of sexual assault.

Table 38–1 • EMERGENCY CONTRACEPTION	
Medication	Regimen
Combined OCPs (Yuzpe method)	Two doses (100 µg EE + 0.5 mg P), 12 hours apart
Single-dose progestin only	Levonorgestrel 1.5 mg
Two-dose progestin only	Levonorgestrel 0.75 mg, 12-24 hours apart
Copper intrauterine device	Nonhormonal, <120 hours after coitus
Ulipristal acetate	One 30 mg pill

Abbreviations: EE = ethynyl estradiol; OCP = oral contraceptive pills; P = progestin (levonorgestrel).

Table 38–2 • POST-EXPOSURE PROPHYLAXIS	
Infection	Regimen
Chlamydia trachomatis	Azithromycin or doxycycline
Neisseria gonorrhea	Ceftriaxone IM
Trichomonas vaginalis	Metronidazole
Hepatitis B*	Hepatitis B vaccine, hepatitis B immune globulin
HIV**	Zidovudine
HPV*	HPV vaccine

*If victim unvaccinated.
**If substantial exposure risk.

Sexual assault leads to a variety of acute emotional reactions ranging from severe distress to numbing of emotions, anger, and denial. There is no universal reaction. Medical providers should emphasize that the victim is not to blame. After the assault, a **rape-trauma syndrome** frequently occurs. This syndrome is characterized by an acute disorganized phase, then a delayed phase of organization. The acute

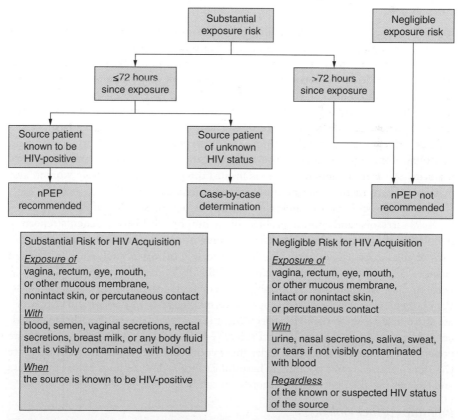

Figure 38–2. Algorithm for evaluation and treatment of possible nonoccupational HIV exposures (CDC 2015 STD Guideline Reference). *Abbreviation: nPEP = non-occupational post-exposure prophylaxis.*

phase lasts days to weeks and is characterized by physical reactions such as body aches, alterations of appetite and sleeping, and a variety of emotional reactions including anger, fear, anxiety, guilt, humiliation, embarrassment, self-blame, and mood swings. The later phase occurs in the weeks to months following and is characterized by flashbacks, nightmares, and phobias as well as somatic and gynecologic symptoms. Victims of sexual assault are at increased risk for post-traumatic stress disorder, major depression, and contemplation of suicide, or actual suicide attempt.

Rape survivors are also at increased risk for some chronic medical problems including chronic pelvic pain, fibromyalgia, and functional gastrointestinal disorders. It is important to consult with social workers and rape crisis counselors to provide immediate intervention, evaluate future emotional and safety needs, and ensure proper follow-up. Rape crisis centers can provide ongoing support to victims, and a list of these types of resources should be provided. In some centers, a sexual assault nurse examiner (SANE), who is extensively trained in this area, is not only responsible for examining the victim and collecting evidence, but also can offer support and community referrals. Close follow-up is important not only for psychological support, but also to ensure that all vaccine schedules are followed and STI testing is performed at appropriate intervals.

Elder Abuse

Elder abuse is a widespread issue that impacts the well-being of approximately **1 in 10 adults over age 60**, with an estimated 4 million older adults affected per year in the United States. Elder abuse can be physical, emotional, psychological, or sexual abuse, or may be in the form of neglect, abandonment, or financial exploitation. Contrary to common assumptions, most incidents of elder abuse do not happen in nursing homes or other institutional settings but **usually take place at home. Often the family, other household members, or paid caregivers** are the abusers. Risk factors for elder abuse include cognitive impairment, depression and anxiety. There is no pathognomonic sign of elder abuse, as signs can vary and may be subtle, and the majority of cases go undetected. It is important to screen all elderly women and men in order to identify victims and provide assistance.

A detailed social history can evaluate family structure, stability of social supports, financial stressors, and substance abuse or mental health history. Patients reporting high levels of stress, depression, anxiety, sleeping or eating difficulties may be the victims of abuse. Special attention should be paid to a **history of multiple falls, frequent emergency room visits or hospitalizations, or difficulty controlling chronic medical problems,** as these may indicate an unstable social or family structure and possibly abuse. **Poor hygiene, weight loss, unkempt appearance, missing assistive devices, and inappropriate attire** may be some signs of neglect. Most states mandate that healthcare providers report confirmed cases to Adult Protective Services, so it is important to educate yourself on the laws in your state. Elder abuse comes in many forms, but the effects are the same. Abuse creates potentially harmful situations and feelings of worthlessness and isolates the elder person from those who can help.

Intimate Partner Violence

Intimate partner violence occurs in every culture, country, and age group, and it affects individuals in all socioeconomic and religious backgrounds. It takes place in same sex as well as heterosexual relationships. According to a 2007 CDC report, 22% of women are physically assaulted by a partner or date during their lifetime, and nearly 25% of women have been raped and/or physically assaulted by an intimate partner at some time. Between 4% and 8% of pregnant women experience physical assault; thus the CDC and ACOG recommend universal screening each trimester and postpartum. Lifelong consequences exist, including physical impairment, emotional trauma, chronic health problems, and even fatality.

Alcohol and/or substance abuse is much more prevalent in women who are victims as well as men who commit violent acts. Because of the high prevalence, the ob/gyn physician must be particularly attuned to this problem. Sensitive, confidential, but direct questioning is the best approach: "Are you being hurt or threatened by anyone?" or "Do you feel safe at home?" It is paramount to assess lethality, such as threats of homicide or suicide, abuse involving severe violence, use and/or access to weapons, pregnancy, or a recent separation. When homicide or child abuse is suspected, it is mandatory to notify the authorities.

Victims of domestic abuse often blame themselves; thus, they should be made aware that they are not responsible for the abuse. They should be empowered to learn about the resources and support services, needs to make their own decisions, and discussions held in confidentiality (to the limits of the law). A safety plan may be discussed including packing a bag in advance, having personal documents ready, having an extra set of car/house keys, establishing a code with friends/family, and having a plan of where to go. They may agree to speak to a social worker or someone at the National Domestic Violence Hotline (1-800-799-SAFE [7233]). Nevertheless, even if the patient denies intimate partner violence, it is beneficial to discuss the issues in a caring manner and offer educational material.

CASE CORRELATION

- See also Case 35 (Acute Pelvic Inflammatory Disease), Case 36 (Ectopic Pregnancy), and Case 37 (Hyperemesis Gravidarum and OB Emergencies).

COMPREHENSION QUESTIONS

38.1 A 22-year-old female college student is sexually assaulted by an unknown male assailant. Penile-to-vaginal intercourse occurred, and the patient states she does not believe a condom was used. The patient is not using any form of birth control and is not sexually active. Prior to prescribing emergency contraception, which of the following is most important to order?

A. Chlamydia assay

B. Pregnancy test

C. Serum alcohol level

D. HIV test

E. Liver function tests

38.2 An 82-year-old woman is being seen for her annual well woman examination. She is brought in by her middle-aged son via wheelchair. The patient has advanced dementia and cannot give a history, but her son says there have been no problems. On examination, you note that the patient is unkempt in appearance. Her BP is 140/85 mm Hg and HR is 90 beats per minute. There are multiple bedsores on the sacral and back area. The patient has a diaper on. A red rash is noted on the introital region, and there is also some bruising on the vulvar and perineal area. Which of the following is the most likely diagnosis?

A. Behcet's disease

B. Chronic alcoholism

C. Elder abuse

D. Lichen sclerosis

E. Squamous cell carcinoma

38.3 A third year medical student is doing research into intimate partner violence in pregnancy. Which of the following statements is most accurate?

A. Although violence does occur against pregnant women, homicide is rare.

B. The CDC recommends screening of intimate partner violence once during the pregnancy, usually at the first prenatal visit.

C. Intimate partner violence can lead to preterm delivery and low birth weight.

D. Usually intimate partner violence lessens during pregnancy due to concern about hurting the fetus.

38.4 A 28-year-old G1P1 woman is the victim of sexual assault. She has recently immigrated to the country and has not been vaccinated against hepatitis B. The assailant is unknown, and his hepatitis B status is unknown. Which of the following is the best management of the patient?

A. Administer HBIG only

B. Administer the hepatitis B vaccine only

C. Administer both HBIG and the hepatitis B vaccine

D. Expectant management since the hepatitis B status is unknown

ANSWERS

38.1 **B.** Prior to emergency contraception (EC), it is vital to obtain an immediate pregnancy test, even for those patients who state that they are not sexually active or have never been sexually active. Because the EC may have a deleterious effect on any current pregnancy, a pregnancy test is mandatory.

38.2 **C.** An elderly patient who has dementia is at risk for elder abuse because they have high needs and also cannot report the abuse. This patient has signs of neglect such as bedsores and unkempt appearance, and likely prolonged soiling without diaper changes. The vulvar bruising is highly suggestive of sexual abuse. Notification of the authorities is mandatory in a situation such as this.

38.3 **C.** Intimate partner violence increases in pregnancy and can lead to preterm delivery, low birth weight, and placental abruption. Homicide, usually in the first trimester, is the second leading cause of injury-related deaths to pregnant women after motor vehicle accidents. The American College of Obstetricians and Gynecologists and the CDC recommend universal screening at the first prenatal visit, each trimester and also postpartum.

38.4 **C.** After a sexual assault, HBIG and the vaccine should be given if the assailant is thought to be hepatitis B positive and the patient has not been vaccinated previously. In a situation when the status of the assailant is unknown, the usual practice is still HBIG for any acute exposure, and then hepatitis B vaccination for longer term immunity.

CLINICAL PEARLS

▶ The most common types of rape are date rape and acquaintance rape.

▶ It is important to screen for sexual assault at every visit.

▶ Sexual assault is a traumatic experience, and allowing the patient to dictate the order of events at evaluation is important.

▶ Emergency contraception is most effective if given within the first 72 hours from the assault.

▶ Post-exposure prophylaxis is indicated to cover *C. trachomatis, N. gonorrhea, T. vaginalis*, and hepatitis B.

▶ If not comfortable with the initial examination and specimen collection, contact a provider who is to ensure property evidence handling.

▶ Repetitive visits, falls, and poor control of medical conditions may be signs of elder abuse.

▶ Intimate partner violence (IPV) is common and is best screened by sensitive and direct questioning.

▶ Mandatory reporting is required in situations where impending homicide or child abuse is suspected.

REFERENCES

American College of Obstetricians and Gynecologists. Intimate partner violence. *ACOG Committee Opinion 518,* 2012.

American College of Obstetricians and Gynecologists. Emergency contraception. Practice Bulletin No. 112. *Obstet Gynecol.* 2010;115:1100-1109.

American College of Obstetricians and Gynecologists. Elder abuse and women's health. Committee Opinion No. 568. *Obstet Gynecol.* 2013;122:187-191.

American College of Obstetricians and Gynecologists. Reproductive and sexual coercion. Committee Opinion No. 554. *Obstet Gynecol.* 2013;121:411-415.

American College of Obstetricians and Gynecologists. Sexual assault. Committee Opinion No. 592. *Obstet Gynecol.* 2014;123:905-909.

Centers for Disease Control and Prevention. The National Intimate Partner and Sexual Violence Survey; 2013a. Available at: cdc.gov/violenceprevention/nisvs. Accessed July 23, 2015.

Federal Bureau of Investigation. Summary Reporting System (SRS) User Manual, version 1.0. Criminal Justice Information Services (CJIS) Division, Uniform Crime Reporting (UCR) Program. DC: FBI; 2013. Available at: http://www.fbi.gov/about-us/cjis/ucr/nibrs/summary-reporting-system-srs-user-manual. Accessed July 30, 2015.

Hoffman BL, Schorge JO, Schaffer JI, eds. *Williams Gynecology.* 2nd ed. New York, NY: McGraw-Hill Education; 2012.

Linden JA. Clinical practice. Care of the adult patient after sexual assault. *N Engl J Med.* 2011;365: 834-841.

Lu MC, Lu JS, Halfin VP. Domestic violence & sexual assault. In: DeCherney AH, Nathan L, Laufer N, Roman AS, eds. *Current Diagnosis & Treatment: Obstetrics & Gynecology*; 2013, Chap. 60, 11e.

Richardson AR, Maltz FN. Ulipristal acetate: review of the efficacy and safety of a newly approved agent for emergency contraception. *Clin Ther.* 2012;34:24-36.

An otherwise healthy 19-year-old man is brought to the emergency department (ED) by his roommate, who states that the patient has "not been acting right" for the past 24 hours. Per the roommate, the patient had complained of a headache 2 days prior to arrival and has been progressively somnolent and confused since then. The patient has no past medical history and does not take any medications. His roommate states that the patient is a college student who does not use any illegal drugs and occasionally drinks alcohol. Review of systems is positive for headache and altered mental status as stated above, as well as a tactile fever for the past 2 days. Additional review of systems is unobtainable, as the patient is unable to answer any questions. On physical examination the patient is noted to be febrile to 38.5°C (101°F) orally, with a heart rate of 120 beats per minute, blood pressure of 114/69 mm Hg, and respiratory rate of 20 breaths per minute. His oxygen saturation is 98% on room air. The head and neck examination are significant for dry mucous membranes and nuchal rigidity. His cardiopulmonary examination is within normal limits, with the exception of tachycardia. The abdomen is soft and nontender. His skin is noted to be warm and well perfused without any rash. The neurologic examination is significant for an altered mental status with a Glasgow coma score (GCS) of 10 (eyes open to voice [3], patient moans to painful stimuli [2], and localizes painful stimuli [5]). The motor examination is symmetric, and the patient appears to be sensate in all extremities. His reflexes are 2+ bilaterally throughout the upper and lower extremities with downgoing toes. Laboratory studies reveal a leukocytosis of 24,000/mm^3 with a left shift and are otherwise unremarkable. A CT scan is completed which shows no mass, shift, bleed, or edema.

► What is the most likely diagnosis?
► What is the next diagnostic study of choice?
► What is the most appropriate treatment of this condition?

ANSWERS TO CASE 39:

Bacterial Meningitis

Summary: This is a 19-year-old man who presents with the classic triad for bacterial meningitis—fever, neck stiffness, and altered mental status.

- **Most likely diagnosis:** Bacterial meningitis.

- **Next diagnostic study:** Lumbar puncture.

- **Appropriate treatment:** Intravenous antibiotics ± steroids.

ANALYSIS

Objectives

1. Understand the diagnostic and therapeutic approach to bacterial meningitis, including when to obtain neuroimaging, when to perform a lumbar puncture, and what empiric therapies to initiate.

2. Recognize the clinical presentation of acute bacterial meningitis.

Considerations

Bacterial meningitis is an inflammation of the leptomeninges (pia/arachnoid/dura-maters) from infection of the arachnoid space, characteristically accompanied by white blood cells and bacteria in the cerebrospinal fluid (CSF). **It is a potentially devastating infection with a mortality rate of 10-30% and persistent neurologic deficit in approximately 10% of those who survive.** It can affect people of all ages but is most commonly seen in the young (children <2 years old) and adults over the age of 50. The emergency physician must consider this diagnosis in patients presenting with any combination of the following signs and symptoms: fever, altered mental status, nuchal rigidity and headache. The classic triad of fever, altered mental status, and nuchal rigidity is present in only 44% to 50% of patients. Almost all patients (99%-100% in the largest study published) have a headache plus at least one of these three clinical signs. Fever is present in 79% to 95% of patients at presentation, and another 4% will develop fever within 24 hours of presentation. Altered mental status (typically confusion or lethargy) is present in 78% to 83% of patients, with 16% to 22% responsive to only painful stimuli and 6% unresponsive to all stimuli. Nuchal rigidity is present in 83% to 94% of patients on initial examination and often persists for more than 1 week after treatment and resolution of infection. However, maneuvers to detect meningismus (eg, Kernig and Brudzinski sign) have been found to have poor sensitivity and should not be used to exclude the possibility of bacterial meningitis.

   Additional findings that may raise concern for the diagnosis of meningitis include seizures, focal neurologic deficits, rash, septic arthritis, papilledema, and photophobia. Seizures have been described in 15% to 30% of patients and are most commonly associated with infections due to *Streptococcus pneumoniae*. Focal neurological deficits are seen in 10% to 35% of patients with *Listeria monocytogenes* as part of a rhombencephalitis syndrome including ataxia (with or without nystagmus) and cranial nerve palsies. *Neisseria meningitidis* may cause palpable purpura in 11% to 64% of patients and concomitant septic arthritis in 7% to 11%. Papilledema and/ or photophobia are rarely present, having been described in less than 5% of cases.

APPROACH TO:
Suspected Bacterial Meningitis

CLINICAL APPROACH

The approach to suspected bacterial meningitis involves appropriate use of diagnostic studies and therapeutic interventions in a timely manner. The best experimental and observational data suggest that time to antibiotics has a profound effect on clinical outcomes. Therefore, our goal in the ED is to maintain a high index of suspicion and **not delay treatment** while diagnostic studies are being completed.

Diagnosis

The cornerstone of the diagnosis of meningitis is the CSF analysis, which is obtained by lumbar puncture (LP). LP can confirm the presence of inflammatory cells in the CSF, identify the causative organism by Gram stain and culture, and evaluate for other potential causes of the patient's symptoms (idiopathic intracranial hypertension, subarachnoid hemorrhage, autoimmune disease, etc.). If a delay in performing the LP is expected, then blood cultures and empiric antibiotics with dexamethasone should be administered PRIOR to obtaining the CSF. A common cause for delay of diagnosis is the time it takes to obtain a computed tomography (CT) scan of the head. CT scanning prior to performing an LP is recommended for any patients with risk factors for having elevated intracranial pressure, which may increase the risk of brain herniation during the procedure. CT scan of the head may also be indicated when searching for alternative causes for altered level of consciousness. See Table 39–1 to review guidelines for which patients should have CT before LP. Approximately 45% of patients with bacterial meningitis will meet one or more of these criteria. All other patients can safely have an LP performed without an antecedent CT scan.

Table 39–1 • INDICATIONS FOR HEAD CT PRIOR TO LP
Altered level of consciousness
Altered mental status
Focal neurologic deficit
Immunocompromised state[a]
History of CNS disease[b]
New-onset seizure (<1 week prior to presentation)
Papilledema
History or evidence of head trauma

[a]Including HIV, AIDS, post-transplant, on immunosuppressant medications.
[b]Including mass lesions, strokes, focal infection, surgery.

Empiric antibiotic therapy should be initiated immediately based on epidemiologic data and local resistance patterns. Administration of antibiotics has minimal effect on chemistry and cytology of CSF but can reduce the yield of Gram stain and culture. In fact, administration of antibiotics can sterilize CSF cultures within an hour. CSF nucleic acid amplification tests, such as polymerase chain reaction, may be considered in cases where antibiotics are given prior to CSF collection. Gram stain of the CSF is successful in identifying the microorganism in approximately 80% of cases. Gram stains can still positively identify an organism in 10% to 15% of patients who have sterile cultures after antibiotic administration. Identification of the causative organism allows clinicians to safely narrow the spectrum of anti-microbial therapy.

As Gram stain results are typically available 1-2 days before culture results, it is helpful to know the Gram-stain pattern of the most common organisms. The presence of gram-positive diplococci suggests *S. pneumoniae* infection, while gram-negative diplococci suggest *N. meningitidis* infection. Small pleomorphic gram-negative coccobacilli suggest *Haemophilus influenzae*, while gram-positive rods and coccobacilli suggest *L. monocytogenes* infection.

Additional cases will be identified by culture of the CSF and blood. Additional CSF analyses should include opening pressure (which can be the only abnormality present in cases of cryptococcal meningitis), CSF protein, CSF glucose, cell count with differential, and CSF lactate. These tests can help to distinguish between the possible causes of meningitis (bacterial, viral, tubercular, neoplasms, autoimmune, etc.), but there is still quite a bit of overlap in results (Table 39–2). Therefore, most patients with a CSF pleocytosis (presence of an elevated number of WBCs) should be admitted to the hospital and treated for bacterial meningitis while awaiting CSF culture results.

Treatment

The most important element of treatment after stabilization of the ABCs is ini-tiation of appropriate antimicrobial therapy. **The most common organisms to cause bacterial meningitis in adult patients are *N. meningitidis* and *S. pneumoniae*.** Initial therapy for adults should include a third-generation cephalosporin (eg, ceftriaxone or cefotaxime) in a sufficient dose (2 g IV) to achieve adequate CSF concentra-tion. These patients should also receive meningitic dosing of vancomycin, given the increasing worldwide prevalence of drug-resistant *S. pneumoniae*.

Patients who are older than 50 years of age, alcoholic, or immunocompromised are at higher risk for additional organisms, including *L. monocytogenes*, *H. influenzae*, and aerobic gram-negative bacilli. Therefore, these patients should have ampicillin added to the empiric antibiotic regimen. Patients less than 1 month of age are at risk for infection with *Streptococcus agalactiae*, *Klebsiella* sp, *E. coli*, and *L. monocytogenes* and require yet another empiric regimen (Table 39–3).

In addition to adequate antimicrobial therapy, a number of recent studies have shown improved outcomes with adjunctive dexamethasone with or before the first dose of antibiotics. Meningitis leads to significant morbidity and mortality as a result of the inflammatory response in the CSF. This response is heightened when antimicrobials are administered, which will lead to bacteriolysis and release of

Table 39–2 • ANALYSIS OF THE CEREBROSPINAL FLUID

Test	Normal Value	Bacterial Meningitis	Viral Meningitis	Fungal Meningitis
Opening pressure	<200 mm H$_2$O	Elevated	Elevated to normal	Elevated to normal (markedly elevated in cryptococcal meningitis)
CSF appearance	Clear (Cloudy CSF indicates the presence of WBCs, RBCs, bacteria, and protein)	Cloudy to purulent	Cloudy	Cloudy
Cell count	<5 WBC/mm³	More marked elevation (>1000 WBC/mm³) unless early infection	Elevated, but usually <2000 WBC/mm³	Elevated
	Differential	PMN predominance	Lymphocytic predominance[a]	Lymphocytic predominance
Gram stain	No organisms	Identifies organisms in 80% of bacterial meningitis; 60% if the patient is pretreated	Negative	Negative
Protein	14-45 mg/dL	More markedly elevated (>100 mg/dL). Elevated in acute bacterial/fungal meningitis; >220 mg/dL is 99% predictive.	Elevated, but usually less than 150 mg/dL	More markedly elevated (>100 mg/dL). Elevated in acute bacterial/fungal meningitis; >220 mg/dL is 99% predictive.
Glucose	50-80 mg/dL	More markedly decreased (<45 mg/dL)	Normal to moderately decreased	Decreased
India ink	Negative	Negative	Negative	Positive in 33% of cryptococcal meningitis
Cryptococcal Ag	Negative	Negative	Negative	90% accuracy for cryptococcal meningitis
Acid-fast stain	Negative	Positive in 80% of tuberculous meningitis	Negative	Negative
CSF lactate	<35 mg/dL	Elevated (rarely normal in bacterial meningitis)	Normal to mild elevation	Normal to mild elevation

Abbreviations: CSF = cerebrospinal fluid; PMN = Polymorphonuclear leukocyte; WBC = white blood cells; Ag = antigen.
[a]Viral meningitis typically has a lymphocyte predominance; however, in the first 48 hours PMNs may predominate.

Table 39–3 • EMPIRIC ANTIMICROBIAL THERAPY BASED ON PATIENT AGE		
Patient Age	**Common Pathogens**	**Empiric Antibiotics**
<1 month	*Streptococcus agalactiae* (Group B streptococcus), *Escherichia coli, Listeria monocytogenes, Klebsiella species*	Ampicillin *plus* cefotaxime *or* ampicillin *plus* an aminoglycoside
1-23 months	*Streptococcus pneumoniae, Neisseria meningitidis, S. agalactiae, Haemophilus influenzae, E. coli*	Vancomycin *plus* a third-generation cephalosporin[a]
2-50 years	*S. pneumonia, N. meningitidis, H. influenzae*	Vancomycin *plus* a third-generation cephalosporin[a]
>50 years	*S. pneumoniae, L. monocytogenes, N. meningitidis,* Group B streptococcus, aerobic gram-negative bacilli	Vancomycin *plus* a third-generation cephalosporin[a] *plus* ampicillin

[a]*Ceftriaxone or cefotaxime.*
Data from Tunkel A, Hartman B, et al. Practice guidelines for the management of bacterial meningitis. Clin Infect Dis. *2004;39:1267-1284 and Thigpen MC, Whitney CG, et al. Bacterial meningitis in the United States, 1998-2007.* N Eng J Med. *2011;364:2016-2025.*

additional inflammatory mediators. Administering a dose of corticosteroids (dexamethasone 0.15 mg/kg IV to max dose of 10 mg every 6 hours) with or before the first dose of antibiotics may attenuate the inflammatory response. It is unclear whether the administration of dexamethasone after the first dose of antibiotics is effective, and some evidence suggests it may cause harm. In children, the greatest benefit was found in patients with *H. influenza* type b; in adults the greatest benefit was found in those with an intermediate GCS of 8-11 and those with *S. pneumoniae* meningitis. Steroids have not been shown to reduce mortality when other causative organisms are responsible for meningitis, but neither have they been shown to cause harm. In general most authorities recommend that a dose of dexamethasone should precede the first dose of antibiotics if you suspect bacterial meningitis.

Family members and close contacts should receive antibiotic prophylaxis to prevent them from developing a similar infection. Current CDC guidelines recommend antibiotic prophylaxis (typically with a fluoroquinolone or rifampin) for close contacts of patients with meningitis due to *N. meningitidis*. "Close contacts" includes anyone in the same household or day-care center, intimate partners, and anyone in direct contact with the patient's oral secretions, including healthcare workers (eg, respiratory therapists). Antibiotic prophylaxis for close contacts of patients with meningitis due to *H. influenzae* is no longer recommended if all contacts 4 years of age or younger are fully vaccinated against Hib disease.

CASE CORRELATION

- See also Case 25 (Altered Mental Status), Case 28 (Stroke), Case 30 (Seizure), and Case 34 (Febrile Seizure).

COMPREHENSION QUESTIONS

39.1 A 30-year-old man presents with altered mental status, fever, and nuchal rigidity. You suspect bacterial meningitis. Which of the following is the appropriate order of your actions?

A. Head CT, lumbar puncture, blood cultures, steroids, antibiotics

B. Blood cultures, head CT, lumbar puncture, steroids, antibiotics

C. Blood cultures, steroids, antibiotics, head CT, lumbar puncture

D. Lumbar puncture, blood cultures, steroids, antibiotics, head CT

E. Head CT, blood cultures, steroids, antibiotics, lumbar puncture

39.2 Which of the following is/are the appropriate empiric antibiotics to administer to a 65-year-old man with suspected bacterial meningitis?

A. Vancomycin alone

B. Vancomycin and ceftriaxone

C. Vancomycin, ceftriaxone, and amoxicillin

D. Vancomycin, ceftriaxone, and ampicillin

39.3 Approximately what percentage of patients with bacterial meningitis present with the classic triad of fever, neck stiffness, and altered mental status?

A. <50%

B. Between 51% and 75%

C. Between 76% and 99%

D. >99%

ANSWERS

39.1 **C.** Neuroimaging is indicated in this patient prior to lumbar puncture given his altered mental status. Given the high suspicion for bacterial meningitis, antibiotic administration should not be delayed for the head CT. It is expected that one would obtain blood cultures and administer dexamethasone prior to the antibiotics in this case.

39.2 **D.** All adults with suspected bacterial meningitis should receive a third-generation cephalosporin, and most institutions advocate for vancomycin to cover drug-resistant *S. pneumoniae*. Ampicillin is added because this patient is older than the age of 50.

39.3 **A.** Although the triad in the question is considered classic, studies have found that it is only present in less than half of the cases. If headache is added to the other 3, then at least 2 of the 4 symptoms are present in approximately 95% of patients.

CLINICAL PEARLS

▶ The classic triad of fever, neck stiffness, and a change in mental status is present in less than 50% of patients with bacterial meningitis.

▶ Younger patients who are otherwise healthy do not require neuroimaging prior to LP if they have a normal neurologic examination, including mental status.

▶ Antibiotic therapy should not be delayed once bacterial meningitis is suspected.

▶ Initial antimicrobial therapy in adults should include a third-generation cephalosporin and vancomycin to cover drug-resistant *S. pneumoniae*.

▶ Dexamethasone prior to or with the first dose of antibiotics has been shown to decrease neurologic sequelae as well as mortality among adults with bacterial meningitis.

REFERENCES

Aronin SI, Peduzzi P, Quagliarello VJ. Community-acquired bacterial meningitis: risk stratification for adverse clinical outcome and effect of antibiotic timing. *Ann Intern Med*. 1998;129:862.

Attia J, Hatala R, Cook DJ, Wong JG. The rational clinical examination. Does this adult patient have acute meningitis? *JAMA*. 1999;282:175.

Brouwer MC, Thwaites GE, Tunkel AR, et al. Dilemmas in the diagnosis of acute community-acquired bacterial meningitis. *The Lancet*. 2012:380(9854):1684-1692.

deGans J, van de Beek D. Dexamethasone in adults with bacterial meningitis. *N Eng J Med*. 2002;347(20):1549-1556.

Hasbun R, Abrahams J, Jekel J, et al. Computed tomography of the head before lumbar puncture in adults with suspected meningitis. *N Eng J Med*. 2001;345(24):1727-1733.

Kanegaye JT, Soliemanzadeh P, Bradley JS. Lumbar puncture in pediatric bacterial meningitis: defining the time interval for recovery of cerebrospinal fluid pathogens after parenteral antibiotic pretreatment. *Pediatrics*. 2001;108:1169.

Thigpen MC, Whitney CG, Messonnier NE, et al. Bacterial meningitis in the United States, 1998-2007. *N Eng J Med*. 2011;364:2016-2025.

Tunkel A, Hartman B, Kaplan S, et al. Practice guidelines for the management of bacterial meningitis. *Clin Infect Dis*. 2004;39:1267-1284.

van de Beek D, Brouwer MC, Thwaites GE, et al. Advances in treatment of bacterial meningitis. *The Lancet*. 2012;380(9854):1693-1702.

van de Beek D, de Gans J, Spanjaard L, et al. Clinical features and prognostic factors in adults with bacterial meningitis. *N Eng J Med*. 2004;351(18):1849-1859.

van de Beek D, de Gans J, Tunkel A, et al. Community-acquired bacterial meningitis in adults. *N Eng J Med*. 2006;354(1):44-53.

Whitney C, Farley M, Hadler J, et al. Increasing prevalence of multidrug-resistant *Streptococcus pneumoniae* in the United States. *N Eng J Med*. 2000;343(26):1917-1924.

A 45-year-old man presents to the Emergency Department (ED) complaining of left shoulder pain. Past history includes numerous skin abscesses, hepatitis C, and injection drug use. He injected black tar heroin into the left upper extremity 2 days ago. On examination the patient is in mild distress. There is a low-grade fever, the heart rate is 115 beats per minute, and blood pressure is 120/60 mm Hg. The dorsum of the upper arm is erythematous, indurated and tender. There is no obvious area of fluctuance. Edema extends to the shoulder and pectoralis region of the trunk.

▶ What is the most likely diagnosis?
▶ What are the next diagnostic and treatment steps?

ANSWERS TO CASE 40:

Skin and Soft Tissue Infections

Summary: This is an injection drug user with a fever and a skin and soft tissue infection (SSTI) of the upper extremity and shoulder.

- **Most likely diagnosis:** Soft tissue abscess from injection drug use. However, necrotizing soft tissue infection (NSTI) is a distinct possibility, and the differential diagnosis also includes cellulitis and septic shoulder joint.

- **Next steps:** Establish IV access. IV antibiotics are generally indicated when a SSTI produces a fever. Establish a definitive diagnosis as quickly as possible, beginning with a careful search for a pus pocket. If an abscess is found, it must be drained. If not, NSTI remains a possibility and immediate surgical exploration is indicated. Search for signs of sepsis, and if present begin early goal directed therapy.

ANALYSIS

Objectives

1. Recognize the range of SSTIs, which can look remarkably similar on first inspection.

2. Become familiar with the usual pathogens responsible for SSTIs and the antimicrobial agents that are commonly used for empirical therapy.

3. Understand that NSTIs can be life threatening, rapidly progressive and difficult to diagnose.

4. Recognize the risk factors associated with necrotizing infections and with unusual pathogens.

5. Appreciate that uncomplicated abscesses often require only incision and drainage, with no antibiotics, for cure.

Considerations

SSTIs are among the most common problems seen in the ED, accounting for 3.4 million annual visits in the United States alone. A rise in the incidence of these infections occurred in the late 1990s, linked to the emergence of community-associated methicillin resistant *Staphylococcus aureus* (MRSA). While simple abscesses are the most common, there is a range of distinct SSTI types, including deep abscesses, nonpurulent cellulitis and NSTIs. NSTIs can be rapidly life-threatening, and timely diagnosis is often difficult. SSTIs of all types are extremely common in injection drug users and thus in emergency departments that serve an injection drug use population. Red flags can alert the astute clinician to a necrotizing infection as well as to unusual pathogens that require special antibiotics. To complicate matters, other diseases affecting the skin and underlying tissues can be confused with infection, particularly gout and other forms of arthritis and bursitis, allergic reactions to insect bites, and deep vein thrombosis.

Diagnosis and management of SSTIs can be tricky. Different types of SSTIs that require different approaches to management can appear similar. While diagnostic tests such as bedside ultrasound, CT scan, and blood lactate levels can be helpful, in most cases the correct diagnosis relies primarily on the bedside examination and judgment of the emergency physician. Many of these infections are primarily a surgical disease. Effective management often requires only the skillful administration of anesthetic and incision and drainage in the ED, but occasionally, immediate exploration and debridement in the operating room is required. Similarly, while judicious use of antibiotics is an important principle in the management of most simple SSTIs, serious SSTIs will occasionally cause sepsis syndrome, in which case immediate intravenous antibiotic administration and aggressive resuscitation is imperative.

APPROACH TO:
Skin and Soft Tissue Infections

DEFINITIONS

SKIN AND SOFT TISSUE INFECTION (SSTI): An infection, usually bacterial, of the skin and/or underlying soft tissues.

NECROTIZING SKIN AND SOFT TISSUE INFECTION (NSTI): A rapidly spreading bacterial infection (monomicrobial or polymicrobial) of the soft tissue below the skin surface including fat, fascia (fasciitis), and muscle (myositis).

PURULENT (CULTURABLE) CELLULITIS: Infection and/or inflammatory changes of the skin surrounding a purulent focus (usually an abscess).

NONPURULENT (NON-CULTURABLE) CELLULITIS: An infection of the skin and underlying dermis without an identifiable purulent focus.

ERYSIPELAS: Nonpurulent cellulitis restricted to the superficial skin layers with a sharply demarcated border.

CLINICAL APPROACH

Diagnosis

Clinical evaluation of SSTIs always begins with a search for a pus pocket because both the differential diagnosis and clinical management depend on whether or not there is pus (Figure 40–1). Circular infections (as opposed to circumferential) on the buttock, groin, and lower extremity almost always harbor pus near the center. First, look for a visible spot of purulence or necrosis. Then palpate carefully for fluctuance, which can be subtle. Fluctuance may be absent if the abscess is deep, as often occurs in the pannus of the buttock or thigh, or if the abscess is early in its course. Very deep intramuscular abscesses can occur with injection drug use.

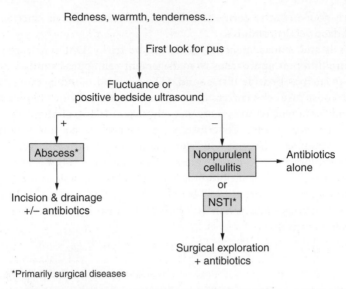

Redness, warmth, tenderness...

First look for pus

Fluctuance or
positive bedside ultrasound

+ → Abscess*

− → Nonpurulent cellulitis → Antibiotics alone

or

NSTI*

Incision & drainage
+/− antibiotics

Surgical exploration
+ antibiotics

*Primarily surgical diseases

Figure 40–1. Algorithm for the management of possibly infectious soft tissue. *Abbreviation: NSTI =
necrotizing skin and soft tissue infection.*

Bedside ultrasound, using a high-frequency linear transducer, can identify deep abscesses that are not appreciated on physical examination. On ultrasound, the abscess cavity typically appears anechoic (black with no echo). CT scan is considered the gold standard for abscess diagnosis and is used to identify those near the neck, groin, and perineum.

Spontaneous, superficial skin abscesses are called furuncles, and patients often assume these are spider bites. Skin abscesses are usually caused by *S. aureus*—over half by MRSA—and less commonly β-hemolytic streptococcal species. Abscesses associated with injection drug use and those occurring near the perineum may contain gram negative and anaerobic bacteria. Abscesses are typically surrounded by a variable amount of cellulitis (so-called purulent cellulitis), and large abscesses may cause fever. If an abscess is not present, the main diagnostic considerations are cellulitis versus NSTI.

Nonpurulent cellulitis tends to occur on the lower extremities in a circumferential pattern, often in an area of preexisting edema. The etiology is usually β-hemolytic streptococcal species, such as *Streptococcus pyogenes*. Cellulitis may be associated with lymphangitis and fever. Nonpurulent cellulitis is sometimes linked to a fungal infection on the foot and may be recurrent in some patients. Erysipelas is a superficial, sharply demarcated cellulitis caused by *S. pyogenes*, which often occurs in young children and elderly patients on the face or lower extremities and which also causes fever and leukocytosis.

Although superficial skin infections can be treated easily, some instances of cellulitis can indicate a high-risk infection in selected settings and unusual circumstances. In such cases there is an increased likelihood of **esoteric or resistant pathogens** and of severe infection requiring admission or an operation. **Infected puncture wounds** of any kind are high risk and likely to involve deep structures like bone, joint, or tendon, and they are likely to respond poorly to conventional antibiotics alone. **Tenosynovitis**, an orthopedic emergency, can complicate puncture wounds on the palmar hand and fingers. **Diabetic foot ulcers**, when infected, tend to harbor multiple resistant pathogens, can lead to NSTI, and generally require specialized podiatric care. Infected mammalian bite wounds, covered elsewhere in this textbook, are high risk, often harbor *Pasteurella* species or *Eikenella* (human bites), and generally require hospital admission. Unusual pathogens that cause SSTIs in the setting of water exposure include *Erysipelothrix*, *Aeromonas*, and *Vibrio vulnificus*, which often causes a necrotizing infection and sepsis.

NSTIs are among the most feared infections in medicine. These infections typically spread rapidly along subcutaneous and muscular facial planes, produce toxins, and trigger an intense cytokine response that leads to septic shock. Classically, NSTIs occur in the setting of devitalized tissue, such as from a shrapnel wound, and the etiology is **polymicrobial**, with **C. perfringens** among the pathogens. A spontaneous, monomicrobial form of NSTI also occurs, typically caused by *S. pyogenes* but occasionally by Clostridial species, *V. vulnificus* or MRSA. Rapid diagnosis requires that the clinician be familiar with the risk factors for NSTI and red flags on physical examination (see Table 40–1).

An important risk factor for community onset necrotizing fasciitis is injection drug use, particularly subcutaneous and intramuscular injection ("skin popping") of black tar heroin. Other infection patterns that should raise a red flag are neglected diabetic foot ulcers and infections of the perineum, particularly in men (leading to Fournier's gangrene). Classic skin signs such as necrosis, bullae, or crepitance are often absent. Clostridial infections associated with injection drug use may produce dramatic tissue edema and extreme leukocytosis. The combination of extreme leukocytosis and hyponatremia is suggestive of an NSTI. Diagnostic imaging can be helpful. Plain x-ray and CT scan may demonstrate gas along facial planes or within muscle, or an unsuspected abscess may be seen. When NSTI is suspected, however, the best diagnostic approach is prompt surgical exploration. The diagnosis is made when subcutaneous devitalized tissue, muscle necrosis, and "dishwater pus" are found.

Table 40–1 • NECROTIZING SKIN SOFT TISSUE INFECTION "RED FLAGS"
Risk Factors
Injection drug use Neglected diabetic foot ulcer Infection of scrotum or perineum
Skin signs
Tense edema Bullae Skin necrosis Crepitus
Diagnostic tests
Gas in tissues on x-ray or CT Extreme leukocytosis Hyponatremia

Table 40–2 • THE THREE MAIN TYPES OF SKIN AND SOFT TISSUE INFECTIONS: USUAL ETIOLOGIC PATHOGENS AND COMMONLY RECOMMENDED ANTIBIOTICS		
SSTI Type	Pathogens	Recommended Antibiotics
Abscess	S. aureus (often MRSA)	TMP-SMX clindamycin vancomycin
Nonpurulent cellulitis	β-hemolytic Streptococcus (such as S. pyogenes)	Cephalexin cefazolin
NSTI	S. aureus (including MRSA) β-hemolytic Streptococcus Clostridial species (often C. perfringens)	Clindamycin vancomycin piperacillin-tazobactam

Abbreviations: MRSA = methicillin-resistant Staphylococcus aureus; NSTI = necrotizing skin and soft tissue infection; SSTI = skin and soft tissue infection.

The bacteriology of the major forms of SSTI are listed in Table 40–2, along with recommended antibiotics.

Management

Abscesses require drainage. Management begins with providing complete analgesia for the procedure. Options include local anesthetic, regional nerve block, and procedural sedation. In most cases, drainage is best accomplished by incision with a scalpel and exploration of the cavity with a clamp, although needle aspiration is a good option for small abscesses on the face. Delaying drainage for a follow-up visit is rarely the right plan. Small abscesses do not require packing. Large abscesses should be packed, and the packing can be changed at 24 hours, either upon emergency department follow-up or by the patient themselves. Loop drainage, in which a vessel loop (sterile rubber band) or Penrose drain is looped loosely through the abscess cavity, is an alternative to traditional packing.

Most simple abscesses resolve completely after incision and drainage, although a recent trial showed a small improvement in cure rate and reduction in recurrent abscesses with routine use of oral trimethoprim-sulfamethoxazole. Antibiotics are generally reserved for complicated abscesses, defined as more than 5 cm, having a large area of surrounding cellulitis, or occurring in an immunosuppressed host. Small and uncomplicated abscesses rarely cause fever. If fever is present in these patients, alternative sources should be considered. Admission for IV antibiotics is recommended for patients with large abscesses accompanied by extensive surrounding cellulitis, particularly if there is a fever. Staphylococcal coverage, including MRSA, is required. Recommended agents include trimethoprim-sulfamethoxazole for oral therapy and vancomycin for IV therapy.

Nonpurulent cellulitis requires antibiotics for cure. Most cases can be treated with oral antibiotics and elevation of the affected part. Good streptococcal coverage is required, usually with a first generation cephalosporin. (Therapy for purulent cellulitis must cover Staphylococcus as well; see above.) Admission for IV antibiotics is usually required if there is fever, lymphangitis or poorly controlled diabetes.

The biggest challenge with NSTIs is timely diagnosis. Once the suspicion for necrotizing infection reaches a reasonable threshold, the emergency physician should immediately consult a surgeon and request operative exploration for both definitive diagnosis and treatment. Immediate broad-spectrum antibiotic therapy is also important and must cover streptococcal species, anaerobes and MRSA. Good choices are vancomycin plus clindamycin or piperacillin-tazobactam. If signs of sepsis are present (hypotension, tachypnea, or lactate >2 mg/dL), aggressive fluid resuscitation should be initiated with ongoing assessment of tissue perfusion.

> ## CASE CORRELATION
>
> • See also Case 41 (Rash with Fever), Case 46 (Facial Laceration), and Case 47 (Rabies/Animal Bite).

COMPREHENSION QUESTIONS

40.1 A 40-year-old woman complains of a spider bite on her leg. It appears to be a necrotic 2 cm lesion on the right leg. What is the most likely diagnosis and etiologic organism?

   A. Spider bite from a dermonecrotic spider species.

   B. Impetigo from Group A *Streptococcus.*

   C. Abscess from a polymicrobial mix of species including *Streptococcus milleri.*

   D. Furuncle from methicillin-resistant *S. aureus.*

40.2 A 35-year-old HIV-positive injection drug user presents, complaining of a hip abscess where he injects heroin. The temperature is 38.1°C, and there is a 10 × 10 cm circular area of erythema and induration on the lateral buttock without fluctuance. Which is the correct management?

   A. Prescribe oral cephalexin for cellulitis and instruct the patient to return in 24 hours to assess whether an abscess has developed.

   B. Attempt needle aspiration at the center of the infection, and if negative, cover with oral antibiotics.

   C. Search for an abscess with bedside ultrasound and establish an IV in anticipation of a drainage procedure and admission for IV antibiotics.

   D. Consult a surgeon immediately for suspected necrotizing SSTI.

40.3 An otherwise healthy young man presents with a 5-cm abscess on the lateral buttock. He is afebrile. The correct management includes all of the following except:

   A. Pack the abscess and have the patient remove the packing himself within 24 hours and soak or bathe twice per day.

   B. Treat with an oral first generation cephalosporin.

   C. Incise with a scalpel and explore and open the cavity with a clamp.

   D. Provide analgesia with oral ibuprofen and a ring of local anesthetic around the abscess.

40.4 Which of the following is true about necrotizing soft tissue infections?

A. Blood pressure in the normal range and normal renal function are strong evidence against this diagnosis.

B. In suspected cases, admission to a medical service for IV antibiotics with surgical consultation as needed is reasonable management.

C. Skin bullae or necrosis or subcutaneous crepitus or tissue gas on x-ray are usually found.

D. Poorly controlled diabetes is the most common risk factor in community onset infection.

E. Vancomycin to cover MRSA is a recommended component of empirical antibiotics.

ANSWERS

40.1 **D.** Necrotic spider bites are unusual, whereas spontaneous furuncles (superficial skin abscesses) are extremely common in emergency practice. Patients with furuncles often complain of a "spider bite." MRSA accounts for 50% to 60% of all SSTIs in US emergency departments and may be even more common in spontaneous furuncles. While most of these simple infections are cured by incision and drainage alone, if antibiotics are deemed necessary, MRSA coverage is a must, with either trimethoprim-sulfamethoxazole, doxycycline or clindamycin.

40.2 **C.** This case is a classic presentation for a deep buttock or thigh abscess related to heroin injection. A septic hip or necrotizing infection should also be considered, although consultation for suspected NSTI is premature at this point. Nonpurulent cellulitis is very unlikely, and simply treating with antibiotics is incorrect management. These abscesses can be very large and may cause a low-grade fever. When there is no obvious fluctuance, imaging should be pursued with ultrasound, or occasionally CT, to confirm the diagnosis and guide drainage. Needle aspiration is reserved for small facial abscesses and has no proven diagnostic role. Given the fever, this patient will likely require IV antibiotics and admission, as well procedural sedation via IV.

40.3 **B.** In a healthy host, an abscess 5 cm or less with only minimal to moderate surrounding cellulitis usually does not require antibiotics. However, if antibiotics are prescribed, doxycycline, trimethoprim-sulfamethoxazole, or clindamycin is the correct choice. Long acting local anesthetic, such as bupivacaine, should be deposited in a ring around the abscess several minutes before incision and drainage. Packing or loop drainage is advised for abscesses that are more than a cm or so below the skin surface, as is commonly encountered in the buttocks, but it can be removed by the patient, with or without repacking. Soaking and scrubbing with soapy water is also recommended.

40.4 **E.** Necrotizing soft tissue infections are uncommon but potentially devastating, and the diagnosis is rarely obvious at first presentation. Shock or organ dysfunction is initially evident in only 0% to 40% of cases. Classic skin signs are important red flags to recognize but are frequently absent, and gas on plain x-ray is seen in 30% of cases, at most. Risk factors include diabetic foot ulcer, infections of the scrotum and perineum in men and injection drug use—which, in urban centers, is the leading cause of community onset necrotizing infections. Group A streptococcal NSTIs can occur spontaneously. Broad-spectrum antibiotic therapy, such as vancomycin plus clindamycin or piperacillin-tazobactam, should be initiated to cover streptococcal species, anaerobes and MRSA.

CLINICAL PEARLS

▶ Different types of SSTIs that require different approaches to management can appear similar.

▶ Abscesses require drainage, and management begins with providing complete analgesia for the procedure.

▶ Admission for IV antibiotics is usually required if there is fever, lymphangitis, or poorly controlled diabetes.

▶ Antibiotics are generally reserved for complicated abscesses, defined as more than 5 cm, having a large area of surrounding cellulitis, or occurring in an immunosuppressed host.

▶ Nonpurulent cellulitis requires antibiotics for cure. Most cases can be treated with oral antibiotics and elevation of the affected part.

▶ The biggest challenge with NSTIs is timely diagnosis.

REFERENCES

Chen JL, Fullerton KE, Flynn NM. Necrotizing fasciitis associated with injection drug use. *Clin Infect Dis*. 2001;33(1):6-15.

Jeng A, Beheshti M, Li J, et al. The role of beta-hemolytic streptococci in causing diffuse, nonculturable cellulitis: a prospective investigation. *Medicine (Baltimore)*. 2010;89(4):217-226.

Moran GJ, Krishnadasan A, Gorwitz RJ, et al. Methicillin-resistant *S. aureus* infections among patients in the emergency department. *N Engl J Med*. 2006;355(7):666-674.

Napolitano LM. Severe soft tissue infections. *Infect Dis Clin North Am*. 2009;23(3):571-591.

Talan DA, Mower WR, Krishnadasan A, et al. Trimethoprim-Sulfamethoxazole versus placebo for uncomplicated skin abscss. *N Engl J Med*. 2016;374(9):823-832.

A 3-year-old boy is brought to the emergency department (ED) by his parents because of a rash that developed yesterday evening. The rash began on his neck and chest, then gradually spread to include his entire body except for his face. It does not seem to be painful or pruritic. Although the child has had a fever and mild cough recently, he states that he "feels fine" and has not had any change in his behavior or oral intake. His parents deny any recent travel, camping or contact with animals. However, the boy does attend daycare, and several other children there have been ill recently. He is an otherwise healthy child with no history of major illness or medication allergies. He is taking acetaminophen as needed for the fever, and his immunizations are up to date.

On examination, his temperature is 38.9°C (102.1°F), blood pressure is 96/50 mm Hg, heart rate ls 112 beats per minute, respiratory rate is 18 breaths per minute, and oxygen saturation is 98% on room air. The boy is sleeping comfortably in his mother's arms but awakes easily during the examination. He does not appear acutely ill. His examination is unremarkable except for an erythematous maculopapular rash covering his neck, torso, and extremities.

▶ What is the most likely diagnosis?
▶ How should this patient be managed?

ANSWERS TO CASE 41:

Rash With Fever

Summary: This is a 3-year-old boy who presents with a rash, fever, and mild upper respiratory symptoms. On examination, he appears well and hydrated. He has a generalized maculopapular rash that spares his face.

- **Most likely diagnosis:** Viral exanthem.

- **Management:** Symptomatic relief (eg, fever control) and follow-up with his primary care physician as needed.

ANALYSIS

Objectives

1. Know the terminology used to describe rashes.

2. Review several causes of rash with fever.

3. Be able to identify "red flags" associated with serious causes of rash.

Considerations

This 3-year-old boy has a maculopapular rash associated with fever and a mild cough. The differential diagnosis is broad but can be focused by taking a detailed history and performing a thorough examination that includes noting the appearance and distribution of the skin lesions. Identifying specific etiologies may be difficult, as multiple organisms and disease processes often cause similar types of rashes. Although most rashes are **not** associated with serious or life-threatening disorders, the ED physician must be able to identify those skin rashes that are more serious.

APPROACH TO:

Rash With Fever

CLINICAL APPROACH

Patients presenting with rash and fever have a broad differential diagnosis that includes relatively minor as well as life-threatening etiologies. A thorough history and physical examination and familiarity with common patterns of skin lesions and their potential causes will help the emergency physician make a quick diagnosis and accurate treatment plan.

Important historical questions include initial appearance and location of skin lesions, direction and rate of progression, duration of rash, and associated features, such as pain or pruritus. The clinician should also inquire about systemic complaints (eg, fever, cough, sore throat, vomiting, diarrhea, seizures, mental status changes, and joint pain) and recent exposures (eg, medications, known allergens,

Table 41–1 • DESCRIPTORS OF COMMON SKIN LESIONS

Macule	Flat, circumscribed area ≤1 cm of discoloration
Patch	Flat, circumscribed area >1 cm of discoloration
Papule	Solid, raised lesion <0.5 cm in diameter
Nodule	Similar to papule but located deeper in the dermis or subcutaneous tissue; >0.5 cm in diameter
Plaque	Solid, raised lesion >0.5 cm in diameter, often formed by confluence of papules
Pustule	Circumscribed, raised, containing purulent fluid
Vesicle	Circumscribed, raised, fluid-containing lesion, <0.5 cm
Bullae	Same as vesicle, except >0.5 cm in diameter
Petechiae	Small (<2-3 mm), flat, non-blanching red or purple spots caused by capillary hemorrhage
Purpura	Larger (>2-3 mm), flat, non-blanching purple discoloration
Wheal	Edematous, transient plaque

animals, chemicals, foods, travel, and sick contacts). Past medical, family, and sexual histories may also provide clues as to the etiology of the rash.

Patients with abnormal vital signs or evidence of toxicity may require initial stabilization before a detailed examination can be performed. If the patient is stable, care should be taken to inspect the entire body, including mucous membranes. It is important to identify the color, morphology (listed in Table 41–1), location, and pattern of arrangement (including symmetry and configuration) of any lesions. A complete physical examination can help elicit additional diagnostic clues (eg, neck examination for nuchal rigidity and neurologic examination in patients with suspected meningococcemia (see Figure 41–1) or pelvic examination in those with possible disseminated gonococcemia). Although laboratory testing is not required for the evaluation of most rashes, it may be useful in some specific circumstances. For example, coagulation

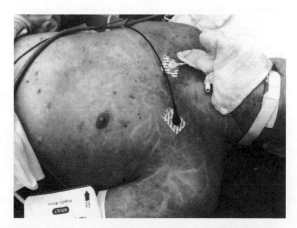

Figure 41–1. Fulminant meningococcemia with extensive purpuric patches.

studies and platelet counts are indicated in patients with petechiae or purpura, and VDRL testing should be performed for suspected syphilis.

When developing a differential diagnosis, the clinician should consider three main categories: infectious, allergic, and rheumatologic. Table 41–2 includes descriptions of several infectious causes of rash with fever. Differentiating an infectious from allergic rash can be difficult. Classically, allergic rashes are pruritic rather than painful. They may be associated with the recent addition of a new medication

Table 41–2 • INFECTIOUS CAUSES OF RASH WITH FEVER		
Disease	**Rash**	**Diagnostic**
Rubella	Pink macular rash beginning on face, spreading to trunk and extremities	Rash before fever Upper respiratory symptoms Forschheimer spots (soft palate petechiae)
Rubeola (Measles)	Red to brown maculopapular rash begins on face, neck, and shoulders, then spreads	The 3 Cs: cough, coryza, conjunctivitis Associated with upper respiratory infection Fever before rash, Koplik spots (bluish-white papules on red base on buccal mucosa)
Roseola (Human herpes virus 6)	Face-sparing pink maculopapular rash	Classically described as sudden onset of rash after resolution of high fever
Fifth disease (Erythema infectiosum)	Bright red facial rash or/with lacy reticular rash	Children: "slapped cheek" appearance Adults: rash after fever associated arthralgias and myalgias May be associated with aplastic crisis Caused by Parvovirus B19
Hand, foot, and mouth disease	Ulcer-like eruption in mouth with macular rash on palms and soles	1 to 2 days of fever followed by mouth ulcers and rash Caused by enteroviruses
Scarlet fever	Erythematous "sandpaper" rash with increased redness in skin folds	Recent acute tonsillar or skin infection "Strawberry tongue," Pastia sign (confluent petechiae in skin folds)
Varicella (chicken pox)	Papules to vesicles ("dewdrops on a rose petal") to pustules that eventually crust	Viral prodrome. Typically starts on trunk and spreads outward Crops of lesions found in different stages. May include mucosal involvement. Consider acyclovir/valacyclovir/famciclovir if complications or in immunocompromised patients
Lyme disease	Erythema migrans primary, macular rash secondary	Initial "bullseye" lesion associated with tick bite (caused by *Borrelia burgdorferi*) Associated fever, arthralgias, myalgias, malaise. Treat with doxycycline, amoxicillin, cefuroxime, IV ceftriaxone, IV penicillin
Rocky Mountain spotted fever	Pink macules to red papules to petechiae. Begins on wrists, forearms, and ankles and spreads	Headache, myalgias, and rash with recent tick exposure Possible bradycardia and leukopenia Treat with doxycycline
Secondary syphilis	Red-pink maculopapular rash Begins on trunk and spreads to palms and soles	Appears 2-3 months after initial chancre Treat with penicillin G

or ingestion of an offending agent, or they may appear in the area of contact with an environmental allergen. Wheals and urticaria are often associated with an allergic reaction. Rheumatologic rashes may appear similar to those of infectious or allergic etiologies but usually present with other systemic symptoms such as fever, fatigue, or arthralgias.

"Red flags" for potentially serious or life-threatening causes of rash include history of immunocompromise, fever, toxic appearance, hypotension, petechiae or purpura, diffuse erythema, severe or localized pain, and mucosal lesions. Petechiae and purpura can be associated with infectious conditions, such as Rocky Mountain spotted fever or meningococcemia, as well as coagulopathies, such as disseminated intravascular coagulation. Diffuse erythema can be a sign of toxic shock syndrome, staphylococcal scalded skin syndrome, or necrotizing fasciitis. Mucosal lesions may be a sign of Stevens-Johnson syndrome (SJS) or toxic epidermal necrolysis (TEN). SJS and TEN are classically associated with drug exposures (such as sulfa, phenytoin, and carbamazepine) or viral infections, although many cases are idiopathic. Both conditions involve systemic symptoms (eg, fever), mucosal erosions, and diffuse cutaneous vesiculobullous lesions with epidermal detachment. They are differentiated by the amount of body surface area (BSA) involved (TEN involves >30% BSA epidermal detachment). Patients with Stevens-Johnson syndrome and TEN are at risk of infection and dehydration.

Treatment

Treatment depends on the underlying process. The specific cause of many viral exanthems remains unidentified. These patients are usually treated symptomatically if they are otherwise well-appearing. Rashes caused by bacteria generally require antibiotic therapy. Table 41–2 lists some common disease processes with their appropriate diagnostic findings and treatments. Mild allergic reactions may be treated with removal of the offending allergen and antihistamines with or without corticosteroids. Patients with Stevens-Johnson syndrome or TEN require admission for IV hydration and other supportive care.

> ## CASE CORRELATION
>
> - See also Case 39 (Bacterial Meningitis) and Case 40 (Skin and Soft Tissue Infections).

COMPREHENSION QUESTIONS

41.1 A 2-year-old boy presents with a 3-day history of fever up to 103.2°F. Although now afebrile for the past 24 hours, he presents today with a maculopapular rash. What is the most likely diagnosis?

A. Rubeola

B. Roseola

C. Hand, foot, and mouth disease

D. Rubella

41.2 An 8-year-old boy presents with a pruritic rash and subjective fever after a weekend camping trip with the local Boy Scout troop. On examination, you notice a linear, confluent maculopapular rash on the child's leg. Which of the following findings is most specific for contact dermatitis secondary to an environmental exposure?

A. Fever

B. Maculopapular appearance

C. Pruritus

D. Linear confluence

41.3 A 2-year-old girl is brought to the ED by her parents for fever up to 103°F, decreased oral intake, and "not acting herself." On examination, the child is lethargic. She has pain with flexion of her neck. She has small, non-blanching red dots on her legs and torso. What is the best management option?

A. PO challenge and reassess

B. Begin IV hydration and empiric antibiotic treatment

C. Fever control and discharge home

D. Obtain laboratory testing to narrow the differential diagnosis

41.4 A 4-year-old girl presents with a fever, desquamating bullous rash covering her torso, and ulcers in her mouth and vaginal area. Her parents want to know what caused her condition. Which is following is the most likely diagnosis?

A. Disseminated gonorrhea

B. Varicella infection

C. Diabetes mellitus

D. Stevens-Johnson syndrome

ANSWERS

41.1 **B.** The boy symptoms are consistent with roseola. Roseola is typically characterized by a history of a high fever followed by a rapid defervescence and a maculopapular rash.

41.2 **D.** Fever, pruritus, and maculopapular rash can be seen with numerous conditions. However, the linear confluence is more consistent with an allergic reaction secondary to an environmental exposure (eg, pattern due to an object, such as poison ivy brushing against the boy's leg).

41.3 **B.** This girl is lethargic. She has fever, meningeal signs, and a rash concerning for meningococcemia. Empiric antibiotic therapy should be started immediately. The other answer choices are reasonable in a patient who is not as ill; thus, astute clinical assessment is critical.

41.4 **D.** The girl presentation is worrisome for Stevens-Johnsons syndrome, which is a rare but serious disorder of mucus membranes and can involve the mouth, nose, eyes, and genitalia. It can be caused medications, viral infections, or can be idiopathic.

CLINICAL PEARLS

▶ A careful history and physical examination are useful in narrowing the differential diagnosis in patients with skin rashes.

▶ Patients with rashes should be examined from head to toe, including mucous membranes.

▶ "Red flags" for potentially serious or life-threatening causes of rash include history of immunocompromise, fever, toxic appearance, hypotension, petechiae or purpura, diffuse erythema, severe or localized pain, and mucosal lesions.

REFERENCES

Centers for Disease Control and Prevention. Diseases and Conditions. Available at: cdc.gov/Diseases Conditions/Accessed: March 31, 2012.

Cydulka RK, Garber B. Dermatologic presentations. In: GL Mandell, JE Bennett, RD Douglas, eds. *Mandell, Douglas, and Bennett's Principles and Practice of Infectious Diseases.* Philadelphia, PA: Churchill Livingstone/Elsevier; 2010.

Kliegman, R, Nelson WE. *Nelson Textbook of Pediatrics.* Philadelphia: Saunders; 2007.

Letko E, Papaliodis DN, Papaliodis GN, et al. Stevens-Johnson syndrome and toxic epidermal necrolysis: a review of the literature. *Ann Allergy Asthma Immunol.* 2005;94(4):419-436.

Marx JA, Hockberger RS, Walls RM, eds. *Rosen's Emergency Medicine: Concepts and Clinical Practice.* 8th ed. Philadelphia, PA: Saunders; 2014.

Schlossberg D. Fever and rash. *Infect Dis Clin North Am.* 1996;10:101-110.

Tintinalli JE, Stapczynski JS, Ma OJ, et al, eds. *Emergency Medicine: A Comprehensive Study Guide.* 8th ed. New York, NY: McGraw-Hill; 2016.

Wolff K, Johnson RA, Fitzpatrick TB. *Fitzpatrick's Color Atlas and Synopsis of Clinical Dermatology.* New York, NY: McGraw-Hill Medical; 2009.

A 39-year-old otherwise healthy man presents to the Emergency Department (ED) with 2 days of fever, headache, abdominal cramping, and muscle aches. He has had nausea and non-bloody, non-bilious emesis, as well as loose stools. He denies neck stiffness, difficulty breathing, and rash. He returned from a trip to Liberia 5 days ago. He appears unwell. His vital signs include: blood pressure 131/72 mm Hg, heart rate 101 beats per minute, respiratory rate 22 breaths per minute, temperature 39.1°C, and oxygen saturation 99% on room air.

▶ What is the most appropriate next step?
▶ What is the most likely diagnosis?
▶ What is the most appropriate treatment?

ANSWERS TO CASE 42:

Emerging Infections

Summary: A 39-year-old man presents to the ED with nonspecific diffuse infectious symptoms (myalgias, fever, headache, nausea, vomiting, diarrhea, and abdominal cramping) following a recent trip to Liberia.

- **Next step: Isolate** the patient. You will certainly pursue treatment of this patient, amelioration of his symptoms, and diagnosis of the infectious source. However, it is critical to ensure a safe environment for providers and the other patients in your ED.

- **Most likely diagnosis:** This patient has nonspecific symptoms; however, his travel history to Liberia puts him at risk for **Ebola Virus Disease (EVD)**.

- **Treatment:** EVD must be contained and confirmed, and patients should be treated with **supportive care.**

ANALYSIS

Objectives

1. Recognize the risk factors for and presentation patterns of emerging infectious diseases.

2. Understand the basis for the severity and mortality associated with these illnesses.

3. Know the treatment pathways for these emerging infectious diseases.

4. Understand the necessary precautions, including isolation measures to contain a potential public health risk.

Considerations

This is a 39-year-old man with the acute onset of nonspecific symptoms, but with recent travel from Liberia. Because of the travel history, there should be a high index of suspicion for a possible serious infectious etiology, which may include traditional or emerging infectious etiologies.

Emerging infectious diseases are those that have come to prominence (or re-emerged) in recent years. While many diseases have been well managed with antimicrobials and vaccines, there are new diseases affecting our species (eg, SARS and MERS), and well-known diseases that are causing new infections (eg, Ebola, methicillin resistant *Staphylococcus aureus*, and extensively drug resistant tuberculosis). Emerging infections do not necessarily cause outbreaks or epidemics, but they are commonly brought to the forefront in lay media when they do occur in such a fashion.

APPROACH TO:
Emerging Infections

DEFINITIONS

CDC: Centers for Disease Control and Prevention, the national public health authority in the United States.

WHO: World Health Organization, the international public health authority of the United Nations.

SARS: Severe Acute Respiratory Syndrome, a viral illness caused by the coronavirus SARS-CoV.

MERS: Middle East Respiratory Syndrome, a viral illness caused by the coronavirus MERS-CoV.

EVD: Ebola Virus Disease, a viral hemorrhagic fever caused by one of the ebola viruses.

Zika Virus Disease: A viral illness due to the Zika virus, which is mostly commonly transmitted via an *Aedes* sp. mosquito bite.

CLINICAL APPROACH

Pathophysiology

Middle East Respiratory Syndrome (MERS) and Severe Acute Respiratory Syndrome (SARS) cause similar illness manifestations in infected individuals. They are caused by related coronaviruses, MERS Coronavirus (MERS-CoV) and SARS-associated Coronavirus (SARS-CoV). Although a large percentage of common colds are likely caused by other coronaviruses, these diseases are severe beyond the typical upper respiratory and gastrointestinal symptoms associated with coronaviruses. The reservoir for the viruses that cause both SARS and MERS is bats.

SARS

SARS-CoV is transmitted from human to human by droplets. Following a 5-day incubation period, it begins with nonspecific illness symptoms (eg, fever, chills, myalgias, headaches, and malaise). Over the next 5 days, the patient develops respiratory symptoms (cough) and often will progress to a viral pneumonia (or bacterial pneumonia due to super-infection). Acute respiratory distress syndrome (ARDS), a life-threatening condition, can also complicate SARS. SARS was responsible for a large outbreak in China from 2002 to 2003 with a case fatality rate just under 10%. SARS-CoV can be identified via serum or respiratory secretion polymerase chain reaction (PCR).

MERS

MERS-CoV is also transmitted from human to human by droplets, but it has a more limited rate of human-to-human transmission when compared to SARS. So far, every primary case of MERS has been traced epidemiologically to the Middle East. Potential reservoirs are camels and bats. Like SARS, MERS infection begins after a 5-day incubation with fever, malaise, myalgias, and other nonspecific symptoms. However, patients with MERS develop pulmonary symptoms more rapidly and more frequently have severe organ dysfunction (eg, ARDS). This emerged in 2012 and has a higher case fatality rate (~35%) than SARS.

Ebola Virus Disease

Ebola Virus Disease (EVD) is the manifestation of infection from one of the ebola viruses. Ebola virus is a genus of viral taxonomy. There are multiple ebola virus species, named geographically (eg, Zaire ebola virus, responsible for the 2014 West Africa outbreak), that cause EVD. The viral reservoirs are likely bats as well as other animals, including primates, serving as hosts. **EVD is a highly contagious and deadly disease that frequently occurs in outbreaks.** This is in part due to spillover from the animal reservoir into humans and the high transmissibility of the disease from person-to-person. Transmission is via bodily fluids; thus, exposure of mucous membranes or broken skin to bodily fluids (eg, blood, saliva, expectorate, semen, or breast milk) of an infected person or other host animal can lead to EVD. After an approximately 10-day incubation period, the symptoms of fever, myalgias, headache, abdominal pain, nausea, vomiting, diarrhea, and bleeding begin. EVD has a high mortality rate, with the WHO reporting an average case fatality of 50% (~40% in the 2014 West Africa outbreak). This is due to severe multiorgan dysfunction, including liver failure, kidney failure, ARDS, distributive and hypovolemic shock, and DIC. Suspicion for the disease is largely based on relevant travel history, and diagnosis can be made with serum antigen PCR or identification of IgM or IgG antibodies. Common laboratory abnormalities include lymphopenia, elevated PTT, elevated PT/INR, thrombocytopenia, and anemia.

Zika Virus Disease

Zika Virus Disease (Zika) manifests as an acute illness with fever, maculopapular rash, arthralgias, and bilateral conjunctivitis. The Zika virus is most commonly transmitted via an *Aedes* sp. mosquito bite. At the time of this writing, active infections are currently present in Mexico, Central America, South America, the Caribbean Islands, the Pacific Islands, and Africa. **Vertical transmission from mother to child can occur both during pregnancy and during childbirth.** At the time of this writing, the consensus for triaging is as follows:

- Ask the pregnant patient about recent travel to Zika-infected countries

- If yes, then ask if symptoms of acute infection (fever, myalgias, rash, and conjunctivitis) are present

- If yes, then offer Zika virus testing

- If positive, then discuss with the patient about amniocentesis versus serial ultrasounds

No cases have been reported of transmission from mother to child from breastfeeding. Zika virus can be spread via **sexual intercourse** (transmission occurs from male partners), as the virus is present in semen longer than blood. Cases of Zika virus transmission via blood transfusion have been reported in countries other than the United States. This infection gained significant attention in 2016, as Zika virus infection during pregnancy has been linked to the development of congenital microcephaly, as well as other brain and eye abnormalities. In 2016, the CDC and WHO issued warnings for pregnant women.

Management

Prevention of disease transmission is very important when it comes to patients with suspected emerging infections. In addition to having an understanding of standard precautions (eg, hand hygiene and the use of personal protective equipment), it is very important to understand transmission-based precautions (Table 42–1). In suspected cases of SARS and MERS, the CDC recommends standard, contact, and airborne precautions. In suspected cases of EVD, the CDC recommends high-level contact precautions and airborne precautions with specialized training in donning and doffing of personal protective equipment (PPE). Zika virus is spread via mosquito bites, vertical transmission from mother to child, sexual intercourse, and blood transfusion, so the use of standard precautions is appropriate.

Treatment

The mainstay of treatment for emerging infections is that of supportive care. Unstable patients should undergo immediate resuscitation following isolation and appropriate precautions. There are multiple paradigms for understanding supportive care, but a straightforward conceptualization centers on evaluating the ABCs (Airway, Breathing, and Circulation) and support of, or application of remedy for, insufficiencies with these if needed. In this way, supportive care is the management of patient-specific parameters rather than disease-specific parameters. For example, supportive care of the **airway** and **breathing** of a patient

Table 42-1 • TRANSMISSION BASED PRECAUTIONS		
Type of Precaution	**Disease Examples**	**Appropriate Actions**
Contact	Rotavirus Norovirus *Clostridium difficile* Methicillin-resistant *S. aureus*	**Caregiver:** gown and gloves **Patient:** single person room
Droplet	Influenza Respiratory syncytial virus Adenovirus *Bordetella pertussis* *Neisseria meningitides*	**Caregiver:** facemask with optional gown, gloves, or face shield **Patient:** facemask when transporting (should be in private room)
Airborne	Tuberculosis Measles Varicella zoster virus	**Caregiver:** fit-tested N-95 respirator +/- gown, gloves, face shield **Patient:** airborne infection isolation room (AIIR) *If unavailable, the patient should wear a facemask and be placed in a closed door room

with MERS or SARS may require endotracheal intubation and mechanical ventilation. Supportive care of **circulation** in a patient with EVD requires careful replacement of fluid losses to maintain normal perfusion parameters (ie, maintain adequate hydration, adequate blood pressure, and adequate perfusion of end organs).

Once the ABCs have been addressed, attention is turned toward the support of ailing or failing body systems. The goals are to treat patient specific endpoints and to uphold vital processes while the body's own defense systems eliminate the viral infection. For example, a patient with failing kidneys may require dialysis, while a patient with a developing bacterial super-infection will require antibiotics. Laboratory abnormalities including electrolyte aberrancies must be thoughtfully addressed. Antipyretics (eg, acetaminophen and ibuprofen) can be given for fever reduction unless a contraindication is present. The use of an antiemetic (eg, ondansetron, metoclopramide, or prochlorperazine) may be helpful if the patient is experiencing nausea and vomiting. The patient's pain should also be addressed and a clinically appropriate medication provided.

Patients with SARS and MERS may present with severe respiratory distress and hypoxia requiring the administration of supplemental oxygen and bronchodilators (eg, albuterol). In the case of ARDS, they are likely to require orotracheal intubation and mechanical ventilation.

Patients with EVD are likely to require intravenous fluids (and possibly vasopressors) for circulatory support, as well as electrolyte supplementation, antipyretics, and analgesics. Serum electrolytes, complete blood counts, and coagulation profiles should be closely monitored. Experimental therapies are currently being developed, including vaccines and blood transfusions containing antibodies to the virus from individuals who survived acute EVD.

Zika is generally a self-limited viral infection that responds to supportive care (ie, antipyretics, analgesics, and oral hydration). Aspirin and NSAIDs should be avoided until Dengue fever is ruled out to reduce the risk of bleeding. Rarely, dehydration or neurologic problems may develop. The most significant risk is to the pregnant patient since congenital microcephaly may ensue. Prevention by avoiding travel to Zika-infected countries is important. Use of permethrin treated long sleeve clothing, EPA-approved mosquito repellent, and staying indoors in screened and air-conditioned areas are helpful.

CASE CORRELATION

- See also Case 39 (Bacterial Meningitis), Case 40 (Skin and Soft Tissue Infections), and Case 41 (Rash With Fever).

COMPREHENSION QUESTIONS

42.1 What is the most common mode of transmission of the Zika virus?

    A. *Aedes* sp. mosquito bite

    B. Vertical transmission from mother to child during breastfeeding

    C. Sexual intercourse

    D. Blood transfusion

42.2 A 66-year-old man presents to the ED with complaints of fever, cough, and malaise for the last 2 days. He is originally from Saudi Arabia and moved to the United States 1 week ago. He is ill-appearing with the following vital signs: blood pressure 110/60 mm Hg, heart rate 120 beats per minute, respiratory rate 26 breaths per minute, temperature 39.0°C, and oxygen saturation of 91% on room air. What is the most likely diagnosis?

    A. Ebola virus disease

    B. Middle East Respiratory Syndrome

    C. Zika Virus

    D. Severe Acute Respiratory Syndrome

42.3 A 22-year-old man presents to the ED with fever, malaise, and arthralgias. He denies cough or runny nose. On examination, he has a mild bilateral conjunctivitis and a maculopapular rash on his torso. He recently returned from a cruise to several Caribbean Islands. What is the most likely cause of his symptoms?

    A. Zika virus

    B. Influenza virus

    C. Coxsackie virus

    D. Ebola virus disease

42.4 What was the mortality rate of the 2014 Ebola virus disease outbreak?

    A. 20%

    B. 40%

    C. 60%

    D. 80%

ANSWERS

42.1 **A.** The most common mode of transmission of the Zika virus is via an *Aedes* sp. mosquito bite. Other modes of transmission include mother-to-child during pregnancy and childbirth, sexual intercourse (transmission occurs from male partners), and blood transfusions in some countries other than the United States. No cases have been reported of transmission from mother to child from breastfeeding.

42.2 **B.** The patient likely has Middle East Respiratory Syndrome (MERS) due to an infection with MERS-CoV. Symptoms of MERS include fevers, cough, and respiratory distress. The incubation period is approximately 5-6 days. This disease is common in the Arabian Peninsula. His recent immigration (1 week ago) to the United States from a high-risk region makes this the most likely diagnosis. Ebola virus disease (EVD) manifests as fever, headache, vomiting, diarrhea, abdominal pain, myalgias, and unexplained hemorrhage. Severe Acute Respiratory Syndrome (SARS) presents in a similar manner; however, there are no currently active outbreaks of SARS, and the most recent (2002-2003) was associated with travel to Asia. Zika virus disease manifests as fever, rash, arthralgia, and conjunctivitis.

42.3 **A.** The patient most likely has Zika virus disease, which manifests as an acute illness of fever, maculopapular rash, arthralgias, and bilateral conjunctivitis. Active infections are present in Mexico, Central America, South America, the Caribbean Islands, the Pacific Islands, and Africa. Influenza is a viral illness that causes abrupt onset of fever, myalgias, arthralgias, and respiratory symptoms (eg, cough, rhinorrhea, and shortness of breath). Coxsackie virus is the cause of the common childhood condition Hand, Foot, and Mouth Disease (HFMD) that presents with fever, malaise, intraoral lesions, and a rash on the palms and soles. Ebola virus disease (EVD) manifests as fever, headache, vomiting, diarrhea, abdominal pain, myalgias, and unexplained hemorrhage.

42.4 **B.** The 2014 outbreak in West Africa was the largest outbreak of Ebola virus disease in history. Two out of five individuals infected with Ebola virus died, resulting in a 40% mortality rate.[3]

CLINICAL PEARLS

▶ A complete social history, including recent travel, is key for the diagnosis, isolation, and treatment of patients who present with a potential emerging infectious disease.

▶ Many of the emerging infections are associated with high morbidity and mortality rates. Early recognition is key to preventing further transmission and saving lives.

▶ In addition to having an understanding of standard precautions (eg, hand hygiene and the use of personal protective equipment), it is very important to understand transmission-based precautions to prevent the spread of disease.

▶ Suspected cases of any of the emerging infectious diseases should be reported to the local health department, who can aid in reporting to the CDC.

REFERENCES

Arabi YM, Arifi AA, Balkhy HH, et al. Clinical course and outcomes of critically ill patients with Middle East respiratory syndrome coronavirus infection. *Ann Intern Med.* 2014;160(6):389-397.

Centers for Disease Control and Prevention. Ebola West Africa 2014 Outbreak Case Counts. Available at: www.cdc.gov/vhf/ebola/outbreaks/2014-west-africa/previous-case-counts.html. Accessed March 23, 2016.

Centers for Disease Control and Prevention. Ebola Virus Disease. Available at: http://cdc.gov/vhf/ebola. Accessed February 26, 2016.

Centers for Disease Control and Prevention. Revised U.S. Surveillance Case Definition for Severe Acute Respiratory Syndrome (SARS) and Update on SARS Cases—United States and Worldwide, December 2003. Available at: **http://www.cdc.gov/mmwr/preview/mmwrhtml/mm5249a2.htm**. Accessed February 27, 2016.

Centers for Disease Control and Prevention. Severe Acute Respiratory Syndrome: Frequently Asked Questions About SARS. Available at: **http://www.cdc.gov/sars/about/faq.html**. Accessed February 27, 2016.

Centers for Disease Control and Prevention. Zika Virus for Health Care Workers: Clinical Presentation and Disease. Available at: **http://www.cdc.gov/zika/hc-providers/clinicalevaluation.html**. Accessed March 8, 2016.

Chan JF. Middle East respiratory syndrome coronavirus: another zoonotic betacoronavirus causing SARS-like disease. *Clin Microbiol Rev.* 2015.

Haagmans BL, Al Dhahiry SH, Reusken CB, et al. Middle East respiratory syndrome coronavirus in dromedary camels: an outbreak investigation. *Lancet Infect Dis.* 2014;14:140-145.

Hui DS. Severe acute respiratory syndrome vs. the Middle East respiratory syndrome. *Curr Opin Pulm Med.* 2014.

Oduyebo T, Petersen EE, Rasmussen SA, et al. Centers for Disease Control and Prevention Update: Interim Guidelines for Health Care Providers Caring for Pregnant Women and Women of Reproductive Age with Possible Zika Virus Exposure—United States, 2016. Available at: **http://www.cdc.gov/mmwr/volumes/65/wr/mm6505e2.htm**. Accessed March 8, 2016.

Zumba et al. Middle East respiratory syndrome. *Lancet.* 2015.

An intoxicated 25-year-old man was brought to the emergency department (ED) by paramedics after he was involved in an altercation and sustained several stab wounds to the torso and upper extremities. His initial vital signs in the ED showed pulse rate of 100 beats per minute, blood pressure of 112/80 mm Hg, respiratory rate of 20 breaths per minute, and Glasgow coma scale of 13. A 2-cm stab wound is noted over the left anterior chest just below the left nipple. Additionally, there is a 2-cm wound adjacent to the umbilicus, and several 1- to 2-cm stab wounds are noted in right arm and forearm, near the antecubital fossa. The abdominal and chest wounds are not actively bleeding and there is no apparent hematoma associated with these wounds. However, one of the wounds in the right arm is associated with a 10-cm hematoma that is actively oozing.

► What are the next steps in the evaluation of this patient?
► What are the complications associated with these injuries?

ANSWERS TO CASE 43:

Penetrating Trauma to the Chest, Abdomen, and Extremities

Summary: A 25-year-old hemodynamically stable, intoxicated man presents with stab wounds to the chest, abdomen, and upper extremities.

- **Next step:** Assess ABCDE: airway, breathing, circulation, disability, and exposure. After completing this survey, consider local exploration of the knife wounds (except chest wounds) to see whether they are superficial or deep.

- **Potential complications from injuries:**

  - Chest wound: Pericardial effusion/tamponade, pneumothorax, hemothorax, diaphragmatic injury.

  - Abdominal wound: Hollow viscus, vascular, or urinary tract injury.

  - Extremities: Vascular, nerve, or tendon injury.

ANALYSIS

Objectives

1. Be able to classify penetrating injuries by location, including chest, thoracoabdominal region, abdomen, flank, back, and "cardiac box."

2. Learn the priorities involved in the initial management of penetrating injuries.

3. Become familiar with the treatments of penetrating truncal and extremity injuries.

Considerations

A systematic approach must be undertaken in the evaluation of this patient. **The clinician must guard against being distracted by injuries not immediately threatening to loss of life or limb.** Likewise, young healthy individuals, particularly those who are intoxicated, may have significant injuries and not manifest many physical examination findings or hemodynamic changes. Advanced trauma life support (ATLS) guidelines stress the initial primary survey to identify and address potentially life-threatening injuries. The primary survey consists of the **ABCDEs (airway, breathing, circulation, disability, and exposure)**. Exposure (removing all of the patient's clothing and rolling the patient to examine the patient's backside) is particularly important in a patient with penetrating trauma because puncture wounds may be hidden in axillary, inguinal, and gluteal folds.

Following the primary survey, preliminary labs, plain x-rays, and a bedside ultrasound should be obtained as clinically indicated. In this case, an upright chest x-ray (CXR), preferably at end expiration, will be needed to assess for pneumothorax and hemothorax. A focused abdominal sonogram for trauma (FAST) examination should be performed to evaluate for pericardial and intraperitoneal free fluid. This patient is hemodynamically stable and possesses minimal abdominal examination findings. Therefore, a reasonable strategy is to perform local wound exploration to determine the depth of the puncture wound. A wound that does not penetrate the abdominal fascia may be irrigated and closed without further diagnostic requirement. However, it is important to note that in an intoxicated patient, the physical examination may not be very sensitive.

APPROACH TO:
Penetrating Trauma

DEFINITIONS

CHEST: Area from clavicles to costal margins, 360 degrees around.

"CARDIAC BOX": Anatomical region bordered by the clavicles superiorly, bilateral midclavicular lines laterally, and the costal margins inferiorly. This box includes the epigastric region between the costal margins. Eighty-five percent of penetrating cardiac stab wounds come from a puncture to the "box."

THORACOABDOMINAL: Area from the inframammary crease (women) or nipples (men), down to the costal margins, 360 degrees around. The clinical significance of a penetrating wound to this region is that there is a risk of injury to the intrathoracic and intra-abdominal contents, as well as to the diaphragm.

ANTERIOR ABDOMEN: Area bordered by the costal margins superiorly, the bilateral midaxillary lines laterally, and the inguinal ligaments inferiorly.

FLANK: Area from the costal margin down to the iliac crest and between the anterior and posterior axillary lines.

BACK: Area between the posterior axillary lines. Because of thick musculature over the back, only about 5% of stab wounds to the back lead to significant injuries.

CLINICAL APPROACH

Initial Management

The primary survey, or ABCDEs, should be addressed first (see Table 1–2 in Section I). The clinician should not be distracted by eye-catching but not immediately life-threatening injuries. In an unstable patient, treatment decisions often need to be made before obtaining diagnostic tests. For example, a patient with a stab wound to the chest and rapidly dropping oxygen saturation or blood pressure will require tube thoracostomy ("B" breathing) prior to confirmatory CXR. Bleeding, even if profuse, is most effectively controlled by direct finger pressure to the bleeding site. Gauze and pressure dressings are generally less effective. All patients should have immediate placement of large-bore IV access at two sites. Volume repletion should be initiated with warm IV fluids or blood products if the patient is showing signs of shock. After completion of the primary survey, a systematic search for other injuries (secondary survey) should be undertaken. Diagnostic tests should be performed expeditiously after the primary survey and often concurrent with the secondary survey (Table 43–1).

In general, gunshot wounds are more likely to cause greater tissue destruction and life-threatening injuries than stab wounds. This is due to the unpredictable path of the bullet, leading to significant tissue destruction. Hence, it is not safe to assume that a bullet has taken a direct path between the entrance and exit wounds.

The management of patients with penetrating injuries has recently undergone significant evolution. During the 1980s and 1990s, most patients underwent invasive diagnostic evaluations, including exploratory laparotomy and angiography based solely on mechanism and location. Currently, selective treatment for some penetrating injuries is acceptable. Selective treatment may involve close observation

Table 43–1 • IDENTIFICATION OF INJURIES

Location	Complications	Signs and Symptoms	Further Studies/ Interventions
Chest	Pericardial effusion/ tamponade Pneumothorax or hemothorax	Distant heart sounds, hypotension, JVD Decreased breath sounds, low oxygen saturation, hypotension	CXR may detect air or fluid in the pleural cavity. FAST is sensitive in detecting fluid within the pericardial sac ED ultrasound is useful in detecting a pneumothorax CT is sensitive in detecting hemothorax, occult pneumothorax Chest tube thoracostomy may yield a rush of air or blood
Abdomen or pelvis	Hollow viscous injury Liver laceration Splenic laceration Vascular injury	Peritonitis Tenderness Shock (hypotension, altered mental status) Bowel evisceration	Local wound exploration CT scan may reveal path of injury and grading of solid organ injuries Angiography may be useful for both diagnosis and treatment FAST—free intraperitoneal fluid Exploratory laparotomy Diagnostic laparoscopy
Back/flank	Retroperitoneal hematoma Urinary tract injury	Hematuria Hypotension	CT is the best diagnostic tool for evaluating retroperitoneal bleeding CT with delayed imaging and intravenous pyelography
Extremities	Vascular injury Nerve damage Tendon disruption	6 Ps (pain, pulselessness, poikilothermia, paresthesias, pallor, paralysis) Hard signs of vascular injury (pulsatile bleeding, absent pulse, expanding hematoma, palpable thrill, audible bruit)	Ankle-brachial indexes (ABIs) CT angiography Angiography Exploration in the OR

and additional minimally invasive diagnostic studies such as ultrasonography, laparoscopy, and thoracoscopy. This option has led to a significant reduction in unnecessary operations. However, selective treatment must be tailored to the clinical situation and balanced against the risk of delay to diagnosis and definitive operative intervention. The decision to proceed with selective treatment is best determined by a qualified surgeon after the initial evaluation.

Specific Anatomical Regions

Chest Injuries Generally, 10% to 15% of patients with penetrating chest trauma require urgent operative intervention. Fortunately, the majority of these patients can be identified within the first minutes by initial hemodynamic instability, the presence of a large hemothorax on CXR, or high chest tube output. The remaining 85% to 90% of patients may require only close observation, diagnostic imaging, or possibly tube thoracostomy.

The upright **CXR** has adequate sensitivity to evaluate for pneumothorax and hemothorax. Obtaining an end-expiratory film may increase the likelihood of detecting a small pneumothorax. In a patient with a high-risk mechanism, the absence of a pneumothorax should be confirmed by a repeat upright CXR in 4-6 hours or by computed tomography (CT). CT of the chest is highly sensitive for the detection of pneumothorax. A small pneumothorax visualized by CT and missed by CXR is referred to as an "occult pneumothorax." An occult pneumothorax should be reevaluated for progression in 4-6 hours by CXR and often does not require a chest tube.

Local wound exploration of a chest injury is not recommended because the procedure itself can penetrate the pleura and cause a pneumothorax. Pneumothorax or hemothorax found by CXR is treated by placement of a 36- or 40-French chest tube. Smaller tubes clot easily with blood and are not indicated in the setting of trauma. If the pneumothorax or hemothorax does not resolve with one adequately-placed chest tube, then a second chest tube should be placed. Early thoracoscopy may also be considered for diagnostic purposes and to establish adequate drainage. There has not been a consensus on the size of traumatic pneumothorax that warrants tube thoracostomy, although recent literature has shown a push toward more invasive procedures, especially when the pneumothorax is 20% or greater. If a **tension pneumothorax** is suspected, **needle decompression** may be useful in the field or in the community setting. In most trauma centers, expedited chest tube placement by an emergency physician has taken the place of needle decompression for tension pneumothorax physiology. Considerations for operative thoracotomy include initial output of 1000-1500 mL of blood, or an output of 200-250 mL per hour for the first 4-5 hours.

Any patient with an injury within the cardiac box should undergo prompt **FAST** examination of the heart by an experienced sonographer. The subxiphoid view may be complemented by a parasternal view. The experienced sonographer can detect pericardial blood with up to 100 percent sensitivity (Figure 43–1). Hemopericardium is an indication for pericardial exploration in the operating room.

Resuscitative (or so-called emergency department) thoracotomy is reserved for patients who are *in extremis* or who have lost vital signs in the ED or within a few minutes prior to arrival. This procedure is associated with a great deal of controversy.

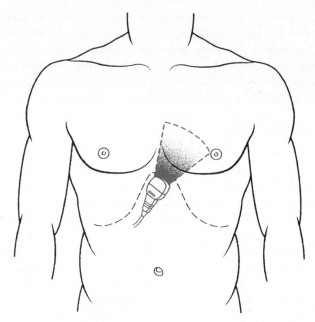

Figure 43–1. FAST examination imaging the subxiphoid region for pericardial fluid.

The practitioner must bear in mind that mortality for these patients exceeds 97%. In addition, this intervention may expose healthcare providers to accidental injury. The best outcomes occur when this procedure is performed in properly selected patients by an experienced physician and in a medical center with the capability to provide definitive treatment.

Thoracoabdominal Thoracoabdominal wounds are of particular interest because injuries to the diaphragm are difficult to detect. Unless the diaphragmatic defect is large, herniation of stomach or intestines is rarely visualized by CXR in the ED. Moreover, CT is not sensitive enough to detect small diaphragmatic injures. Surgical consultation should be obtained when diaphragmatic injury is suspected because the definitive diagnostic study is surgical evaluation by **laparoscopy or thoracoscopy**. If these injuries go untreated, herniation of intra-abdominal contents into the chest may eventually occur due to the presence of negative intrathoracic pressure.

Anterior Abdomen Immediate indication for **laparotomy** includes evidence of **shock** (hypotension, tachycardia, cold and clammy skin, or diaphoresis), **peritonitis**, **gun-shot wound** with a suspected bullet trajectory through the abdominal cavity, or **evisceration** of abdominal contents. In the absence of these findings, further radiographic evaluation or observation is indicated.

Local wound exploration is the best initial evaluation for a stable patient with an abdominal stab wound. This procedure is performed after preparing the skin with an antiseptic agent, creating a sterile field and anesthetizing the skin and soft tissues. The skin laceration is enlarged, and the wound tract is gently followed until either its termination or its violation of the anterior abdominal fascia. An intact fascia makes it highly unlikely that there is an intra-abdominal injury, and therefore the wound may be irrigated and dressed or loosely closed, depending on its size.

If the anterior abdominal fascia has been penetrated, then it is critical that a surgeon becomes involved in the patient's care in order to help facilitate observation with serial abdominal examinations or surgical intervention. Historically, diagnostic peritoneal lavage (DPL) was performed at the bedside to further investigate potential intra-abdominal injuries. However, DPL has been largely replaced by ultrasound (FAST) in addition to CT scan or diagnostic laparoscopy in the hemodynamically stable patient and by laparotomy in the unstable patient.

Back/Flank The physical examination, FAST, and DPL are insensitive in diagnosing injuries to the retroperitoneum, including the colon, kidneys, and ureters. The only clue to a retroperitoneal process irritating the psoas muscles may be the patient's need to flex their hips. Hematuria is the most reliable sign of injury to the kidneys, ureters, and bladder. If gross or microscopic hematuria is present or if a high degree of suspicion exists for possible injury, further evaluation is needed. CT with delayed images, intravenous pyelography (**IVP**), and perhaps retrograde cyst-urethrography are useful imaging modalities. Recent literature suggests that most renal injuries without associated hemodynamic compromise or urinary collection system leaks do not mandate exploration. These patients require hospital admission, bedrest, and serial laboratory studies. Laparotomy may be necessary for high-grade renal lacerations in an unstable patient.

Extremities The six Ps of arterial insufficiency (pain, paralysis, paresthesia, pallor, pulselessness, and poikilothermia) and the hard signs of vascular injury (pulsatile bleeding, expanding hematoma, absent distal pulses, palpable thrill, or audible bruit) should be evaluated. Their presence is an indication for immediate operative or angiographic evaluation. A careful pulse examination should be performed to look for a deficit. If pulses are not palpable, then Doppler can be used to identify arterial flow. Sites of injury should be auscultated for a bruit that can represent a traumatic arteriovenous fistula. Ankle-brachial indexes (ABIs) can be a useful measurement for evaluating lower extremity vascular trauma. An ABI value of less than 0.9 may represent vascular injury and therefore warrants further investigation. However, in long-standing diabetics, ABIs are less sensitive due to stiffened diseased vasculature leading to spurious values. Additionally, a motor or sensory deficit can represent nerve or tendon injury that is best evaluated and treated in the operating room.

CASE CORRELATION

- See also Case 1 (Airway Management/Respiratory Failure), Case 2 (Hemorrhagic Shock), Case 4 (Critical Care Resuscitation), Case 44 (Extremity Fracture and Neck Pain), and Case 45 (Trauma and Extremes of Age).

COMPREHENSION QUESTIONS

43.1 A 23-year-old man is involved in an altercation in the parking lot after a base-ball game. He suffers a single stab wound 2-cm medial and superior to the left nipple. His blood pressure is 110/80 mm Hg and heart rate is 80 beats per minute. Which of the following management options is most appropriate for this patient?

A. CXR, wound exploration, and ECG

B. CXR and CT scan of the abdomen

C. CXR and cardiac ultrasound

D. CXR, cardiac ultrasound, and laparoscopy

E. Wound exploration, chest radiograph (CXR), cardiac ultrasound, CT scan of the chest

43.2 For which of the following patients is CT imaging an appropriate diagnostic option?

A. A 38-year-old man with diffuse abdominal pain, involuntary guarding, and a 6-in knife impaled just below the umbilicus

B. A 22-year-old man with a single stab wound to the back, pulse rate of 118 beats per minute, blood pressure of 94/80 mm Hg, and gross hematuria

C. A 16-year-old adolescent boy with a single stab wound 2 cm above the left inguinal crease, with heart rate of 120 beats per minute and blood pressure of 90/78 mm Hg

D. A hemodynamically stable, 34-year-old woman, who is 26 weeks preg-nant and has a single stab wound to the back and no other abnormalities on physical examination

E. A hemodynamically stable, 40-year-old man with a single stab wound to the right chest, respiratory rate of 38 breaths/min and diminished breath sounds on the right

43.3 A 34-year-old man is brought into the ED after a motor vehicle accident. He complains of dyspnea and initially had an oxygen saturation of 88%. On examination, he has decreased breath sounds of the right chest and now has an oxygen saturation of 70% on room air. Which of the following is the most appropriate next step?

A. Chest radiograph

B. CT of the chest

C. Tube thoracostomy

D. Heparin anticoagulation

E. Anterior lateral thoracotomy

ANSWERS

43.1 **C.** CXR is sensitive in identifying hemothorax and pneumothorax, while cardiac ultrasound is useful in identifying pericardial fluid. Wound exploration of the chest is not recommended because the information gained is limited and the procedure is associated with the potential of producing a pneumothorax. An ECG provides limited information regarding cardiac injury and is generally not done. A stab wound above the nipple line is rarely associated with intra-abdominal injury; therefore, CT scan of the abdomen or diagnostic laparoscopy is unnecessary.

43.2 **D.** CT of the abdomen may be useful in identifying injuries to the retroperitoneal structures in a patient with a stab wound to the back. The patient being 26-week pregnant does not contraindicate CT scan. Further diagnostic studies would not be beneficial in patients listed in choices A, B, and C because these patients are exhibiting signs of significant injury that would necessitate urgent exploratory laparotomy.

43.3 **C.** The constellation of clinical signs points toward a pneumothorax. The presence of significant hypoxia requires immediate placement of a chest tube prior to chest radiograph confirmation, as further delay may progress to cardiovascular collapse.

CLINICAL PEARLS

▶ The systematic approach to the trauma patient is ABCDE (airway, breathing, circulation, disability, exposure).

▶ A wound that does not penetrate the abdominal fascia may be irrigated and closed without further diagnostic studies.

▶ Penetrating trauma to the chest below the nipple line may cause thoracic, intra-abdominal, and occult diaphragmatic injuries.

▶ The FAST (focused abdominal sonogram for trauma) is fairly accurate in assessing intraperitoneal free fluid.

▶ Approximately 85% of penetrating cardiac stab wounds originate from a puncture to the "cardiac box."

REFERENCES

Cameron JL, Cameron AM, ed. *Current Surgical Therapy*. 11th ed. St. Louis, MO: Mosby; 2013.

Como JJ, Bokhari F, Chiu WC, et al. Management of penetrating abdominal trauma, selective non-operative. *J Trauma*. 2010;68:721-733.

Mowery NT, Gunter OL, Collier BR, et al. Management of hemothorax and occult pneumothorax. *J Trauma*. 2011;70:510-518.

Townsend CM, Beauchamp RD, Evers BM, Mattox KL, eds. *Sabiston Textbook of Surgery*. 19th ed. Philadelphia, PA: W.B. Saunders; 2012.

Trunkey DD, Asensio JA, eds. *Current Therapy of Trauma and Surgical Critical Care*. 2nd ed. St. Louis, MO: Mosby; 2015.

A 26-year-old waiter was serving food at a social function when he tripped and fell down a flight of stairs. He did not lose consciousness following the event but complains of severe neck pain and right wrist and hand pain. He was placed in a C-collar and transported by EMS to the emergency department (ED) with appropriate C-spine precautions. His vital signs and cardiopulmonary examinations are within normal limits, Glasgow coma scale (GCS) is 15, and he is able to move all extremities. Palpation of his neck reveals tenderness at the midline, and his right distal forearm/wrist/hand is swollen and exquisitely tender to touch.

► What are the appropriate steps in the evaluation of his neck pain?
► What are the important elements in the evaluation of his right upper extremity?

ANSWERS TO CASE 44:

Extremity Fracture and Neck Pain

Summary: A 26-year-old man tripped and fell down some stairs and now complains of neck and right upper extremity pain. His history and presentation are concerning for cervical spine and right upper extremity injuries.

- **Evaluation of neck pain:** Computed tomography (CT) of the cervical spine. If the CT does not demonstrate any bony fractures or dislocation and his midline tenderness persists, then obtain flexion/extension x-rays or MRI of the C-spine to help differentiate ligamentous injury/spinal instability from soft tissue contusion.

- **Evaluation of upper extremity:** Given the soft tissue swelling and the location of pain, physical examination of the affected extremity should include detailed evaluation of the hand, wrist, and forearm, and this should include clinical assessments of tissue perfusion and functionality. Although vascular injuries are uncommon with this patient's injury mechanism, arterial inflow needs to be evaluated based on capillary refill and presence or absence of pulses. If the perfusion status is in doubt, Doppler evaluation of pulse quality and pressures should be obtained. X-rays of the humerus, radius, ulna, wrist, and hand should be obtained to assess for possible bone injuries.

ANALYSIS

Objectives

1. Learn the common cervical spine injuries associated with the various injury mechanisms.

2. Learn the decision rules that guide the use of cervical spine radiography in trauma patients.

3. Learn the current role of corticosteroids in patients with spinal cord injuries.

4. Learn the ED management of elbow, forearm, wrist, and hand injuries.

Considerations

The neck pain associated with midline tenderness on palpation in this patient raises the concern for C-spine injury; therefore, radiographic evaluations must be obtained for further assessment. Either three views of the C-spine (AP, lateral, and odontoid views) or CT can be performed. CT is preferable over three views and is the preferred diagnostic study in many centers because it is associated with much lower rates of false-negative examinations than plain radiography. CT would be especially helpful in this patient who exhibits concerning symptoms and physical findings. If the neck pain and midline C-spine tenderness persist despite negative CT findings, additional imaging to determine C-spine stability or to identify ligamentous injuries should be obtained. C-spine precautions should be maintained until the possibility of unstable injury can be eliminated based on imaging. Only when imaging studies indicate the absence of flexion/extension instability or the absence of ligamentous injuries on MRI can the patient be assumed to have neck pain related to soft tissue injuries only.

This patient also exhibits findings in the right distal forearm/wrist/hand that suggest the possibility of bony injuries. The initial evaluation should be directed toward evaluations of hand and digit functions—namely, motor/sensory functions and ligamentous integrity. Careful palpation of the hand, wrist, and forearm should also be performed to localize areas of concern for bony injuries. Two-view radiographs should be obtained to assess the bony integrity of the humerus, radius, ulna, carpal bones, and phalanges. When identified, fractures and dislocations should be reduced to minimize neurovascular compromises. Further assessments and management of all bony, ligamentous injuries and functional abnormalities should be discussed with an orthopedic or hand specialist.

APPROACH TO:

Cervical Spine and Upper Extremity Orthopedic Injuries

DEFINITIONS

NEXUS LOW-RISK CRITERIA: This C-spine clearance approach was derived based on a 1998 publication by Hoffman et al (*Ann Emerg Med.* 1998;32:461-469). The recommendations are that C-spine radiography is indicated for asymptomatic trauma patients unless they meet all of the following criteria: (1) No posterior midline cervical tenderness, (2) No evidence of intoxication, (3) Normal level of alertness, (4) No focal neurologic deficits, and (5) No painful distracting injuries. The major limitation of this approach is that no precise definition for painful distracting injuries was provided.

THE CANADIAN C-SPINE RULE (CCR): This is a guideline to determine the need for radiographic evaluations of **alert and stable trauma patients.** In comparison to the NEXUS criteria, the CCR has been shown to have slightly greater sensitivity and specificity for identification of patients who do not have C-spine injuries (Figure 44–1).

PARTIAL CORD SYNDROMES: Compression or contusions to the spinal cord can develop with or without concomitant bony injuries. Compression of the **anterior cord** can produce complete motor paralysis and loss of pain and temperature perceptions. **Posterior cord** syndrome (Brown-Sequard) causes paralysis, loss of vibratory sensation and proprioception ipsilaterally and loss of pain and temperature sensations contralaterally. **Central cord** syndrome is produced by injuries to the corticospinal tract, which produces great upper extremities weakness in comparison to the lower extremities.

CLINICAL APPROACH

Millions of adults at risk for cervical spine injuries and/or upper extremity orthopedic injuries are evaluated in EDs throughout the United States and

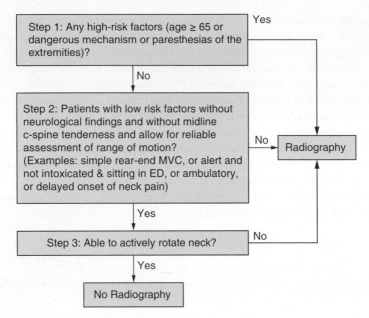

Figure 44-1. Sample algorithm for assessing neck injury.

Canada every year. Among patients presenting with intact neurological status to the ED, the incidence of acute C-spine fracture or spinal injury is less than 1%. Even though spinal injury incidences are low, there are great consequences associated with mismanagement. Similarly, mismanagement of upper extremity injuries can lead to potential employment and functional compromises.

Clearing the C-spine in the Blunt Trauma Patient

The goal of C-spine clearance is to establish that injuries are not present, and based on statistics, probabilities for injuries are low. The approach to patients is based on patient classifications, where individuals are classified as **asymptomatic, temporarily non-assessable, symptomatic**, and **obtunded. Asymptomatic patients** can be approached using the CCR, which has been shown to lead to the reduction in unnecessary radiography and has been demonstrated to be superior in comparison to the NEXUS criteria. For **temporarily non-assessable patients (either due to intoxication or distracting injuries)**, the approach is to assess the patient as an obtunded patient or reassess the individual after treatments of distracted injuries or return of normal mentation. **Symptomatic patients** are recognized by the presence of neck pain, midline tenderness, or neurologic signs and symptoms. Symptomatic patients need to be initially evaluated with either 3-view C-spine x-rays or preferably CT; symptomatic patients with negative CT who are suspected of having ligamentous injuries need to be further evaluated with MRI of the C-spine, and if both CT and MRI are negative, then the patients can be discharged with a collar for comfort; however, if the patient has persistent neck pain after 2 weeks, flexion/extension films are recommended to assess C-spine stability. **All symptomatic patients should be evaluated by a spine specialist prior to discharge from the ED.**

For **obtunded trauma patients** (altered mental status or prolonged intubation, psychiatric disturbances or uncooperative), the initial evaluation is CT of the C-spine. If this is negative, there are two options; one option is to clear the C-spine, and the second option is to perform MRI to rule out ligamentous injuries. The major argument against MRI is the cost of the study paired with the very low incidence in the literature of stable C-spine injuries with a negative CT scan. The main argument for use of MRI is the severity of possible consequences of C-collar clearance in a patient with a rare, unstable C-spine injury, which may include neurologic damage or even paralysis. It should be pointed out that current trauma guidelines support clearing the C-collar in the obtunded patient after negative high-quality CT alone. Still, all obtunded trauma patients should be evaluated by trauma and/or spine specialists, as this is still a controversial area, and clinical judgment is an important factor.

Emergency Department Management of C-spine Injuries

The **initial management of any patient with C-spine injuries is to prioritize the ABCs, as most C-spine injuries do not occur as isolated injuries**. Early definitive airways may be required for some patients who develop soft tissue swelling of the neck that lead to airway compromise. Similarly, definitive airway and mechanical ventilation may be required in patients with paralysis or muscle weakness associated with C-spine injuries. Definitive airway management in these patients is best accomplished by in-line C-spine stabilization and orotracheal intubations, following rapid-sequence induction. It is important to bear in mind that most of the respiratory accessory muscles receive their motor innervations from the thoracic level, and the diaphragm receives its innervations from C3-C5; therefore, patients with compromised ventilation secondary to C-spine injuries generally do not exhibit any external signs of respiratory distress, **and the most reliable way to detect hypoventilation is by $Paco_2$ measurements on arterial blood gas**. Estimation of neurologic deficits can be determined based on physical examinations and radiographic evidence of fracture and/or dislocation. From C1 to C7, nerve roots exit above the level of the vertebrae, and from C8 and below, nerve roots exit below the vertebrae.

If possible, it is always preferable to perform a thorough motor-sensory examination prior to intubation. For patients with spinal cord injuries, a mean arterial pressure of 85-90 mm Hg should be maintained to maximize spinal cord perfusion. If needed, patients with isolated spinal cord injuries may benefit from initiation of vasopressors, such as dopamine or norepinephrine. Bradycardia associated with neurogenic shock can be addressed with atropine.

The priorities for any spinal cord injury patients are to address the life-threatening injuries first followed by management of the limb and quality-of-life threatening injuries.

Role of Corticosteroids for Spinal Cord Injuries

In the past, corticosteroids were a mainstay of therapy in the early management of spinal cord injury patients; however, more recent studies show they have high risks without clinical benefit. Treatment with corticosteroids is associated with increased rates of sepsis and other steroid-associated medical complications. In light of these published data, the application of corticosteroids for spinal cord injured patients is discouraged, and steroids should not be initiated for these patients.

Management of Upper Extremity Injuries

Upper extremity injuries are commonly encountered in the ED. Inappropriate diagnosis and management in the ED can lead to chronic pain and threaten recreational and vocational activities. Orthopedic injuries to the upper extremities are categorized by the bone, location (proximal, midshaft, or distal), presence or absence of joint involvement, degree of angulation, extent of comminution, and whether the fracture is open or closed.

Forearm fractures: Rotation of the forearm is crucial for hand function and activities of daily living. Normally, the radius rotates around the fixed ulna, and the ability of these bones to rotate around each other depends on the shape of the bones and their positions in relationship to each other. Initial evaluations of patients require careful determination of neurovascular status of the extremity followed by x-rays. Injuries that involve only one of the two bones are generally stable and are treated by closed manipulation, cast immobilization under conscious sedation, or ultrasound-guided regional nerve blocks. **Most displaced fractures that involve both the ulna and radius are considered unstable fractures** and are less amendable to closed fixations; therefore, many of these fractures are managed by open-reduction and internal fixations.

Distal radius fractures: This is one of the most common fractures encountered in children and adults. The bimodal distribution of this injury demonstrates a peak in late childhood (predominantly males) and after the sixth decade of life (predominantly females). The most common mechanism associated with this injury is a ground-level fall with outstretched hand. The **Colles-Pouteau fracture** is a fracture of the distal radial metaphysis with dorsal displacement of the distal fragment, and this represents the most commonly encountered distal radial fracture. In children, distal radius fractures are grouped as **metaphyseal and physeal fractures.** Physeal fractures demonstrating involvement of the growth plate and can be further classified by the **Salter-Harris classifications.** Most of distal radius fractures in children are treated by closed reduction and cast fixation. The goals of a management in adults are to restore bone alignment and avoid shortening of the radius. The decision to treat patients by closed reduction and fixation versus operative reduction and fixation are determined by the degree of alignment, age, and functional status of the patients. Common complications associated with these injuries are malunion, nerve injury, tendon injury, stiffness, and chronic pain.

Carpal bone fractures: There are eight carpal bones in the hand. Carpal bones in general have limited blood supply and are susceptible to avascular necrosis following injuries. Often, details of fractures and/or dislocations of the carpal bones are difficult to visualize by plain radiography; therefore, CTs or MRIs are sometimes used to determine the location and extent of injuries. Most displaced fractures are managed by operative reduction and fixation. Some of the stable, non-displaced carpal fractures can be initially approached with cast fixation.

The management of any carpal injuries should be discussed with an orthopedic or hand specialist.

Metacarpal and phalangeal fractures: These fractures can be sometimes overlooked, especially in a patient with multisystem injuries. The failure to identify and treat these injuries could lead to potential finger misalignment, pain, and functional loss. The goal of management of metacarpal fractures is to preserve bone length, rotational functions, and articular functions, which can be accomplished by either immobilization or internal fixation. The goal of managing phalangeal fractures is to minimize angulation and rotational deformities. Functional recoveries in most cases require patients' participation in rehabilitation programs. Early involvement of a hand or orthopedic specialist is vital in the management of these patients.

CASE CORRELATION

- See also Case 1 (Airway Management/Respiratory Failure), Case 2 (Hemorrhagic Shock), Case 43 (Penetrating Trauma to the Chest, Abdomen, and Extremities), and Case 45 (Trauma at Extremes of Age).

COMPREHENSION QUESTIONS

44.1 A 78-year-old man is brought to the emergency center from an extended care facility. The patient reportedly was found to have fallen down in the bathroom. He has contusions over his face and is confused. According to reports by his caretakers, this is his baseline mental status. How would you clear his C-spine?

    A. Palpation of his C-spine for tenderness; if it is not tender, then ask him to turn his head and if no pain is reported, the C-spine is cleared.

    B. Keep him in C-spine precaution and reexamine him later when his mental status is improved.

    C. Obtain CT, MRI; if these are negative, obtain flexion/extension films.

    D. CT of the C-spine.

    E. Remove the collar if he denies neck pain.

44.2 Which of the following approaches is most appropriate for the clearance of the C-spine in a 25-year-old man who is the driver of a car struck from behind? He is hemodynamically stable, nonintoxicated, and has a GCS of 15.

    A. NEXUS criteria

    B. Canadian C-spine rule

    C. CT of the C-spine

    D. 3-view x-ray of the C-spine

    E. Remove the collar because he does not have any pain

44.3 A 22-year-old man has a C5 fracture and C5-C6 subluxation, absence of motor or sensory functions below the C4 level, heart rate of 45 beats per minute, and blood pressure of 100/60 mm Hg. Which of the following is the most appropriate next step in management?

A. Maintain mean arterial pressure >85-90 mm Hg

B. Surgical airway

C. Orotracheal intubation with rapid sequence induction

D. Blind nasotracheal intubation

E. Administer atropine 1 mg intravenously

44.4 Which of the following patients' presentations is most compatible with the Brown-Sequard syndrome?

A. A 20-year-old man with absence of all motor/sensory functions in all extremities

B. A 20-year-old man with greater weakness in the upper extremities than the lower extremities

C. A 20-year-old man with complete motor paralysis, loss of vibratory sensation and proprioception on the ipsilateral side, and contralateral loss of pain and temperature sensation

D. A 20-year-old man with fracture/dislocation of C5-C6 and intact motor/sensory functions throughout

E. A 20-year-old man with normal CT of the C-spine and motor and sensory deficits below the C6 level

ANSWERS

44.1 **D.** For this patient with chronic altered mental status due to underlying medical conditions, the approach to clear his C-spine is one directed toward obtunded patients, since the patient's responses are not reliable. His C-spine can be cleared based on a normal CT of the C-spine alone, which is sufficient to identify greater than 99% of all vertebral bony fractures/dislocations. An MRI can be considered following the CT results, depending on the clinical judgment of the trauma and neurosurgical physicians.

44.2 **B.** The Canadian C-spine rule (CCR) is an approach developed for the clearance of C-spines in asymptomatic patients following low-mechanism events. The CCR has been compared to the NEXUS criteria and found to be more specific and sensitive in clearance of the C-spine.

44.3 **C.** This patient has signs consistent with neurogenic shock following a high spinal cord injury. The first concerns are his airway and ventilation. The airway appears to be clear, but he needs a definitive airway to maintain optimal ventilation. Orotracheal intubation with rapid sequence induction and in-line C-spine stabilization is the optimal airway strategy for this patient. Maintenance of adequate pulse and blood pressure is important to maintain spinal cord perfusion, but these steps should be delayed until a secured airway is established. Remember the ABCs.

44.4 **C.** The Brown-Sequard syndrome is caused by posterior spinal cord injury, characterized by paralysis, loss of vibratory sensation and proprioception on the ipsilateral side, and loss of pain and temperature sensation on the contralateral side. Patient described in A is compatible with complete cord injury. The patient described in B is compatible with central cord injury. The patient in D appears to have vertebral fractures/dislocation without neurologic compromises. The patient in E has a spinal cord injury without radiographic abnormality (SCIWORA); SCIWORAs occur more commonly in children than adults.

CLINICAL PEARLS

▶ The initial management of any patient with C-spine injuries is to prioritize the ABCs and includes assuring an effective airway.

▶ The Canadian C-spine rule is an effective evaluation system to clinically clear C-spines in asymptomatic patients.

▶ Symptomatic patients need to be initially evaluated with either 3-view C-spine x-rays or preferably CT; symptomatic patients with negative CT who are suspected of having ligamentous injuries need to be further evaluated with MRI of the C-spine.

▶ Cervical spine injuries occur in 1% to 3% of all victims following blunt trauma.

▶ Distal radius fractures have a bimodal pattern with peaks in late childhood and after the sixth decade of life.

REFERENCES

Abraham MK, Scott S. The emergent evaluation and treatment of hand and wrist injuries. *Emerg Med Clin N Am*. 2010;28:789-809.

Anderson PA, Gugala Z, Lindsey RW, et al. Clearing the cervical spine in the blunt trauma patient. *J Am Acad Orthop Surg*. 2010;18:149-159.

Como JJ, Diaz JJ, Dunham C, et al. Cervical spine injuries following trauma. *J Trauma*. 2009;67: 651-659.

Congress of Neurological Surgeons. Guidelines for the Management of Acute Cervical Spine and Spinal Cord Injuries. 2013;72:1-259.

Heggeness MH, Gannon FH, Weinberg J, et al. Orthopedic surgery. In: Brunicardi FC, Andersen DK, Billiar TR, et al, eds. *Schwartz's Principles of Surgery*. 9th ed. New York, NY: McGraw-Hill; 2010:1557-1608.

Lifchez SD, Sen SK. Surgery of the hand and wrist. In: Brunicardi FC, Andersen DK, Billiar TR, et al, eds. *Schwartz's Principles of Surgery*. 9th ed. New York, NY: McGraw-Hill; 2010:1609-1645.

Petel MB, Humble SS, Cullinane DC, et al. Cervical spine collar clearance in the obtunded adult blunt trauma patient. *J Trauma*. 2015;78:430-441.

It is approximately 2 AM when a woman presents to the emergency department (ED) with her 3-year-old son. According to the mother, the patient was playing and fell off the upper level of his bunk bed earlier in the evening. On examination, the child is somnolent. His pulse rate is 110 beats per minute, blood pressure is 100/85 mm Hg, respiratory rate is 28 breaths per minute, and Glasgow coma scale (GCS) score is 11 (eye opening 2, verbal 5, motor 4). There is presence of soft-tissue contusion over the left frontal scalp and ecchymosis over the left periorbital region. The lungs are clear with bilateral breath sounds. The abdomen is mildly distended and tender throughout. The patient's left thigh is markedly swollen and tender, and all his extremities are mottled and cool.

▶ What is the most likely mechanism responsible for this patient's clinical picture?
▶ What are the next steps in the management of this patient?

ANSWERS TO CASE 45:

Trauma and Extremes of Age

Summary: A 3-year-old boy presents several hours after an unwitnessed fall, with somnolence and external signs of head injury. In addition to the contusions on the scalp, his abdomen is distended and tender, left thigh is swollen and tender, and his skin is mottled and cool.

- **Most likely responsible mechanism:** This child has multiple injuries, possibly secondary to intentional trauma.

- **Next steps in management:** Pediatric trauma resuscitation and evaluation to include administration of intravenous fluids, a thorough examination, and a computed tomography (CT) scan of the head and abdomen. **Protection of the child by reporting potential child abuse, and admission to the hospital.**

ANALYSIS

Objectives

1. Become familiar with the evaluation and management of pediatric and geriatric patients with multiple severe injuries presenting in shock.

2. Recognize the signs in the presentation of children and elderly patients that are consistent with abuse and become familiar with the appropriate response.

Considerations

The presentation of this child should raise concerns for multiple reasons, and it is vitally important to appropriately prioritize your attention to these concerns. The first priority should be to address his medical condition and not the mechanism of the injury. This patient's vital signs presented in the case scenario are not out of the range of normal for his age (Table 45–1). Despite the normal vital signs, his general presentation indicates the potential for multisystem injuries, and combined with the findings of mottled and cool skin, it is indicated that this child is in **hemorrhagic shock until proven otherwise.** The vital signs of an injured child can be within normal ranges for an extended period of time due to an excellent ability to compensate physiologically for hypovolemia. However, when the limits of that compensatory

Table 45–1 • NORMAL VITAL SIGNS BY AGE GROUP			
Age Group (Years)	Heart Rate (Beats/Min)	Blood Pressure (mm Hg)	Respiratory Rate (Breaths/Min)
0-1	120	80/40	40
1-5	100	100/60	30
5-10	80	120/80	20

reserve are reached, the ability of a child to tolerate shock is poor and his condition will likely decline very rapidly.

The secondary concern regarding this child is the manner in which he presented, suggesting potential abuse. Factors that raise these concerns include the **delay in presentation**, the extent of **the injuries that appear much more severe than can be accounted for by the history**, the age of the child, and the **unwitnessed report** of the injury. All 50 states have mandatory child abuse reporting laws for the treating physician. Regardless of the management plan, this child should be placed in a protected environment (admission to the hospital), and a report of suspected abuse should be submitted. However, the treating physician's suspicions or emotions should not delay the child's medical care (which is the first responsibility). Accurate and complete evaluations and documentation of your findings in an unbiased manner are the first important steps. Confrontations with family members in the midst of a trauma room evaluation are rarely fruitful and can hamper your efforts to care for the child.

APPROACH TO:

Trauma at Extremes of Age

CLINICAL APPROACH

A **systematic and expeditious approach** to children with unknown injury mechanisms or mechanisms capable of producing multisystem injury should include a rapid survey for all potential injuries, **consideration of the need for intubation, administration of intravenous fluids, and the prevention of heat loss. CT scan of the head and abdomen** may be obtained for further evaluation as needed, and the patient should be prepared for operative care as indicated. In those patients with multiple injuries identified, prioritizing the most life-threatening problem is of paramount importance. Even when intracranial hemorrhage may be suspected on the basis of physical presentation, the immediate threat to most children with multisystem injury is hypovolemic shock from abdominal injury and other hemorrhagic sources. Addressing blood loss source is critical not only for the correction of hemorrhagic shock but also for the prevention of secondary brain injury in these patients.

The guidelines found in the advanced trauma life support (ATLS) and advanced pediatric life support (APLS) manuals should be followed in the initial management of injured children. The **initial priorities** are the assessment and maintenance of **airway, oxygenation, and ventilation**. Determination for immediate intubation is dependent on the initial evaluation of the child and the resources available. Certainly, if there is any **airway compromise**, or if the **neurological status** raises concern of airway protection (a **GCS score <9;** Table 45–2), then **intubation is mandatory**. If the airway is not compromised and the GCS score is adequate, then the decision for elective intubation may be determined by the level of patient cooperation for the timely completion of potentially lifesaving diagnostic studies, such as CT imaging.

The circulation and neurological status should be the next priorities. Approximately 90% of pediatric patients presenting with blunt trauma are successfully

Table 45–2 • PEDIATRIC GCS VERBAL SCORES	
5	Appropriate words or social smile, fixes and follows
4	Cries, but consolable
3	Persistently irritable
2	Restless, agitated
1	None

managed without operative intervention. However, the **initial signs of shock, including tachycardia, skin changes, and lethargy, represent a loss of approximately 25% of the child's blood volume** (Table 45–3). The likelihood of injury requiring operative control of hemorrhage is much greater in these children, and careful attention should be paid to the amount of fluid or blood that is required to maintain stable vital signs. A large-bore IV should be started, and two sequential boluses of **20 mL/kg of warmed crystalloid solution** should be administered. If further fluids are required beyond this, then administration of packed red blood cells (10 mL/kg) should be considered. Evaluation of the **abdomen by ultrasound (if unstable) or CT scan** should be performed to determine the extent of injuries. **If the vital signs worsen** during the attempt to obtain a head and abdominal CT scan, this should be abandoned and a **laparotomy performed** to control any hemorrhage.

There is no doubt that the child in this case often presents a considerable challenge. Not only does the possibility of abuse evoke strong emotions that are difficult to ignore during the evaluation, but there is also potential of multiple life-threatening injuries that must be prioritized. A systematic and efficient approach, with focus on the most immediate of concerns, cannot be emphasized enough (Table 45–4).

Table 45–3 • SYSTEMIC RESPONSES TO BLOOD LOSS IN THE PEDIATRIC PATIENT		
<25% Blood Volume Loss	25%-45% Blood Volume Loss	>45% Blood Volume Loss
Weak, thready pulse; increased heart rate	Increased heart rate	Hypotension, tachycardia to bradycardia
Lethargic, irritable, confused	Change in the level of consciousness, dulled response to pain	Comatose
Cool, clammy	Cyanotic, decreased capillary refill, cold extremities	Pale, cold
Minimal decrease in urinary output; increased specific gravity	Minimal urine output	No urine output

Data from ATLS Manual, American College of Surgeons. 1997:297.

Table 45–4 • INITIAL MANAGEMENT OF THE INJURED CHILD
Primary survey • Establishment of a reliable airway • Ventilation • Establishment of large-bore IV lines • Support of circulation • Rapid assessment of neurological status
Secondary survey • Diagnostic studies • Establishment of surgical priorities • Mass lesion in the brain • Chest and abdominal injuries • Peripheral vascular injuries • Fractures

Data from O'Neill JA. Principles of Pediatric Surgery. St Louis, MO: Mosby; 2003:783.

THE BATTERED CHILD

There are very few things encountered by physicians that will evoke as strong, distasteful emotions as child abuse, making one think that reporting of these cases would not be a significant problem. However, to report a case of child abuse, the physician must first recognize that it is child abuse. The subtleties of recognizing child abuse, as well as the fear of making incorrect accusations of caregivers who appear well-meaning, can make this a difficult issue. The reporting and protection of the battered child is further confounded by the legal requirements for appropriate and complete documentation by the physician, which often is lacking if suspicions of abuse were not entertained upon initial presentation.

Intentional injury accounts for approximately 10% of all trauma cases in children younger than 5 years old. While this figure may be alarming, it also suggests that the vast majority of trauma in children is actually accidental. There are several key aspects of the history, physical examination, and presentation of the child that should alert the practitioner to the possibility that the trauma was not accidental. Table 45–5 lists suggestive characteristics that should alert the practitioner to abuse. Skin and soft-tissue injuries are the most common injuries encountered in child abuse cases. This is followed by fractures, which often are multiple or repetitive. The third most common problem with child abuse is head injury. Unfortunately, this is also the injury with the highest mortality.

Currently, there is no federal standard regarding the legal requirements for reporting of child abuse. However, all states have mandatory reporting legislation for suspected child abuse that includes healthcare workers, school personnel, social workers, and law enforcement officers. Very few states recognize the physician-patient communication privilege as exempt from these reporting requirements. Most states impose either a fine or imprisonment penalty to individuals who knowingly or willfully fail to report abuse. However, several states also impose penalties for false reports of child abuse.

When intentional injury is suspected in a pediatric trauma case, the appropriate child protective agency should be notified after the child's medical condition is addressed.

Table 45–5 • PATTERNS SUGGESTING PHYSICAL ABUSE	
Presentation	Age younger than 3 years (limited ability to communicate) Significant delay between injury and presentation Presence of risk factors • Chronic illness • Premature birth • Congenital deficiencies • Mental delay
History	Unwitnessed injury Injuries not consistent or more significant than suggested by the history Evasive responses Reported self-injury not consistent with the child's stage of development
Physical Examination	Multiple injuries Signs of prior injuries and fractures Injuries and different stages of healing Pattern of injuries • Demarcated buttock-scalding injuries • Retinal hemorrhage • Multiple bruises • Hand or whip marks • Cigarette burns

During the investigational process, it is often incumbent on the medical personnel to provide a high-visibility protected environment for the child. Although it is often emotionally tempting for the physician to become involved in the investigational process, it is important at this stage to **maintain focus on the medical condition.** This becomes particularly important in terms of adequate documentation. A **complete, unbiased, and well-recorded history and physical** examination can be vital in the protection of the child at a later date.

Particularly important information includes detailed descriptions of the reported mechanism of the injury, the time of the injury and any delay in presentation, the presence of witnesses, conflicts, and inconsistencies. A complete physical examination should be documented and should include pictures or diagrams of all bruises, documentation of the color of each bruise, a complete neurological examination, and a genital examination. An eye examination for retinal hemorrhages should be performed because this is often encountered with cerebral trauma and the "shaken baby syndrome." Radiographic evaluations should be performed on all extremities to search for patterns of previous injury (Table 45–6). Any reports from previous admissions (including from other hospitals) should be referenced.

GERIATRIC TRAUMA

Older patients often have coexisting medical problems that may impact the response to acute injuries. Details surrounding the initial injuring events are frequently relevant (eg, medication reactions, chest pains, and strokes). Nevertheless, the basic approach to trauma in the elderly patient is the same as the approach to the adult patient.

Table 45–6 • MUSCULOSKELETAL MANIFESTATIONS OF ABUSE
Spiral fractures attributed to falls
Subperiosteal calcification with no history of injury
Multiple fractures in various stages of healing
Bucket-handle fractures or epiphyseal–metaphyseal separation and fragmentation from pulling or shaking forces
Unexplained fractures associated with chronic subdural hematomas

Data from, O'Neill JA. Principles of Pediatric Surgery. *St Louis, MO: Mosby; 2003.*

When assessing the geriatric trauma patient, the possibility of elder abuse must be taken into consideration. If elder abuse is suspected, practitioners should follow the same steps used when assessing suspected child abuse.

Physiological Changes

The older age group is one of the fastest growing population sectors in the United States. Thus, the number of geriatric trauma incidents, arbitrarily defined as affecting those older than age 65-70 years, is expected to likewise increase. Injuries in these individuals are associated with a higher mortality and longer hospital stay. Many physiological changes occur with aging (Table 45–7), including the progressive loss of myocyte number and increase in myocyte volume, resulting in ventricular stiffness and cardiac diastolic dysfunction. Furthermore, atherosclerotic changes cause large vessel stiffness and increased afterload. Additionally, aging contributes to diminution of cardiac β-adrenergic response, leading to diminished heart rate response.

Table 45–7 • PHYSIOLOGICAL ALTERATIONS ASSOCIATED WITH AGING
Cardiovascular
• Loss of myocyte with reciprocal increase in myocyte volume and diminution in cardiac diastolic volume
• Large vessel calcification with increase in afterload
• Diminished cardiac chronotropic response to β-adrenergic stimulation
• Intimal hyperplasia and decreased vascular compliance result in decreased arterial perfusion
Pulmonary
• Decrease in forced expiratory volume in 1 second (FEV_1) due to decrease in respiratory muscle strength and increase in chest-wall rigidity
• Decrease in functional respiratory alveolar surface area
Renal
• Diminution in renal size after age 50
• Glomerulosclerosis may occur as the result of degenerative processes such as hypertension and diabetes, leading to loss of glomerular filtration rate (GFR)
Hepatic
• Decrease in liver size after age 50
• Diminished and delayed regenerative capacity of the liver
Immunological
• Impairment in T-lymphocyte–mediated immunity resulting in increased infection risks
• Inflammatory mediated responses are diminished (TNF-alpha, IL-1, IL-6, and leukocyte adhesion molecule expression) leading to diminished inflammatory responses

Because of the age-related cardiovascular changes, **the elderly patient is much less capable of responding to increases in cardiac output demands. Myocardial infarction is the leading cause of death among 80-year-old patients in the postoperative and post-injury settings.** The elderly patient's limited ability to respond to stress and injuries has prompted some groups to apply age (>70 years) as the sole criteria for trauma-team activation, and by adapting to this approach, these investigators have demonstrated significant reduction in geriatric trauma mortality.

Outcome Predictors in Geriatric Patients

Various groups have attempted to identify outcome predictors in geriatric trauma patients (Table 45–8). "High-risk" patients can be identified based on mechanism, physiological parameter, and laboratory parameters. In the management of "high-risk" patients, early admission to the ICU with earlier initiation of invasive hemo-dynamic monitoring, along with aggressive resuscitation based on hemodynamic parameters, are associated with a reduction in geriatric trauma patient mortality. Thus, **expedited patient disposition to allow early invasive monitoring** and **resuscitation** is helpful. Scalea and colleagues (1990) showed that early resuscitation of the "high-risk" elderly trauma patients with **goals directed** at attaining **cardiac output** of more than 3.5 L/min and/or a **mixed venous saturation of greater than 50%** led to an improvement in survival from 7% in historical control patients to 53% in the aggressively managed patients. More recent observations have not supported aggressive resuscitation measures based on predetermined parameters because overly aggressive fluid resuscitation can contribute to pulmonary and cardiovascular complications. Close observations and monitoring directed toward the avoidance of tissue hypoperfusion and minimizing stresses related to hypothermia and pain are the important priorities during the initial management of older victims of traumatic injuries.

Given the overall poorer survival of geriatric trauma patients, some questions have been raised regarding the quality of life of the survivors. Long-term studies of

Table 45–8 • PREDICTORS OF MORBIDITY AND MORTALITY
MORBIDITY PREDICTORS
Mechanisms
• Automobile-pedestrian collision
• Diffuse beating
Physiological parameters
• SBP <150
Laboratory parameters
• Base deficit (≤6 mEq/L)
• Lactic acid (>2.4 mmol/L)
Anatomical injuries
• Blunt chest trauma with rib fractures
MORTALITY PREDICTORS
• SBP <90
• Hypoventilation (respiratory rate <10/min)
• GCS = 3

geriatric trauma patients indicate that the majority of survivors return to a level of previous independence. Factors associated with long-term **reduced independence** include **hemodynamic shock upon admission, GCS score <7, age >75 years, head injury, and sepsis.**

CASE CORRELATION

- See Case 2 (Hemorrhagic Shock), Case 43 (Penetrating Trauma to the Chest, Abdomen, and Extremities), and Case 44 (Extremity Fracture and Neck Pain).

COMPREHENSION QUESTIONS

45.1 A 3-year-old boy is brought into the ED with multiple bruises, abrasions, and several deep lacerations over the flank region. The parents state that he fell out of his bed. Which of the following is the most important next step in this patient?

A. Reporting these injuries to child protective services

B. Firmly, but without judgment, confront the parents with the discrepancy of the story and the injuries

C. Take accurate pictures of the injuries and seal them in an evidence envelope

D. Evaluate the ABCs and any urgent injuries

E. Station guards in front of the exits of the building to prevent the parents from leaving

45.2 An 11-month-old infant is brought into the ED after rolling down a staircase while still buckled into the infant car seat. The baby is crying but is consolable by his mother. His heart rate is 116 beats per minute and blood pressure 80/40 mm Hg at rest. The physical examination reveals only slight bruising over the knees. The abdomen is nontender. Which of the following is the best next step?

A. CT scan of the abdomen to assess for intraperitoneal hemorrhage

B. Chest radiograph to assess for pleural hemorrhage

C. Continued observation and reassurance

D. IV access and infusion of normal saline 10 mL/kg

E. Transfuse 10 mL/kg PRBC

45.3 An 80-year-old woman was a pedestrian struck by an automobile travel-ing at a speed of 20 miles per hour. An evaluation identified right tibia and fibula fracture, right pubic ramus fracture, and facial lacerations. Her vital signs are a pulse of 80 beats per minute, blood pressure of 120/70 mm Hg, respiratory rate of 20 breaths per minute, and a GCS score of 15. Which of the following sequences of events is the most appropriate in management of this patient?

A. Computed tomography (CT) scan of the abdomen; plain x-rays of the pelvis, lower extremities, and spine; splinting of fractures; and invasive monitoring in the ICU

B. CT scan of the abdomen; splinting of fractures; invasive monitoring in ICU; and x-rays of the pelvis and lower extremities

C. Invasive monitoring in ICU; splinting of the fractures; and CT of abdomen

D. Splinting of fractures; invasive monitoring in the ICU; CT of abdomen; and x-rays of the extremities and pelvis

E. Exploratory laparotomy, splinting of the femur fracture, and pelvic fixation

ANSWERS

45.1 **D.** The first and foremost priority is the patient's medical condition and as normal, initially addressing the ABCs. Child protective services probably do need to be notified, and the injuries do need to be documented. In general, the parents should not be confronted but rather asked about their story.

45.2 **C.** The normal heart rate and blood pressure levels of a child are substan-tially different from that of any adult. These values are normal for this infant; therefore, more aggressive measures are not indicated at this time.

45.3 **B.** This sequence of events outlined is most appropriate for immediate iden-tification of a possible intra-abdominal hemorrhagic source in a patient with injury mechanism capable of producing multiple injuries. When this life-threatening problem is ruled out, the next steps are early invasive monitor-ing in the ICU and stabilization of fractures to decrease pain and injuries to adjacent soft tissue, while simultaneous efforts are made to identify other non—life-threatening injuries. Exploratory laparotomy is not indicated in this patient at this time because she is hemodynamically stable and without clear signs of intra-abdominal injuries.

CLINICAL PEARLS

▶ The first priority in evaluating a pediatric or geriatric trauma patient is the ABCs.

▶ The most life-threatening injury in intentional child injury is head injury.

▶ Soft-tissue and skin injuries are the most common child injury.

▶ Myocardial infarction is the leading cause of death among 80-year-old patients in the postinjury setting.

▶ Early management of the geriatric trauma patient should be directed toward early monitoring of patients to avoid hypovolemia, inadequate treatment of pain, and hypothermia.

REFERENCES

Committee on Pediatric Emergency Medicine Council on Injury, Violence, and Poison Injury, Section on Critical Care, Section on Orthopaedics, Section on Surgery, Section on Transport Medicine, Pediatric Trauma Society, and Society of Trauma Nurses Pediatric Committee. *Pediatrics*. 2016;138: 1516-1569.

Cooper A. Early assessment and management of trauma. In: Whitefield Holcomb III G, Murphy JP, Ostlie DJ, eds. *Ashcraft's Pediatric Surgery*. 5th ed. Philadelphia, PA: Saunders Elsevier; 2010: 167-181.

Reske-Nielsen C, Medzon R. Geriatric trauma. *Emergency Med Clin North Am*. 2016;34:483-500.

Victorino GP, Chong TJ, Pal JD. Trauma in the elderly patient. *Arch Surg*. 2003;138:1093-1098.

A 32-year-old man, involved in a motor vehicle collision (MVC), is brought to the emergency department (ED). He lost control of his car and hit a utility pole with the front end of his car while traveling at approximately 35 MPH. He was thrown against the windshield of the car, hitting his face and forehead against the windshield. There was no loss of consciousness. His blood pressure is 125/79 mm Hg, heart rate is 92 beats per minute, respiratory rate is 16 breaths per minute, and pulse oxygenation is 99% on room air. On examination, he has a 7-cm laceration on the right side of his face that courses from his right ear to just below the lower lip. He is alert and has no focal neurologic deficits on examination. When he is asked to smile, the right side of his mouth droops.

▶ What is the most likely diagnosis?
▶ What is the most appropriate therapy?

ANSWERS TO CASE 46:
Facial Laceration

Summary: A 32-year-old man presents to the ED after an MVC. There is no evidence of injury except for a 7-cm laceration on the right side of his face, which courses from his ear to across the cheek and ends just below the right lower lip. His neurologic examination is normal except for the inability to smile on the right side.

- **Most likely diagnosis:** Right facial nerve laceration.

- **Most appropriate therapy:** Microsurgical repair of right facial nerve and closure of skin laceration.

ANALYSIS

Objectives

1. Understand the critical structures that can be injured in facial lacerations.

2. Understand the need for tetanus immunization in trauma patients.

3. Know the basic principles of facial laceration repair.

Considerations

This patient suffered a laceration across his right cheek after being involved in an MVC. The **mainstay in trauma management includes managing the airway, breathing, and circulation (ABCs).** Once the primary survey is complete, the physician then performs the secondary survey, which includes a head-to-toe physical examination that evaluates for non-life-threatening injuries. **Any trauma to the head, face, or neck should raise concern for a cervical spine (C-spine) injury.** If there is suspicion for a C-spine injury, the patient should be placed in a rigid cervical collar until either appropriate imaging can be performed or appropriate clinical evaluation completed. Facial trauma often results in bony injuries to the orbits and mandible. Injury to cranial nerves (CN) V and VII are common. The facial nerve (CN VII) exits the stylomastoid foramen and branches into motor and sensory branches to the temporal, zygomatic, buccal, and mental regions. Lacerations to the **buccal branch** are associated with injury to the **parotid duct.** Identification of a **facial nerve injury** is critical because **delayed diagnosis results in poor outcome.** Microsurgical techniques give fairly good results. After repair of the injury, the patient needs a **tetanus immunization** if the last time the patient received a tetanus vaccine was longer than 5 years ago.

> # APPROACH TO:
> ## Facial Lacerations

DEFINITIONS

FACIAL TRAUMA: Any soft or deep tissue injury secondary to physical force, burns, or foreign objects to the following structures: the scalp, forehead, nose, eyes, lips, cheeks, tongue, oral cavity, and jaw.

VERMILLION BORDER: The junction between the lip and facial skin. An injury to this area can result in a significant cosmetic defect if not repaired correctly.

AURICULAR HEMATOMA: Collection of blood in the ear that results from the traumatic interruption of the perichondrium and cartilage. If left untreated, it can evolve into a fibrous mass, leaving the affected ear with a cauliflower-like appearance.

SADDLE NOSE DEFORMITY: Nasal injury secondary to the necrotic breakdown of the septal cartilage. It is caused by a traumatic injury to the nose resulting in a nasal septal hematoma. If the hematoma is left untreated, it separates the septal cartilage from its perichondrium, depriving it of its nutrient supply.

TETANUS: An often fatal infectious disease caused by the bacteria *Clostridium tetani*, which usually enters the body through a puncture, cut, or open wound.

CLINICAL APPROACH

The basic approach to wound care includes assessment for other injuries, probing the depth of the wound, irrigation, a neurovascular examination, and deciding on whether primary closure is advisable (ie, leave open if infection is likely, such as contamination or delay in presentation). The length of time the suture stays in place and the type of suture depends on the body location (Table 46–1). Additionally, the need to update the patient's tetanus vaccination should be assessed.

Table 46–1 • SUTURE SIZE FOR CORRESPONDING ANATOMIC REGION	
Anatomic Region	**Suture Size**
Face	5-0 to 6-0
Scalp	3-0 to 5-0
Chest	3-0 to 4-0
Back	3-0 to 4-0
Abdomen	3-0 to 4-0
Extremities	4-0 to 5-0
Joints	3-0 to 4-0
Oral	3-0 to 5-0 absorbable

Irrigation

When the decision to suture is made, a stepwise preparation must take place. All wounds must first be irrigated and explored for foreign bodies and environmental debris. Proper irrigation can significantly reduce the risk of wound infection. High-pressure and large-volume irrigation remains the gold standard to reduce or eliminate particulate matter and bacterial loads from the wound. This is usually established with a 35- to 60-mL syringe and 16- to 19-gauge catheter using constant hand pressure. This generates a pressure of 5-8 psi, which is adequate to irrigate a wound. Sterile saline is the most commonly used irrigant. Application of povidone iodine, hydrogen peroxide, and detergents should be avoided because of their toxic effects on tissue.

Anesthesia

Once irrigation is complete and the wound is examined, anesthesia should be administered. Delaying anesthesia until irrigation is completed allows the patient to reveal any sensation of a retained foreign body that might dislodge during irrigation. Local anesthetics are divided into two major groups, amides and esters. Although it is rare, some patients are allergic to anesthetics. However, if a patient is allergic to one class, the other class can be safely administered. It is thought that the allergy is to the preservative in the anesthetic, rather than the anesthetic itself (Table 46–2).

Local anesthesia can be attained in many ways, including injection directly into the wound, topical application, and nerve block. The most common method is local infiltration. Several techniques are available to reduce pain experienced by the patient during injection. These include using smaller gauge needles, injecting at a slow rate, infiltrating the wound edge instead of surrounding skin, adding sodium bicarbonate

Table 46–2 • COMMONLY USED LOCAL ANESTHETICS				
Class	Name	Onset	Duration of Action (h)	Maximal Dose (mg/kg)
Amides	Bupivacaine (w/epinephrine)	Slow	4-5 7-8	2 3
	Ropivacaine (w/epinephrine)	Medium	3-4 6-7	3 3
	Mepivacaine (w/epinephrine)	Rapid	2-3 5-6	5 7
	Lidocaine (w/epinephrine)	Rapid	1-2 2-4	5 7
Esters	Procaine (w/epinephrine)	Slow	0.5-1 1-1.5	8 10
	Tetracaine (w/epinephrine)	Slow	3-4 9-10	1.5 2.5
	Prilocaine (w/epinephrine)	Medium	0.5-1 5-6	5 7.5
	Chloroprocaine (w/epinephrine)	Rapid	0.5-1 1-1.5	10 15

to the anesthetic solution at a 1:10 dilution, and warming the solution. Some authors recommend first applying topical anesthetic. This is particularly useful in the pediatric population. Initially TAC (tetracaine, 0.25%-0.5%; adrenaline, 0.025%-0.05%; cocaine, 4%-11%) was commonly used, but it was associated with seizure, arrhythmia, and cardiac arrest. LET (lidocaine, 4%; epinephrine, 0.1%; tetracaine, 0.5%) is generally safer than TAC and is used for anesthesia of the face and scalp. EMLA (eutectic mixture of local anesthetics) consists of lidocaine and prilocaine and is also commonly used. Because of the possibility for systemic absorption of lidocaine and tetracaine, these anesthetics should be avoided in large wounds and mucus membranes.

Epinephrine is added to many anesthetic solutions. This augments hemostasis and prolongs the duration of action of the anesthetic by decreasing systemic absorption through local vasoconstriction. Although it is controversial, it is recommended to **avoid injecting solutions with epinephrine into sites such as digits, the tip of the nose, ears, and penis due to the risk of necrosis. It is also advisable to avoid epinephrine in the case of a skin flap repair, as this may cause necrosis of the flap and poor healing.**

Suture Placement

To reduce scarring, sutures on the face should be placed approximately 1-2 mm from the wound edge and 3 mm apart. Cosmesis is less of a concern with other body areas.

Wound Closure

Once the wound is irrigated, explored, and anesthetized, closure can begin. Below are several methods and approaches for wound closure depending on the site of injury.

Scalp and Forehead

These lacerations are usually caused by a combination of blunt and sharp trauma. Careful inspection of the wound is critical, with care to palpate for depressed skull fractures and assess the integrity of the galea aponeurosis, which covers the periosteum. Repair usually follows the skin lines for the best cosmetic result. The **scalp should be closed with a 4-0 monofilament suture of different color than the patient's hair,** or **staples** can be used. Sutures and staples should be **removed after 7-10 days.** Because scalp lacerations can be associated with significant hemorrhage, rapid closure with staples may decrease the blood loss. If the galea is involved, it should be repaired with long-lasting absorbable suture material (eg, Vicryl and Monocryl). **Closing the galea helps to control heavy bleeding associated with scalp wounds and limits the spread of potential infection. Forehead** lacerations should be repaired in layers. The skin should be approximated with **6-0 nonabsorbable interrupted sutures, which should be removed after 5 days.** Care should be taken to precisely approximate hair lines.

Eyelids

The eyelid is thin, delicate, and functionally and cosmetically important. Because of the risk of periorbital trauma, the emergency physician should have a **low threshold to refer to an oculoplastic specialist or ophthalmologist** for evaluation and repair. This includes **lacerations to upper and lower lid margins** and those **involving the lacrimal duct.** Any laceration **medial to the puncta** should be highly concerning for a canalicular **system injury.** Staining the laceration with fluorescein dye can be used to determine damage to the canaliculus. In addition, damage to the levator palpebrae superioris muscle should be ruled out with traumatic lacerations of the upper lid.

This commonly manifests as ptosis. A majority of eyelid lacerations can be managed without suture repair, including lacerations that are superficial and involve less than 25% of the eyelid. When sutures are indicated, repair is generally undertaken **with 6-0 or 7-0 interrupted sutures, with care to stay superficial; the suture is removed after 3-5 days.**

Nose

The nose is commonly injured and is the most common fracture in domestic violence victims. It is the focal point of the face; thus, it is important to ensure proper management of nasal lacerations for optimal cosmesis. Inspection for the depth of injury is important. Infection can occur when all of the layers are penetrated or when cartilage is exposed. **Septal trauma may lead to hematoma formation, which can lead to necrosis of the septum** or **chronic obstruction of the nasal passageway.** Untreated hematoma separates the septal cartilage from its perichondrium, depriving it from the nutrient supply. The septal cartilage can necrose, resulting in a **saddle nose deformity.** Therefore, septal hematomas require drainage. Anesthesia in this area is difficult because of the tightness of skin over the cartilage, but it can be obtained via a dorsal nerve block. Injection directly into a wound can distort wound edges for repair and is extremely uncomfortable. Epinephrine must be avoided in this area. Topical lidocaine is generally helpful. Cartilage lacerations should be repaired with 4-0 or 5-0 absorbable sutures, and the skin closed with 6-0 nonabsorbable suture for 3-5 days. Lacerations to the nasal alae are usually complex and difficult to anesthetize; these wounds often require consultation of a plastic or ear, nose, and throat (ENT) surgeon.

Lips

The junction between the skin and the red portion of the lip, the vermillion border, is of vital cosmetic importance. Additionally, the orbicularis oris muscle that surrounds the mouth is critical for facial expression, speech formation, and the retention of saliva. Lacerations involving the lip that do not cross the vermillion border can be closed in layers with **6-0 nonabsorbable suture and left in place for 5 days.** If the vermillion border is disrupted, the first stitch in repair should exactly approximate the border using 6-0 nonabsorbable suture. This first suture needs to be precise **because even a 1-mm discrepancy is noticeable** (Figure 46–1). A plastic surgeon can be consulted for these injuries. Regional anesthesia is helpful, as local anesthetic infiltration can obscure the anatomy. The most common regional blocks include the mental nerve block and infraorbital block for the lower and upper lip, respectively. If a lip laceration is through and through, prophylactic penicillin, amoxicillin, cephalexin, or clindamycin is indicated. Otherwise, antibiotics are not typically indicated.

Ears

In patients with trauma to the ear region, the physician should evaluate the patient for a **basilar skull fracture** or tympanic membrane rupture. Signs of basilar skull fracture include periorbital ecchymosis (raccoon eyes), mastoid ecchymosis (Battle's sign), or hemotympanum. After inspection, cotton can be placed into the ear canal during irrigation of any lacerations. Regional auricular block is effective, and again, epinephrine should be avoided. Lacerations of the ear should be approached with

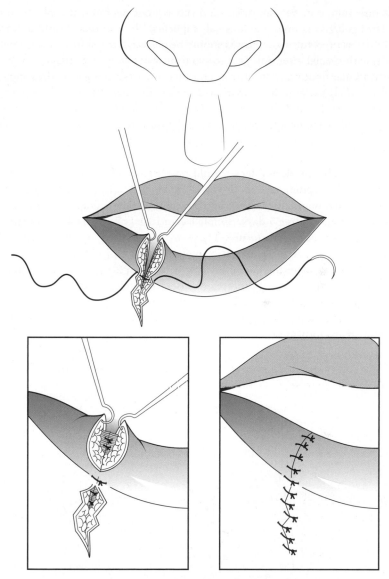

Figure 46–1. Lip laceration crossing the vermillion border. The first step is to approximate the vermillion-skin junction. The orbicularis muscle is then approximated and, finally, the skin is repaired.

the following goals: cosmesis, avoidance of hematoma, and infection prevention. Repair of lacerated ear tissue should mirror its symmetric counterpart as much as possible for the best cosmetic results. Superficial lacerations should be repaired with 6-0 nonabsorbable sutures and removed in 5 days. Meticulous hemostasis is important to prevent hematoma formation. If an auricular hematoma is present and is left unaddressed, the ear is prone to abnormal cartilage production and subsequent calcification commonly referred to as a "cauliflower ear." Auricular hematoma, avulsed tissue, or crushed cartilage is probably best handled by a plastic surgeon or otolaryngologist. Any cartilage that is exposed should be covered to reduce infection, erosive chondritis, and subsequent necrosis. If a plastic surgeon or otolaryngologist is unavailable, small superficial lacerations should be repaired with uninterrupted sutures. Sutures should be placed in the skin surrounding these wounds, with special attention paid to avoid suturing the ear cartilage, which could lead to avascular necrosis. After the laceration is repaired, a **pressure dressing should be applied to help prevent the formation of an auricular hematoma.** It is imperative to place gauze both behind the auricle and within its crevices. A gauze roll or elastic bandage should then be applied, encircling the head to produce adequate pressure.

Cheeks and Face

Lacerations of the **cheek and face** should be repaired after investigating the vital structures in the region, such as the facial nerve and parotid duct (Figure 46–2). Generally, a **6-0 monofilament interrupted suture technique is appropriate for repair. Sutures are removed after 5 days. Simple lacerations (<2 cm) isolated to the buccal cavity typically do not need closure.** These areas are highly vascularized and heal well without sutures. Proper irrigation is important to prevent complications of infection. **Lacerations in the buccal cavity greater than 2 cm have the propensity to collect food,** which can lead to infection. These typically require closure. Absorbable 5-0 sutures are preferred. All intraoral wounds are dirty wounds and are at high risk for infection. Therefore, prophylactic penicillin, amoxicillin, cephalexin, or clindamycin is indicated.

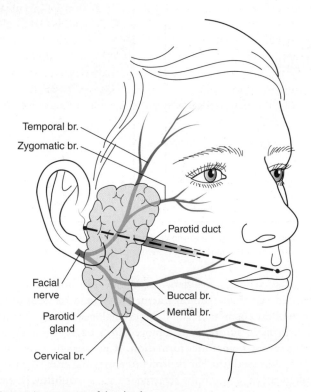

Figure 46–2. Anatomic structures of the cheek.

TETANUS IMMUNIZATION

Tetanus is an acute, often fatal, but preventable disease caused by the gram-positive bacterium *Clostridium tetani*. The **spores are ubiquitous in soil** and animal manure. Contamination of a wound with *C. tetani*, particularly in **devitalized, crushed, or infected tissue**, can lead to its proliferation and expression of the neuroexotoxin **tetanospasmin**. This powerful exotoxin acts on the motor endplates of skeletal muscle, the spinal cord, the sympathetic nervous system, and the brain, leading to generalized muscle rigidity, autonomic nervous system instability, and severe muscle contractions. **The most common presentation of tetanus is muscle spasm of the masseter muscles,** known as "lockjaw," but the back, arms, diaphragm, and lower extremities can also be affected. The diagnosis is made clinically. In up to 10% of tetanus cases, the patient does not recall a wound. The usual incubation period varies from 7 to 21 days but can extend from 3 to 56 days.

Patients with tetanus should be **admitted to the intensive care unit.** Wound debridement, respiratory support as needed, and muscle relaxants or neuromuscular blockade may be helpful. **Patients with a tetanus infection should receive passive immunization and tetanus immunoglobulin (TIG) 3000-6000 units IM on the side opposite of the tetanus toxoid injection.** TIG clearly reduces morbidity and mortality by neutralizing unbound toxin (toxin binds irreversibly, so only unbound toxin can be neutralized). Metronidazole or penicillin is usually given, but its efficacy is questionable.

Prevention of tetanus is accomplished with regular active immunization of all individuals. The dose of tetanus toxoid (TT) or diphtheria/tetanus toxoid (dT) is 0.5 mL IM, regardless of age (see Table 46-3). It is frequently given in combination with the vaccination for acellular pertussis (TDaP). **TIG is given to patients with a possible tetanus exposure (a wound that is not considered clean or minor) and incomplete tetanus immunization** (<3 injections) (see Figure 46–3). The dosage varies with age. Tetanus immunoglobulin and tetanus toxoid should be administered in different body sites with different syringes.

Table 46–3 • A GUIDE TO TETANUS PROPHYLAXIS IN BASIC WOUND MANAGEMENT				
History of Adsorbed Tetanus Toxoid (# of Doses)	**Clean, Minor, Wound**		**All Other Wounds**	
	TDaP, TD or DTaP	TIG	TDaP, TD or DTaP	TIG
Unknown or <3	Yes	No	Yes	Yes
≥3	No[a]	No	No[b]	No

Abbreviations: *TDaP = tetanus, diphtheria, acellular pertussis; DTaP = diphtheria, tetanus, acellular pertussis; Td = tetanus, diphtheria; TIG = tetanus immunoglobulin.*
[a]*Yes, if >10 years since the last tetanus toxoid containing vaccine dose.*
[b]*Yes, if >5 years since the last tetanus toxoid containing vaccine dose.*
Note: *Please refer to CDC guidelines for more complete recommendations (CDC Health Information for International Travel 2008, Chapter 4: Prevention of Specific Infectious Diseases).*

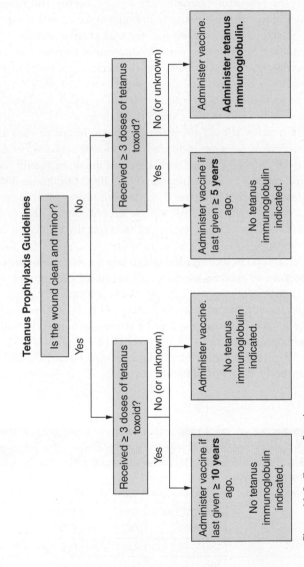

Figure 46–3. Tetanus flowchart.

> ## CASE CORRELATION
>
> - See also Case 43 (Penetrating Trauma to the Chest, Abdomen, and Extremities), Case 44 (Extremity Fracture and Neck Pain), and Case 45 (Trauma and Extremes of Age).

COMPREHENSION QUESTIONS

46.1 A 31-year-old man sustains a slash wound to the superior eyelid during an altercation. The globe appears intact, and the patient's extraocular movements are normal. He is able to keep the affected eye closed with adequate strength against resistance. However, you notice marked ptosis of the affected eyelid at rest. The most likely damaged structure is:

  A. Facial nerve

  B. Levator palpebrae superioris muscle

  C. Orbicularis oculi muscle

  D. Trigeminal nerve

46.2 You are the EM physician working the night the man in the above question arrives. You note that the laceration extends medially, and this raises your suspicion for canalicular injury. In this case you should:

  A. Suture the wound, including the medial canthus carefully in perfect alignment.

  B. Anesthetize and further dissect the area of concern and explore for injury.

  C. Apply methylene blue dye to the eye to examine for injury to the canalicular system.

  D. Consult ophthalmology.

46.3 The man in Question 46.1 tells you he cannot recall if he received all of his childhood vaccinations and is unable to remember if he ever had a tetanus vaccination. This patient should receive:

  A. Tetanus toxoid now.

  B. Tetanus immunoglobulin now.

  C. Tetanus toxoid and tetanus immunoglobulin now.

  D. Tetanus toxoid now, and tetanus immunoglobulin as needed, if concerning symptoms develop.

46.4   A 24-year-old mechanic presents via EMS with a long, deep scalp laceration sustained by hitting his head on a metal car part while attempting to stand up from a laying position. The wound is bleeding profusely. The blow has lacerated the galea, but there is no obvious skull deformity. Direct pressure does not stop the bleeding adequately. Which of the following is most appropriate method to achieve hemostasis?

A.   Continued direct pressure to the area.

B.   Suture the galea aponeurotica with vicryl suture.

C.   Attempt to locate the bleeding vessels and tie them off.

D.   Approximate the galea aponeurotica with staples.

46.5   An 18-year-old man presents to you after sustaining a blow to the upper lip during an altercation. The wound is shallow but gaping. It is 2 cm long and involves the vermillion border. The appropriate management of this patient includes:

A.   Suture the mucosa with chromic gut and the skin with nylon.

B.   Suture the mucosa with chromic gut and the skin with nylon, and discharge with antibiotics.

C.   Leave the wound open, and discharge with antibiotics.

D.   Leave the wound open, discharge with antibiotics and recommend patient follow-up with an oral surgeon the next day.

ANSWERS

46.1   **B.** The levator palpebrae superioris is a skeletal muscle that elevates and retracts the eyelid. It is innervated by a branch of the oculomotor nerve (CN III). The adjoining superior tarsal muscle, which is comprised of smooth muscle and is sympathetically innervated, also assists with elevation of the upper eyelid. Given the mechanism of injury, these are likely to have been affected. The orbicularis oculi muscle (C) is innervated by the temporal and zygomatic branches of the facial nerve (CN VII) (A). These are unlikely to be affected in this patient, as he has the ability to close his eye against resistance. The trigeminal nerve (CN V) (D) has sensory branches responsible for facial sensation as well as a motor component which innervates the muscles of mastication.

46.2 **D.** When there is any suspicion for canalicular injury, it is necessary to immediately consult a reconstructive specialist, most likely ophthalmology or oculoplastics. These repairs are outside of the typical scope of practice for an emergency medicine physician (A). Failure to correctly repair a canalicular injury will cause a failure of tears to drain appropriately through the nasolacrimal system. This causes tears to overflow onto the face, a condition known as epiphora. Dissecting the area of concern (B) may cause inadvertent damage to the lacrimal duct. Fluorescein dye, not methylene blue (C), may be used to evaluate for a canalicular injury. Methylene blue is irritating to the eye and may cause chemical conjunctivitis. One instills fluorescein into the affected eye and checks for the appearance of dye in the nose (may ask patient to blow his or her nose and examine tissue for the dye). However, this is best done in conjunction with the specialist.

46.3 **C.** Given the degree of complexity of the wound as well as the possibility of a substantially non-clean blade, this patient requires both tetanus toxoid and tetanus immunoglobulin, as he cannot recall if he has ever had a tetanus vaccination (see Figure 46–3 for details [Tetanus Flow Chart]). Per the CDC, wounds not considered clean and minor include, but are not limited to, wounds contaminated with dirt, feces, soil, and saliva; puncture wounds; avulsions; and wounds resulting from missiles, crushing, burns, and frostbite.

46.4 **B.** In a profusely bleeding scalp laceration, the galea aponeurotica should promptly be sutured with absorbable suture to achieve hemostasis. It is inappropriate to use non-absorbable materials (D). Attempting to locate the various, tiny bleeding vessels and tie them off (C) is not a feasible option. In addition, closing the galea prevents the spread of infection, should the wound become infected. Direct pressure (A) is an appropriate initial effort, but it is not adequately stopping the bleeding; therefore, continued pressure is not the best option.

46.5 **A.** A lip laceration involving the vermillion border can be cosmetically detrimental if not repaired properly. Even a 1 mm discrepancy in alignment is readily noticeable. It is well within the scope of practice of the emergency medicine physician to repair these wounds (D). In addition, there is no indication for antibiotics in a shallow lip laceration (B, C, D). Antibiotic use may be considered in through and through lacerations. The skin should be closed with non-absorbable (nylon) sutures, the first being placed to approximate the vermillion border. The mucosa should be closed with absorbable (chromic gut) sutures.

CLINICAL PEARLS

▶ The vermillion border must be precisely approximated because of its important cosmetic characteristics. Even a small discrepancy in lining up the tissue is noticeable.

▶ The facial nerve courses from the mastoid region across the cheek area and is prone to injury in facial lacerations. Care must be taken to identify an injury to the nerve to prevent permanent deformity.

▶ Complex lacerations of the face, eye, ear, nose, and mouth, including lacerations associated with focal neurologic deficits (eg, facial droop or ptosis) should be cared for with expert consultation, such as an ENT surgeon or ophthalmologist.

▶ Meticulous hemostasis is important in repairing ear lacerations to avoid "cauliflower ear."

▶ Tetanus is an acute disease of wound contamination, which is largely preventable with immunization. All patients at risk for tetanus and not up-to-date on their tetanus vaccination should receive tetanus immunoglobulin or tetanus toxoid.

REFERENCES

Brown DJ, Jaffe JE, Henson JK. Advanced laceration management. *Emerg Med Clin N Am.* 2007;25: 83-99.

Brunicardi FC, Anderson DK, Billiar TR, et al, eds. *Schwartz's Principles of Surgery.* 9th ed. New York, NY: McGraw-Hill; 2009.

Centers for Disease Control and Prevention. Vaccines and Immunizations: Tetanus, http://www.cdc.gov/vaccines/pubs/pinkbook/downloads/tetanus.pdf. Accessed July 31, 2016.

Kretsinger K, Broder KR, Cortese MM, et al. Preventing tetanus, diphtheria, and pertussis among adults: use of tetanus toxoid and acellular pertussis vaccine recommendations of the Advisory Committee on Immunization Practices (ACIP) and recommendation of ACIP, supported by the Healthcare Infection Control Practices Advisory Committee (HICPAC), for use of TDaP among health-care personnel. *MMWR Recomm Rep.* 2006;55(RR-17):1-37.

Roberts JR, Hedges JR. *Clinical Procedures in Emergency Medicine.* 6th ed. Philadelphia, PA: Saunders; 2013.

Tintinalli JE, Kelen GD, Stapczynski JS, eds. *Emergency Medicine.* 8th ed. New York, NY: McGraw-Hill; 2015:302-304.

Updated recommendations for use of tetanus toxoid, reduced diphtheria toxoid and acellular pertussic (TDaP) vaccine from the Advisory Committee on Immunization Practices, 2010. *MMWR Morb Mortal Wkly Rep.* 2011;60(01)13-15.

A 15-year-old adolescent boy was cleaning some items in the shed in his backyard in the middle of the afternoon when he saw a bat in middle of the shed. The bat bit the boy on his dominant hand, after which the teenager ran into the house. His parents brought the boy to the emergency department. His vital signs on arrival were a blood pressure of 115/70 mm Hg, heart rate of 105 beats per minute, respiratory rate of 14 breaths per minute, pulse oximetry of 99% on room air, and temperature of 37.1°C (98.9°F). Inspection of the wound shows deep bite marks with a laceration close to the proximal interphalangeal joint. The bat escaped after the boy was bitten and was not found.

▶ What is the most likely diagnosis?
▶ What is the next step in treatment?

ANSWERS TO CASE 47:

Rabies/Animal Bite

Summary: A teenager complains of a deep bite to his dominant hand by a bat acting strangely. The bite is fresh, and the bat cannot be located.

- **Most likely diagnosis:** Unprovoked attack by a rabies-infected bat.

- **Best initial treatment:** Notify animal control to locate the animal, then clean the wound and administer both passive and active rabies immunization to the patient. Administer tetanus toxoid if not received within the last 5 years.

ANALYSIS

Objectives

1. Recognize that bat bites are a common vector for rabies.

2. Know the treatment of common bite injuries.

3. Know the clinical presentation of rabies.

4. Know the treatments for rabies and when treatment should be given.

5. Understand the basic principles of snakebite management.

Considerations

This 15-year-old teenager encountered a **bat exhibiting abnormal behavior.** The bat, normally a nocturnal animal, is active in the afternoon. This is suspicious for a rabies-infected bat. Other important considerations in this case are the location of the **bite near a joint space,** the patient's **tetanus status,** and the possibility of **retained teeth.**

In this patient's case, postexposure prophylaxis for rabies and delayed primary closure to observe for infection are reasonable. **Postexposure prophylaxis** for rabies should include a combination of immediate **passive (rabies immunoglobulin)** immunization and **active immunization** (human diploid cell vaccine [HDCV]). **Tetanus vaccine** should be administered if the patient has not received it **within the last 5 years.**

APPROACH TO:

Animal Bites

DEFINITIONS

HYDROPHOBIA: The violent contraction of respiratory, diaphragmatic, laryngeal, and pharyngeal muscles initiated by consumption of liquids.

VENOM: A specialized form of saliva that is rich in proteins, polypeptides, peptidases, and nucleases. Its effects can range from paralysis, digestion, or incapacitation to death.

CLINICAL APPROACH

General Bite Management

Good wound care is the mainstay of bite management. A detailed history of the bite, including type of animal, whether provocation occurred, location of bite, and time since the bite, should be followed by a careful physical examination. Physical examination should focus on the patient's neurovascular status, the potential for tendon involvement, any evidence of cellulitis, and the potential for joint space violation. **The wound should be irrigated, tetanus booster updated if more than 5 years has elapsed since the last administration and antibiotics administered if the bite is high risk for infection or already infected.** A radiograph should also be obtained to evaluate for a fracture and retained teeth. For bites with potential tendon injury, the involved extremity should be splinted. Simple bites of the trunk and extremities (except for hands and feet) less than 6 hours old can generally be closed primarily. Simple bites of the head and neck area less than 12 hours old also can be repaired primarily. However, puncture wounds, bites of the hand or foot, wounds more than 12 hours old, and infected tissues are usually left open.

With any bite injury, the appropriate authorities should be notified to find the animal and observe it for abnormal behavior. Prior to arriving to the ED, any open wound or bite should be thoroughly washed with soap and water. In the ED, **irrigation of the wound with saline removes debris and lowers bacterial counts.** There is no added benefit to the addition of hydrogen peroxide or povidone iodine to the irrigant. Any foreign body or devitalized tissue should be removed. Administering prophylactic antibiotics in the case of simple bites is left to physician preference, as there is no conclusive evidence that it reduces infection rates.

The clenched-fist injury, also called a **"fight bite,"** is especially important to assess because a small bite injury may deeply embed bacteria into the joint spaces or tendon sheaths of the hand. This can lead to a serious infection. A radiograph to assess for fracture or foreign body should be performed. The wound should be irrigated, the tendons examined, and antibiotics administered. In cases of delayed evaluation, look for signs of infection including cellulitis, abscess formation, or tenosynovitis. Due to the high risk of infection, these cases typically require admission to the hospital for IV antibiotics or surgery.

Bacterial Infections

Dogs, cats, and humans account for almost all mammalian bite injuries. Oral flora in dogs and cats include *Staphylococcus aureus*, **Pasteurella spp**, *Capnocytophaga canimorsus*, *Streptococcus*, and oral anaerobes. Humans usually have mixed flora, including *S. aureus*, *Haemophilus influenzae*, **Eikenella corrodens** and beta-lactamase–positive oral anaerobes. In cat bite wound infections, *Pasteurella multocida* is the most commonly isolated bacteria. Human bite infections are typically polymicrobial. Good initial-choice antibiotics include amoxicillin–clavulanic acid, ticarcillin–clavulanic acid, ampicillin–sulbactam, or a second-generation cephalosporin. Duration of administration for established infections is **10-14 days and 3-5 days for prophylaxis.** Failed outpatient treatment of wound infections is an indication for admission and IV antibiotics.

Rabies

Rabies is a single-stranded ribonucleic acid (RNA) **rhabdovirus** that attacks the central nervous system and causes an encephalomyelitis that is almost always fatal. It has a variable incubation period, averaging 1-2 months, but it may be as short as 7 days or as long as 1 year. Clinical presentation begins with a **1- to 4-day prodrome** with fever, headache, malaise, nausea, emesis, and a productive cough. An encephalic stage follows with hyperactivity, excitation, agitation, and confusion. Brainstem dysfunction follows with cranial nerve involvement and excessive salivation, followed by coma and respiratory failure. **Hydrophobia** (the violent contraction of respiratory, diaphragmatic, laryngeal, and pharyngeal muscles initiated by consumption of liquids) is a late sign of infection.

A bite is the most common means of transmission of rabies. Although animal vaccination programs have decreased the incidence of rabies, they have not completely eliminated it. Risk factors for transmission include unprovoked attacks, unknown or unobserved animals, and animals displaying unusual behavior. Animals with increased lacrimation, salivation, dilated irregular pupils, unusual behavior, or hydrophobia are particularly suspected. Bites to the face or hands confer the highest risk of rabies transmission, but any breakage of the skin can transmit the virus. Worldwide, in locations with incomplete animal vaccination, dogs are the most frequent vector for rabies transmission to humans. In the United States, dogs are largely rabies free. No rabies cases have been recorded in animals having received two injections, but animals only receiving one vaccine have been infected. **Healthy dogs, cats, or ferrets that bite humans should be confined and observed for at least 10 days for signs of illness;** with any sign of illness, the animal should be euthanized and its head shipped refrigerated to a laboratory qualified to assess for rabies.

Rabies Prophylaxis

A thorough history and physical examination in the context of the geographical location will give important clues for treatment. Identification of the animal and observation will help guide treatment as described earlier. Preexposure prophylaxis with active vaccination may be given to individuals at risk (animal trainers, animal control field workers, etc). This does not obviate the need for postexposure prophylaxis. **Postexposure prophylaxis is indicated for any person possibly exposed to a rabid animal.** Postexposure prophylaxis is a medical urgency, not an emergency, but time is essential. **Rabies immunoglobulin** can give a rapid, **passive immunity that will last for 2-3 weeks.** Passive immunization with human rabies immunoglobulin 20 IU/kg should be injected around the wound site as soon as possible. Active immunization should then be given intramuscularly with a different syringe at a different site. The active vaccines include HDCV, purified chick embryo cell vaccine (PCEC), and rabies vaccine adsorbed (RVA). They and should be administered on days 0, 3, 7, and 14. Active immunization will lead to antibody formation in about 1 week and should last for several years.

Snakebites

Venomous snakes are found throughout the United States except in Maine, Alaska, and Hawaii. There are two main families of venomous species: the Crotalinae and the Elapidae. The Crotalinae, also called pit vipers because of the presence of a pitlike depression on their face, includes rattlesnakes, copperheads, and water moccasins. The Elapidae includes the coral snakes.

Not every snakebite results in the release of venom into the victim; "dry bites" occur up to 20% of the time. When venom is injected, it usually occurs in subcutaneous tissue and is absorbed via the lymphatic and venous system. Clinical manifestations of envenomation will vary depending on the toxin, depth of envenomation, location of the bite, and size and underlying health of the victim. Pit viper envenomation ranges from minor local swelling and discomfort at the injection site to marked swelling, pain, blisters, bruising, and necrosis at the incision site; systemic symptoms include fasciculations, hypotension, and severe coagulopathy. In contrast, Elapid envenomation usually begins as minor pain at the incision with a delayed serious systemic reaction that may lead to respiratory distress secondary to neuromuscular weakness.

The primary objectives in snakebite management are to determine if envenomation occurred, to provide supportive therapy, to treat the local and systemic effects of envenomation, and to limit tissue loss and disability. If the species can be identified, the appropriate antivenin can be administered if required. Treatment of envenomations is varied. If it is a "dry bite," general wound care is usually sufficient. Radiographs should be performed to evaluate for retained teeth. Signs of envenomation can be broadly classified into either **hematologic or neurologic**. Hematologic effects of envenomation include **disseminated intravascular coagulopathy, ecchymosis, and bleeding disorders**. If there are signs of envenomation, laboratory studies including, but not limited to, clotting studies, liver enzymes, and complete blood counts with platelets are necessary. Giving blood products to an envenomated patient with a coagulopathy will not correct the problem. The circulating venom responsible for the coagulopathy is still present and will likely inactivate the blood products. Therefore, the mainstay in treatment in venom-induced coagulopathy is antivenin, preferably type specific, not blood products. Nonetheless, if the patient is bleeding, it is prudent to administer both antivenom and blood products. The most commonly available antivenom for treatment of North American Crotalid envenomations is **Crotalidae polyvalent immune fab (CroFab). Surgical debridement or fasciotomy in the setting of envenomation should not be done,** as this may lead to further bleeding. Neurologic effects include weakness, **paresthesia, paralysis, confusion, and respiratory depression**. Asymptomatic patients who were bit by a pit viper should be observed for 8-12 hours after the bite. This should be extended to 24 hours for coral snakebites because of the absence of early symptoms. The local poison control center should be contacted early in all symptomatic snakebites and will be able to help with management and location of antivenin. The national phone number for the **poison control center is 1-800-222-1222**. While the American Heart Association has recommended the use of pressure dressings in the treatment of snakebites, correct application of these is extremely difficult, and incorrect application may result in harm. Their position is still being debated at this time.

CASE CORRELATION

- See also Case 40 (Skin and Soft Tissue Infections), Case 41 (Rash With Fever), and Case 46 (Facial Laceration).

COMPREHENSION QUESTIONS

Match the single best therapy (A to E) to the clinical scenarios in Questions 47.1 to 47.4.

 A. Identify the species, clean and immobilize the site, and administer antivenin.

 B. Clean the bite site and treat with prophylactic antibiotics.

 C. Clean the site, observe the animal, and watch for signs of secondary infection.

 D. Clean the site and begin rabies prophylaxis with active and passive immunization.

 E. Admit for radical surgical debridement in the operating room.

47.1 Your dog, who was immunized against rabies within the last year, bites your neighbor.

47.2 A woman arrives in your ED with a human bite to her breast that occurred earlier in the day. There is a small puncture wound and no signs of cellulitis.

47.3 A scoutmaster brings a boy scout to the ED with a snakebite to his left foot. He says he heard the snake's rattle just before it bit him. His entire foot is purple, swollen to his mid-calf, and very painful to the touch.

47.4 While raking leaves under his fruit tree at dusk, a man says a bird flew into his face. When he checked his face in the mirror he saw a bite mark under blood streaks.

ANSWERS

47.1 **C.** This is a low-risk bite. The dog is a house dog with a low risk of ever contracting rabies. You have it immunized every year and can observe it for 10 days. As always, clean the bite thoroughly and consider radiographs to be sure that no broken teeth are in the wound and that the bone has not been penetrated. Administer tetanus if indicated, and watch for secondary bacterial infection. Prophylactic antibiotics are indicated. Although answer B (clean bite and treat with antibiotics) is a possible answer, it is better to observe the animal (Answer C).

47.2 **B.** Human bites have high rates of infectivity. This wound does not appear to be infected. Nonetheless, the wound should be cleaned and a 3- to 5-day course of prophylactic antibiotics should be initiated. Human bites rarely lead to retained teeth, so a radiograph is not indicated. If this bite occurred on the hand or across a joint space, a radiograph should be performed. Tetanus toxoid should be given if indicated. TDaP has now been approved for use in patients over 65 years old.

47.3 **A.** This is a high-risk snakebite. The authorities should immediately be notified to search for the snake. Although some percent of venomous snakebites fail to inject venom, this bite is clearly envenomed. The rapid swelling, pain, and discoloration demands immediate attention. First responders should immobilize the site and place constriction bands that *do not* obstruct arterial flow. The swelling is not a compartment syndrome unless elevated pressures are measured. **Avoid incisions and fasciotomies** or packing in ice. Immediate antivenin injection in and around the site should be a priority. Remember that species-specific antivenin is important and that administration time is critical. Best results are obtained within 4 hours. Mark the swelling every 15 minutes, evaluate coagulation profiles, electrocardiogram (ECG), renal function, and liver function, and consider ICU admission to ensure adequate perfusion and to avoid disseminated intravascular coagulation (DIC). An index of antivenin can be obtained from the American Zoo and Aquarium Association (301-562-0777) as well as your local poison control center (800-222-1222).

47.4 **D.** This injury is at high risk for rabies transmission. Dusk is the usual time for bat activity, and although this man did not feel a bite, he discovered bite marks under his injury site. Bats carry high rates of rabies, and this man was bitten on the face. Because the animal cannot be examined, immediate passive and active immunization should be initiated and tetanus vaccination administered, if indicated. As always, watch for secondary bacterial infection.

CLINICAL PEARLS

- ▶ In the United States, rabies transmission by dogs is nearly zero, whereas transmission by bats is more often seen. Worldwide, dog transmission is still common.

- ▶ Rabies prophylaxis is indicated for uncaught wild animals and animals that start behaving abnormally.

- ▶ Bites that are more than 6 hours old are, in general, left open because of the risk of infection.

- ▶ Snakebites should be treated like other bites, with special attention paid to species identification and rapid administration of antivenin if required.

REFERENCES

Ball V, Younggren BN. Emergency management of difficult wounds: part I. *Emerg Med Clin North Am.* 2007;25:101-121.

Campbell BT, Corsi JM, Boneti C, et al. Pediatric snakebites: lessons learned from 114 cases. *J Pediatr Surg.* 2008;43(7):1338-1341.

Gold BS, Dart RC, Barish RA. Bites of venomous snakes. *N Engl J Med.* 2002;347(5):347-356.

Leung AK, Davies HD, Hon KL. Rabies: epidemiology, pathogenesis, and prophylaxis. *Adv Ther.* 2007;24(6):1340-1347.

Markenson D, Ferguson JD, Chameides L, et al. Part 13: First aid: 2010 American Heart Association and American Red Cross International consensus on first aid science with treatment recommendations. *Circulation.* 2010;122(16 Suppl 2):S582-S605.

Ruha A. Pizon AF. Native (US) venomous snakes and lizards. In: *Goldfrank's Toxicologic Emergencies.* 10th ed. New York, NY: McGraw-Hill; 2014.

Rupprecht CE, Briggs D, Brown CM, et al. Use of a reduced (4-dose) vaccine schedule for postexposure prophylaxis to prevent human rabies. *MMWR Recomm Rep.* 2010;59(RR-2):1-9.

Schalamon J, Ainoedhofer H, Singer G, et al. Analysis of dog bites in children who are younger than 17 years. *Pediatrics.* 2006;117(3):e374-e379.

A 13-year-old adolescent boy presents to the emergency department with a chief complaint of sore throat and fever for 2 days. He reports that his younger sister has been ill for the past week with "the same thing." The patient has pain with swallowing but no change in voice, drooling, or neck stiffness. He denies any recent history of cough, rash, nausea, vomiting, or diarrhea. He denies any recent travel and has completed the full series of childhood immunizations. He has no other medical problems, takes no medications, and has no allergies.

On examination, the patient has a temperature of 38.5°C (101.3°F), a heart rate of 104 beats per minute, a blood pressure of 118/64 mm Hg, a respiratory rate of 18 breaths per minute, and an oxygen saturation of 99% on room air. His posterior oropharynx reveals erythema with tonsillar exudates without uvular deviation or significant tonsillar swelling. Neck examination is supple without tenderness of the anterior lymph nodes. Chest and cardiovascular examinations are unremarkable. His abdomen is soft and nontender with normal bowel sounds and no hepatosplenomegaly. Skin is without rash.

► What is the most likely diagnosis?
► What are the dangerous causes of sore throat you don't want to miss?
► What is your diagnostic plan?
► What is your therapeutic plan?

ANSWERS TO CASE 48:

Streptococcal Pharyngitis ("Strep Throat")

Summary: This is a 13-year-old adolescent boy with pharyngitis. He has fever, tonsillar exudate, no cough, and no tender cervical adenopathy. There is no evidence of airway involvement.

- **Most likely diagnosis:** Streptococcal pharyngitis.

- **Dangerous causes of sore throat:** Epiglottitis, peritonsillar abscess, retropharyngeal abscess, and Ludwig's angina.

- **Diagnostic plan:** Use Centor criteria to determine probability of bacterial pharyngitis and rapid antigen testing when appropriate.

- **Therapeutic plan:** Evaluate the patient for need of antibiotics versus supportive care.

ANALYSIS

Objectives

1. Recognize the different etiologies of pharyngitis, paying close attention to those that are potentially life threatening.

2. Be familiar with widely accepted decision-making strategies for the diagnosis and management of group A beta-hemolytic streptococcal (GABS) pharyngitis.

3. Learn the treatment of GABS pharyngitis and understand the sequelae of this disease.

4. Recognize acute airway emergencies associated with upper airway infections.

Considerations

This 13-year-old patient presents with a common diagnostic dilemma: sore throat and fever. The first priority for the physician is to assess whether the patient is more ill than the complaint would indicate: **stridulous breathing, air hunger, toxic appearance, or drooling with inability to swallow would indicate impending disaster.** The ABCs (airway, breathing, circulation) must always be addressed first. This patient does not have those types of "alarms." Thus, a more relaxed elicitation of his history can take place, and examination of the head, neck, and throat can be performed. In instances suggestive of epiglottitis, such as stridor, drooling, and toxic appearance, examination of the throat (especially with a tongue blade) may cause upper airway obstruction in children, leading to respiratory failure. During the examination, the clinician should be alert for complications of upper airway infection; however, this patient presents with a simple pharyngitis.

Overall, the most common etiology of pharyngitis is viral organisms. This teenager has several features that make group A streptococcus more likely: **age less than 15 years, fever, absence of cough,** and **the presence of tonsillar exudate.** Of note, the patient does not have "tender anterior cervical adenopathy." The diagnosis of group A streptococcal pharyngitis can be made clinically or with the aid of rapid antigen testing. Rapid streptococcal antigen testing can give a fairly accurate result immediately; treatment or nontreatment with penicillin can be based on this result. If the rapid streptococcal antigen test is positive, antibiotic therapy should be given; if the rapid test is negative, throat culture should be performed and antibiotics should be withheld. The **gold standard for diagnosis is bacterial culture,** and if positive, the patient should be notified and given penicillin therapy.

APPROACH TO:
Pharyngitis

CLINICAL APPROACH

The **differential diagnosis of pharyngitis**is broad and includes:

- **Viral Etiologies** (rhinovirus, coronavirus, adenovirus, herpes simplex virus [HSV], influenza, parainfluenza, Epstein-Barr virus [EBV], and cytomegalovirus [CMV] [causing infectious mononucleosis], coxsackievirus [causing herpangina], and the human immunodeficiency virus [HIV]).

- **Bacterial Causes** (group A beta-hemolytic streptococcus [GABS], group C. *streptococci, Arcanobacterium haemolyticum*, meningococcal, gonococcal, diphtheritic, chlamydial, *Legionella*, and *Mycoplasma* species), specific anatomically related conditions caused by bacterial organisms (peritonsillar abscess, epiglottitis, retropharyngeal abscess, and Ludwig's angina), candidal pharyngitis, aphthous stomatitis, thyroiditis, and bullous erythema multiforme. **Viruses** are **the most common cause of pharyngitis.**

Group A streptococcus causes pharyngitis in 5% to 10% of adults and 15% to 30% of children who seek medical care with the complaint of sore throat. It is often clinically indistinguishable from other etiologies, yet it is the major treatable cause of pharyngitis. Infectious mononucleosis is important to exclude because of the risk of splenomegaly and splenic rupture. Other **bacterial etiologies** may also be treated with antibiotics. Studies suggest that certain symptoms and historical features are suggestive of streptococcal pharyngitis and may help guide the provider in generating a reasonable pretest probability of GABS. The Centor criteria, modified by age, are helpful in assessing for GABS (Table 48–1). The McIsaac score adds one point to the Centor score for those <15 years, and subtracts one point for those >45 years.

Of note, recent epidemiologic data suggest *Fusobacterium necrophorum* causes pharyngitis at a rate similar to GABS in young adults and if not treated is implicated

Table 48–1 • CENTOR CRITERIA FOR PREDICTING STREPTOCOCCAL PHARYNGITIS		
Criteria	Score	Rationale
Presence of tonsillar exudate	1 point	More likely bacterial etiology
Tender anterior cervical adenopathy	1 point	More likely bacterial etiology
Fever by history	1 point	More likely bacterial etiology
Absence of cough	1 point	More likely viral etiology
Age less than 15 years[a]	Add 1 point to score	Common age for Streptococcal pharyngitis
Age more than 45 years[a]	Subtract 1 point from score	Less common age for Streptococcal pharyngitis

[a]Modifications to the original Centor criteria. See interpretation of the score in text.
Data from Centor RM, Witherspoon JM, Dalton HP, et al. The diagnosis of strep throat in adults in the emergency room. Med Decis Making. 1981;1:239-246; and McIsaac WJ, White D, Tannenbaum D, Low DE. A clinical score to reduce unnecessary antibiotic use in patients with sore throat. CMAJ. 1998;158(1):75-83.

in causing LeMierre Syndrome (septic thrombophlebitis of the jugular vein), a life-threatening suppurative complication.

Throat cultures remain the gold standard for the diagnosis of GABS pharyngitis, but they have several limitations in use for daily practice. False-negative throat cultures may occur in patients with few organisms in their pharynx or as a result of inadequate sampling (improper swabbing method or errors in incubation or reading of plates). False-positive throat cultures may occur in individuals who are asymptomatic carriers of GABS. Throat cultures are costly and, perhaps more importantly, require 24-48 hours for results. Although it may be reasonable to delay therapy for this period of time (delay will not increase likelihood of development of rheumatic fever), it requires further communication with the patient and perhaps an uncomfortable latency in therapy for the concerned parent.

The rapid-antigen test (RAT) for GABS, despite having some limitations, has been embraced by many experts and incorporated into diagnostic algorithms. The **RAT is 80% to 90% sensitive** and exceedingly specific when compared to throat cultures. Results are point-of-care and available in minutes. Many experts recommend **confirmation of negative RAT with throat culture.** Individuals with **positive RAT results should be treated.** Newer technologies, such as the optical immunoassay, may prove to be as sensitive as throat cultures while providing results within minutes; its cost-effectiveness has not been established.

- Patients with 4 points from the Centor and/or McIsaac criteria should be empirically treated because their pretest probability is reasonably high (although this practice may result in over treatment in as many as 50% of patients).

- Patients with 0 or 1 points should NOT receive antibiotics or diagnostic tests (the criteria have been shown here to yield a negative predictive value of roughly 80%).

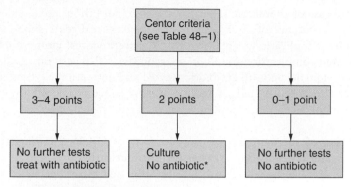

Figure 48–1. Algorithm when RAT unavailable.

- Patients with 2 or 3 points should have RAT, and those with positive RAT results should be treated. Negative RAT results should warrant withholding antibiotics and should be followed with a throat culture.

For instances when **RAT is unavailable**, one accepted algorithm is given in Figure 48–1.

- Patients with 3 or 4 points should be empirically treated with antibiotics.

- Patients with 0 or 1 point should NOT receive antibiotics or diagnostic tests.

- Patients with 2 points should NOT receive antibiotics. The possible exceptions to this 2-point rule are in the setting of a GABS outbreak, patient contact with many children, an immunocompromised patient, or a patient with recent exposure to someone with confirmed GABS.

Of note, **antibiotic therapy in GABS** pharyngitis has been **de-emphasized** because complications have become increasingly rare and the data to support the efficacy of antibiotic therapy in prevention of these complications is sparse and many decades old.

The complications of GABS can be classified into nonsuppurative and suppurative processes. The **nonsuppurative complications of GABS pharyngitis** include **rheumatic fever, streptococcal toxic shock syndrome, poststreptococcal glomerulonephritis, and PANDAS** (pediatric autoimmune neuropsychiatric disorder associated with group A streptococci). Rheumatic fever is now rare in the United States (an incidence of <1 case per 100,000) and is thought to be caused by only a handful of strains of GABS. Despite its rarity, rheumatic fever can result in highly morbid cardiac and neurological sequela; it also remains the most common cause of acquired heart disease in children and adolescents in some developing countries. Published literature suggests the GABS number needed to treat (NNT) to prevent one case of rheumatic fever is between 53 and thousands, depending on the endemic incidence of rheumatic fever. Streptococcal toxic shock syndrome is a very rare complication of pharyngitis. Poststreptococcal glomerulonephritis, another feared complication of GABS pharyngitis, is also very rare, and it occurs with equal frequency in both antibiotic-treated and nonantibiotic-treated groups. It is unclear if antibiotic therapy reduces the incidence of PANDAS, which is a clinical entity in development and presents with episodes of obsessive-compulsive behavior.

Prevention of the suppurative complications of GABS pharyngitis remains perhaps the most compelling reason for antibiotic therapy. These processes include **tonsillopharyngeal cellulitis, peritonsillar and retropharyngeal abscesses, sinusitis, meningitis, brain abscess, and streptococcal bacteremia.** The precise incidence of these complications is unclear, but what remains clear is that these are often preventable sequela that can have devastating consequences. Ultimately, the current practice is to treat suspected GABS pharyngitis with an appropriate antibiotic.

Treatment of GABS

Penicillin is the antibiotic of choice for GABS pharyngitis. A Cochrane review of the literature concluded that penicillin is the first choice antibiotic in patients with acute throat infections. The antibiotic is inexpensive, well-tolerated, and has a reasonably narrow spectrum. **Oral therapy requires a 10-day course,** although multiple daily doses for this duration may pose an issue with respect to compliance; penicillin V 500-mg bid dosing for 10 days in adults (as opposed to 250 mg tid or qid) is a reasonable alternative. For patients in whom compliance may be a significant issue, **a single IM shot of 600,000 units of penicillin G benzathine in patients weighing less than 27 kg (1.2 million units if patient weighs >27 kg)** is another option, although it requires an uncomfortable injection and, more significantly, it cannot be reversed or discontinued should an adverse reaction occur. All patients, regardless of final diagnosis, should be given adequate analgesia and reassurance. It has been shown that individuals who are perceived to want antibiotics may ultimately just want pain relief.

While somewhat controversial, some physicians recommend steroids as an anti-inflammatory agent to decrease the pain and swelling associated with GABS. A meta-analysis of over a thousand patients showed improvement 4.5 hours faster with steroids compared to placebo with a minimal reduction in pain scores. If clinically indicated, the standard agent is **dexamethasone 0.6 mg/kg up to 10 mg PO or IM.** (Higher doses are recommended for children, consult resources for guidance).

Airway Complications

There are several life-threatening causes of sore throat. Patients may suffer airway obstruction from acute epiglottitis, peritonsillar abscess, retropharyngeal abscess, and Ludwig's angina (Table 48–2); the latter requires prompt diagnosis and treatment to avoid spread of this highly infectious condition. Management of

Table 48–2 • COMPLICATED UPPER AIRWAY INFECTIONS			
	Clinical Presentation	**Diagnosis**	**Treatment**
Epiglottitis	Sudden onset of fever, drooling, tachypnea, stridor, toxic appearing	Lateral cervical radiograph (thumb-printing sign)	Urgent ENT (ear, nose, throat) consultation for airway management Helium-O_2 mixture Cefuroxime antibiotic therapy
Retropharyngeal abscess	Usually child (or if adult due to trauma) Fever, sore throat, stiff neck, no trismus	Lateral cervical radiograph or CT imaging	Stabilize airway Surgical drainage Antibiotics (penicillin and metronidazole)
Ludwig's angina	Submaxillary, sublingual, or submental mass with elevation of tongue, jaw swelling, fever, chills, trismus	Lateral cervical radio-graph or CT imaging	Stabilize airway Surgical drainage Antibiotics (penicillin and metronidazole)
Peritonsillar abscess	Swelling in the peritonsillar region with uvula deviation, fever, sore throat, dysphagia, trismus	Cervical radiograph or CT imaging Aspiration of the region with pus	Abscess drainage Antibiotic therapy (penicillin and metronidazole)

the airway in these conditions (see Table 48–2) sometimes necessitates emergency cricothyroidotomy (Figure 48–2) because the pharynx and larynx may be edematous, distorted, or inflamed. Prompt identification of acute retroviral syndrome from recent HIV infection can allow for early antiretroviral therapy. Infectious mononucleosis should be identified so that potentially serious sequela can be considered. These complications include splenomegaly that predisposes the patient to traumatic rupture of the spleen with relatively minor trauma or that may cause splenic sequestration and thrombocytopenia.

CASE CORRELATION

- See also Case 1 (Airway Management/Respiratory Failure).

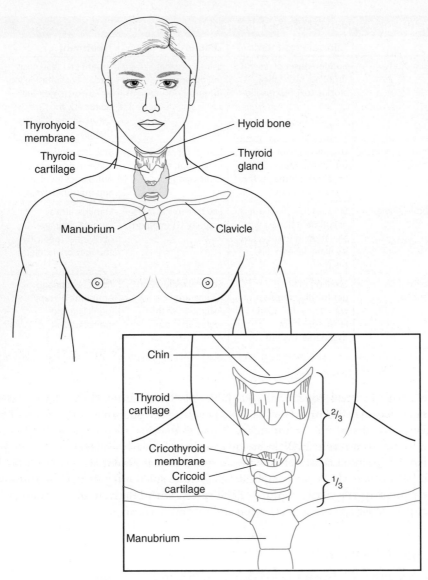

Figure 48–2. Anatomy of the neck for emergency cricothyroidotomy. Note the location of the thyroid and cricoid cartilages.

COMPREHENSION QUESTIONS

48.1 A 48-year-old man is noted to have a 2-day history of sore throat, subjective fever at home, and no medical illnesses. He denies cough or nausea. On examination, his temperature is 38.3°C (101°F), and he has some tonsillar swelling but no exudate. He has bilateral enlarged and tender lymph nodes of the neck. The rapid streptococcal antigen test is negative. Which of the following is the best next step?

A. Oral clindamycin

B. Perform throat culture and treat based on results

C. Observation

D. Begin amantadine

48.2 Which of the following patients is most likely to have group A streptococcal infection?

A. An 11-month-old male infant with fever and red throat

B. An 8-year-old girl with fever and sore throat

C. A 27-year-old man with a temperature of 38.9°C (102°F), pharyngitis, and cough

D. A 52-year-old woman who complains of fever of 39.2°C (102.5°F) and sore throat

48.3 A 19-year-old college student has had a sore throat, mild abdominal pain, and fever for 5 days. He was playing football with some friends and was tackled just short of the goal line, hitting the grass somewhat forcibly. He experienced some abdominal pain and passed out. The EMS (emergency medical services) was called, and his vital signs revealed the heart rate as 140 beats per minute and blood pressure as 80/40 mm Hg with a distended abdomen. Which of the following is the most likely etiology?

A. Vasovagal reaction

B. Ruptured aortic aneurysm

C. Complications of Epstein-Barr infection

D. Ruptured jejunum

48.4 An 18-year-old woman presents with fever and a sore throat. She meets criteria for treatments for GABS pharyngitis. Which medication would you prescribe (in addition to penicillin)?

A. Clindamycin

B. Erythromycin

C. Acyclovir

D. Dexamethasone

E. Methotrexate

ANSWERS

48.1 **B.** This individual has a modified Centor score of 2 (history of fever, tender adenopathy, no cough, age >45). The rapid antigen test is negative, but a definitive culture should be performed for a Centor score of 2 or 3, and treatment should be based on culture results.

48.2 **B.** GABS is most common in patients younger than 15 years (although not in infants). McIsaac added age as a criterion because patients older than age 45 years have a much lower incidence of streptococcal pharyngitis.

48.3 **C.** This patient most likely suffered from splenic rupture caused by mononucleosis (EBV). He is hypotensive because of the massive hemoperitoneum. Aortic aneurysm is rare in teenagers.

48.4 **D.** Dexamethasone has been shown to decrease the amount of symptomatic time of pharyngitis and also to decrease pain. However, penicillin alone is sufficient, and no other medications are needed.

CLINICAL PEARLS

▶ The most common cause of pharyngitis is viral.

▶ The Centor criteria suggestive of GABS pharyngitis include tonsillar exudate, tender anterior cervical adenopathy, history of fever, and absence of cough.

▶ GABS pharyngitis is more common in patients younger than 15 years of age and is less common in those older than 45 years of age.

▶ Overtreatment of pharyngitis with antibiotics is common and is a major source of antibiotic overuse.

▶ Glomerulonephritis is a rare complication of GABS pharyngitis (but not GABS infections of other tissues) that is not clearly prevented by antibiotic therapy.

▶ Rheumatic fever is an exceedingly rare complication of GABS pharyngitis that can be prevented by antibiotic therapy.

▶ Complicated upper airway conditions should be considered when a patient presents with "sore throat."

▶ In general, cricothyroidotomy is the safest method of surgically securing an airway in the ED.

REFERENCES

Bisno AL. Acute pharyngitis. *N Engl J Med*. 2001;344(3):205-211.

Bisno AL, Gerber MA, Gwaltney JM, Kaplan EL, Schwartz RH. Practice guidelines for the diagnosis and management of group a streptococcal pharyngitis. *Clin Infect Dis*. 2002;35:113-125.

Centor RM. Expand the pharyngitis paradigm for adolescents and young adults. *Ann Intern Med*. 2009;151(11):812-815.

Lee JL, Naguwa SM, Cesma GS, Gerhwin ME. Acute rheumatic fever and its consequences: a persistent threat to developing nations in the 21st century. *Autoimmunity Reviews*. 2009;9:117-123.

Linder JA, Chan JC, Bates DW, et al. Evaluation and treatment of pharyngitis in primary care: the difference between guidelines is largely academic. *Arch Intern Med*. 2006;166:1374.

McIsaac WJ, Kellner JD, Aufricht P, et al. Empiric validation of guidelines for the management of pharyngitis in children and adults. *JAMA*. 2004;291(13):1587.

Snow V, Mottur-Pison C, Cooper RJ, Hoffman, JR. Principles of appropriate antibiotic use for acute pharyngitis in adults. *Ann Intern Med*. 2001;134:506-508.

Van Driel ML, De Sutter AI, Keber N, et al. Different antibiotic treatments for group A streptococcal pharyngitis. *Cochrane Database of Systematic Reviews*. 2010;10. Art. No.:CD004406. DOI: 10.1002/14651858.CD004406.pub2.

Van Driel ML, Sutter AD, Deveugele M, et al. Are sore throat patients who hope for antibiotics actually asking for pain relief. *Ann Fam Med*. 2006;4(6):494.

Wing A, Villa-Roel C, Yeh B, et al. Effectiveness of corticosteroid treatment in acute pharyngitis: a systematic review of the literature. *Acad Emer Med*. 2010;17:476-483.

A 60-year-old woman presents to the emergency department (ED) with severe left eye pain, redness, and blurred vision for 3 hours. She reports that her symptoms began while watching a movie at the local cinema. She initially thought that she had eyestrain, but then her eye began to progressively ache. She denies any symptoms in her right eye. The patient denies preceding trauma, photophobia, ocular discharge, increased tearing, or prior eye surgery. She occasionally wears non-prescription reading glasses because she is farsighted. There are no prior similar events. She also reports seeing colored halos around the light fixtures in the ED and having a headache over her left brow, some nausea, and one episode of vomiting. She denies dizziness, weakness, imbalance, abdominal pain, or chest pain.

On examination, her blood pressure is 135/85 mm Hg, pulse is 90 beats per minute, respirations are 18 breaths per minute, and temperature is 37°C (98°F). She is alert and in obvious discomfort, but she is able to tolerate ambient light. She has no periorbital signs of trauma. The left conjunctiva has **ciliary flush** (circumferential reddish ring around the cornea) but no discharge or visible foreign body. Visual acuity is 20/30 in the right eye but only finger counting in the left eye. Visual fields are grossly intact. Gentle palpation of the closed left eye reveals that it is much firmer than the right. Her left pupil is 5 mm, fixed, and unreactive. Her right eye appears normal; the pupil is 3 mm and briskly reactive. She does not experience pain in the left eye when direct light is applied to the right eye (absent consensual photophobia). Extraocular movements are intact and non-painful. The left cornea is slightly edematous (cloudy–steamy), which makes fundoscopy difficult. The right fundus appears normal. Her temporal arteries are pulsatile and nontender. The rest of the physical examination, including the remainder of the neurological examination, is normal.

- ▶ What is your next diagnostic step?
- ▶ What is the most likely diagnosis?
- ▶ What is your next therapeutic step?

ANSWERS TO CASE 49:

Red Eye

Summary: This is a 60-year-old woman with acute onset of left eye redness, pain, and markedly decreased visual acuity. The left eye feels firmer to palpation than the right eye. The left cornea is edematous with a fixed and dilated pupil.

- **Next diagnostic step:** Slit-lamp examination should be performed, and intra-ocular pressures must be measured in both eyes. The intraocular pressures, measured using a Tono-Pen, are 16 and 52 mm Hg in the right and left eye, respectively. Cell and flare (inflammatory changes) are absent. Both anterior chamber depths are shallow. There is no evidence of hyphema (blood) or hypopyon (white cells) in the anterior chamber. Fluorescein staining is unremarkable.

- **Most likely diagnosis:** Acute angle-closure glaucoma.

- **Next step:** Preserve vision using measures to lower the intraocular pressure (IOP) as quickly as possible. Consult ophthalmology as soon as possible.

ANALYSIS

Objectives

1. Become familiar with the vision-threatening causes of a painful red eye.

2. Understand the basic treatment modalities and disposition options for vision-threatening causes of a painful red eye.

3. Recognize the clinical settings, signs, and symptoms, as well as complications, of acute angle-closure glaucoma.

4. Understand the key treatment modalities for angle-closure glaucoma.

Considerations

This 60-year-old woman complains of non-traumatic acute onset of left eye pain, redness, and vision loss with a significant increase in IOP noted on examination. This case is an example of acute angle-closure glaucoma (AACG), a true oph-thalmologic emergency characterized by rapidly elevated intraocular pressure, which compromises blood flow to the optic nerve **and can result in permanent vision loss.** It is likely that her underlying narrow anterior chamber angle, plus the combination of being in dim lighting, limited outflow of aqueous humor as the cornea and iris apposed one another. Careful questioning eliminated the use of prescribed medications or over the counter drugs as additional potential triggers of AACG.

APPROACH TO:
Red Eye

ACUTE ANGLE-CLOSURE GLAUCOMA

The **mechanism of AACG or primary angle-closure glaucoma is pupillary block** of the trabecular meshwork obstructing the outflow of the aqueous humor. Normally, aqueous humor is produced by the ciliary body in the posterior chamber and diffuses through the pupil into the anterior chamber, where it is drained via the trabecular meshwork. A balance exists between aqueous humor production and outflow to maintain a normal IOP. However, some individuals are predisposed to acute angle closure glaucoma secondary to anatomical and environmental factors. Many other forms of glaucoma have a far more insidious, benign presentation, with an inexorable loss of vision. The provider must always consider the diagnosis of AACG because it is possible to get sidetracked evaluating the associated symptoms of headache, nausea, vomiting or abdominal pain by looking for neurologic or gastrointestinal etiologies. Risk factors include age-related lens thickening and hyperopia (far-sightedness), which results in a shortened eyeball and a relatively shallow anterior chamber. There is a 75% risk of a similar attack in the fellow eye if left untreated. Medications which cause pupil dilatation and pupillary block can also trigger AACG, including anticholinergics, tricyclic antidepressants, adrenergic agonists, and topical mydriatics. Non-pupillary block AACG has been associated with sulfur-containing drugs such as topiramate, hydrochlorothiazide, and even acetazolamide, but the mechanism is unclear.

Acute angle-closure glaucoma can occur with stress, fatigue, dim lighting, or sustained work at close range. The patient may present with mild unilateral eye ache or intense pain, blurring, nausea, vomiting, abdominal pain, diaphoresis, and frontal headache. The **hallmarks of the physical examination** include a **fixed, dilated, midposition** pupil, diffuse conjunctival injection, **corneal edema** (clouding), and a shallow anterior chamber (Figure 49–1). Slit-lamp examination may reveal mild cell and flare but no hyphema or hypopyon. The IOP will be elevated (normal is 9-21 mm Hg); pressures can reach 80 mm Hg in AACG. The other eye must always be examined for anterior chamber depth (the angle is usually narrow) and IOP.

Management

The therapeutic goal of the initial management of acute angle-closure glaucoma is to decrease IOP by decreasing aqueous production and increasing outflow. The principal treatment modalities include aqueous suppressants, osmotic agents, and miotic agents. After corneal edema subsides, **the definitive treatment is a laser peripheral iridectomy** performed by an ophthalmologist.

Treatment to lower the intraocular pressure should be initiated in the ED in **consultation with an ophthalmologist**. Intraocular pressure is first lowered by decreasing aqueous humor production with agents such as topical **beta-blocker (timolol 0.5%), an α-2-agonist (apraclonidine), and a carbonic anhydrase inhibitor (acetazolamide 500 mg orally or IV).** Patients with a sulfa allergy may not tolerate

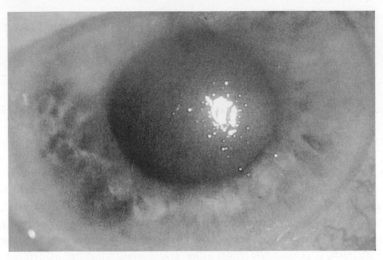

Figure 49–1. Acute angle-closure glaucoma. Pupil is mid-dilated, fixed, and the cornea is cloudy. (*Reproduced with permission, from Tintinalli JE, Kelen GD, Stapczynski JS, eds.* Emergency Medicine. *6th ed. New York, NY: McGraw-Hill; 2004:1460.*)

acetazolamide. **Osmotic agents,** such as mannitol and glycerol, can be used instead of acetazolamide to dehydrate the vitreous humor, which decreases intraocular fluid volume and thus lowers IOP. Mannitol may induce hypotension in patients with poor cardiac function, and glycerol should be avoided in diabetic patients. **Miotics (pilocarpine)** enhance trabecular outflow by constricting the pupil to disrupt the corneal-iris apposition. Intraocular pressure should be first lowered by the administration of topical beta-blockers and acetazolamide prior to the administration of pilocarpine, as the ischemic iris sphincter may be unresponsive to pilocarpine at extremely high intraocular pressures (>50 mm Hg). Pilocarpine is only used in patients with native lenses since pilocarpine will induce movement in artificial lens. Systemic concerns related to topical beta-blocker administration include asthma, severe chronic obstructive pulmonary disease (COPD), bradycardia, heart block, congestive heart failure, and myasthenia gravis. Systemic absorption of topical agents can be reduced up to 70% by instructing the patient to close his or her eyes while occluding the lower tear ducts at the root of the nose after applying the drops. Punctal occlusion for at least 10 seconds decreases drug absorption by the nasal mucosa. The patient should also receive analgesic and antiemetic medications.

Differential Diagnosis of the Red Eye

Other vision-threatening and painful causes of a red eye include severe conjunctivitis, keratitis, corneal ulcer, anterior uveitis, endophthalmitis, orbital cellulitis, scleritis, and temporal arteritis (Table 49–1). Causes of acute vision loss are outlined in Table 49–2.

In this case, the absence of any discharge makes the possibility of **conjunctivitis** highly unlikely, but discharge can be scant. However, gonococcal conjunctivitis (the most serious form of bacterial conjunctivitis) produces a copious purulent

Table 49–1 • DIFFERENTIAL DIAGNOSIS OF THE RED EYE	
Processes That Usually Do Not Impair Vision	**Processes That Can Impair Vision**
• Viral conjunctivitis/allergic conjunctivitis • Nongonococcal or nonchlamydial conjunctivitis • Subconjunctival hemorrhage • Dacrocystitis • Blepharitis • Episcleritis • Peripheral corneal pterygium • Preseptal cellulitis	• Corneal infection (gonococcal infection/chlamydia/herpes simplex virus/herpes zoster virus) • Keratitis • Corneal ulcer • Anterior uveitis • Scleritis • Pterygium (encroaching on the paracentral cornea) • Orbital cellulitis • Endophthalmitis

discharge with an intensely red eye and may potentially perforate the cornea. With chlamydial conjunctivitis the clinical course is more chronic; although the conjunctivae are very red, there is scant discharge. The incidence of sexually transmitted chlamydial conjunctivitis is increasing.

Distinguishing between bacterial and viral conjunctivitis can be challenging. A recent literature review suggests that a bacterial etiology is more likely if the patient has a diffusely red conjunctivum, which renders the tarsal (eyelid) vessels indistinguishable, a purulent discharge, and bilaterally matted eyelids in the morning (morning gluing). A bacterial etiology is less likely if the eye redness is not noticeable at 20 feet or if the eyelids are not matted in the morning.

Most conjunctivitis is viral and is often caused by adenovirus species. Epidemic keratoconjunctivitis is especially severe. Patients have profound conjunctival redness and swelling (chemosis), a watery discharge, and lymphadenopathy.

Corneal inflammation, or **keratitis**, may be due to viral, bacterial, or protozoal infection, contact lenses, trauma, or ultraviolet light. Severe keratitis can progress to a **corneal ulcer**, which may be visible to the unaided eye as a white defect. Distinguishing an **ulcer** from a corneal abrasion is clinically significant and can be challenging. Examination with the slit lamp is required. The major distinction is the hazy/cloudy stroma that lies beneath the ulcer in contrast to the clear stroma deep to most abrasions. A slit-lamp examination is a necessary part of the evaluation of all patients with a red eye. Fluorescein staining should be included

Table 49–2 • DIFFERENTIAL DIAGNOSIS OF ACUTE VISION LOSS	
Painful Vision Loss	**Painless Vision Loss**
AACG	Retinal detachment
Corneal ulcer	Vitreous hemorrhage
Anterior uveitis	Posterior vitreous detachment
Scleritis	Central retinal artery occlusion
Endophthalmitis	Central retinal vein occlusion
Optic neuritis	
Temporal arteritis	

in every examination and may be the only way to identify the classic dendrite with terminal bulb markings found in herpes simplex keratitis. Herpes zoster dendrites taper at their ends and may be associated with periorbital dermatomal vesicular eruptions or lesions at the tip of the nose (Hutchinson sign of nasociliary involvement). Patients with HIV are at risk for complications of herpes zoster virus (HZV) and must undergo careful corneal and retinal evaluation to prevent vision loss.

Anterior uveitis (iritis) is associated with pain, blurred vision, photophobia (direct and consensual), circumcorneal redness, and anterior chamber cells and flare. A hypopyon (layer of white cells) may be visible along the inferior rim of the anterior chamber. The affected pupil may be smaller, irregular, and minimally reactive. IOP can be elevated. Etiologies include idiopathic, infectious (tuberculosis, syphilis, herpes simplex/zoster, toxoplasmosis, cytomegalovirus [CMV]), autoimmune (sarcoidosis, collagen-vascular diseases, human leukocyte antigen [HLA] B27-associated), and post-traumatic causes. Uveitis due to herpes simplex virus (HSV) and HZV is common in HIV positive patients. Because treatment involves topical corticosteroids with their attendant risk of glaucoma, cataracts, or reactivation of herpes simplex infections, patients should be referred to an ophthalmologist.

Endophthalmitis is inflammation of the vitreous humor and can be endogenous, secondary to hematogenous spread from a distant site, or exogenous from inoculation after penetrating trauma. Traumatic endophthalmitis usually develops within 3 days of a penetrating injury, retained foreign body, or ocular surgery. Hallmarks include decreased vision, eye pain, hypopyon, anterior chamber cells and flare, an absent red reflex, and a hazy vitreous. Varying degrees of eyelid swelling, chemosis (conjunctival swelling), and severe conjunctival injection will also be present. Causative organisms include *Bacillus cereus*, coagulase-negative *Staphylococcus*, *Streptococcus*, gram-negative rods, and fungi. Any patient with a hypopyon requires an emergent ophthalmology consult. Orbital CT or ultrasound B-scan microscopy (UBM) may help diagnose a foreign body. Systemic and intravitreal antibiotics will be necessary to preserve any remainder of vision.

Orbital cellulitis, defined as infection deep to the orbital septum, is usually associated with blurred vision, diplopia, conjunctival injection, lid swelling, proptosis, fever, toxicity, and limited or painful ocular motility. An orbital computed tomography (CT) (axial and coronal cuts) is diagnostic and will often reveal sinusitis (often ethmoid). Admission and parenteral antibiotics are indicated because the infection can potentially spread to the brain. Preseptal or periorbital cellulitis is a superficial and far less serious entity, but it can be difficult to distinguish from orbital cellulitis. In general, these patients are less toxic appearing and have less pain. Most of these patients can be discharged on oral antibiotics with close follow-up to make sure they did not have an early presentation of the more serious orbital cellulitis.

Subconjunctival hemorrhages should be **painless and not affect vision**. These hemorrhages are often spontaneous but may be associated with minor trauma, including coughing and sneezing. In the setting of blunt trauma, continue evaluating for hyphema, globe rupture, or retrobulbar hemorrhage if the patient complains of pain or vision changes. Patients should be informed that the redness (bruise) might take weeks to spontaneously resolve.

Blunt trauma to the eye may result in a **hyphema** (blood in the anterior chamber) and painful, blurred vision. Blood may be visible to the unaided eye if it layers, or it may only be seen with the slit-lamp in the anterior chamber (microhyphema) on maximum magnification. Initial treatment includes elevating the head 30 degrees, an eye shield to prevent additional trauma, mydriatics to paralyze the ciliary body allowing the iris to rest, pain medication, antiemetics, and consultation. Complications include staining of the cornea by the red cells, producing a partially opaque cornea, elevated IOP secondary to red blood cells occluding the trabecular outflow tract, and rebleeding.

Scleritis symptoms include severe eye pain, redness, and decreased vision. Frequently, the cause is an underlying systemic disorder, such as a connective tissue disease, autoimmune disorder, HSV, HZV, HIV, Lyme disease, or syphilis. Rheumatoid arthritis is the most common systemic cause of scleritis. HZV is the most common infectious cause of scleritis. The conjunctival, episcleral, and scleral vessels are inflamed, either diffusely or focally. While episcleral vessels blanch with topical vasoconstrictors and move under cotton swabs, scleral vessels do not. Additionally, the entire sclera may have a bluish or violaceous hue and may be very tender upon palpation. Treatment of the underlying disorder may involve systemic corticosteroids, immunosuppressive therapy, and nonsteroidal anti-inflammatory drugs (NSAIDs).

CASE CORRELATION

- See also Case 27 (Bell Palsy) and Case 29 (Headache).

COMPREHENSION QUESTIONS

49.1 A 40-year-old man complains of acute onset of left eye redness with circumcorneal injection (ciliary flush), blurred vision, and pain with bright lights. On examination, his pupil is small and minimally reactive with cell and flare noted on slit lamp examination. He also has pain in the affected eye when light is directed in the unaffected eye (consensual photophobia). Which of the following is the most likely diagnosis?

    A. Acute angle-closure glaucoma

    B. Acute anterior uveitis

    C. HZV infection

    D. Corneal abrasion

49.2 A 52-year-old woman with Type 2 diabetes presents with 2 days of right eye pain, foreign body sensation, redness, and decreased vision. These symptoms began after she sustained a scratch to her eye when she was trying to pick up her 2-year-old grandchild, who was throwing a tantrum. Visual acuity is 20/200 in her right eye and 20/30 in her left eye. The right pupil is 3 mm and sluggishly reactive, and the left pupil is 3 mm and briskly reactive. The right eye has a ciliary flush; the left conjunctiva is normal. A large, dense white defect is visible on the right cornea, and a hypopyon is also present. Cell and flare are noted. Fluorescein uptake is large and extends deep below and beyond the margins of the ulcer. The right fundus cannot be visualized. Which of the following is the most next most appropriate action?

A. Prescribe a topical ophthalmic steroid medication as well as a return to ED in 24 hours.

B. Prescribe a topical ophthalmic antibiotic medication and a return to ED in 12 hours.

C. Arrange an emergent ophthalmology consultation.

D. Check the blood glucose, and if it is normal recommend timely visit to her doctor.

49.3 A 40-year-old woman presents with a 2 week history of redness, severe pain, and decreased vision in her right eye. She denies conjunctival discharge. Visual acuity is 20/40 in the right eye and 20/20 in the left. The pupils are 3 mm and reactive bilaterally. Extraocular movements are intact but increase the right eye pain. The temporal aspect to the right eye is reddish blue. A drop of phenylephrine is applied to the right eye, but the reddish blue area does not blanch. The right eye is soft but tender to palpation. An ophthalmologist might order all of the following tests except:

A. HLA B 27 marker

B. Rheumatoid factor

C. RPR for syphilis

D. Conjunctival culture

49.4 A 39-year-old man with a history of migraines presents to the ED with a headache over both brows, nausea, and blurry vision for the past 6 hours. He recently started taking topiramate for his migraines and admits to taking a second dose 12 hours ahead of schedule today. The current headache began gradually but is slightly worse than usual, and the blurry vision is new. His vision is usually normal. He denies trauma or fever. Visual acuity is 20/200 in both eyes, and the pupils are each 4 mm and minimally reactive. The conjunctivae are normal, and the anterior chambers are clear but shallow. There is no fluorescein uptake. Fundoscopy is normal. The neurological examination is non-focal. Which of the following is the next most appropriate immediate test?

A. CT head without contrast

B. CT of orbit

C. MRI head

D. Measure intraocular pressures

ANSWERS

49.1 **B.** Acute anterior uveitis usually presents as photophobia, blurred vision, and a painful red eye. A ciliary flush and cells with flare are noted on slit-lamp examination.

49.2 **C.** An emergent ophthalmology consult is appropriate for a diabetic patient with a deep corneal ulcer and a hypopyon in order to assess for endophthalmitis. This patient will require IV and intravitreal antibiotics and hospital admission.

49.3 **D.** When the clinical pattern suggests scleritis, as in this example, a conjunctival culture would not be typically ordered in the absence of discharge. Studies which evaluate systemic diseases such as rheumatoid arthritis, sarcoidosis, syphilis, inflammatory bowel disease, and reactive arthritis would be appropriate. Rheumatoid arthritis is the most common systemic disease associated with scleritis.

49.4 **D.** Tonometry. Acute angle closure glaucoma is an uncommon but significant side effect of topiramate (Topamax), an anticonvulsant and antimigraine medication. Patients typically present with bilateral blurry vision, headache, nausea, and vomiting. However, eye redness is minimal or absent, unlike most cases of AACG. Topiramate-induced AACG usually occurs within several weeks of beginning the medication or within several hours if the dosage is doubled.

CLINICAL PEARLS

▶ A useful working differential diagnosis for vision-threatening causes of red eye includes acute angle-closure glaucoma, anterior uveitis, endophthalmitis, corneal ulcer, corneal infection, chlamydial/gonococcal conjunctivitis, orbital cellulitis, hyphema, retrobulbar hemorrhage, and scleritis.

▶ Subconjunctival hemorrhages should be painless and do not affect vision. In the setting of blunt trauma, continue evaluating for hyphema, hypopyon, globe rupture, endophthalmitis, or retrobulbar hemorrhage if the patient complains of pain or vision changes since emergent ophthalmologic consultation would be indicated.

▶ Penlight pupil assessment, slit-lamp examination, fluorescein staining, measurement of intraocular pressure, and ophthalmoscopy are essential elements of a thorough evaluation of the red eye.

▶ Beware of systemic complications from topical ophthalmologic medications. Allergic reactions and complications such as bradycardia and bronchospasm from topical beta-blockers are common.

REFERENCES

AhKee EY, Egong E, Shafi A, et al. A review of drug-induced acute angle closure glaucoma for non-ophthalmologists. *Qatar Med J*. 2015:6 (online).

Azari A, Barney NP. Conjunctivitis. A systematic review of diagnosis and treatment. *JAMA*. 2013;16:1721-1729.

Bagheri N, Wajda BN, eds. *The Wills Eye Manual*, 7th ed. Philadelphia, PA: Lippincott Williams & Wilkins; 2016.

Narayana S, McGee S. Bedside diagnosis of the 'Red Eye': a systematic review. *Am J Med*. 2015;128: 1220-1224.

Romaniuk VM. Ocular trauma and other catastrophes. *Emergency Med Clin N Am*. 2011;31:399-411.

Uhr JH, Mishra K, Wei C, et al. Awareness and knowledge of emerent ophthalmic disease among patient in an Interna Medicine Clinic. *JAMA Ophthalmol*. 2016.

A 28-year-old man with a history of sickle cell disease (SCD) presents to the emergency department (ED) complaining of lower leg pain and lower back pain for 2 days. He states that the pain is more severe than his usual "pain crisis" and is burning and throbbing. He just finished a bike ride 2 days before. He denies fevers, shortness of breath, vomiting, hemoptysis, or lower extremity swelling, headaches, sick contacts, recent travel, changes in medications, and drug or alcohol use. His last pain crisis was 3 months ago. He usually takes acetaminophen and hydrocodone for pain control during his crises; however, neither has provided relief during this episode. On physical examination, his temperature is 37.5°C (99.5°F), blood pressure is 126/65 mm Hg, heart rate is 98 beats per minute, respiratory rate is 22 breaths per minute, and oxygen saturation is 98% on room air. Lung examination reveals scant crackles in the right lower lung field. He does not have any jugular venous distension, calf tenderness, or lower extremity edema.

His initial workup includes a normal chest x-ray, and normal labs: venous blood gas (VBG), complete blood count, reticulocyte count, lactate dehydrogenase level, haptoglobin, type and screen, liver function tests, and basic metabolic panel. He is given morphine for pain control and a 2 L bolus of intravenous fluids. The patient is admitted for pain control. Approximately 24 hours later, the patient develops shortness of breath and chills. Repeat vital signs show: temperature 38.4°C (101.2°F), blood pressure is 132/73 mm Hg, heart rate is 100 beats per minute, respiratory rate is 28 breaths per minute, and oxygen saturation is 94% on room air. The patient is placed on 3 liters/min by nasal cannula, which improves his hypoxia and tachypnea, and a repeat chest x-ray is done, which shows bilateral infiltrates.

▶ What is the most concerning issue regarding this patient?
▶ What is the next step in management?

ANSWERS TO CASE 50:

Sickle Cell Crisis

Summary: This is a 28-year-old man with a history of SCD who presents initially with a painful episode but later becomes febrile, tachypneic, and hypoxic.

- **Most concerning issue:** Acute chest syndrome (ACS).

- **Next step in management:** Pain control, arterial blood gas, and evaluate for other causes of hypoxia such as pulmonary embolism, pneumonia, or pulmonary edema.

ANALYSIS

Objectives

1. Understand the treatment of simple pain crises in patients with SCD.

2. Understand the diagnosis and treatment of ACS.

3. Understand other life-threatening complications of SCD and their initial management.

4. Understand pain management for sickle cell.

Considerations

The patient in this case, a 28-year-old man with known SCD, has acute onset of back and limb pain and subtle findings on the pulmonary examination. The initial concern is for acute pain crisis. His initial vital signs are stable; however, 24 hours later on repeat examination after he develops respiratory distress, his oxygen saturation is 94% on room air, his respiratory rate is 28 breaths per minute, he is febrile to 101.2°F, and his heart rate is increased to 100 beats per minute. These findings are concerning and should be followed up with a VBG to assess for severe sepsis (ie, lactic acidosis). Pulmonary embolism, pneumonia, **sepsis**, and **ACS** should be considered as possible diagnoses. These are not mutually exclusive diagnoses and frequently overlap in individuals with SCD. ACS is a clinical phenomenon in which individuals with SCD become critically ill and develop progressive respiratory failure in a pattern similar to acute respiratory distress syndrome (ARDS). Before development of fulminant ARDS, individuals often manifest findings identical to pneumonia (pulmonary infiltrate, fever, and dyspnea), as does the patient in this case. Criteria for the diagnosis of ACS in the literature are identical to the diagnosis of pneumonia because the initial phases are identical, but **it is the development of progressive respiratory failure and non-response to antibiotics that truly defines ACS.** The first step is to look at the patient. Assess for signs of increased work of breathing, vital sign abnormalities, and signs of Systemic Inflammatory Response Syndrome (SIRS), Sepsis, or Septic Shock. All patients with SIRS should receive early IV antibiotics. Making the diagnosis of ACS and distinguishing from pneumonia is somewhat arbitrary and based largely on the presence of findings consistent with pneumonia but with failure to improve clinically with antibiotics. The etiology of ACS is poorly understood, but recent research suggests that autoamplifying inflammatory cascades are triggered via the same mechanism as super-antigen, LPS-mediated sepsis because hemoglobin breakdown products activate toll-like receptor 4. When ACS and pneumonia are on the differential diagnosis, initial management is supportive and includes oxygen, antibiotics, gentle intravenous fluid (preferably hypotonic fluid), and analgesia. If the patient continues to deteriorate, exchange transfusion and simple transfusion must be initiated early, as these are the only therapies thought to reduce mortality from ACS. Thus, it is important to consult the hematology team early into the patient's presentation to the ED, especially if the patient's clinical course is not improving, which may indicate they need an exchange transfusion.

DEFINITIONS

ACUTE CHEST SYNDROME: The presence of a new lobar or segmental infiltrate on chest radiography in the presence of fever, respiratory symptoms, and/or chest pain in a patient with SCD. The underlying causes are varied but may be exacerbated by infectious causes (eg, pneumonia) or non-infectious causes (eg, pulmonary embolism or asthma).

VASOOCLUSIVE CRISIS: Occlusion of blood flow causing regional hypoxia and acidosis. The underlying etiology for vasooclusion is multifactorial, but inflammation is a pivotal component. Dehydration leads to the distorted sickle cell shape of RBCs and results in their abnormal adhesion to the vascular endothelium that in turn triggers an inflammatory response. This inflammatory response results in vasoocclusion and tissue infarction. These processes alone contribute to the pain, but most likely it is the secondary inflammatory response caused by tissue infarction that results in the severe pain seen in SCD.

SPLENIC SEQUESTRATION: Occurs when red cells become trapped in the spleen, resulting in a rapidly enlarging spleen, a sudden drop in hemoglobin, and the potential for shock.

TRANSIENT RED CELL APLASIA: A transient cessation of erythropoiesis resulting in the acute onset of anemia and reticulocytopenia. The most common cause of aplasia appears to be infection, specifically parvovirus B19.

CLINICAL APPROACH

SCD, an autosomal recessive disorder of hemoglobin, affects approximately 100,000 individuals in the United States. SCD is caused by abnormal hemoglobin production. In humans, hemoglobin is composed of two alpha and two beta chains. However, in SCD, hemoglobin S (HbS) results when a valine is substituted for glutamine in the sixth position of the beta chain. Under hypoxic or acidotic conditions, this abnormal hemoglobin polymerizes inside the red cell, creating a sickled shape. The resulting damage to the red cell initiates a cascade of hemolysis, abnormal cell adhesion and endothelial dysfunction that leads to progressive organ damage.

The gene for HbS is autosomal recessive. Patients who are **heterozygous** (HbAS) have sickle trait and are generally asymptomatic except under extreme stress (eg, severe dehydration, temperature, or pressure change). Those who are **homozygous**

(HbSS) have SCD and are highly susceptible to vasoocclusion and pain crises. In addition to HbS, hundreds of other known beta globin mutations exist. The combination of one HbS with another variant hemoglobin (the most common is HbSC) also results in SCD; however, these typically manifest a milder course.

Potential triggers for sickle cell crises are numerous. Some common triggers include infections (bacterial and viral), dehydration, exposure to cold temperatures, and low oxygen environments. It should be recognized, however, that spontaneous, unexplained crises are common. Because these patients are functionally asplenic after early childhood, they are also at significant risk for bacterial infections, especially by **encapsulated organisms** such as *Salmonella typhi, Haemophilus influenza* type B, *Streptoccoccus pneumoniae, Neisseria meningitidis*, and Group B *streptococci*. Penicillin prophylaxis has significantly decreased the morbidity and mortality secondary to bacterial infections.

COMMON COMPLICATIONS

SCD can affect multiple organ systems (Table 50–1). During the assessment of patients with SCD, the history should focus on **identifying any precipitating causes and complications.** Pain that is different from previous pain crises may be an indicator of a potentially life-threatening event. A rapid assessment of the vital signs and a careful physical examination are important because severe complications in sickle cell crisis often present with nonspecific manifestations. The clinician's concern should be heightened if the patient has a fever, severe abdominal pain, respiratory or neurological symptoms, joint swelling, priapism, or pain that is not relieved by usual measures.

Vasoocclusive Crisis

Acute vasoocclusive events (VOEs), or "painful crises," are the **most common complications of SCD** and the most frequent cause of ED visits in this patient population. Polymerization of the sickle cell hemoglobin causes the red blood cells to become rigid and sticky and formed into shapes that sometimes have the appearance of a sickle, hence the name. This sickle shape of the RBCs was once thought to be the key component in occlusion of microvasculature and therefore the cause of VOE. We now know, however, that VOE is a result of a multitude of factors including: red cell function, blood viscosity, adherence of sickled cells to endothelium, and environmental factors. In fact, a study by Frenette et al (2002) published in PNAS demonstrated that WBCs adhere to the endothelium wall and RBCs then stick to the WBCs, causing vascular occlusion. This model helps to show how those patients with sickle cell may live in a homeostatic balance with circulating sickle cells, but a seemingly minor event such as a viral illness, dehydration, trauma, or exercise may tip this balance, resulting in VOE.

Dactylitis

The first manifestation of VOE in infants may present as dactylitis, or hand-foot syndrome. Infarctions in the metacarpals result in episodes of pain and swelling involving the hands and feet. Infants and toddlers with dactylitis may become irritable, refuse to walk, or cry when touched or held. As children with SCD get older, pain shifts to the arms, legs, back, and pelvis, whereas adolescents may also

Table 50–1 • SICKLE CELL CRISES

Type of Crisis	Comments	Diagnosis	Treatment
Vasoocclusive crises: Precipitants are infection, dehydration, stress, fatigue, cold, high altitude			
Musculoskeletal pain	Commonly in low back, femur, tibia, humerus	Examination: Normal or may have local tenderness	Hydration, analgesia
Abdominal pain	Pain usually acute onset, poorly localized, and recurrent; broad differential includes hepatobiliary, splenic, or renal disease	Examination: No peritoneal signs; complete blood count, liver function tests	Treat underlying etiology, supportive care[a]
Acute chest syndrome	Pleuritic chest pain, cough, dyspnea	Examination: Fever, tachypnea, rales; pulse oximetry, chest x-ray, arterial blood gas, V/Q scan, angiography	Treat underlying etiology, supportive care, supplemental oxygen, antibiotics, anticoagulation
Central nervous system crisis	Headache, neurological deficit, seizure, mental status changes; usually infarct in children and hemorrhage in adults	CT scan, lumbar puncture, MRI	Exchange transfusion
Priapism	Painful erection without sexual stimulation caused by sickling in corpus cavernosum	Examination: engorged, painful penis	Supportive care, exchange transfusion, aspiration of corpus cavernosum, intrapenile injection of vasodilator, urologic consultation
Dactylitis	Swelling of hands and/or feet; usually occurs before 2 years of age	Painful edema of hands and/or feet	Supportive care, warm compresses
Renal crisis	Usually asymptomatic; may have flank pain	Urinalysis shows hematuria or tissue	Supportive care
Hematological crises			
Splenic sequestration	Rapid onset of fatigue, listlessness, pallor, abdominal pain; most common in children <6 years of age	Examination: hypovolemia, splenomegaly; severe anemia or significant drop in hemoglobin	Correction of hypovolemia, PRBC transfusion, exchange transfusion, splenectomy
Aplastic crisis	Precipitants: Parvovirus B19 infection, folic acid deficiency, phenylbutazone	Significant drop in hemoglobin with low reticulocyte count	IV fluids, PRBC transfusion; usually self-limited
Infectious crises			
	Common organisms: encapsulated (*Haemophilus influenzae, Streptococcus pneumoniae*), *Salmonella typhi, Mycoplasma pneumoniae, Escherichia coli, Staphylococcus aureus*	Examination: fever; complete blood count, urinalysis, blood and sputum and urine cultures (as indicated), chest x-ray	Broad-spectrum antibiotics

Abbreviations: CT = computed tomography; IV = intravenous; V/Q ventilation = perfusion; PRBC = packed red blood cell.
[a]Supportive care includes hydration and analgesia.

complain of involvement of the chest and abdomen. These vasoocclusive episodes usually last from 3 to 9 days, but it is not atypical for those patients with longer episodes to continue to have patterns where their episodes remain prolonged.

Infection

Infection is the major cause of mortality in SCD. Virtually all patients with SCD are asplenic, predisposing them to overwhelming infections from **encapsulated microorganisms.** In addition to sepsis, patients are susceptible to other infections, such as pneumonia, meningitis, and osteomyelitis. Although prophylactic penicillin and vaccines for pneumococci and *Haemophilus influenzae* type B have reduced the incidence of sepsis in this patient population, **pneumococcal sepsis remains a significant cause of death in children with SCD.** Adults are less vulnerable because their immune systems have matured to allow for type-specific antibody production; however, they are still at risk for infectious from atypical organisms, and fever must be taken very seriously in all patients with SCD.

Acute Chest Syndrome

ACS is defined in the literature as the presence of two of the following: a **new lobar or segmental pulmonary infiltrate or focal abnormality on CXR, fever higher than 38.5°C** (101.3°F), **respiratory symptoms, hypoxemia, or chest pain.** Clinically, ACS is differentiated from pneumonia when patients continue to deteriorate despite antibiotics and supportive care. In these individuals, immediate transfusion (preferably exchange transfusion) may be lifesaving. **ACS is a serious, life-threatening condition that should be recognized early, and management should be initiated as early as possible.** ACS is thought to result from an auto-amplifying cascade of inflammation triggered initially by an increase in hemolysis. Infection, hemolysis, pulmonary infarction due to vasoocclusion, and fat emboli from marrow infarction may all contribute to ACS. Hemolysis plays a role in inflammation more specifically through activation of the TLR4 pathway. Hemin is released with hemolysis and is a potent agonist of the TLR4 pathway, which results in a catastrophic vascular leak in the lungs, very similar to that seen in sepsis-triggered ARDS. These similarities in inflammatory-mediated mechanisms correlate with the similarity in management of ACS with pneumonia-mediated sepsis. Infectious organisms associated with ACS include *S. pneumoniae* in younger children and atypical organisms, such as *Mycoplasma* or *Chlamydia*, in adolescents.

Chest pain from vasoocclusion may cause splinting and hypoventilation, leading to atelectasis and subsequent development of ACS in a patient who initially presents with a painful episode. Therefore, pain management and monitoring of respiratory status are paramount, as ACS carries a high risk of progression to respiratory failure, with **approximately 13% requiring mechanical ventilation and 3% resulting in death.**

ACS usually manifests on hospital days 3-5. The finding of an infiltrate on chest radiograph is diagnostically significant, but it should be recognized that it is common for the initial radiograph to be normal. Laboratory evaluation should include a CBC, reticulocyte count, blood cultures, and type and screen. A baseline VBG measurement should be obtained, followed by serial VBG measurements to evaluate for worsening lactate. In patients with ACS and concern for hypoxia (O_2 Sat <94%),

supplemental oxygen should be administered as needed. **Exchange (or conventional) transfusion** should be initiated in patients with hypoxia, hypoxemia (Pao_2 <70-80 mm Hg), a drop in hemoglobin more than 2 g below baseline, or any other signs of progressive deterioration despite antibiotics. Exchange transfusion replaces a patient's sickled RBCs with exogenous non-sickled RBCs and overall decreases blood viscosity. If exchange transfusion is not available or a patient's hemoglobin and/or hematocrit is decreased, then a simple transfusion is an alternative option that gives a patient exogenous blood without removing any of the patient's blood. If considering exchange transfusion, a hematology consult should be considered. All patients should receive **empiric antibiotics** that cover typical and atypical microorganisms; most commonly a macrolide and third generation cephalosporin is given. Analgesia for chest pain should be provided but managed carefully to prevent hypoventilation. Regular use of an incentive spirometer has shown to significantly reduce the frequency of subsequent episodes of chest pain. Hypotonic intravenous fluids such as D5 1/2 NS should most likely be used for hydration and should not exceed 1.5 times maintenance in order to prevent volume overload.

Stroke (Cerebrovascular Accidents)

Patients with SCD are at **greatly increased risk for both ischemic and hemorrhagic stroke.** Most strokes in children are ischemic events, usually involving large arteries, whereas hemorrhagic strokes are more common in adults. Common presenting signs and symptoms include hemiparesis, aphasia, dysphasia, cranial nerve palsies, seizure, or coma. A non-contrast enhanced CT scan should be obtained as soon as possible, followed by MRI and MRA with diffusion weighted imaging. The treatment for ischemic stroke in **children is exchange transfusion**, as conventional therapies (tissue plasminogen activator and antiplatelet agents) are not indicated. Ischemic strokes in **adults** with SCD are thought to be more likely the result of common ischemic stroke mechanisms; therefore, **conventional therapies are recommended.**

Splenic Sequestration

Acute splenic sequestration is the **most dangerous cause of acute exacerbation of anemia in patients with SCD.** This occurs when red cells become trapped in the spleen, resulting in a sudden drop in hemoglobin and the potential for shock. It typically occurs between the ages of 3 months to 5 years. Patients typically present with sudden weakness, pallor, tachycardia, or abdominal fullness. The mortality of this condition is high, and death can occur within a matter of hours without aggressive management. All patients should be transfused with packed red blood cells emergently. **Splenectomy may be necessary** in children with recurrent splenic sequestration.

Aplastic Crisis

Patients with SCD are susceptible to transient red cell aplasia (TRCA). The majority of TRCA are caused by Parvovirus B19 infection. The virus is directly cytotoxic to erythroid precursors, which can cause transient suppression of erythropoiesis and reticulocytopenia. This will present as significant anemia after an illness without signs of hemolysis, usually 5 days postexposure and continuing 7-10 days. Intravenous immunoglobulin (IVIG) infusion is the standard treatment once the diagnosis is made.

Priapism

Priapism, a prolonged painful erection of the penis, is a well-recognized complication of SCD that can result in fibrosis and impotence. Approximately 50% of men with SCD reported having at least one episode of priapism before 21 years of age. In addition to pain management, effective strategies for immediate and sustained detumescence consist of aspiration of blood from the corpora cavernosa followed by irrigation of the corpora cavernosa with dilute epinephrine. In all cases, early urologic consultation should be obtained.

Pain Management

It is important to note that **pain** is often the primary presenting complaint of all sickle cell–associated crises. It is thought that pain is caused by ischemia secondary to a multitude of factors resulting in vasooclusion. This vasooclusion results in local acidosis, which in turn engenders more endothelial cell dysfunction, and the pain worsens.

Unfortunately, recent evidence shows that **patients with SCD are regularly undertreated for their pain.** This is likely due to sociocultural factors as well as the challenges of navigating the subjectivity of pain. Adequately treating pain is a vital component in the treatment of sickle cell patients who present to the ED.

The mainstay of **treatment for a pain crisis** is **supportive care: supplemental oxygen (only if hypoxic),** *gentle* **hydration (hypotonic fluids at maintenance WITHOUT a fluid bolus), and analgesia.** Due to the chronicity of these pain crises and the long-standing pain that results from sickle cell complications (eg, avascular necrosis), adequate analgesia plays a pivotal role in patient care. Patients with moderate to severe pain typically require **intravenous opioids.** In patients with poor vascular access secondary to chronic intravenous line placement, subcutaneous (intramuscular is more painful and carries no pharmacologic advantage) administration is a suitable alternative. Oral opioids are used for patients in less severe pain. Although there are no definitive studies that show which opioid is superior in treating a pain crisis, morphine sulfate or hydromorphone are commonly used as first-line agents. Hydromorphone is a good option for patients who cannot tolerate the side effects of morphine (eg, nausea and pruritus). Meperidine, a commonly prescribed opioid, should be avoided due to its increased risk of causing seizures via its renally cleared metabolite, normeperidine. Dosing of analgesics should be individualized for each patient and should be titrated to pain relief. Adjunctive therapy with nonsteroidals (NSAIDs), particularly ketorolac, should be considered as a second line therapy. However, long-term use of NSAID medications increases the risk of renal failure and peptic ulcer disease. Hydroxyurea is another adjunctive therapy indicated in all individuals with HbSS; however, it has no use in the acute setting. It is a myelosuppressive agent that stimulates the production on fetal hemoglobin, HbF, which ultimately leads to less sickling episodes and perhaps mitigates other factors associated with development of pain crises. Its use, however, should be monitored, as leukopenia, neutropenia, and thrombocytopenia are common side effects. Overall, personalized pain management should involve active patient participation, as many will know their medication, dose, and frequency of administration that is most beneficial to them.

> ### CASE CORRELATION
>
> - See also Case 13 (Acute Exacerbation of Asthma), Case 14 (Pulmonary Embolism), Case 15 (Bacterial Pneumonia), and Case 51 (Transfusion Complications).

COMPREHENSION QUESTIONS

50.1 A 3-year-old girl is brought into the ED by her mother for being pale and irritable. The girl is known to have SCD. Which of the following tests would help to differentiate an aplastic crisis from a vasoocclusive crisis?

A. Reticulocyte count

B. Bone marrow biopsy

C. Peripheral smear

D. Hemoglobin level

E. Haptoglobin level

50.2 A 2-year-old boy with SCD is being seen by his pediatrician. Which of the following would make the most impact on mortality risk?

A. Screening urine culture

B. Bone radiograph to assess for osteomyelitis

C. Pneumococcal vaccination

D. Chest radiograph to assess for ACS

E. Bone marrow biopsy to assess anemia

50.3 A 12-year-old girl is brought into the ED at the direction of her pediatrician. The patient's mother informs you that the patient has SCD. Which of the following findings would be most concerning to you?

A. Fever

B. Pain that is typical of past crises

C. Mild abdominal pain

D. Hematuria

E. Strabismus

50.4 Which of the following is most accurate concerning ACS?

A. It is an uncommon complication of SCD.

B. It can be caused by pulmonary infection or infarct.

C. It can be ruled out with a normal chest x-ray.

D. Antibiotics should not be given until the patient is proven to have an infection.

ANSWERS

50.1 **A.** The reticulocyte count is low in aplastic crisis but elevated or normal with a vasoocclusive crisis. A bone marrow biopsy is invasive and causes a delay in diagnosis. Neither a smear nor a haptoglobin level would differentiate between the two diagnoses. A hemoglobin level may not show a difference in the acute setting.

50.2 **C.** Pneumococcal sepsis is the leading cause of death in children aged 1-3 years. Thus, pneumococcal vaccine is critical in its prevention.

50.3 **A.** The clinician should be worried if the patient has a fever, severe abdominal pain, respiratory or neurological symptoms, joint swelling, pain that is not relieved by usual measures, or priapism. The other signs and symptoms here require additional workup but are not harbingers of the same level of morbidity as a fever.

50.4 **B.** ACS is caused by pulmonary infection or infarct. It is a common complication of SCD that is difficult to confirm simply by a chest radiograph. Because it is difficult to differentiate from infectious pneumonia, patients should be empirically started on antibiotics.

CLINICAL PEARLS

▶ SCD can manifest in any organ system and has a variety of clinical presentations, ranging from mild to life threatening.

▶ Because patients with SCD are functionally asplenic after early childhood, they are at risk for infection by encapsulated organisms (eg, *Haemophilus influenzae, Streptococcus pneumoniae*) and therefore must be immunized with the appropriate vaccines.

▶ ACS is the leading cause of premature death in patients with SCD. Having a low threshold of suspicion in patients presenting with respiratory complaints, abnormal oxygen saturation, or findings on lung examination is critical.

▶ Treatment of ACS involves supplemental oxygen, hydration, analgesia, empiric antibiotics, and exchange transfusion.

▶ Splenic sequestration has a very high mortality. Patients present with an abrupt drop in hemoglobin and the potential for shock, requiring emergent transfusion and splenectomy.

▶ Aplastic crisis occurs from a transient suppression of erythropoiesis. It is characterized by significant anemia accompanied by a low reticulocyte count. It is most commonly caused by parvovirus B19.

▶ Patients in pain crises require prompt attention and treatment of their pain. Intravenous opioids, such as morphine or hydromorphone, are the mainstay of pain management in the ED.

REFERENCES

Ballas SK. Pain management of sickle cell disease. *Hematol Oncol Clin North Am*. 2005;19(5): 785-802, v. Epub 2005/10/11. doi: S0889-8588(05)00089-4 [pii]10.1016/j.hoc.2005.07.008. PubMed PMID: 16214644.

DeBaun MR, Vichinsky E. Sickle cell disease. In: *Nelson Textbook of Pediatrics*. 18th ed. New York, NY: Saunders; 2007:2026-2031.

Ghosh S, Adisa OA, Chappa P, et al. Extracellular hemin crisis triggers acute chest syndrome in sickle mice. *J Clin Invest*. 2013;123(11):4809-4820. Epub 2013/10/03.doi: 10.1172/JCI64578. PubMed PMID: 24084741; PubMed Central PMCID: PMC3809772.

Givens M, Rutherford C, Joshi G, et al. Impact of an emergency department pain management protocol on the pattern of visits by patients with sickle cell disease. *J Emerg Med*. 2007;32:239-243.

Glassberg J. Current guidelines for sickle cell disease: management of acute complications. *Emergency Medicine Practice Guidelines Update*. 2009;1(3):1-3.

Hassell KL. Population estimates of sickle cell disease in the U.S. *Am J Prev Med*. 2010;38(4 Suppl): S512-21. Epub 2010/04/02.doi: S0749-3797(09)00960-X [pii]10.1016/j.amepre.2009.12.022. PubMed PMID: 20331952.

Knight-Madden J, Serjeant GR. Invasive pneumococcal disease in homozygous sickle cell disease: Jamaican experience 1973-1997. *J Pediatr*. 2001;138(1):65-70. Epub 2001/01/10.doi: S0022-3476(01)09636-6 [pii]10.1067/mpd.2001.109709. PubMed PMID: 11148514.

Lee A, Thomas P, Cupidore L, Serjeant B, Serjeant G. Improved survival in homozygous sickle cell disease: lessons from a cohort study. *BMJ*. 1995;311(7020):1600-1602. Epub 1995/12/16. PubMed PMID: 8555802; PubMed Central PMCID: PMC2551498.

McClish DK, Penberthy LT, Bovbjerg VE, et al. Health related quality of life in sickle cell patients: the PiSCES project. *Health Qual Life Outcomes*. 2005;3:50. Epub 2005/09/01.doi: 1477-7525-3-50 [pii]10.1186/1477-7525-3-50. PubMed PMID: 16129027; PubMed Central PMCID: PMC1253526.

McClish DK, Smith WR, Dahman BA, et al. Pain site frequency and location in sickle cell disease: the PiSCES project. *Pain*. 2009;145(1-2):246-251. Epub 2009/07/28.doi: 10.1016/j.pain.2009.06.029. PubMed PMID: 19631468; PubMed Central PMCID: PMC2771372.

McCreight A, Wickiser J. Sickle cell disease. In: Strange GR, Ahrens WR, Schfermeyer R, Wiebe R, eds. *Pediatric Emergency Medicine*. 3rd ed. 2009:Chapter 100.

Rees DC, Williams TN, Gladwin MT. Sickle-cell disease. *Lancet*. 2010;376(9757):2018-2031. Epub 2010/12/07.doi: 10.1016/S0140-6736(10)61029-X. PubMed PMID: 21131035.

Swerdlow PS. Red cell exchange in sickle cell disease. *Hematology Am Soc Hematol Educ Program*. 2006:48-53. Epub 2006/11/25. doi: 2006/1/48 [pii]10.1182/asheducation-2006.1.48. PubMed PMID: 17124039.

Turhan A, Weiss LA, Mohandas N, Coller BS, Frenette PS. Primary role for adherent leukocytes in sickle cell vascular occlusion: a new paradigm. *Proc Natl Acad Sci U S A*. 2002;99(5):3047-3051. Epub 2002/03/07.doi: 10.1073/pnas.05252279999/5/3047 [pii]. PubMed PMID: 11880644; PubMed Central PMCID: PMC122470.

Vichinsky EP, Neumayr LD, Earles AN, et al. Causes and outcomes of the acute chest syndrome in sickle cell disease. National Acute Chest Syndrome Study Group. *N Engl J Med*. 2000;342(25): 1855-1865. Epub 2000/06/22. PubMed PMID: 10861320.

Zempsky W. Evaluation and treatment of sickle cell pain in the emergency department: paths to a better future. *Clin Pediatr Emerg Med*. 2010;11:265-273.

A 10-year-old boy with sickle cell disease presents to the emergency department (ED) in the midst of presumed sickle cell crisis manifested as severe abdominal pain, pleuritic chest pain, dyspnea, and fever. His initial hemoglobin is 9 g/dL, white blood cell count (WBC) is 15,500 cells per mm^3, and chest x-ray reveals a nonspecific infiltrate in the left lung field with a small left pleural effusion. The electrocardiogram reveals sinus tachycardia. Following treatment with intravenous fluid, supplemental oxygen by nasal cannula, parenteral analgesics, and empiric broad-spectrum antibiotics therapy, the patient complained of worsening dyspnea and chest pain, requiring increased oxygen supplementation by facemask and eventual endotracheal intubation. At this juncture, exchange transfusion therapy is contemplated.

▶ What are the complications associated with blood transfusions in this setting?
▶ What are the ways to reduce the incidence of transfusion-related complications?

ANSWERS TO CASE 51:

Transfusion Complications

Summary: A 10-year-old boy presents with sickle cell crisis associated with severe respiratory symptoms (acute chest syndrome). The patient continues to have significant respiratory symptoms despite supportive care, and therefore exchange transfusion therapy is considered.

- **Transfusion complications:** Transfusion reactions and transfusion-related infections.

- **Ways to reduce transfusion complications:** Strict adherence to patient identification, specimen handling, and blood product storage protocols, and thorough review of transfusion history. Transfuse blood products based on need rather than arbitrary transfusion triggers.

ANALYSIS

Objectives

1. Develop an understanding of the epidemiology and basic pathophysiology of transfusion reactions.

2. Learn the evaluation and treatment of acute, life-threatening transfusion complications.

3. Learn the indications for blood product transfusion.

Considerations

Because sickle cell disease predisposes the patient to chronic anemia, it is very likely that this particular patient has had an extensive history of transfusions; therefore, a thorough review of the transfusion history is vital. If the patient or the medical records indicate prior occurrence of minor transfusion reactions, then premedication with antihistamines and/or antipyretics may be useful. As a group, patients who are homozygous for sickle hemoglobin are at markedly increased risk of suffering complications from transfusion therapy, including transfusion-related infectious (approximately 10% are infected with hepatitis C virus), and noninfectious complications related to alloimmunization (affecting up to 50% of sickle cell patients). The increased risks of alloimmunization are primarily related to recurrent antigen exposure and phenotypic dissimilarities between blood cells in the predominately white-donated blood supply and African American sickle cell patients.

To reduce the risk of transfusion-related complications, blood banks have intensified the cross-matching process for transfusions in sickle cell patients, with a demonstrable decrease in rates of alloimmunization. **Leukocyte-reduced packed red blood cells (PRBC) are recommended for patients with sickle cell disease and other patients requiring recurrent transfusions.** Additional benefits include a reduced rate of human leukocyte antigen (HLA) alloimmunization and possible decreased rates of febrile nonhemolytic transfusion reactions (FNHTRs).

APPROACH TO:
Transfusion Complications

CLINICAL APPROACH

Conceptually, transfusion complications are best categorized into acute immune-mediated reactions, delayed immune-mediated reactions, nonimmunologic complications, and infectious complications.

ACUTE IMMUNE-MEDIATED REACTIONS

Acute Hemolytic Transfusion Reactions

Acute hemolytic transfusion reactions occur in 1:25,000 transfusions and cause death in 1:470,000 transfusions. The **majority of acute hemolytic transfusion reactions** are due to **errors made during the processing of the blood**, usually a failure of patient identification at specimen collection or during the transfusion process. The majority of these reactions may be avoided with meticulous specimen processing, patient identification, and adherence to transfusion guidelines. Onset of reaction is **immediate, presenting with a combination of hypotension, tachypnea (often with the sensation of chest constriction), tachycardia, fever, chills, nausea, hemoglobinuria, and flank pain (from renal capsular stretch) and body pain (joints and legs)**. Hemolysis can be either intravascular (more severe) or extravascular and is directed toward donor red blood cells (RBCs), usually mediated by preformed antibodies (anti-A and anti-B) within the recipient's serum. Because the causative antibodies to ABO group antigens are preexisting in susceptible individuals, no prior alloantigen exposure is necessary for acute hemolysis to occur. However, recent sensitization to other alloantigens (such as an Rh-negative patient being exposed to Rh-positive blood) can result in similar pathology if a subsequent blood transfusion contains the same alloantigen(s). Given the potential for new alloantibody formation, a blood sample from the recipient should only be used for cross-matching assays within 48 hours from the time of collection.

Immediate management of suspected cases includes stopping the transfusion and changing the IV tubing or using alternative access sites to initiate aggressive crystalloid infusions, aiming to **maintain urine output above 1-1.5 mL/kg/h for 24 hours.** The remainder of the transfusion and a sample of the patient's blood should be sent to the blood bank for testing. The sequelae of acute hemolysis include **acute tubular necrosis (ATN), disseminated intravascular coagulation (DIC), and shock.** DIC may be confirmed by the presence of **hemoglobinuria and plasma-free hemoglobin.** The definitive diagnosis of acute hemolytic transfusion reactions is made with **direct antiglobulin test** (DAT, also known as the direct Coombs assay), which detects antibody or complement bound to the surface of donor RBCs in a sample of the recipient's blood.

Febrile Nonhemolytic Transfusion Reactions

These reactions occur with approximately 0.5% to 1% RBC units, 2% apheresis platelet unit, and 5% to 30% donor-pooled platelets. Febrile nonhemolytic transfusion reactions (**FNHTR**) **constitute the most common and least-worrisome complications of blood product transfusion.** Patients may present with fever, chills, rigors, headache, malaise, and tachycardia but **without hemodynamic instability and respiratory compromise.** Because prior history of transfusion is required for this reaction, **fever in a first-time transfusion recipient should be treated as an acute hemolytic reaction until proven otherwise.** Conversely, prior episodes of FNHTR indicate an increased risk of recurrence.

FNHTR is a diagnosis of exclusion, so the first step in management is to **rule out a hemolytic reaction or bacterial contamination.** Samples of the patient's blood and the transfusate should be sent for analysis. Once assured that the reaction is non-hemolytic and non-septic, treatment includes stopping the transfusion, administration of an antipyretic, and patient reassurance. Patients with a history of febrile reactions can be premedicated with antipyretics. **Antipyretic premedication is a matter of preference but should be generally avoided in first-time transfusion recipients because fever is more likely to represent serious sequelae in these patients.**

Allergic Transfusion Reactions

The incidence of allergic reactions is 1% to 3% of transfusions, and the reactions are caused by recipient antibodies (immunoglobulin [Ig] E) against donor serum proteins; symptoms may range from urticaria to frank anaphylaxis. Urticaria can be managed symptomatically with antihistamines and by briefly stopping the transfusion until symptoms resolve. Mild allergic reactions do not necessitate discontinuing the transfusion, as symptoms are not strictly dose related. Patients prone to develop these reactions can be premedicated with antihistamines to prevent the development of mild allergic reactions.

Frankly, anaphylactic reactions to blood products are rare (1:20,000 to 1:170,000) and can occur within seconds of transfusion initiation. Anaphylactic reactions are IgE-mediated and occur, in most cases, as the result of **genetic deficiency of IgA in the recipient**, resulting in the production of anti-IgA, IgE. Other less-common causes of anaphylaxis include reactions caused by IgE against allergens in the transfused blood, and the passive transfer of reactive IgE from donor to the recipient. **Patients with known IgA deficiency should be given RBCs and platelets that have been thoroughly washed free of plasma proteins. Plasma component transfusions in IgA-deficient patients should be obtained from IgA-deficient donors.**

Anaphylaxis should be managed by immediately addressing the ABCs (airway, breathing, circulation), accompanied by the administration of **epinephrine, antihistamines, bronchodilators and corticosteroids**, along with the immediate discontinuation of the transfusion. **Patients taking angiotensin-converting enzyme (ACE) inhibitors** will have more severe anaphylactic reactions (ie, severe angioedema) because of their **inability to degrade bradykinin.**

Transfusion-Related Acute Lung Injury

Transfusion-related acute lung injury (TRALI), with an estimated incidence of 1:4500 transfusions, is an under-recognized **life-threatening complication of transfusion.**

TRALI is thought to be **mediated by anti-leukocyte antibodies**, resulting in systemic inflammation and neutrophil-mediated lung injury. The onset is generally within 6 hours of exposure to plasma-containing transfusion products, with most cases occurring within 1-2 hours. Random donor platelet transfusions (pooled platelets) are responsible for the majority of cases. Patients with hematological malignancies and cardiac disease are at increased risk of developing TRALI. Fever, tachycardia, and dyspnea are the most common presenting symptoms. **The hallmark of this complication is respiratory distress with the presence of diffuse, bilateral alveolar and interstitial infiltrates on radiographic imaging.** TRALI may be easily confused with acute pulmonary edema secondary to volume overload. Because **TRALI patients have normal to low left-heart pressures, echocardiography may be useful to differentiate between TRALI and pulmonary edema.** The management of this condition consists of stopping the transfusion and immediate attention to the "ABCs," which may include intubation and mechanical ventilation, restrictive tidal volumes, and restrictive fluid resuscitation. Respiratory compromise is usually self-limiting within 48-72 hours. The mortality rate associated with TRALI is about 10%.

DELAYED IMMUNE-MEDIATED REACTIONS

Delayed Hemolytic Transfusion Reactions

Delayed hemolytic transfusion reactions (DHTRs) are notably less severe than their acute hemolytic counterparts. The incidence is about 1:1000 transfusions in the general population but is up to 11% in patients with sickle cell disease. The mechanisms of DHTR are related to recipients having developed antibodies against RBC alloantigens from prior foreign RBC exposures, most often through prior transfusions or pregnancies. These antibodies may not be fully expressed until a repeat transfusion induces their production and thus can go undetected on initial blood typing.

Unlike acute hemolytic reactions, which require high circulating levels of reactive antibodies, the **alloantibodies responsible for DHTR are present only at low levels prior to transfusion.** Following exposure to these alloantigens, antibody generation is slowly increased over the following days, resulting in hemolysis of the donor RBCs. **Symptoms associated with DHTR are mild to nonexistent.** Patients typically present with a mild fever and recurrent anemia. No specific therapy is warranted aside from repeat transfusion. The best treatment is prevention, which is made possible with a carefully maintained blood bank database that is accessible across healthcare systems.

Graft-Versus-Host Disease

Transfusion-related graft-versus-host disease (GVHD) is a rare disorder where donor lymphocytes engraft and proliferate in the recipient's bone marrow, which over time may lead to a severe graft-mediated reaction against the recipient's tissues, including the bone marrow. It is **fatal in more than 90% of cases.** Symptoms of GVHD develop on average 1-2 weeks following transfusion and include fevers, maculopapular rashes, hepatitis, diarrhea, nausea, vomiting, weight loss, and pancytopenia leading to sepsis and death. **Immunocompromised recipients are especially** at risk for GVHD; therefore, blood products administered to these patients should be subjected to gamma irradiation to render remaining leukocytes incapable of proliferation. Blood products donated by first-degree relatives or between patients with partially matched HLA haplotypes have an increased risk of donor lymphocyte engraftment because of homology between donor and recipient HLA genes; therefore, blood product donated by first-degree relatives should be irradiated prior to transfusions. The highest incidence of GVHD has been from regions where the population is racially homogeneous with high likelihood of shared HLA haplotype (eg, Japan). GVHD is most problematic when patients receive fresh blood that is processed within 7 days from time of collection. In the United States, blood products that are older than 7 days generally do not contain viable lymphocytes.

Post-Transfusion Purpura

Post-transfusion purpura is a rare complication, characterized by sudden thrombocytopenia occurring 5-10 days following transfusion of any blood product. The pathophysiology involves native platelet destruction, mediated by antibodies to the platelet antigen (PLA)1. Anti-PLA1 antibodies develop in patients previously exposed to foreign platelets through transfusion or pregnancy. Patients usually present with spontaneous bleeding (mucous membranes, epistaxis, hematochezia, or hematuria). Nine percent of patients may develop intracranial hemorrhage. The diagnosis is confirmed by the detection of anti-platelet antibodies. Treatment may be supportive alone in mild cases, or it may require the administration of intravenous immunoglobulin, corticosteroids, plasma exchange therapy, and transfusion with PLA1-negative platelets. If left untreated, the thrombocytopenia usually resolves spontaneously within 2 weeks of onset.

Alloimmunization

Alloimmunization refers to the formation of new antibodies against antigens on donated cells. The formation of alloantibodies against HLA surface molecules may render patients refractory to platelet transfusions, thus supporting the administration of leukoreduced blood for patients who will likely need exogenous platelets in the future. The presence of alloantibodies is primarily responsible for the increased rates of transfusion complications seen in repeat transfusion recipients like patients with hemoglobinopathies.

INFECTIOUS COMPLICATIONS

The most frequent and concerning infectious complication of transfusion therapy is bacterial contamination, which can be detected in up to 2% of blood products. Typically, a contaminated transfusion will result in fevers, chills, hypotension and rigors within 4 hours of blood product administration. The most commonly isolated organism in refrigerated products (ie, RBCs) is *Yersinia enterocolitica*, which can grow at temperatures as low as 1°C (33.8°F). Other cryophilic organisms include *Pseudomonas*, *Enterobacter*, and *Flavobacterium*. Platelets, which are stored at room temperature (22°C-24°C [71.6°F-75.2°F]) and may be pooled from multiple donors, are more likely to develop gross contamination than refrigerated products like PRBCs and plasma. *Staphylococcus* and *Salmonella* are often reported in fatal cases of platelet transfusion-mediated sepsis. Signs and symptoms may include fevers, rigors, chills, rash, hypotension, and even shock accompanied by sepsis. Symptoms may develop immediately or over several hours. Suspected cases of contamination should be managed with respiratory and circulatory support, immediate discontinuation of the transfusion, and broad-spectrum antibiotic therapy including coverage of *Pseudomonas* species. It is often difficult to distinguish some of the immune-mediated transfusion reactions from bacterial contamination; thus **any transfusion that causes hypotension in the setting of fever warrants immediate testing of the donor blood with Gram stain and culture, in addition to standard workup for hemolytic reactions.**

Indications for Blood Products

Given the potential complications from blood product transfusion, it is imperative that physicians understand and follow the indications for blood transfusion. The transfusion of blood products is indicated in patients with acute blood loss associated with hemodynamic instability and those with a large amount of ongoing blood loss in hemodynamically stable individuals. The use of transfusion triggers had been a common practice in the past; however, based on the findings of a randomized controlled clinical trial (TRICC trial), hospitalized patients maintained at a hemoglobin values of 7-9 g/dL had lower in-hospital mortality than those maintained at hemoglobin values of 10-12 g/dL. The findings of the TRICC trial demonstrated that critically ill patients (with the exception of patients with acute coronary syndrome) can tolerate much lower hemoglobin levels than previously believed. The transfusion of packed RBC should be determined based on patients' needs rather than an arbitrary laboratory value. Since the publication of the TRICC trial, multiple other randomized trials comparing liberal versus restrictive transfusion triggers in a wide variety of clinical settings have demonstrated that patients fare equally well if not better when a restrictive strategy for transfusion is maintained.

Platelet transfusion is generally indicated in patients with platelet count of less than 10,000 µL, 10,000 to 20,000 µL with bleeding, less than 50,000 µL with a severe trauma, and those with bleeding time greater than 15 minutes. Fresh-frozen plasma transfusion is considered appropriate in bleeding patients with a prothrombin time more than 17 seconds; it is also indicated following massive transfusion where replacement of 1 unit of fresh-frozen plasma and one single donor platelet unit for each unit of PRBC transfused is recommended as a strategy to improve clotting and hemostasis (hemostatic resuscitation).

CASE CORRELATION

- See also Case 4 (Resuscitation and Critical Care in the Emergency Department) and Case 50 (Sickle Cell Crisis).

COMPREHENSION QUESTIONS

51.1 A hemodynamically stable 40-year-old man with gastrointestinal (GI) bleeding and a hemoglobin of 6 g/dL is receiving packed RBC transfusion. Soon after the initiation of blood transfusion, the patient becomes confused, develops urticaria, and is subsequently unresponsive with a systolic blood pressure of 60 mm Hg. Which of the following agents may have worsened this patient's condition?

A. Lisinopril (an ACE inhibitor)

B. Atenolol

C. Lactated Ringer solution

D. Morphine sulfate

E. Salicylate

51.2 A 55-year-old homeless male presents to the ER with fatigue, dark stools, and a hemoglobin level of 4 mg/dL. While awaiting GI evaluation, he receives 2 units of PRBC. During the transfusion, he develops rigors, his temperature is 38.5°C, and his blood pressure is 100/60 mm Hg. Appropriate therapy includes all of the below except:

A. Cessation of the transfusion

B. Confirmation of blood type compatibility with the blood bank

C. Broad spectrum antibiotics

D. Fluid restriction

E. Gram stain of the transfusate

51.3 A 60-year-old woman with chronic anemia caused by a myelofibrosis presents to the emergency room from her oncologist's office with a hemoglobin of 6 g/dL. She notes feeling very lethargic over the past week and had some mild chest discomfort while climbing stairs in her house last night. A type- and cross-match is performed for 2 units of packed erythrocytes, which are given without incident, and marked improvement in her symptoms is seen. While going over discharge instructions with the emergency physician, the patient notes that she feels feverish and slightly short of breath. Over the next several minutes her dyspnea worsens markedly. Vital sign measurement reveals an oxygen saturation of 93%, a heart rate of 120 beats per minute, and a blood pressure of 95/55 mm Hg. The patient continues to deteriorate from a respiratory standpoint despite supplemental oxygen, requiring endotracheal intubation. A portable chest radiograph shows evidence of diffuse bilateral infiltrates. Which of the following statements is most accurate regarding this patient's condition?

A. This patient's left ventricular end-diastolic pressure is likely to be elevated.

B. This condition has a mortality rate of up to 90%.

C. Diuretic therapy is unlikely to be effective.

D. Radiographic abnormalities develop several days after the onset of clinical manifestations.

E. Mechanical ventilatory support is generally not helpful.

ANSWERS

51.1 **A.** Patients taking ACE inhibitors may experience a more severe anaphylactic reaction than other patients because of their inability to degrade bradykinin; however, these agents do not confer an increased risk of anaphylaxis. Patient misidentification is the leading preventable cause of transfusion reactions.

51.2 **D.** The differential for the change in this patient's vital signs includes an acute hemolytic transfusion reaction, an allergic reaction (though a fever to this degree would be uncommon), or a contaminated transfusion. It is appropriate to stop the transfusion and recheck the crossmatch. Antihistamines and antibiotics may be appropriate, but fluid restriction would not be the preferred treatment for either an acute hemolytic reaction or a septic transfusion reaction.

51.3 **C.** Patients with TRALI are not volume overloaded but rather suffer from increased capillary permeability at the level of the pulmonary vasculature. As such, they have normal to low left-side heart pressures and will only be harmed by diuretic therapy because of the potential to cause organ hypoperfusion. Mortality rates are around 10%. Radiographic abnormalities are present almost immediately and persist for several days after the resolution of clinical manifestations. Mechanical ventilatory support is a mainstay of therapy for patients with suspected TRALI, as the process is generally self-limiting.

CLINICAL PEARLS

▶ Allergic transfusion reactions are common. They are generally mild and consist of fever and itching.

▶ Hemolytic transfusion reactions are less common and may feature hemodynamic instability and hematuria.

▶ TRALI, thought to be mediated by antileukocyte antibodies, presents with fever, tachycardia, and dyspnea as the most common presenting symptoms.

▶ The hallmark of TRALI is respiratory distress with the presence of diffuse, bilateral alveolar and interstitial infiltrates on radiographic imaging.

REFERENCES

Chan AW, de Gara CJ. An evidence-based approach to red blood cell transfusions in asymptomatically anaemic patients. *Ann R Coll Surg Engl*. 2015;97:556-562.

Delaney M, Wendel S, Bercovitz RS, et al. Transfusion reactions: prevention, diagnosis and treatment. *Lancet*. 2016;388(10061):2825-2836. doi: 10.1016/S0140-6736(15)01313-6.

Herbert PC, Wells G, Blajchman MA, et al. A multicenter, randomized, controlled clinical trial of transfusion requirement in critical care. Transfusion requirements in critical care investigators, Canadian Critical Care Trials Group. *N Engl J Med*. 1999;340:409-417.

Leo A, Pedal I. Diagnostic approaches to acute transfusion reactions. *Forensic Sci Med Pathol*. 2010;6:135-145.

Vamvakas EC, Blajchman MA. Blood still kills: six strategies to further reduce allogeneic blood transfusion-related mortality. *Transfus Med Rev*. 2010;24:77-124.

A 74-year-old man is found in his small apartment after having a seizure on a hot summer afternoon. The EMS providers state that they found him in a poorly ventilated apartment without any air conditioning. They established an IV of normal saline prior to arrival and obtained a finger stick glucose of 146 mg/dL. Because he was postictal during transport, they were unable to obtain any other history about past medical problems, medications, or allergies.

On arrival in the emergency department (ED), his temperature is 41.1°C (106°F), blood pressure is 157/92 mm Hg, heart rate is 156 beats per minute, and respiratory rate is 28 breaths per minute. He is extremely warm to touch. He is combative, moaning, and flailing his arms and legs at staff. His pupils are midrange and reactive to light. His mucous membranes are dry. His neck is supple. His skin is flushed, hot, and dry.

▶ What is the most likely diagnosis?
▶ What is the best initial treatment?

ANSWERS TO CASE 52:

Heat-Related Illnesses

Summary: This is a 74-year-old man who is found to be hyperthermic, tachycardic, tachypneic, and with altered mental status following a seizure.

- **Most likely diagnosis:** Seizure secondary to heat stroke, but it is essential to rule out other causes, such as sepsis and medication overdose.

- **Best initial treatment:** Management of the ABCs and rapid cooling.

ANALYSIS

Objectives

1. Learn the clinical signs and symptoms associated with heat-related illness.

2. Learn the management and treatment of heat-related illness.

Considerations

When evaluating hyperthermic patients, the clinician must first determine if the patient has a fever or is suffering from heat stroke. The presumptive diagnosis of heat stroke can be made on the basis of environmental conditions and circumstantial evidence (hot day, enclosed apartment without air conditioning or adequate ventilation), and the next step is to determine the severity of the patient's heat-related illness, which could be useful in guiding his treatment. Because **heat stroke has a mortality of 10% to 20% even with treatment**, it is essential to diagnose and begin therapy immediately. This patient has severe heat stroke, as evidenced by his altered mental status and seizure. Simultaneously, laboratory and radiographic studies should be performed to rule out infectious etiologies and drug overdoses.

APPROACH TO:

Heat-Related Illnesses

DEFINITIONS

HEAT STRESS: Patients have sensations of discomfort and physiologic strain with normal core temperatures. These patients exhibit decreased exercise tolerance and no other symptoms.

HEAT EXHAUSTION: Mild dehydration, with or without sodium abnormalities. Patients have profuse sweating, thirst, nausea, vomiting, confusion and headache, and may have collapsed. Core temperatures range from 38°C to 40°C (100°F-104°F). Generally, the victim is not able to continue his/her activities as the result of the environmental conditions.

HEAT STROKE: Severe dehydration with core temperature greater than 40°C. Patients are flushed, with hot, dry skin. Symptoms include those associated with central nervous system (CNS) disturbances, such as dizziness, vertigo, syncope, confusion, delirium, and unconsciousness. Classically, heat strokes develop slowly over days and occur more frequently in older individuals with chronic illnesses.

EXERTIONAL HEAT STROKE: Heat stroke affecting individuals involved in strenuous physical activities. This type of heat stroke can have a more rapid onset than non-exertional heat strokes. Weather conditions, including high humidity and increased temperatures, are risk factors. The at-risk individuals are highly motivated athletes, laborers, and military personnel and recruits.

CLINICAL APPROACH

The primary abnormality in heat-related illnesses is the individual's inability to adequately transfer heat (produced from normal metabolic activities) to the environment, resulting in an increase in core temperature. Risk factors for developing heat illness include ambient heat and humidity, extremes of age, strenuous exercise, cardiovascular disease, dehydration, obesity, and impaired mentation. Additional risk factors include medications (eg, diuretics, anticholinergics, antihistamines, phenothiazines, cyclic antidepressants, sympathomimetics, and alcohol).

The spectrum of heat-related illness varies in severity from benign to severe. Table 52–1 describes the minor syndromes. In contrast to these benign entities, **heat stroke is characterized by a loss of thermoregulation, tissue damage, and**

Table 52–1 • MINOR HEAT ILLNESSES			
Diagnosis	Cause	Symptoms	Treatment
Heat edema	Vasodilation and pooling of fluids in dependent areas	Mild swelling of hands and feet	Self-limited; elevate legs, use of support hose; no diuretics
Heat rash	Blockage of sweat gland pores, may have secondary staphylococcal infection	Pruritic, erythematous, maculopapular rash on clothed areas	Antihistamines for itching, loose-fitting clothing; chlorhexidine cream, dicloxacillin, or erythromycin if infected
Heat cramps	Salt depletion (often from drinking only water)	Severe muscle cramps in fatigued skeletal muscles (usually calves, thighs, shoulders) during or after strenuous exercise	Fluid and salt replacement, rest
Heat syncope	Vasodilation, decreased vasomotor tone, volume depletion	Postural hypotension and syncope	Removal from heat source, rehydration, rest
Heat exhaustion	Water and salt depletion	Sweating, weakness, fatigue, headache, nausea, dizziness, malaise, light-headedness, temperature usually <40°C (104°F)	Rest, volume, and salt replacement

multiorgan failure. Classically, patients present with **hyperpyrexia (temperature >41°C [105.8°F])**, CNS dysfunction (eg, altered mental status, seizure, and focal neurological deficits), and anhidrosis.

Diagnosis

Heat stroke, a diagnosis of exclusion, is hyperthermia with concomitant CNS dysfunction. The differential diagnosis includes alcohol withdrawal, salicylate toxicity, phencyclidine, cocaine, or amphetamine toxicity, tetanus, sepsis, neuroleptic malignant syndrome, encephalitis, meningitis, brain abscess, malaria, typhoid fever, malignant hyperthermia, anticholinergic toxicity, status epilepticus, cerebral hemorrhage, diabetic ketoacidosis, and thyroid storm.

Laboratory studies should include complete blood count, electrolytes, blood urea nitrogen (BUN)/creatinine, glucose, liver enzymes, coagulation studies, urinalysis, urine myoglobin, and arterial blood gas. An electrocardiogram (ECG) should be considered if the patient has syncope or a history of cardiovascular disease. Chest radiographs are useful to rule out aspiration or pulmonary infections. CT scan of the head and/or lumbar puncture may also be helpful in individuals suspected of having CNS lesions and/or infections.

Treatment

In treating heat stroke, the clinician should strive to stabilize the **ABCs, commence rapid cooling, replace fluid and electrolyte losses, and treat complications.** The goal is to cool the patient to 40°C (104°F) to avoid overshoot hypothermia. There are a number of cooling methods that are applied and these can be divided categorically as *evaporative* techniques and *conduction* techniques. **Although there are strong proponents for the different cooling methods, there is no current consensus regarding which of the techniques is most effective. In all patients, the initial measures consist of removing the patient from the hot environment if possible and removing clothing.** Evaporative cooling using cool mist and fans is simple and effective approach to cooling in the field; the evaporative approach is advocated by a number of investigators because the physical cooling principle suggests that the evaporation of 1 mL of water is associated with seven times the amount of heat dissipation when compared to melting 1 g of ice. Alternative cooling methods also include ice packs placement to the groin and axillae, cooling blankets, ice water immersion, peritoneal lavage, and cardiopulmonary bypass. Antipyretics are not effective in reducing the temperature in these individuals.

Shivering can be controlled with benzodiazepines or phenothiazines. Benzodiazepines can also be helpful to prevent or treat seizure activities that these patients may develop. If the laboratory studies reveal evidence of rhabdomyolysis, mannitol administration and alkalinization of the urine are additional treatment considerations. The most common complications of heat stroke are rhabdomyolysis, renal failure, liver failure, disseminated intravascular coagulation, heart failure, pulmonary edema, and cardiovascular collapse.

The following independent negative prognosticators for survival have been identified, and these include age more than 80 years, cardiac disease, cancer, core temperature more than 40°C, living in an institution, previous diuretic use, systolic BP <100 mm Hg, GCS <12, and transport to hospital by ambulance.

CASE CORRELATION

- See also Case 53 (Lightning and Electrical Injury), Case 54 (Frostbite and Hypothermia), and Case 55 (Drowning).

COMPREHENSION QUESTIONS

52.1 A 70-year-old man is brought into the ED complaining of headache and fatigue. His blood pressure is 100/70 mm Hg, heart rate is 100 beats per minute, and core temperature is 40.3°C (104.5°F). Upon using ice bags, his core temperature is down to 38°C (100.4°F). Which of the following is the best next step?

   A. Observation for 4-6 hours and then, if stable, discharge home

   B. Continue ice bags until the core temperature is 36.7°C (98°F)

   C. Admission to the hospital for observation of complications

   D. Administer cold gastric lavage

   E. Discharge the patient only if he can be placed in a different environment after discharge

52.2 A 33-year-old man is found comatose at a construction site in the noon-hour on a hot summer day. His core temperature is 41.7°C (107.1°F). The ED physician orders evaporative cooling measures and ice packs. The patient begins to exhibit intense shivering. Which of the following is the best next step?

   A. Continued observation

   B. Short-acting benzodiazepine

   C. Begin intravenous cooling solution

   D. Increase the number of ice bags

   E. Stop the cooling

52.3 A 38-year-old man was found after a drug overdose unconscious on the side of a field in the middle of summer. He was found to have a core temperature of 42°C and was significantly volume depleted. His blood pressure is 90/60 mm Hg and heart rate 120 beats per minute. IV fluids are administered, and active cooling measures are undertaken. The patient's CPK levels are 3000 IU/L. Which of the following is the best treatment?

   A. Alkylanization of the urine

   B. Insulin

   C. Tissue plasminogen activator

   D. Steroids

ANSWERS

52.1 **C.** All patients with severe heat exhaustion or heat stroke, particularly those who are older, should be admitted to the hospital.

52.2 **B.** This patient most likely has exertional heat stroke, in which core temperature elevations may occur rapidly; therefore, measures directed at reducing his core temperature are appropriate and must be continued. Benzodiazepines are first-line therapy for shivering or seizures in heat stroke.

52.3 **A.** This patient has rhabdomyolysis, as evidenced by the markedly elevated CPK levels. The best treatment is IV hydration and alkylanization of the urine to prevent renal damage. With such high CPK levels, a large amount of IV fluids is usually required. Urine alkylanization is important to prevent precipitation of myoglobin and uric acid crystals within the renal tubule. Other treatments include mannitol and loop diuretics.

CLINICAL PEARLS

▶ Heat stroke is distinguished from other heat illnesses by a loss of thermoregulation, tissue damage, and multiorgan failure. Classically, these patients present with hyperpyrexia and CNS dysfunction.

▶ Heat stroke has a mortality of 10% to 20% even with treatment; therefore, it is essential to diagnose and begin therapy immediately.

▶ The treatment of heat stroke consists of stabilizing the ABCs, rapid cooling, replacing fluid and electrolyte losses, and treating any complications (eg, shivering, seizures, and rhabdomyolysis).

REFERENCES

Becker JA, Stewart LK. Heat-related illness. *Am Fam Physician*. 2011;83:1325-1330.

Hausfater P, Megarbane B, Dautheville S, et al. Prognostic factors in non-exertional heatstroke. *Intensive Car Med*. 2010;36:272-280.

Leon LR, Bouchama A. Heat stroke. *Compr Physiol*. 2015;5:611-647.

Pryor RR, Bennett BL, O'Connor FG, Young JM, Asplund CA. Medical evaluation for exposure extremes: heat. *Wilderness Environ Med*. 2015;26(4 Suppl):S69-75.

Two men in their twenties are brought to the emergency department by para-medics. Per report, they were victims of lightning injury while playing golf. Eye-witnesses at the scene report that the victims were standing several feet apart, when one of the men was struck directly by lightning that resulted in both men falling to the ground immediately and becoming unconscious. One of the victims was found pulseless at the scene, and cardiopulmonary resuscitation (CPR) was initiated by a bystander. The second man was noted to be unconscious for several minutes after the incident and has remained confused. On examination, the first victim has extensive soft-tissue burns over his back and legs. He is intubated and being ventilated without spontaneous respirations. No palpable pulse is identi-fied, and fine ventricular fibrillation appears on the electrocardiogram (ECG) mon-itor. The second victim is awake with a pulse rate of 80 beats per minute, blood pressure of 130/80 mm Hg, respirations of 18 breaths per minute, and Glasgow coma scale (GCS) score of 13, with no identifiable external sign of injury.

▶ What are the complications of lightning injury?
▶ How are the complications identified?
▶ What are the basic treatment modalities for the sequelae of lightning injuries?

ANSWERS TO CASE 53:

Lightning and Electrical Injury

Summary: Two adult victims present to the emergency department following lightning injuries. One patient who presents in cardiac arrest appears to have been a victim of direct lightning strike, while the second victim appears to have minimal external signs of injury.

- **Lightning-related complications:** Cardiac injury (usually in the form of arrhythmia), respiratory arrest, neurological damage, spinal cord injury, burns, skin, and muscle injury.

- **Identification of complications:** Thorough and careful physical examination and electrocardiography will identify arrhythmia and cutaneous burns. The extent of potential multi-system injury should be determined. Computed tomography (CT) scan of the head is indicated in all patients with severe lighting injury and those with abnormal neurological examination. Radiographs for associated skeletal injury should be performed as indicated.

- **Treatment of sequelae:** Aggressive, persistent resuscitation according to advanced life support protocol is indicated, including airway control and ventilatory support until spontaneous circulation and respiration is restored. Spinal protection and immobilization are necessary until injury is ruled out. Related injuries such as burns are treated expectantly.

ANALYSIS

Objectives

1. Learn the spectrum of injury associated with lightning and electrocution.
2. Understand the relationship between Ohm law and injuries produced by electric current.
3. Learn to recognize and treat the immediate and late complications associated with electrical injury and lightning injury.

Considerations

One patient suffered a direct lightning strike and is in cardiac arrest. Because of the massive direct current countershock, lightning strike can induce depolarization of the entire myocardium, leading to cardiac standstill. **Immediate cardiac arrest is the most common cause of death after a lightning strike.** However, respiratory arrest may also occur, either due to paralysis of the respiratory center in the medulla or as a result of tetany of the respiratory muscles from electric current passing through the thorax. Many patients will regain cardiopulmonary function if timely and appropriate resuscitation efforts are able to sustain oxygenation and circulation while the organ systems recover.

Given the first patient's young age and lack of comorbid factors, there is a greater likelihood for response to resuscitation efforts than in victims with cardiac arrest from other traumatic causes. The heart's inherent automaticity renders spontaneous recovery possible if immediate defibrillation and tissue oxygenation is maintained. The second patient, although hemodynamically stable, has suffered a high-risk electrical injury with loss of consciousness. Head and/or spinal injury could be present as a consequence of being "thrown" by the lightning strike. He requires evaluation with CT scan of the head, ECG, spinal immobilization, and evaluation and initial observation in the ICU for close monitoring of the cardiopulmonary status. The extent of burn injuries make him susceptible to infections, metabolic compromise, compartment syndrome, and renal insufficiency.

APPROACH TO:

Lighting and Electrical Injury

CLINICAL APPROACH

Although lightning strike is a rare phenomenon, **it is associated with a 25% fatality rate.** Lightning strike accounts for approximately 100 deaths annually in the United States, and **more than 70% of those who survive have permanent injuries.** Electrical injury, excluding lightning, is responsible for more than 500 deaths annually, with approximately 20% of victims younger than 18 years of age. The effects of electrical injury are related to the intensity and magnitude of the electric current. According to **Ohm law**, the current flow (amperage) is directly related to the voltage and inversely related to the resistance in the current's pathway, represented by the following formula: **current (amperage) = voltage/resistance.** Because of low resistance, **nerves, blood vessels, mucous membranes, and muscle are the preferred pathways for electric current passage and are most susceptible to injury.** Bones, fat, tendon, and skin have relatively high resistance and therefore sustain less damage during electric and lightning injuries. The probable path of the electrical current should be assessed during the physical examination; for example, burns on both hands indicate a path likely through the heart, which has a poor prognosis.

Electrical current exists in two forms: **alternating current (AC)** and **direct current (DC).** AC involves electrons flowing back and forth in cycles, whereas in DC, the electron flow occurs in only one direction. Alternating current (AC) is more dangerous because it may cause tetanic muscle contractions and a "locking on" phenomenon, preventing the victim from releasing the electrical source and resulting in prolonged exposure to the current. Lightning strike is a form of DC electrical injury with extremely high voltage and amperage but short exposure duration. During lightning injury, the electrons flow in only one direction, typically inducing a single intense muscle contraction that "throws" the victim and causes simultaneous fractures and spinal injury. There are four types of lightning injury (Table 53–1).

Pathophysiology

Cardiac effects of electrical injury include (a) direct necrosis of the myocardium, (b) ischemic injury as a result of vasoconstriction caused by excess catecholamine release, or (c) disturbances in the cardiac rhythm. Even low currents can produce arrhythmias, including asystole and ventricular tachycardia. Late dysrhythmias are

Table 53–1 • TYPES OF LIGHTNING INJURY
Direct strike: The most serious type; when the major path of lightning current travels through the victim
Side flash (splash): When the current is discharged from a victim or object of direct strike onto a nearby person. In these cases, the current is traveling through paths of least resistance to the victim
Ground current or stride potential: When the lightning strikes the ground and then enters the victim's body from one foot and exits via the opposite foot
Flashover phenomenon: When the force of nearby lightning causes expansion and implosion of surrounding air, causing a blast effect
Blunt injury: This type of injury may occur when the victim is in close proximity to the shockwave produced by lightning, and the forces may result in the victim being thrown, causing tympanic membrane ruptures and other contusive injuries

uncommon in previously healthy patients but can be produced by patchy myocardial necrosis and injury to the sinoatrial (SA) node. Lightning can induce cardiac standstill by depolarizing the entire myocardium. Because of the inherent automaticity of the heart, normal sinus rhythm often spontaneously returns.

Clinical Considerations

Cardiovascular Effects All victims of lightning strike and high-voltage electric injury should have immediate ECG monitoring and cardiopulmonary support to maintain tissue perfusion as needed. This includes basic and advanced cardiac life support with defibrillation as needed. Aggressive resuscitation should be performed due to reports of excellent recovery even after cardiac arrest. Victims of electrical injury with no loss of consciousness or physical findings who are asymptomatic and have a normal ECG can be safely discharged home.

Neurological Effects Nerve damage is common after electrical injury, but there are no pathognomonic findings. Approximately 75% of patients struck by lightning will have transient loss of consciousness and brief extremity weakness or paresthesia. Lightning strike victims often have temporary paralysis with loss of sensation that typically involves lower limbs known as **keraunoparalysis.** Strength and sensation return to normal within a few hours. Other common neurological findings in electrical injury are confusion, amnesia, headache, visual disturbances, and seizures. Direct spinal cord injury has been reported after hand-to-hand flow with damage to C_4-C_8.

The most serious neurologic effect is injury to the respiratory control center in the medulla, resulting in respiratory arrest. This is especially common after lightning strike and high-voltage electrical injuries. In addition, lightning and electrical injury victims often have fixed and dilated pupils as a result of autonomic responses, which should not be interpreted as a sign of non-survival until cerebral function is fully assessed.

As in any apneic trauma victim, the **airway, oxygenation, and ventilation** should be restored immediately. **CT scan of the head** is indicated in patients with neurological findings or loss of consciousness to evaluate for possible intracranial pathology. **Spinal immobilization** should be continued until neurological examination is normal or injury is ruled out radiographically. Most victims of electrical and lightning injury without cardiac arrest will survive but should be counseled that persistent sequelae, including memory deficit, sleep disturbances, dizziness, fatigue, headaches, and attention deficits, may occur.

Skin Burns are common after high-voltage electrical injury but are less often seen after lightning strike because of the instantaneous exposure time. Victims of electrical injury have "flush burns" caused by heat generated by the electrical current, or "flame burns," usually as a consequence of ignition of clothing. Lightning strike can cause partial-thickness linear burns in areas of high sweat concentration and low resistance, which result in a transient fern-like skin pattern called the **Lichtenberg figure** (Figure 53–1) that is pathognomonic of lightning. In children, the most common mode of electrical injury is from chewing or biting electrical cords, which manifests as perioral edema and eschar formation. **Children may have excessive bleeding from the labial artery as a consequence of perioral burns.**

Thorough **physical examination** will reveal any cutaneous manifestations of electrical injury. Early **intravenous access** should be established for fluid management as soon as possible in any burned patient. Fluids should be titrated to a targeted urine output of 0.5 mL/kg/h in adults, 1 mL/kg/h in children under 20 kg, and 1-2 mL/kg/h in patients with rhabdomyolysis. Severe injuries will require admission to a specialized burn unit.

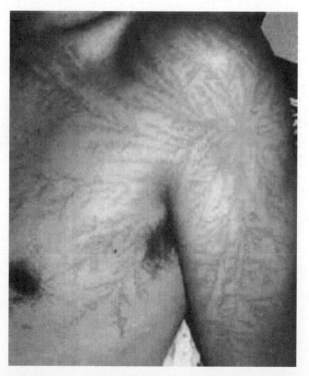

Figure 53–1. Lichtenberg figure—branching fern-like electrical discharge pattern.

Special Considerations

Extensive muscle injury with tissue damage and necrosis is possible with high-voltage electrical injuries. A cool extremity with diminished sensation or pulse may be caused by vasospasm and nerve ischemia, which may resolve spontaneously with time. This should be differentiated from extremity compartment syndrome by reexamination with **compartment pressure** measurements as indicated in selected patients. Aggressive treatment by **fasciotomy** is indicated when elevated compartment pressures are identified.

The kidneys are particularly vulnerable to anoxic damage that accompanies electrical injury, where **rhabdomyolysis** is common. However, rhabdomyolysis is rare after lightning injury. Patients with myoglobinuria should be treated with aggressive fluid resuscitation to maintain kidney perfusion and function.

Lightning strike may lead to ophthalmologic and otologic injuries. Rupture of the tympanic membrane occurs in up to 50% of lightning victims, while sensorineural deafness or vestibular injury less commonly result. **Cataracts, corneal burns, optic nerve injury, intraocular hemorrhage, and uveitis** are additional problems that can present as late sequelae of lightning strike. **Curling ulcers** are common in burn victims, and preventative treatment for these stress ulcers should be initiated at admission. Other injuries associated with electrical and lightning injuries include **fractures** from severe muscle contraction or blunt trauma after exposure. Upper limb and spinal fractures are common.

Some victims of lightning injury are simply found down without a witnessed event. When the history is unclear, thorough evaluations should be initiated to look for other causes such as cerebral vascular accident, toxic ingestions, spinal cord injuries, closed head injuries, myocardial infarctions, and primary seizure disorders which may be responsible for the unexplainable neurologic and cardiovascular deficits.

CASE CORRELATION

- See also Case 44 (Cervical Spine and Upper Extremity Orthopedic Injuries), Case 52 (Heat-related Illness), and Case 54 (Frostbite and Hypothermia).

COMPREHENSION QUESTIONS

53.1 A 40-year-old man employed as an electrician is brought to the ED after accidentally grabbing a high-voltage wire, causing him to fall from an 8-ft ladder onto his back on the pavement below. He was ambulatory at the scene but because of persistent left hand and arm pain, he presents to the ED for treatment. He is conscious and conversant but complains of intense pain at the site of a 3-cm burn wound on his left hand and pain throughout his left forearm. His GCS is 15, and he is stable from the cardiopulmonary view. He has dry eschar over the hand wound, the sensation and motor activities are diminished in his left hand, and he has firmness and tenderness throughout the left forearm. Which of the following next steps is most appropriate?

A. Obtain x-rays to rule out fractures.

B. Measure forearm compartment pressures.

C. Administer systemic antibiotics to prevent skin infection.

D. Obtain electromyograms (EMGs) to rule out peripheral nerve injury.

E. Obtain a CT scan to evaluate the muscle and nerves.

53.2 A 49-year-old man was fixing the electrical wiring in his house as a remodeling project and neglected to shut off the electricity at the electrical box. He suffered a substantial electrical injury primarily on the right hand and was taken by paramedics to the ED. Which of the following is most likely to be true regarding electrical injury?

A. Cataract formation usually only occurs when there is a contact point on the head.

B. Renal failure is usually a result of direct electrical injury to the kidney.

C. With high-voltage injuries, dysrhythmia usually develops 24-48 hours after injury.

D. Electrical burns commonly produce a fern-like skin burn pattern.

E. Even with minor cutaneous involvement, major internal injury can occur.

53.3 Two 13-year-old boys were curious about the inner workings of high-voltage transformers. After scaling the fence around a complex near their school, one of the boys touched the transformer, believing he would be immune to electrical shock because he was wearing rubber-soled tennis shoes. He suffered a 10,000 V jolt of electricity. Which of the following organ systems is most susceptible to high-voltage injuries?

A. Bones, tendons, and muscles

B. Skin, brain, and fat

C. Fat, heart, and skeletal muscle

D. Blood, nerves, and mucous membranes

E. Hair

53.4 A 45-year-old accountant was suddenly struck by lightning and thrown to the ground while getting into his car atop his high-rise office building during a thunderstorm. Which of the following is most accurate regarding complications to his injuries?

A. Tetanic contractions are commonly caused by DC current.

B. The instantaneous duration of exposure lessens cutaneous burn risk compared to other high-voltage electrical injuries.

C. Rhabdomyolysis is a common delayed sequela.

D. Respiratory arrest is caused by paralysis of thoracic muscles.

E. Lightning strike carries 80% mortality.

ANSWERS

53.1 **B.** This patient's history of high-voltage injury and current complaint of intense forearm pain, diminished motor and sensory function of the hand, and forearm tenseness are highly suspicious for compartment syndrome secondary to myonecrosis. Direct compartment measurement is the most rapid and reliable approach to diagnosis. Even though fracturing can occur from the fall, bony injury would not account for motor and sensory changes in the hand. Treatment of burn wounds with systemic antibiotics is not indicated. CT scan is not sensitive for identification of compartment syndrome.

53.2 **E.** Even with minor cutaneous involvement, major internal injury can occur. The renal failure following electrical shocks generally occurs as a result of myoglobinuria. Although dysrhythmia is common after electrical injury, it almost always develops *immediately* after exposure. Cataract formation may occur even without a contact point on the head. Lichtenberg figure is the transient fern-like pattern that occurs on the skin of lightning strike victims because the electricity is splashed onto skin based on the vascular and nerve distribution patterns of the skin.

53.3 **D.** In high-voltage injuries, electricity tends to follow the path of least resistance. Blood, nerves, and mucous membranes are frequently injured after electrical exposure because of their low resistance. Fat, bones, and tendon have high resistance.

53.4 **B.** Because of brief electrical exposure length, burns are relatively rare in lightning injury. Lightning is DC current, and respiratory arrest is usually a result of injury to the respiratory control center in the medulla. Rhabdomyolysis is common after high-voltage electrical injury but rare after lightning strike. Contrary to popular beliefs, the mortality associated with lightning injuries is low, with most recent series reporting rates of 5% to 10%.

CLINICAL PEARLS

► Major injuries associated with lightning and electrical exposure include cardiac, pulmonary, neurologic, CNS, and burns.

► Victims of lightning strike should be treated with aggressive ventilatory and circulatory support until cerebral function can be assessed because many patients will recover function with time.

► Typical signs of brain death, such as fixed/dilated pupils and apnea, do not necessarily indicate brain death in electrical victims. Typical triage criteria for mass casualty situations do not apply to electrical injury because of the rates of favorable outcomes despite concerning clinical findings.

► Major internal damage is common with electrical injury, even with small outward signs of injury. Workup should include a broad assessment for less immediately obvious injuries, such as compartment syndrome.

► Associated burns should be evaluated and treated according to burn protocols, with transfer to a specialized burn center when appropriate.

REFERENCES

Davis C, Englen A, Johnson EL, et al. Wilderness Medical Society Practice Guidelines for the Prevention and Treatment of Lightning Injuries: 2014 update. *Wild Env Med*. 2014;25:S86-95.

Fish RM, Geddes LA. Conduction of electrical current to and through the human body: a review. *Journal of Plastic Surgery*. 2009. Available at: www.eplasty.com.

Gottlieb LJ, Nguyen TQ, Lee RC. Electrical trauma. In: Hall JB, Schmidt GA, Kress JP, eds. *Principles of Critical Care*. 4th ed. New York, NY: McGraw-Hill Education; 2015:1175-1180.

Katz RD, Deune EG. Electrical and lightning injuries. In: Cameron JL, Cameron AM, eds. *Current Surgical Therapy*. 10th ed. Philadelphia, PA: Elsevier Saunders; 2011:1047-1057.

O'Keefe Gatewood M, Zane RD. Lightning injuries. *Emerg Med Clin N Am*. 2004;22:369-403.

Ritenour AE, Morton MJ, McManus JG, et al. Lightning injury: a review. *Burn*. 2008;34:585-594.

Zimmermann C, Cooper MA, Holle RL. Lightning safety guidelines. *Ann Emerg Med*. 2001;39: 660-664.

A 44-year-old homeless man is found on a park bench in the middle of the winter. He is cold and covered in snow. A concerned citizen calls 911, and EMS transports the patient to the Emergency Department. The patient is minimally responsive. A pack of cigarettes and a small bottle of whiskey are found in his jacket pocket. On examination, he is thin and disheveled. His extremities are pale and cold with clear fluid-filled blisters on his hands and several of his fingers. His blood pressure is 110/70 mm Hg, heart rate is 90 beats per minute and irregular, respiratory rate is 18 breaths per minute, and his rectal temperature is 30°C. He is not shivering.

▶ What is your next step?
▶ What is the most likely diagnosis?
▶ What are your first steps in treatment?

ANSWERS TO CASE 54:

Frostbite and Hypothermia

Summary: A 44-year-old homeless man with a history of ethanol use and cigarette smoking was exposed to freezing temperatures and now has a decreased level of consciousness. The patient has an irregular heart rhythm, likely atrial fibrillation. He is not shivering, and his rectal temperature is 30°C. Additionally, he has frostbite on his hands and several fingers.

- **Next step:** The patient presents with altered mental status (AMS). His ABCs (airway, breathing, and circulation) should be assessed, and reversible causes of AMS (eg, hypoglycemia) should be considered.

- **Most likely diagnosis:** Cold exposure injury leading to hypothermia and frostbite.

- **First steps in treatment:** Begin rapid core rewarming and prevent further systemic heat loss. Remove any wet or constrictive clothing. Wrap the patient in warm, dry blankets, and consider using a forced-air warming blanket. Additionally, administer warm intravenous fluids. His frostbitten hands will also need to be rewarmed.

ANALYSIS

Objectives

1. Recognize the spectrum of cold exposure injuries.

2. Understand the pathophysiology of frostbite.

3. Understand the pathophysiology of hypothermia and how it affects various organ systems.

4. Know the treatments for frostbite and hypothermia.

Considerations

Accidental hypothermia is a multifaceted entity encompassing a range of clinical features. Risk factors associated with the development of hypothermia include advanced age, diabetes mellitus, tobacco use, alcoholism, peripheral vascular disease, peripheral neuropathy, Raynaud's disease, and exposure to windy weather, which increases the rate of heat loss from the skin. Frostbite occurs when the skin and body tissues are exposed to cold temperature for a prolonged period of time. Evaluation of core body temperature is necessary to determine if hypothermia exists and to what degree. Once his wet and constrictive clothing are removed, passive rewarming techniques can be used to increase the core body temperature. The patient should be examined to determine if clinically significant frostbite exists. To minimize soft tissue injury in this patient, the rewarming process should not be delayed.

APPROACH TO:

Frostbite and Hypothermia

DEFINITIONS

HYPOTHERMIA: Core body temperature below 35°C, which is below what is required for normal metabolism.

FROSTNIP (First-degree frostbite): Deposition of superficial ice crystals on the skin with partial skin freezing. Typically, this is a retrospective diagnosis because it is defined by the absence of tissue damage upon rewarming.

FROSTBITE: Occurs when the skin tissue freezes. Second and third degree frostbite involve the skin. Fourth degree frostbite involves deeper structures such as muscle, tendon, and bone.

TRENCH FOOT: Condition that results from prolonged exposure of the extremities to a cool and wet environment, without freezing. Prolonged exposure to this environment leads to decreased peripheral circulation. This was common in trench warfare during World War I.

CHILBLAINS (PERNIO): A non-freezing cold-related injury that occurs in cool, humid environments. It is characterized by red, scaly lesions, often on the face, hands, or feet.

CLINICAL APPROACH

Hypothermia

Pathophysiology The human cold response is aimed at maintaining the core body temperature and the viability of the extremities. The skin's thermoreceptors are densest on the upper torso. These peripheral thermoreceptors signal a central thermostat, located in the preoptic region of the anterior hypothalamus, to activate autonomic and behavioral heat regulation mechanisms. Peripheral cooling of the blood leads to catecholamine release, sympathetic stimulation, thyroid stimulation, shivering thermogenesis, and peripheral vasoconstriction. Heat loss is therefore reduced via peripheral vasoconstriction. Powered by stored glycogen, **shivering thermogenesis** can provide several hours of heat and stops when glycogen stores are depleted. The extremities are protected by the **hunting reaction**, which consists of irregular, 5-10 minute cycles of alternating vasodilation and vasoconstriction that protect the extremities against sustained periods of vasoconstriction. If the body is exposed to cold for a prolonged duration or of significant magnitude, then the core body temperature is threatened and this mechanism is abandoned (the so-called "life-versus-limb" mechanism). Once the body has physiologically lost the ability to compensate for the cold, injury is inevitable. The physiologic consequences of cold injury are thus considered by a systems approach.

Heat loss occurs through four basic mechanisms: conduction, convection, radiation, and evaporation. Conduction occurs through heat transfer from the warmer body to a cooler object. In a wet environment, this occurs at a much greater rate. Convection is the transfer of heat from movement, where wind acts as a confounding factor that draws heat away from the body. Radiation is heat transfer by electromagnetic waves from the non-insulated areas on the body. Evaporation of water leads to heat loss through exhalation of warm air.

There are many predisposing factors for the development of hypothermia (Table 54–1). These can be generalized into four overlapping categories: disrupted circulation, increased heat loss, decreased heat production, and impaired thermoregulation.

Two high-risk populations include individuals who consume ethanol and the elderly. Ethanol use predisposes to hypothermia in many ways. First, it impairs judgment and thermal perception, which in turn increases the risk of cold exposure. Ethanol predisposes to hypoglycemia, impedes shivering (eg, lack of fuel interferes with shivering), and causes peripheral vasodilation (eg, increases heat loss). In addition, ethanol lowers the hypothalamic thermoregulatory set point, resulting in a reduction of core temperature. The elderly exhibit age-related impairments in many of the systems of thermoregulation. The elderly often have an impaired shivering response, decreased mobility, and malnutrition. They are less able to discriminate cold environments and often lack the ability of adequate vasoconstriction. The risk is also increased secondary to medications (particularly cardiac medications) which impede thermoregulation. The risk of fall is also increased in the elderly. It is critical to rule out sepsis as the cause of hypothermia in the elderly, particularly if the patient is found indoors.

Table 54–1 • HYPOTHERMIA RISK FACTORS	
Disrupted Circulation	**Increased Heat Loss**
Tight-fitting clothing	Cold, windy environments
Medications	Medications
Smoking	Ethanol
Diabetes	Extremes of age
Peripheral vascular disease	Burns
Dehydration	
Decreased Heat Production	**Impaired Thermoregulation**
Hypothyroidism	Stroke
Hypoadrenalism	Tumor
Hypoglycemia	Ethanol
Malnutrition	Benzodiazepines
Beta-blockers	Opioids
Neuroleptics	Barbiturates
Extremes of age	Phenothiazines Atypical antipsychotics Alpha-blockers Extremes of age

Table 54–2 • SYSTEMIC EFFECTS OF HYPOTHERMIA		
Stage	Core Temp (°C)	Characteristics
Mild	37.6	Normal rectal temperature
	36	Increase in metabolic rate, BP, and preshivering muscle tone
	35	Maximal shivering response
	34	Development of the "umbles: bumble, stumble, tumble;" amnesia, dysarthria, poor judgment, maximum respiratory stimulation, tachycardia
	33.3	Development of ataxia and apathy, decreasing minute ventilation, cold diuresis
Moderate	32	Stupor, 25% decrease in oxygen consumption
	31	Extinguished shivering reflex
	30	Development of atrial fibrillation
	29	Progressive decrease in level of consciousness, pupils dilated
Severe	28	Decreased ventricular fibrillation threshold; decrease in oxygen consumption and pulse, hypoventilation
	27	Loss of reflexes and voluntary movement
	26	Anesthesia and areflexia
	25	Cerebral blood flow and cardiac output falls
	24	Hypotension and bradycardia
	23	Loss of corneal reflexes, areflexia
	22	Maximal risk of ventricular fibrillation
Profound	20	Lowest resumption of cardiac electromechanical activity
	19	EEG silent
	18	Asystole
	13.7	Lowest adult accidental hypothermia survival
	15	Lowest infant accidental hypothermia survival
	9	Lowest therapeutic hypothermia survival

Abbreviations: BP = blood pressure; CT = computed tomography; EEG = electroencephalogram.

Hypothermia has effects on many organ systems. The systemic effects of hypothermia vary based on the degree of hypothermia (Table 54–2).

Cardiovascular Cardiovascular complications are common throughout the spectrum of cold injury. The body's initial response to mild cold stress is **tachycardia.** However, as temperatures decline, the response of the cardiovascular system shifts from tachycardia to progressive **bradycardia**, which is **refractory to standard treatments** (eg, atropine). A multitude of cardiac dysrhythmias are seen in hypothermia. The most common is **atrial fibrillation.** The **Osborn (or J wave)** is a well-known manifestation of hypothermia seen on electrocardiogram (ECG) (Figures 54–1 and 54–2). It is characterized by elevation at the junction of the QRS complex and the ST-segment and is typically seen at temperatures below 32°C. As temperatures drop below 28°C, **ventricular fibrillation** occurs. As the core body temperature drops, so does oxygen consumption. It is theorized that this decline in oxygen consumption explains why some profoundly hypothermic patients have been successfully resuscitated.

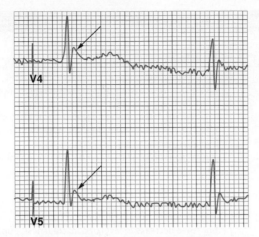

Figure 54–1. The J (Osborn) wave (arrows) appears on electrocardiograms of approximately 80% of hypothermic patients. In general, the amplitude and duration of the Osborn wave are inversely related to core temperature. (Reproduced, with permission, from Hall JB, Schmidt GA, Wood LDH. *Principles of Clinical Care.* 3rd ed. New York, NY: McGraw-Hill Education; 2005:1681.)

Respiratory The initial response to mild cold is an increase in respiratory rate. With continued or severe cold exposure, the stimulation of this system begins to slow down. **Respiratory depression** occurs with resultant respiratory acidosis from carbon dioxide retention. Protective airway mechanisms are impaired

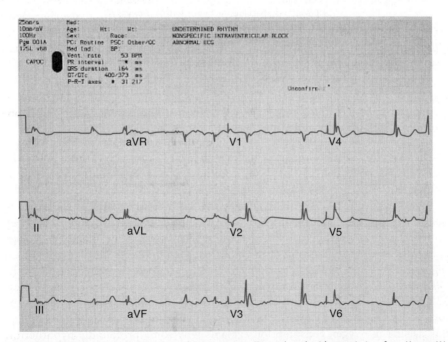

Figure 54–2. ECG shows J waves in a hypothermic patient. (Reproduced, with permission, from Knoop KJ, Stack LB, Storrow AB. *Atlas of Emergency Medicine.* 2nd ed. New York, NY: McGraw-Hill Education; 2002:516.)

due to decreased ciliary motility, bronchorrhea, and thickening of respiratory secretions.

Renal Hypothermia leads to dehydration and hypotension, which causes a decrease in renal blood flow and glomerular filtration rate. However, peripheral vasoconstriction leads to shunting of blood centrally, causing a central hypervolemia, inhibition of ADH, impaired renal tubular function, and the loss of concentrating abilities. This results in large-volume cold diuresis and further dehydration.

Gastrointestinal Poor perfusion to the liver results in the inability to clear toxins, the retention of lactate, and a metabolic acidosis.

Neurologic As temperature declines, an individual's level of conscious also declines. Pupillary light response and deep tendon reflexes decline. Muscular tone tends to increase.

Hematologic Hypothermia leads to many hematologic changes. The most common includes a progressive hemoconcentration, resulting in an increase in hematocrit. In addition, hypothermia inhibits enzymatic reactions of the clotting cascade, leading to a progressive coagulopathy.

Frostbite

Maintenance of core temperature takes precedence over rewarming of the extremities. When the body is exposed to a magnitude or duration of cold that is significant enough to disrupt the core body temperature, continuous and intense vasoconstriction occurs, promoting frostbite to the exposed tissue. **Frostbite occurs when tissue temperatures are below 0°C.** There are two mechanisms for tissue damage: architectural cellular damage from ice-crystal formation and microvascular thrombosis and stasis.

The initial phase of frostbite, the **pre-freeze phase**, is characterized by tissue temperatures dropping below 10°C and cutaneous sensation loss. There is microvascular vasoconstriction and endothelial leakage of plasma into the interstitial tissues. Crystal formation does not occur until tissue temperatures drop below 0°C. Areas of skin that experience a slow rate of cooling will develop ice crystals in the extracellular matrix, whereas cells that undergo rapid cooling develop intracellular ice crystals. Extracellular matrix ice crystals are more favorable to cell survival. During the **freeze–thaw phase**, extracellular ice crystals form. In an attempt to maintain osmotic equilibrium, water leaves the cells, causing cellular dehydration and intracellular hyperosmolality. This leads to cellular collapse and demise. The third phase is the **progressive microvascular collapse phase.** Red cells form sludge and microthrombi during the first few hours after the tissues are thawed. The exact mechanism is unclear; however, hypoxic vasospasm, hyperviscosity, and direct endothelial damage all adversely affect flow. Ultimately, there is plasma leakage and arteriovenous shunting resulting in thrombosis, increased tissue pressure, ischemia, and necrosis (known as the **late ischemic phase**). These mechanisms result in three zones of injury in frostbite (Table 54–3).

TABLE 54–3 • FROSTBITE ZONES OF INJURY	
Zone of hyperemia	Least severe Most superficial and proximal Recovers without treatment in 10 days
Zone of stasis	Moderately severe Possibly reversible cell damage Treat by restoring circulation
Zone of coagulation	Most severe Deepest Occurs distally Irreversible cell damage

The clinical presentation of frostbite varies based on the depth of injury. There are four degrees of frost bite injury based on tissue depth (Table 54–4).

MANAGEMENT

The ultimate goal of prehospital treatment is preservation of life. **Frostbite and hypothermia often coexist, and prevention of further systemic heat loss is the priority. Field rewarming should not be performed if there is any potential for interrupted or incomplete thawing**, unless the possibility of evacuation does not exist. This is because **tissue refreezing is disastrous.** However, it is appropriate to remove wet,

TABLE 54–4 • DEGREES OF FROSTBITE		
Degree of Frostbite	**Tissues Involved**	**Clinical Presentation**
1st degree (Frostnip)	Superficial skin	Numbness, erythema, edema, desquamation, dysesthesia No blisters Full recovery expected
2nd degree	Full-thickness skin	Edema and erythema progressing to blistering within 6-24 hours Blisters desquamate and form black eschars over several days Good prognosis with appropriate treatment
3rd degree	Full-thickness skin, subdermal plexus	Tissue loss involving entire thickness of skin Hemorrhagic blisters, skin necrosis, blue-gray discoloration Poor prognosis; often requires grafts or partial amputation
4th degree	Muscle, tendon, bone	Tissue loss involving entire thickness of skin plus deeper structures Mottled, dry, black, mummified eschar with deep aching joint pain Extremely poor prognosis; requires amputation

constricting clothing and replace with dry clothing or blankets. There is a direct relationship between the length of time the tissue is frozen and the extent of cellular damage.

As with all patients who present to the ED with a life-threatening condition, the ABCs should always be promptly addressed, followed by simultaneous evaluation and stabilization. The patient should be placed on a cardiac monitor and have an intravenous catheter placed. Most patients are **dehydrated**. Warm intravenous fluids (crystalloid) should be administered. A core temperature needs to be rapidly determined. This is best achieved by obtaining a rectal temperature. Most standard hospital thermometers only read as low as 34°C. Therefore, in patients suspected to be hypothermic, it is critical to measure core temperature using a specialized thermometer capable of reading low temperatures. Once this occurs, a thorough history should be obtained including ambient temperature, wind velocity, duration of exposure, type of clothing worn, medication history, substance use history, and preexisting medical problems that could affect heat loss.

Diagnostic testing is important. A bedside capillary blood glucose should be obtained early in the resuscitation of hypothermic patients. Correcting hypoglycemia early in presentation may prevent the need for more invasive rewarming techniques. As temperature declines, pulse oximetry may not be reliable, so an arterial or venous blood gas can determine oxygen saturation. An ECG should be obtained to evaluate for cardiac dysrhythmia. Laboratory studies may reveal an elevated hematocrit and low platelet count. **Hyperkalemia** is indicative of cellular acidosis and is a marker for a poor prognosis. Elevation in the blood urea nitrogen (BUN) and creatinine (Cr) is common. Low thyroid hormone and cortisol levels may reveal a medical condition that predisposed to hypothermia. A high index of suspicion for occult traumatic injury is necessary, as trauma and hypothermia commonly occur together. Consider a CT scan of the head and other radiographic studies on patients who have an altered mental status or who do not improve with rewarming.

Based on the severity of hypothermia, various rewarming schemes are followed. These include passive rewarming, active external rewarming for moderate hypothermia, and active core rewarming in severe hypothermia.

Passive external rewarming allows patients to warm by endogenous heat production. This requires the ability to shiver. Individuals who are malnourished, hypoglycemic, or have a core temperature below 30°C are not candidates for passive external rewarming. Therefore, this is a good option in healthy patients with a mild degree of hypothermia. The patient should be removed from the cold or wet environment and wrapped in blankets, sleeping bags, or other insulating materials.

The decision to actively rewarm a patient implies a greater degree of hypothermia and possibly a coexisting medical condition. **Active external rewarming** involves the application of heat directly to the skin by way of forced-air surface warming blankets, warm water immersion, radiant heat sources, and warm water bottles. In the hospital setting, forced-air rewarming is most practical.

Active core rewarming refers to techniques that warm the patient from the inside out and are used to rewarm severely hypothermic patients. There are several methods used in active core rewarming, including positive pressure ventilation using warm air, peritoneal, bladder and pleural irrigation with warmed saline, and extra-corporeal blood rewarming. These methods are reserved for severely hypothermic patients and those presenting with cardiac arrest.

Hypothermic patients may experience complications secondary to rewarming. **After drop** refers to the continual decline in core body temperature after the patient is removed from the cold environment. The current theory holds that rewarming causes disequilibrium across a gradient such that the body is cooled from the periphery to the inside and the core body temperature will continue to drop until core temperature is equal to peripheral temperature. This was thought to predispose to ventricular fibrillation. However, there is little evidence to support this.

For patients who are pulseless and show no signs of life, death pronouncement only occurs when the individual's core body temperature is above 35°C. Since the physiologic response to hypothermia is extremely varied, the well-known adage, "no one is dead until they are warm and dead" is often valid. Ventricular fibrillation is typically resistant to defibrillation until core temperatures are above 28°C. Therefore, continuous chest compressions should be administered until the patient has been rewarmed to a temperature above 35°C.

After stabilizing the core temperature and addressing associated conditions, **rapid thawing** should be initiated. For frostbite, **rapid rewarming of frozen or partially thawed tissue is accomplished by immersion in a gently circulating water bath that is carefully maintained at a temperature of 37°C to 39°C.** Rewarming is continued until the tissue is pliable and distal erythema is noted, usually about 10-30 minutes. Active, gentle motion is encouraged, but direct tissue massage should be avoided. Parenteral analgesics should be administered, as tissue rewarming causes throbbing, burning pain, and tenderness. Sensation is often diminished after thawing and then disappears with bleb formation. Sensation does not normalize until healing is complete.

After thawing, the injured extremities should be elevated to minimize swelling. Sterile dressings should be applied and involved areas handled gently. Digital exercises are encouraged to help avoid venous stasis. Treatment also includes NSAIDs, topical aloe vera, debridement of clear blisters (hemorrhagic blisters should be left alone), and tetanus vaccination if indicated. Antibiotics are also often given. In cases of gangrene, amputation is often delayed for up to 3 weeks because the extent of tissue injury is difficult to assess initially.

CASE CORRELATION

- See also Case 52 (Heat Related Illnesses), Case 53 (Lightning and Electrical Injury), and Case 55 (Drowning).

COMPREHENSION QUESTIONS

54.1 A 72-year-old woman with a history dementia is reported missing by nursing home staff late one December night. The patient is found 2 hours later, lying on a park bench, soaking wet, wearing only a thin night gown and no shoes. EMS has arrived on the scene. Which of the following is the most appropriate next step in management?

A. Check capillary blood glucose

B. Immediately establish intravenous access and administer intravenous fluids

C. Assess the ABCs

D. Cover the patient with any available materials

54.2 A 14-year-old boy wandered into the woods while chasing after his dog and lost his bearings. He was not wearing any shoes. He was found approximately 12 hours later and presents to the ED with clear, fluid-filled blisters on his toes and feet. What is the most likely diagnosis?

A. Second-degree frostbite

B. Trench foot

C. First-degree frostbite

D. Chilblains

54.3 A homeless man of unknown age presents to the ED unresponsive. Bystanders believe he was outside all night in a snow storm. His core temperature is 30°C. What is the most common cardiac dysrhythmia seen in hypothermia?

A. Sinus tachycardia

B. Sinus bradycardia

C. Ventricular fibrillation

D. Atrial fibrillation

ANSWERS

54.1 **C.** The first step in emergency care is always to address and stabilize the ABCs. Checking a capillary glucose is important in a patient with altered mental status but should be done after ABCs are addressed. The patient's wet clothing should be removed and dry, warm blankets should be used to cover the patient. Intravenous access should also be established and warm intravenous fluids should be given. However, none of these measures should occur until the ABCs have been assessed.

54.2 **A.** The patient has clear, fluid-filled blisters on his toes and feet consistent with a diagnosis of second-degree frostbite. First-degree frostbite, also known as frostnip, is more superficial and not associated with blister formation. Chilblain, also known as pernio, occurs on skin that is exposed to cold, but non-freezing conditions. It is most common on the face, ears, and hands and is characterized by red, scaly lesions. Trench foot occurs from chronic exposure of the feet to cool, damp conditions.

54.3 **D.** Atrial fibrillation is the most common dysrhythmia in hypothermia and is characteristic at a core temperature of 30°C. Prolongation of any interval, bradycardia, asystole, atrial fibrillation and flutter, and ventricular tachycardia may also be seen. In this patient a 12-lead ECG was obtained showing an Osborne (J) wave, which is indicative of a junctional rhythm and is consistent with hypothermia. J waves may be seen at any temperature below 32.2°C, most frequently in leads II and V6. Below a core temperature of 25°C, they are most commonly found in the precordial leads (especially V3 and V4) and their size increases. J waves are usually upright in aVL, aVF, and the precordial leads.

CLINICAL PEARLS

▶ Hypothermia and frostbite often occur simultaneously.

▶ Ethanol use and advanced age are risk factors for cold-exposure injury.

▶ Field rewarming for frostbite is rarely warranted because of the potential for incomplete or interrupted rewarming. The injured parts should be protected, core temperature stabilized, and patient transfer to the ED arranged.

▶ Frostbitten areas should be treated with immersion in a circulating water bath maintained at a temperature of 37°C to 39°C.

▶ Standard hospital thermometers only read as low as 34°C. Specialized low-temperature thermometers are required to obtain an accurate core body temperature.

▶ A severely hypothermic patient can present with rigidity, asystole, and with fixed pupils; however, he or she should not be pronounced deceased until the core body temperature has been warmed to at least 35°C.

▶ Hypoglycemia, sepsis, and hypothyroidism are conditions that may mimic or coexist with hypothermia.

REFERENCES

Ahya SN, Flood K, eds. *The Washington Manual of Medical Therapeutics*, 33rd ed. St Louis, MO: Lippincott Williams & Wilkins; 2010.

Brown D. Hypothermia. In: Tintinalli JE, et al, eds. *Emergency Medicine: A Comprehensive Study Guide*. 8th ed. New York, NY: McGraw-Hill; 2016.

Brown DJ, Brugger H, Boyd J, Paal P. Accidental hypothermia. *N Eng J Med*. 2012;367:1930.

Danzl DF, Zafren K. Accidental hypothermia. In: Rosen P, et al, eds. *Emergency Medicine, Concepts and Clinical Practice*. 8th ed. Philadelphia, PA: Saunders; 2014.

Freer L, Imray CHE. Frostbite. In: Auerbach PS, ed. *Wilderness Medicine*. 6th ed. Philadelphia, PA: Mosby Elsevier; 2012.

Hermann L, Weingart S. Hypothermia and other cold-related emergencies. *Emerg Med Pract*. 2003;5(12):1-22.

Olin JW. Other peripheral arterial diseases. In: Goldman L, Bennett JC, eds. *Cecil Textbook of Medicine*. 24th ed. Philadelphia, PA: WB Saunders; 2011.

Paddock MT. Cold Injuries. In: Tintinalli JE, et al, eds. *Emergency Medicine: A Comprehensive Study Guide*. 8th ed. New York, NY: McGraw-Hill; 2016.

Van der Ploeg GJ, Goslings JC, Walpoth BH, Bierens JJ. Accidental hypothermia: rewarming treatments, complications and outcomes from one university medical centre. *Resuscitiation*. 2010;81(11): 1550-1555.

Zafren K, Danzl DF. Frostbite. In: Rosen P, et al, eds. *Emergency Medicine, Concepts and Clinical Practice*. 8th ed. Philadelphia, PA: Saunders; 2014.

A group of teenagers was swimming at the lake when one of the boys failed to surface after diving off a platform. He was quickly found and rescued by another swimmer from the lake bottom. The patient was noted to be apneic, and cardiopulmonary resuscitation (CPR) was initiated by one of the bystanders. After the paramedics arrived, the patient was noted to have spontaneous shallow respirations, a weak palpable pulse, and Glasgow coma scale (GCS) score of 7 (eyes 1, verbal 2, motor 4). The paramedics intubated the patient and transported him to the emergency department (ED). In the ED, the patient has an initial pulse of 70 beats per minute, blood pressure of 110/70 mm Hg, temperature of 35.6°C (96.1°F), GCS score of 6 (eyes 1, verbal 1, motor 4), and oxygen saturation of 92% on 100% Fio_2.

▶ What are the complications associated with this condition?
▶ What is the best treatment for this patient?

ANSWERS TO CASE 55:

Drowning

Summary: A teenage boy presents with drowning following a diving accident at a lake.

- **Complications:** Drowning results in global hypoxia and tissue ischemia primarily affecting the brain, lungs, and heart. Early complications include noncardiogenic pulmonary edema, hypoxic encephalopathy, respiratory and metabolic acidosis, dysrhythmias, and renal impairment. Coagulopathy, electrolyte abnormalities, and hemodilution or hemoconcentration are rare but possible sequelae. Pneumonia and acute respiratory distress syndrome can occur later in the patient's hospital course.

- **Best treatment:** The most important treatment to optimize outcome is rapid initiation of resuscitation in the prehospital setting (ie, stabilizing the ABCs [airway, breathing, and circulation]). To this end, bystander CPR can be vitally important. Victims of drowning often require aggressive respiratory support, which may range from administration of supplemental oxygen to intubation. If cervical spine injury is suspected (as in this patient who dove off a platform), cervical spine stabilization should be maintained until spinal trauma is ruled out.

ANALYSIS

Objectives

1. Learn the pathophysiology of drowning.
2. Become familiar with the epidemiology and prevention of drowning.
3. Learn the specific problems associated with cold-water-drowning.

Considerations

The initial management of patients with drowning is stabilization of the ABCs and correction of hypoxemia. In the ED, all of these patients require continuous cardiac monitoring and pulse oximetry. Initial diagnostics may include a complete blood count, blood glucose, electrolytes, creatinine, arterial blood gas, and chest x-ray. This intubated patient will need to be admitted to the ICU, where continued cardiopulmonary monitoring and mechanical ventilation support can be provided.

When encountering a patient with drowning, the ED physician must always consider whether any precipitants exist that also require treatment. These precipitants may include alcohol or drug intoxication, seizures, hypoglycemia, dysrhythmias, cardiac arrest, attempted suicide or homicide, intracerebral hemorrhage, and child abuse or neglect. In addition, if the submersion is associated with a history of trauma (eg, diving into water and motor vehicle collision), cervical spine and head injuries are considerations that may require further evaluation. Hypothermia should also be considered if the patient is submersed in cold water.

APPROACH TO:
Drowning

DEFINITIONS

DIVING REFLEX: Physiologic response to submersion to reduce the utilization of oxygen, including bradycardia and peripheral vasoconstriction.

DROWNING: Primary respiratory impairment due to submersion/immersion in a liquid medium. The patient may live or die after this event.

DROWNED: A person who died from drowning.

SUBMERSION: The entire body, including the airway, is under water.

IMMERSION: A portion of the body is covered in water. For drowning to occur, usually at least the face and airway are immersed.

CLINICAL APPROACH

Epidemiology and Prevention

Drowning is the fourth most common cause of accidental death in the United States. It is responsible for more than 500,000 deaths annually worldwide. In children less than 19 years old, it is the second leading cause of death (behind motor vehicle collisions). Risk factors for drowning include age, gender, and race. The incidence of drowning peaks in toddlers and young children, adolescents and young adults, and in the elderly. However, drowning deaths are most common in toddlers and older teenagers. Males account for 80% of drowning victims older than 12 months.

Alcohol use and some medical conditions have also been associated with an increased risk of drowning. Among teenagers and adults, **alcohol use may be a contributing factor in 30% to 50% of cases.** Seizures, autism, and other developmental and behavioral disorders also increase the risk of drowning. **In patients with prolonged QT syndrome, immersion in cold water may further extend the QT interval, causing dysrhythmias.**

Drowning can occur in natural bodies of water (freshwater and saltwater) as well as in domestic settings (such as bathtubs and swimming pools). Infants may even drown in toilets or buckets of water. However, if the **infant is less than 6 months old or has an atypical presentation, healthcare providers should maintain a high suspicion for abuse.** Efforts to decrease the incidence of drowning have focused on educating the public and increasing awareness of preventive measures. Preventive measures include adequate fencing around pools, decreasing the use of alcohol when engaged in water sports, increasing the supervision of children playing in or near water, and increasing the number of citizens trained in CPR. Water safety education for children, teenagers, and parents that encourages wearing flotation devices and never swimming alone should be reinforced in the school, community, and physician's office.

Pathophysiology of Drowning

Victims of drowning initially hold their breaths. As hypoxia and air hunger develop, they eventually involuntarily swallow and aspirate water. After aspiration of 1-3 mL/kg of water, dilution and washout of surfactant occurs, resulting in atelectasis, decreased gas exchange across the alveoli, non-cardiogenic pulmonary edema, and ventilation-perfusion mismatch. This leads to worsening hypoxia and respiratory and metabolic acidosis. If this process continues, neuronal death and cardiovascular collapse ensue.

"Dry drowning" is a term that was traditionally used to refer to drowning deaths that occurred without aspiration of a significant amount of water (perhaps due to severe laryngospasm, hypoxia, and loss of consciousness). However, the medical literature does not support this mechanism of injury. Dry drownings are probably due to causes besides simple submersion.

Management

Patients with drowning may present with signs of pulmonary and central nervous system dysfunction or dysrhythmias. The patient may arrive in extremis with hypoxia, cyanosis, hypothermia, severe respiratory distress, or respiratory arrest. Other pulmonary findings may include tachypnea, wheezes, rales, or rhonchi. Neurologically, patient presentations may range from a mild alteration of consciousness to coma. **Neurological deficits at the time of initial evaluation do not necessarily portend a poor patient outcome.** Dysrhythmias are mainly the result of hypoxemia and acidosis and may include ventricular fibrillation, ventricular tachycardia, and bradycardia asystole. Patients with severe drowning may develop acute respiratory distress syndrome, hypoxic encephalopathy, or cardiac arrest.

All patients should be placed **on continuous cardiac monitoring and pulse oximetry** in the ED. An **ECG** is useful to rule out QT prolongation and dysrhythmias. A **chest x-ray** should also be performed to identify any infiltrates or pulmonary edema with the caveat that initial x-ray findings may progress over time. Although they are often normal at first, a baseline complete blood count, electrolytes, creatinine, and glucose should be obtained. Arterial blood gases may be helpful in monitoring for acidosis, hypercarbia, and hypoxemia.

The most critical element in the treatment of drowning victims is prompt and effective basic life support delivery in the prehospital setting, specifically correcting hypoxia by ventilation. **Prompt rescue breathing increases the victim's chance of survival.** Chest compressions should be initiated if the patient has no pulse. It is also important to note that the majority of patients receiving ventilation or chest compressions will have subsequent vomiting. The **Heimlich maneuver is not recommended** to expel fluid from the lungs because of the high rate of aspiration induced by this maneuver and the delay it causes in initiation of ventilation. An awake patient with mild respiratory symptoms may benefit from noninvasive positive pressure ventilation (NIPPV), although a risk of gastric distention and vomiting does exist with the use of NIPPV. Indications for intubation include a lack of protective airway reflexes, respiratory distress, hypercarbia, hypoxia (despite noninvasive oxygen delivery), and apnea.

Intravenous fluids consisting of lactated Ringer solution or normal saline should be initiated in most of these patients. **Glucose-containing solutions are generally contraindicated**, except in hypoglycemic patients. Scientific investigations indicate that glucose solutions may worsen the neurological outcome in animals that have incomplete cerebral ischemia. In general, empiric antibiotics are not indicated for patients with drowning. Antibiotics may benefit patients who were submerged in grossly contaminated water or manifest signs of infection.

Patients who are asymptomatic may be observed in the ED for 4-6 hours. If they maintain normal oxygen saturations on room air and have normal pulmonary examinations and chest x-rays, they may be discharged home. Admission is required for patients who are symptomatic, have been unconscious, hypoxic, apneic, have an abnormal chest x-ray, or have evidence of dysrhythmia.

Cold Water Drowning

Drowning in cold water may be more advantageous than drowning in warm water due to induction of hypothermia. **Hypothermia has been theorized to be neuroprotective** because of the induction of a global hypometabolic state, leading to the conservation of oxygen and glucose for brain metabolism. Cold water also has potentially deleterious effects, most significantly cardiac irritability (leading to dysrhythmias), exhaustion, and altered mental status. Although some case reports have described patients who survived prolonged submersion in cold water, hypothermia is usually a poor prognostic indicator.

CASE CORRELATION

- See also Case 52 (Heat-related Illnesses), Case 53 (Lightning and Electrical Injury), and Case 54 (Frostbite and Hypothermia).

COMPREHENSION QUESTIONS

55.1 Each of the following patients is being treated for drowning. Which one of the following is most appropriate for discharge from the ED after several hours of observation?

    A. A 3-year-old boy found face-down in the swimming pool required 4 minutes of CPR, had a return of normal vital signs with GCS score of 15 and mild respiratory distress.

    B. A 12-year-old boy was found unconscious and submerged in a swimming pool after striking his head on the bottom. His chest x-ray (CXR) and head CT are normal. His GCS score is 14. He is complaining of headache and no respiratory symptoms.

    C. A 6-year-old boy was washed into the ocean by a large wave and was rescued by a bystander. No CPR was required, and the boy had an initial GCS score of 14 and normal vital signs. CXR and physical examination are normal. Room air O_2 saturation is 95%.

    D. A 3-month-old infant was brought to the ED after accidental submersion in the bathtub. The physical examination is unremarkable except for bruising over both arms and ankles. His CXR is normal, and his room air O_2 saturation is 98%.

55.2 Which of the following is a correct statement regarding drowning?

A. Antibiotics may benefit patients who were submersed in grossly contaminated water.

B. The diving reflex is neuroprotective for adults who are submersed in cold water.

C. Neurological deficits on initial evaluation portend a poor prognosis.

D. A normal initial chest x-ray rules out pulmonary injury.

55.3 A 24-year-old patient is brought to the ED after drowning in a local lake. Upon arrival to the ED, he has a heart rate of 98 beats per minute, blood pressure of 90/56 mm Hg, respiratory rate of 34 breaths per minute, and oxygen saturation of 84%. He opens his eyes to pain, responds to questions with grunts, and withdraws from pain. Auscultation of the chest reveals diffuse rales. What is the next best step in management?

A. Aggressive deep suctioning

B. Endotracheal intubation

C. IV fluid bolus

D. Noninvasive positive pressure ventilation

ANSWERS

55.1 **C.** The child described in Answer C is stable, alert, and has normal vital signs and pulmonary status, and can be safely discharged. Although the boy described in choice A is stable, his initial requirement for 4 minutes of CPR places him at a great risk for pulmonary and neurological sequelae. The patient described in B has mild respiratory symptoms, but his mechanism of injury and neurological findings are concerning for a closed head injury that requires further observation. The patient described in D is stable from the standpoint of drowning, but the physical findings suggest possible intentional injury that may need further investigation.

55.2 **A.** Antibiotics may benefit patients who were submersed in grossly contaminated water or who have signs of infection on examination. The diving reflex is strongest in infants and children. Neurological deficits at the time of initial evaluation do not rule out the possibility of neurological recovery. Initial chest x-ray findings may progress over time.

55.3 **B.** This patient has findings of severe respiratory distress with tachypnea as well as a marked hypoxia. Additionally, the mental status is depressed. This patient would be best served by endotracheal intubation for ventilation and also airway protection.

CLINICAL PEARLS

▶ Precipitants (such as alcohol use, seizures, and hypoglycemia) and associated cervical spine and head injuries must be considered in any patient with drowning.

▶ The most common complications of drowning involve pulmonary or central nervous system dysfunction and dysrhythmias.

▶ The most important treatment to optimize outcome is rapid initiation of resuscitation in the prehospital arena. Victims of drowning often require aggressive respiratory support.

REFERENCES

Bowers RC, Anderson TK. Disorders due to physical and environmental agents. In: Stone CK, Humphries RL, eds. *Current Diagnosis and Treatment: Emergency Medicine.* 6th ed. Available at: http://www.accessmedicine.com/content.aspx?aID=3113673. Accessed May 1, 2016.

Causey AL, Tilelli JA, Swanson ME. Predicting discharge in uncomplicated near-drowning. *Am J Emerg Med.* 2000;18:9-11.

Kuo DC, Jerrard DA. Environmental insults: smoke inhalation, submersion, diving, and high altitude. *Emerg Med Clin N Am.* 2003;21:475-497.

Marx JA, Hockberger RS, Walls RM, eds. *Rosen's Emergency Medicine: Concepts and Clinical Practice.* 8th ed. Philadelphia, PA: Saunders; 2014.

Tintinalli JE, Stapczynski JS, Ma OJ, et al, eds. *Emergency Medicine: A Comprehensive Study Guide.* 8th ed. New York, NY: McGraw-Hill; 2016.

Volturo GA. Submersion injuries. In: Aaron CK, Abujamra L, eds. *Harwood Nuss' Clinical Practice of Emergency Medicine.* 4th ed. Lippincott Williams & Wilkins; 2005.

Weinstein MD, Kriegr BP. Near-drowning: epidemiology, pathophysiology, and initial treatment. *J Emerg Med.* 1996;14:461-467.

A 25-year-old woman is brought to the emergency department (ED) by police after attempting to break into a grocery store. When she was apprehended, EMS noted that her pupils were large and that she seemed "high." The patient states that she has been "smoking" for the past year. She admits she recently lost her job due to tardiness and stealing to continue "smoking," which she states makes her feel more energetic. She notes that without her "smokes," she craves the drug, becomes very sleepy, depressed, and has a huge appetite. She comments that even though she was not trying to lose weight, she lost 30 pounds in the past 6 months. In the ED, she complains of chest pain. The patient has a temperature of 38°C (100.4°F), heart rate of 120 beats per minute, and blood pressure of 160/90 mm Hg. Her pupils are both dilated at 6 mm and reactive. Her thyroid is normal to palpation. The heart and lung examinations reveal tachycardia but are otherwise normal. Neurologic examination is unremarkable.

▶ What is the most likely diagnosis?
▶ What is the best treatment for the probable condition?

ANSWER TO CASE 56:

Cocaine Intoxication

Summary: This 25-year-old woman was arrested while attempting to burglarize a grocery store. Further questioning reveals she lost her job because she was habitually late and stealing, secondary to her desire to "smoke." She has required more and more of the drug to get high and has been unsuccessful in her attempts to quit "smoking." She suffers from cravings, sleepiness, depression, and hyperphagia when she is unable to "smoke." While high, the patient feels euphoric and a sense of heightened energy. Her pupils are dilated; she has a low-grade fever, tachycardia, and hypertension. She has unintentionally lost 30 lbs over 6 months.

- **Most likely diagnosis:** Cocaine intoxication.

- **Best treatment:** Benzodiazepines for anxiety and phentolamine for blood pressure control.

ANALYSIS

Objectives

1. Recognize the clinical manifestations of cocaine intoxication.

2. Know the treatment for acute cocaine intoxication.

Considerations

This patient has many of the clinical signs and symptoms of cocaine intoxication. Cocaine is a sympathomimetic with local anesthetic and vasoconstrictive properties. Complications of cocaine intoxication include severe hypertension (with concomitant end organ damage), hyperthermia, myocardial infarction, intracerebral hemorrhage, seizures, dysrhythmias, and kidney injury caused by rhabdomyolysis. The mainstays of treatment are benzodiazepines (often in large dosages) and supportive measures. Acute cocaine intoxication may be difficult to distinguish from other conditions such as heat stroke, sedative-hypnotic withdrawal, intoxication with other sympathomimetics/anticholinergics, thyrotoxicosis, and infections or structural lesions of the central nervous system.

APPROACH TO:

Cocaine Intoxication

CLINICAL APPROACH

After marijuana, cocaine is the second most commonly used illicit drug. With such widespread use, ED visits related to cocaine intoxication and its complications have risen substantially. A recent study shows that 14% of people older than 12 years have tried cocaine. The routes of administration include intranasal, intravenous, and inhalation by smoking. Frequently, cocaine is combined with other drugs such as heroin ("speedball") or alcohol ("liquid lady").

Cocaine causes release of norepinephrine, epinephrine, serotonin, and dopamine. This leads to a sympathomimetic state. Cocaine also acts as a local anesthetic through sodium channel blockade. This effect is responsible for many of the dysrhythmias and conduction abnormalities associated with cocaine use.

Symptoms of cocaine intoxication include euphoria, feelings of power or aggression, agitation, anxiety, hallucinations (classically formication, a tactile sensation of insects crawling on the skin), and delusions. Physical examination may reveal mydriasis, tachycardia, hypertension, hyperthermia, diaphoresis, tremors, or seizures. Coingestants or contaminants may result in atypical presentations (eg, cocaine plus heroin: mixed sympathomimetic-opioid presentation).

Table 56–1 summarizes the acute complications of cocaine intoxication. The effects on the cardiovascular and neurologic systems are of major concern.

Chest pain is a frequent complaint of those who present to the ED after cocaine use. Cocaine causes coronary vasoconstriction while also increasing the myocardial oxygen demand and platelet aggregation. The ED physician must maintain a high index of suspicion for myocardial ischemia and infarction, even with an atypical history and normal initial ECG; between 0.7% and 6% of these patients will have an acute myocardial infarction. These patients are typically younger, nonwhite cigarette smokers without other risk factors for coronary artery disease. Benzodiazepines, often in large doses, are useful in treating cocaine-induced chest pain. Administration of aspirin, nitrates, and morphine are advisable. The use of beta-**blockers is controversial due to the risk of an unopposed alpha-adrenergic effect, leading to increased hypertension and coronary vasoconstriction.** Thrombolytic therapy of an ST elevation myocardial infarction should be avoided if coronary vasospasm or dissection is suspected or severe, uncontrolled hypertension exists (due to the risk of intracerebral hemorrhage). Emergent coronary artery catheterization may provide the best diagnostic information.

Table 56–1 • ACUTE COMPLICATIONS OF COCAINE INTOXICATION	
Autonomic	Hyperthermia, rhabdomyolysis, hypertension, dehydration
Cardiac	Dysrhythmia, myocarditis, endocarditis, cardiomyopathy, myocardial infarction or ischemia, coronary artery dissection, aortic rupture
Central nervous system	Seizures, intracranial hemorrhage or infarction, altered mental status, spinal cord infarction, intracranial abscess, acute dystonia
Pulmonary	Pulmonary hemorrhage, barotrauma (pneumothorax, pneumomediastinum, pneumopericardium), pneumonitis, asthma, pulmonary edema
Gastrointestinal	Intestinal ischemia, bowel necrosis, splenic infarction, ischemic colitis, gastrointestinal bleeding
Renal	Renal insufficiency or failure, renal infarction
Miscellaneous	Deep venous thrombosis, nasal perforation, sinusitis, oropharyngeal burn, infection (local or systemic), placental abruption, spontaneous abortion

For patients with hyperthermia or agitation, evaluation of acute cocaine intoxication should also include a basic metabolic panel and creatine kinase to assess for renal failure, metabolic acidosis, and rhabdomyolysis. Patients with altered mental status or seizures should have a computed tomography (CT) of the head performed to assess for intracerebral hemorrhage.

In general, patients with acute cocaine intoxication require only supportive care, including monitoring and intravenous fluids. **Agitation and sympathomimetic effects are best controlled using benzodiazepines such as lorazepam or diazepam.** Phenothiazines (such as haloperidol) should be avoided because they may lower the seizure threshold, contribute to hyperthermia, and have dysrhythmic effects. Atrial dysrhythmias may respond to benzodiazepines or calcium channel blockers. Intravenous sodium bicarbonate administration may be useful for wide-complex tachycardias (or lidocaine if the dysrhythmia is refractory to bicarbonate). The drug of choice to treat severe hypertension is the alpha-antagonist phentolamine. Intravenous nitroglycerin or nitroprusside may also be used. Again, beta-blocking agent use is controversial. Seizures are treated with benzodiazepines. Hyperthermia requires continuous monitoring of core temperature and rapid cooling. Patients with rhabdomyolysis require increased fluid resuscitation in order to maintain 1-3 mL/kg/h of urine output.

Asymptomatic body packers may be carefully monitored and given activated charcoal and polyethylene glycol (whole bowel irrigation) to hasten the passage of the packets of cocaine. These packets usually contain lethal doses of cocaine and can be rapidly fatal if ruptured. If the patient becomes acutely hypertensive, hyperthermic, or agitated, or if the patient manifests other signs of cocaine intoxication, benzodiazepines should be given and surgery emergently consulted for operative removal of the packets. Endoscopy is usually avoided due to a risk of packet perforation. Packets will not necessarily be visible on plain radiographs.

The patient presenting with cocaine intoxication responds to benzodiazepine administration and has no further complications may be discharged from the ED after a period of observation. Patients with ongoing chest pain, ECG changes, enzyme elevations or requiring ongoing pharmacologic treatment should be admitted to a monitored bed for further observation. Body packers need to be observed until all packets have passed.

CASE CORRELATION

- See also Case 57 (Acetaminophen Toxicity), Case 58 (Ethanol Withdrawal), and Case 59 (Anti-muscarinic Toxidrome).

COMPREHENSION QUESTIONS

56.1 A 25-year-old man is brought to the emergency room by police because of suspected cocaine intoxication. He is noted to be very agitated (fighting against five burly policemen) and wild eyed. On examination, his blood pressure is 180/100 mm Hg and heart rate is 110 beats per minute. He is noted to have rotatory nystagmus. The neurologic examination reveals no focal abnormalities. Which of the following is the most likely diagnosis?

A. Amphetamine intoxication

B. Cocaine intoxication

C. Opiate intoxication

D. Phencyclidine intoxication

56.2 A 28-year-old man is noted to have extremely elevated blood pressure (210/130 mm Hg) associated with chest pain and dyspnea. His urine drug screen is positive for cocaine metabolites. Which of the following is the best next step?

A. Albuterol intravenously

B. Ephedrine intravenously

C. Labetalol intravenously

D. Lorazepam intravenously

56.3 A 35-year-old man is brought to the ED with altered level of consciousness, drowsiness, and pinpoint pupils. Which of the following is the most appropriate initial therapy for this patient?

A. Activated charcoal

B. Bicarbonate

C. Lorazepam

D. Naloxone

56.4 A 34-year-old male presents after ingesting several packets of cocaine 6 hours ago. He reports that he feels well and has no complaints. His vital signs are within normal limits. An abdominal radiograph reveals a tubular foreign body within the patient's mid-abdomen. The most appropriate next step in treatment is:

A. Activated charcoal

B. Nasogastric lavage

C. Surgical retrieval

D. Whole bowel irrigation

ANSWERS

56.1 **D.** Phencyclidine intoxication often presents with agitation, superhuman strength, and rotatory or vertical nystagmus.

56.2 **D.** Benzodiazepines should be used as the first-line agent for nearly all cocaine toxicities. The hypertension is caused by sympathetic stimulation. Beta-blockers are contraindicated because they can result in unopposed alpha-adrenergic stimulation and exacerbation of the chest pain and hypertension. Hypertension unresponsive to benzodiazepines may require intravenous phentolamine, an alpha-adrenergic antagonist.

56.3 **D.** This patient likely has an opiate intoxication (drowsiness and pinpoint pupils). Cocaine intoxication usually causes agitation and dilated pupils. Naloxone counteracts the effect of opioids.

56.4 **D.** Whole bowel irrigation is recommended to decrease intestinal transit time. Surgery is indicated only in symptomatic patients. The utility of giving activated charcoal more than 1 or 2 hours after ingestion is not well established.

CLINICAL PEARLS

▶ The clinical manifestations of cocaine intoxication result from sympathetic overstimulation and vasoconstriction.

▶ Cocaine intoxication can cause life-threatening complications, such as dysrhythmias, hyperthermia, and hypertensive emergencies.

▶ Beta-blockers are controversial in patients with cocaine intoxication because of the risk of unopposed aplha-adrenergic stimulation.

▶ Benzodiazepines are a mainstay of treatment for cocaine toxicity and many of its complications.

REFERENCES

Aghababian RV, Bird SB, Braen GR, et al, eds. *Essentials of Emergency Medicine*. Sudbury, MA: Jones and Bartlett Learning; 2011:820-822.

Marx JA, Hockberger RS, Walls RM, eds. *Rosen's Emergency Medicine: Concepts and Clinical Practice*. 8th ed. Philadelphia, PA: Saunders; 2014.

McCord J, Jneid H, Hollander JE, et al. Management of cocaine-associated chest pain and myocardial infarction: a scientific statement from the American Heart Association Acute Cardiac Care Committee of the Council on Clinical Cardiology. *Circulation*. 2008;117;1897-1907.

Prosser JM. Special considerations. In: Hoffman RS, Howland M, Lewin NA, Nelson LS, Goldfrank LR, et al, eds. *Goldfrank's Toxicologic Emergencies*. 10th ed. New York, NY: McGraw-Hill; 2015.

Schaider JJ, Barkin RM, Hayden SR, Wolfe R, et al, eds. *Rosen and Barkin's 5-Minute Emergency Medicine Consult*. 4th ed. Philadelphia, PA: Lippincott Williams & Wilkins; 2011.

Tintinalli JE, Stapczynski JS, Ma OJ, et al, eds. *Emergency Medicine: A Comprehensive Study Guide*. 8th ed. New York, NY: McGraw-Hill; 2016.

An 18-year-old woman is brought by a friend to the emergency department (ED) about 30 minutes after she took "a bunch" of Tylenol. The patient states she was upset with her parents, who grounded her after she came home late from a party. She swallowed half a bottle of extra-strength Tylenol in order to "make them feel sorry." She is tearful, says she was "stupid," and denies any true desire to hurt herself or anyone else. She has no other complaints and denies any past attempts to hurt herself. On examination, her blood pressure is 105/60 mm Hg, heart rate is 100 beats per minute, and respiratory rate is 24 breaths per minute (crying). Her pupils are equal and reactive bilaterally. Her sclera are clear, and her mucous membranes are moist. The lungs are clear, and heart sounds are regular. The abdominal examination is benign with normal bowel sounds. She is awake and alert without any focal neurologic deficits.

► What is the most appropriate next step?
► What are the potential complications of this ingestion?
► What is the mechanism of acetaminophen toxicity?

ANSWERS TO CASE 57:

Acetaminophen Toxicity

Summary: This is an 18-year-old woman with an acute acetaminophen overdose 30 minutes prior to arrival in the ED. She is alert and oriented with stable vital signs.

- **Most appropriate next step:** Obtain IV access; send appropriate laboratory studies; administer activated charcoal; evaluate need for *N*-acetylcysteine (NAC).

- **Potential complications:** Hypoglycemia, metabolic acidosis, hepatic failure, and renal failure.

- **Mechanism:** Production of toxic metabolite, *N*-acetyl-*p*-benzoquinoneimine (NAPQI).

ANALYSIS

Objectives

1. Learn the general approach to the poisoned patient.

2. Recognize the clinical signs and symptoms of acetaminophen toxicity.

3. Understand the evaluation and treatment of patients with acetaminophen toxicity.

Considerations

Acetaminophen (APAP) is one of the most commonly used analgesics and anti-pyretics. It is available in a variety of prescription, over-the-counter, and combination medications labeled for fever, cold, cough, and pain relief. As a result, it is the most common over-the-counter agent reported in accidental and intentional over-doses, leading to more hospitalizations after overdose than any other pharmaceutical agent. A toxic exposure to APAP is suspected when more than 200 mg/kg or more than 10 g is ingested in a single dose or over the course of 24 hours. In addition, an ingestion of more than 150 mg/kg or more than 6 g/day for at least 2 consecutive days is potentially toxic. Hepatotoxicity is the most life-threatening complication but may be indolent. Thus, serum APAP level and a precise time of ingestion are important to plot on the Rumack Matthew nomogram to assess likelihood of toxicity. This patient was forthcoming about the medication used in the overdose; however, many patients will underreport or deny the use of APAP. Consequently, an APAP level should be drawn on all suspected overdose patients. Although clinical evidence of hepatotoxicity may be delayed for 24-72 hours, NAC therapy is most effective if started within 8 hours of ingestion. Because this patient reported the ingestion within 30 minutes, there is time for a serum APAP level, activated charcoal decontamination, and then NAC therapy. If time is an issue, NAC treatment should be initiated without delay. Emesis should not be induced because of the possible delay in therapy. After medical stabilization, assessment of suicide potential is important.

APPROACH TO:

Acetaminophen Toxicity

DEFINITIONS

TOXIDROMES: Signs and symptoms associated with poisoning.

RUMACK-MATTHEW NOMOGRAM: Acetaminophen toxicity nomogram based on serum acetaminophen concentration versus time after ingestion.

CLINICAL APPROACH

Under normal circumstances, most APAP is metabolized in the liver and excreted by the kidneys. Of the remainder, approximately 5% is excreted unchanged in urine, and another 5% is metabolized by the hepatic cytochrome P450 system to form NAPQI. This toxic intermediate is then detoxified by conjugation with glutathione. In acute APAP overdose, glutathione becomes depleted and leads to the accumulation of NAPQI, which then binds to hepatocyte intracellular proteins, causing hepatocellular necrosis. APAP toxicity can be divided into four clinical phases (Table 57–1).

Clinical Evaluation

When approaching the poisoned or overdose patient, the clinician's priorities are to stabilize the ABCs, decontaminate, minimize absorption, and administer any antidotes. Important historical information includes type, amount, and timing of ingestion; current symptoms; circumstances of ingestion (accidental or intentional); and possible coingestants. The physical examination should focus on the airway, abdomen (RUQ tenderness) and mental status. A complete physical examination is important to search for any concomitant toxic syndromes (toxidromes) (Table 57–2). Table 57–3 lists common antidotes. Consulting with the local poison control center is also recommended for any suspected ingestion or overdose.

Diagnostic studies include serum electrolytes, blood urea nitrogen (BUN)/creatinine, glucose, liver enzyme levels, coagulation studies, and urinalysis (as well as

Table 57–1 · CLINICAL PHASES OF APAP TOXICITY			
Phase 1	Phase 2	Phase 3	Phase 4
Preinjury period (30 min to 24 h after ingestion)	Onset of liver injury (24-72 h after ingestion)	Maximum liver injury (72-96 h after ingestion)	Recovery period (4-10 d after ingestion)
Nonspecific symptoms: anorexia, nausea, vomiting, malaise, diaphoresis, anxiety; may be asymptomatic	Nausea, vomiting, right upper quadrant and epigastric pain and tenderness, elevated liver enzymes	Anorexia, nausea, vomiting, peak liver enzyme abnormalities; fulminant liver failure (encephalopathy, coagulopathy, hypoglycemia, metabolic acidosis), renal failure, and death	Resolution of hepatic dysfunction

Table 57–2 • COMMON TOXIDROMES		
Toxidrome	Clinical Findings	Common Agents
Anticholinergic	Tachycardia, hyperthermia, dry skin and mucous membranes, delirium, urinary retention, mydriasis, flushed skin, absent bowel sounds	Antihistamines, phenothiazines, tricyclic antidepressants, scopolamine, Jimson weed, belladonna
Cholinergic	Salivation, lacrimation, urination, diarrhea, miosis, bradycardia, emesis	Organophosphate insecticides, pilocarpine, betel nuts
Opioid	Coma, respiratory depression, pinpoint pupils	Codeine, heroin, morphine, meperidine, hydrocodone
Sedative-hypnotic	Decreased level of consciousness, respiratory depression, hypotension, variable pupillary changes, hypothermia, seizures	Barbiturates, benzodiazepines
Sympathomimetic	Hypertension, tachycardia, mydriasis, hyperpyrexia, arrhythmias	Cocaine, methamphetamine, ephedrine, ecstasy

pregnancy test if appropriate). Because coingestion is common, a toxicology screen and salicylate level should be obtained. An ECG should be obtained to evaluate for dysrhythmias associated with other ingestants and electrolyte abnormalities. If the patient's mental status is altered, a computed tomography (CT) scan of the head is also recommended. However, the single best predictor of the risk of hepatotoxicity is a serum APAP level. This should be drawn 4 hours postingestion or immediately if the time of ingestion is unknown. Using the APAP level and the Rumack-Matthew nomogram, the clinician can then predict the severity of toxicity and determine the need for NAC therapy (Figure 57–1). The APAP level between 4 and 24 hours of ingestion is plotted; if the level falls above the lower line, known as the treatment line, NAC should be initiated. This nomogram is not applicable for chronic ingestions, delayed ingestions, unknown time or duration of ingestion, extended release APAP, or coingestions.

Treatment

Initial treatment of the patient with an APAP overdose consists of stabilizing the ABCs, obtaining IV access, and placing the patient on cardiac and oxygen saturation monitors.

Gastric lavage is rarely necessary due to the rapid gastrointestinal absorption of APAP. Activated charcoal can reduce gastric absorption of the drug but may also adsorb oral NAC. Thus, if activated charcoal is given, separating the first dose of NAC and activated charcoal by 1-2 hours may be preferable. Activated charcoal is recommended in patients who present within 4 hours of a known or suspected APAP ingestion. Activated charcoal should not be given in patients who have altered mental status, are sedated or are otherwise unable to protect their airway secondary to a risk of aspiration.

NAC, the antidote for APAP toxicity, acts by replenishing glutathione stores and combining with NAPQI as a glutathione substitute. It is most effective when

Table 57–3 • COMMON ANTIDOTES: DOSES AND INDICATIONS

Antidote	Pediatric	Adult	Poison
N-acetylcysteine	140 mg/kg PO, then 70 mg/kg PO q4h for 18 total doses OR 150 mg/kg IV over 15 min-1 h, then 50 mg/kg IV over 4 h, then 100 mg/kg over 16 h		Acetaminophen
Activated charcoal	1 g/kg PO		Most ingested poisons
Crotalidae polyvalent immune Fab	4-6 vials IV initially over 1 h; may be repeated 2 vials every 6 h for 18 h	Same as pediatric dose	Envenomation by Crotalidae
Calcium gluconate 10% (9 mg/mL elemental calcium)	0.2-0.25 mL/kg IV	10 mL IV	Hypermagnesemia, hypocalcemia (ethylene glycol, hydrofluoric acid), calcium-channel antagonists, black widow spider venom
Calcium chloride 10% (27.2 mg/mL elemental calcium)	0.6-0.8 mL/kg IV	10-30 mL IV	
Cyanide antidote kit			
Amyl nitrate	Not typically used	1 ampule in oxygen chamber of ambu-bag 30 sec on/30 sec off	Cyanide poisoning
Sodium nitrite (3% solution)	0.33 mL/kg IV	10 mL	Hydrogen sulfide (use only sodium nitrite)
Thiosulfate (25% solution)	1.65 mL/kg IV	50 mL IV	
Deferoxamine	Initial dose: 20 mg/kg IM/IV (15 mg/kg/h IV); 1 g max	Initial dose: 1 g IM/IV (15 g/kg/h IV); 6 g/d max	Iron
Dextrose	0.5 g/kg IV	1 g/kg IV	Hypoglycemia
Digoxin immune Fab	(Empiric)	(Empiric)	
Acute	10-20 vials IV	10-20 vials IV	Digoxin and cardiac glycosides
Chronic	1-2 vials IV	4-6 vials IV	
Ethanol 10% for IV administration	10 mL/kg over 30 min, then 1.2 mL/kg/h[a]	Ethylene glycol, methanol	
Folic acid/leucovorin	1-2 mg/kg q4-6h IV	Methotrexate (only leucovorin)	
Fomepizole	15 mg/kg IV, then 10 mg/kg q12h	Methanol, ethylene glycol, disulfiram	
Flumazenil	0.01 mg/kg IV	0.2 mg IV	Benzodiazepines
Glucagon	50-150 µg/kg IV	3-10 mg IV	Calcium channel blocker, β-blocker
Hydroxycobalamin (may be used with sodium thiosulfate)	70 mg/kg IV over 30 min (5 g max)	5 g IV over 30 min	Cyanide, nitroprusside

(Continued)

Table 57–3 • COMMON ANTIDOTES: DOSES AND INDICATIONS (CONTINUED)

Antidote	Pediatric	Adult	Poison
IV lipid emulsion 20%	1.5 mL/kg IV over 1 min (may repeat × 2), then 0.25 mL/kg/min IV	100 mL IV over 1 min, then 400 mL IV over 20 min	Calcium channel blocker, β-blocker (rescue therapy)
Methylene blue	1-2 mg/kg IV Neonates: 0.3-1 mg/kg	1-2 mg/kg IV	Oxidizing chemicals (eg, nitrites, benzocaine, sulfonamides)
Octreotide	1 µg/kg SC q6h	5-100 µg SC q6h	Refractory hypoglycemia after oral hypoglycemic agent ingestion
Naloxone	As much as is needed. Typical starting dose 0.01 mg/kg IV	As much as is needed. Typical starting dose 0.4-2 mg IV	Opioid, clonidine
Physostigmine	0.02 mg/kg IV	0.5-2 mg IV	Anticholinergic substances (not cyclic antidepressants)
Pralidoxime (2-PAM)	20-40 mg/kg IV, then 20 mg/kg/h	1-2 g IV, then 500 mg/h	Cholinergic substances
Protamine	1 mg neutralizes 100 U of unfractionated heparin; administered over 15 min		Heparin
	0.6 mg/kg IV (empiric)	25-50 mg IV (empiric)	
Pyridoxine	Gram for gram of ingestion if amount of isoniazid is known		Isoniazid, Gyromitra esculenta, hydrazine
	70 mg/kg IV (5 g max)	5 g IV	
Sodium bicarbonate	1-2 mEq/kg IV bolus then 2 mEq/kg/h IV		Sodium channel blockers, alkalinization of urine or serum
Thiamine	5-10 mg IV	100 mg IV	Wernicke syndrome, "wet" beri-beri
Vitamin K₁	1-5 mg/d PO	20 mg/d PO	Anticoagulants (eg, warfarin)

^aThis is an approximation. Doses should be titrated to ethanol level of 100-150 mg/dL.
Reproduced, with permission, from Tintinalli JE, Kelen GD, Stapczynski JS, eds. Emergency Medicine. 6th ed. New York, NY: McGraw-Hill; 2004:1017.

given within 8 hours of ingestion. The indications for NAC include a toxic level as determined using the Rumack-Matthew nomogram or evidence of hepatic failure. NAC can be empirically started if a toxic APAP ingestion is suspected and an APAP level will not be available within 8 hours of the ingestion; NAC can then be discontinued if the APAP level is nontoxic and the patient is asymptomatic. Any patient who requires NAC treatment should be admitted to the hospital. Although the nomogram is not applicable for ingestions greater than 24 hours prior to ED arrival, NAC therapy may still be helpful.

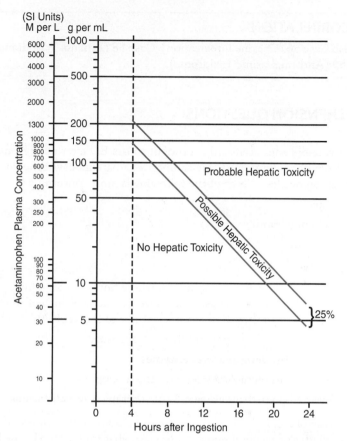

Figure 57–1. Acetaminophen toxicity nomogram based on serum acetaminophen concentration versus time after ingestion.

The standard 72-hour NAC regimen is an oral loading dose of 140 mg/kg, followed by maintenance doses of 70 mg/kg every 4 hours for 17 additional doses. Because of its acrid smell and taste, oral NAC often induces nausea and vomiting. Dilution in fruit juice or a chilled drink and the administration of antiemetics can be helpful.

If the patient has intractable vomiting, altered mental status, or fulminant hepatic failure, intravenous NAC may be indicated (150 mg/kg loading dose, followed by 50 mg/kg over 4 hours, followed by 100 mg/kg over 16 hours). Patients receiving intravenous NAC should be closely observed, as rate-related anaphylactoid reactions can occur.

A small fraction of patients will develop fulminant hepatic failure, which is associated with a 60% to 80% mortality rate. Most deaths associated with liver failure occur 3-5 days postingestion and are attributed to cerebral edema, sepsis, hemorrhage, multiorgan failure, or acute respiratory distress syndrome.

> ## CASE CORRELATION
>
> - See also Case 56 (Cocaine Intoxication), Case 58 (Ethanol Withdrawal), and Case 59 (Anti-muscarinic Toxidrome).

COMPREHENSION QUESTIONS

57.1 A 16-year-old adolescent girl is brought to the ED after taking a number of pills from her parents' medicine cabinet. The parents have brought in all the medication bottles. Which of the following is most concerning for toxicity?

A. Ampicillin

B. Diphenhydramine

C. Fluoxetine

D. Theophylline

57.2 A 34-year-old man admits taking "the whole bottle" of acetaminophen over the course of 36 hours because of a severe headache. Which of the following is the best guide to determine whether or not to initiate NAC therapy?

A. Initiate NAC due to potentially toxic exposure

B. Serum APAP level and liver enzymes

C. Plotting the serum APAP level on the nomogram

D. If over 24 hours have elapsed, NAC therapy is not efficacious

57.3 A 25-year-old man is brought into the ED 1 hour after a witnessed overdose of 20-25 pills of acetaminophen tablets. At what time would be the best time to draw the APAP level?

A. As soon as the patient arrives in the ED

B. At 2 hours postingestion

C. At 4 hours postingestion

D. At 8 hours postingestion

57.4 A 38-year-old school teacher took a "large number of Tylenol tablets" and is found to have an APAP level of 200 µg/mL. The estimated time postingestion is 8 hours. The first dose of NAC is given. Which of the following is the next step to guide therapy?

A. Check APAP level 4 hours after the first NAC dose, and if it is below the toxicity line, no further NAC is needed.

B. Check the APAP level 12 hours after the first NAC dose, and if it is below the toxicity line, no further NAC is needed.

C. Check the APAP level and liver function tests at 8 hours after the first NAC dose, and if it is in the normal/nontoxic range, then no further NAC is needed.

D. Give the entire course of NAC, and no further APAP levels are necessary.

Match the following antidotes (A to H) to the clinical situations (Questions 57.5 to 57.8):

    A. Calcium gluconate

    B. Deferoxamine

    C. Digoxin Fab

    D. Glucagon

    E. N-acetylcysteine

    F. Naloxone

    G. Physostigmine

    H. Vitamin K

57.5 A 45-year-old man takes too many of his antihypertensive pills and is noted to have a heart rate of 40 beats per minute.

57.6 A 22-year-old pregnant woman with preeclampsia receiving intravenous medication to prevent seizures develops weakness and difficulty breathing.

57.7 A 24-year-old man is brought into the ED with somnolence, pinpoint pupils, and track marks on his arm.

57.8 A 56-year-old woman taking tablets to "thin her blood" is noted to be bleeding from her gums and has multiple bruises on her arms and legs.

57.9 A 37-year old man presents with an acetaminophen overdose. He has also taken a large number of benzodiazepines and is lethargic. Which of the following is the best next step in treatment?

    A. Activated charcoal

    B. Gastric lavage

    C. N-acetylcysteine therapy IV

    D. N-acetylcysteine therapy orally

ANSWERS

57.1 **D.** Theophylline has a very narrow therapeutic index, with toxic effects of tachycardia, nausea, vomiting, and seizures. It is a methylxanthine medication used in asthma and COPD, and pharmacologically has similarities to caffeine. Activated charcoal and whole bowel irrigation should be considered. Seizures due to theophylline toxicity is best treated by lorazepam.

57.2 **A.** At 24 hours postingestion, NAC therapy may still be useful. Due to the historically toxic exposure, NAC should be started while a serum APAP level and liver enzymes are checked. If the APAP level is undetectable and the liver enzymes are normal, subsequent doses of NAC can be discontinued. The Rumack-Matthew nomogram is not applicable for ingestions more than 24 hours prior to evaluation.

57.3 **C.** A serum APAP should be drawn 4 hours postingestion; the nomogram has relevance between 4 hours and 24 hours postingestion. The value at 4 hours can provide guidance regarding the aggressiveness of treatment.

57.4 **D.** Once it is determined by the nomogram that the APAP dose is potentially toxic, the entire NAC regimen is given. No further APAP levels need to be drawn.

57.5 **D.** Glucagon is effective in treating calcium-channel blocker or beta-blocker overdose, which are the most likely medications causing a bradycardia. Glucagon stimulates cAMP synthesis independent of the beta-adrenergic receptor, enabling calcium to enter intracellularly. Patients with symptomatic bradycardia needing immediate therapy benefit from atropine or in dire circumstances, transcutaneous pacing.

57.6 **A.** This patient is likely receiving magnesium sulfate for seizure prophylaxis, and the antidote for hypermagnesemia is calcium gluconate.

57.7 **F.** Naloxone is the treatment of choice for opiate overdose. This individual likely is a heroin abuser based on the pinpoint pupils and the track marks suggestive IV drug use. Naloxone is available IV, IM, or intranasal.

57.8 **H.** This patient likely has warfarin overdose, which is treated by vitamin K. Life-threatening bleeding can be addressed with transfusion with clotting factors.

57.9 **C.** IV NAC is indicated because the patient has altered mental status. Activated charcoal may be given through a nasogastric tube if the patient is intubated.

CLINICAL PEARLS

▶ Because the devastating effects of APAP toxicity may be delayed for 24-72 hours and antidotal therapy is most effective if started within 8 hours of ingestion, the clinician must have a high level of suspicion of APAP toxicity in any poisoned patient.

▶ APAP toxicity is caused by the formation of a toxic metabolite, *N*-acetyl-*p*-benzoquinoneimine (NAPQI).

▶ *N*-acetylcysteine (NAC) is the antidote for APAP toxicity and should be given if a toxic ingestion is suspected (based on ingested dose or APAP level and Rumack-Matthew nomogram). It is most effective if given within 8 hours of ingestion.

▶ The priorities when dealing with a patient with an APAP overdose are to perform a rapid assessment, stabilize the ABCs, decontaminate, minimize absorption, and administer NAC if appropriate.

▶ In general, an APAP level should be drawn on any patient with an overdose history, even when APAP ingestion is denied.

REFERENCES

Aghababian RV, Bird SB, Braen GR, et al, eds. *Essentials of Emergency Medicine.* Sudbury, MA: Jones and Bartlett Learning; 2011.

Marx JA, Hockberger RS, Walls RM, eds. *Rosen's Emergency Medicine: Concepts and Clinical Practice.* 8th ed. Philadelphia, PA: Saunders; 2014.

Schaider JJ, Barkin RM, Hayden SR, Wolfe R, et al, eds. *Rosen and Barkin's 5-Minute Emergency Medicine Consult.* 4th ed. Philadelphia, PA: Lippincott Williams & Wilkins; 2011.

Tintinalli JE, Stapczynski JS, Ma OJ, et al, eds. *Emergency Medicine: A Comprehensive Study Guide.* 8th ed. New York, NY: McGraw-Hill; 2016.

Wolf SJ, Heard KH, Sloan EP, Jagoda AS. Clinical policy: critical issues in the management of patients presenting to the emergency department with acetaminophen overdose. *Ann Emerg Med.* 2007;50:292-313.

A 50-year-old man presents to the emergency department (ED) with anxiety, insomnia, and nausea. He denies having any hallucinations or seizures. He states that he had been drinking about a half bottle of hard liquor each day for years. After his wife threatened to divorce him and he was fired as a result of his alcoholism, he decided to stop drinking "cold turkey." His last alcohol intake was 2 days ago. He has a history of hypertension for which he takes hydrochlorothiazide. He does not smoke or use illicit drugs.

On examination, his temperature is 100.4°F, blood pressure is 175/95 mm Hg, heart rate is 120 beats per minute, and respiratory rate is 24 breaths per minute. He is tremulous, diaphoretic, and appears mildly dehydrated with dry mucous membranes. The lungs are clear to auscultation, and he is tachycardic with normal heart sounds. He is alert and oriented and does not have any focal neurologic deficits except for bilateral distal sensory loss in the hands and feet (in a stocking-glove distribution).

▶ What are the potential complications in this patient?
▶ What is the best treatment for this patient?

ANSWERS TO CASE 58:

Ethanol Withdrawal

Summary: This is a 50-year-old man with acute alcohol withdrawal as evidenced by his anxiousness, tremor, and signs of autonomic hyperactivity (hyperthermia, hypertension, tachycardia, tachypnea, and diaphoresis). He does not currently exhibit the more serious signs of alcohol withdrawal, such as seizures, hallucinations, or delirium.

- **Potential complications:** Seizures, hallucinations (auditory, visual, or tactile), delirium (delirium tremens [DTs]).

- **Treatment:** Intravenous (IV) fluids, repletion of electrolytes as needed, benzodiazepines to control symptoms and prevent more serious manifestations of withdrawal (listed above).

ANALYSIS

Objectives

1. Recognize the clinical signs and symptoms of ethanol withdrawal (including seizures, hallucinations, and delirium).

2. Understand the evaluation and treatment of patients with ethanol withdrawal.

Considerations

Because ethanol abuse is prevalent, emergency physicians should be prepared to treat patients who present with alcohol withdrawal. Symptoms may range from mild anxiety, nausea or vomiting, insomnia, and tremor to hallucinations, seizures, and delirium. Mild cases of withdrawal may be treated with oral benzodiazepines; however, patients with more serious symptomatology may require large doses of IV benzodiazepines, IV hydration, repletion of electrolytes, and hospital admission.

APPROACH TO:

Ethanol Withdrawal

CLINICAL APPROACH

Among patients presenting to the ED for any complaint, the prevalence of alcoholism or inappropriate drinking is estimated to be between 8% and 40%. Some patients arrive at the ED due to a desire to stop drinking, while others have already stopped their alcohol intake and require treatment of the symptoms of withdrawal. In addition, alcohol-dependent patients with prolonged ED stays may be unable to maintain their usual ethanol intake and begin to manifest withdrawal symptoms. As such, emergency physicians must be prepared to treat this syndrome.

Because ethanol has a depressant effect on the central nervous system (CNS), withdrawal leads to CNS excitation. Symptoms may range from mild anxiety, nausea or vomiting, insomnia, and tremor to agitation, hallucinations, seizures, and delirium. Patients often manifest signs of **autonomic hyperactivity** (hyperthermia, hypertension, tachycardia, tachypnea, diaphoresis, and hyperreflexia). Withdrawal may occur as soon as the blood alcohol level starts to decline following an abrupt change in alcohol intake. Minor withdrawal tends to begin early, peaking at 24-36 hours, while major withdrawal usually occurs after 24 hours and peaking after 48 hours.

Alcohol withdrawal hallucinations may be auditory, visual, or tactile, although auditory hallucinations are most common. Alcohol withdrawal seizures are tonic-clonic (generalized) and may occur once or multiple times. Up to one-third of these patients progress to delirium tremens, the most severe form of alcohol withdrawal. It is characterized by fluctuating levels of consciousness, cognitive disturbances, profound confusion, and severe autonomic hyperactivity. With aggressive treatment, the mortality of DTs is currently about 5%.

The differential diagnosis of alcohol withdrawal is broad and includes infection (eg, meningitis and encephalitis), other seizure disorders (eg, epilepsy), endocrine disorders (eg, thyrotoxicosis or thyroid storm), trauma (eg, intracranial hemorrhage), metabolic abnormalities (eg, hypoglycemia), psychiatric disorders (eg, schizophrenia), drug intoxication (eg, sympathomimetics and antihistamines), and other types of withdrawal syndromes (eg, benzodiazepines). Benzodiazepines are widely used as anxiolytics, sleep aids, anticonvulsants, and muscle relaxants. **Because benzodiazepines are also CNS depressants, withdrawal from these agents may be clinically indistinguishable from alcohol withdrawal.** A history of prolonged or high dose benzodiazepine use may help differentiate between the two. Abrupt discontinuation of short-acting benzodiazepines may cause symptoms after 2-3 days, while withdrawal from long-acting agents may present up to 7 days after cessation.

Important patient history includes current symptomatology, daily alcohol intake, timing of last alcohol intake, comorbidities, and any other medication or other drug use. The initial evaluation of the patient should include the assessment (and stabilization if necessary) of the ABCs. A complete set of vital signs is necessary in order to identify any autonomic hyperactivity. The patient should be examined from head to toe, looking for evidence of alternative etiologies for the patient symptoms (eg, signs of trauma associated with intracranial hemorrhage, nuchal rigidity with meningitis, thyromegaly with thyrotoxicosis, etc). In addition, a thorough neurologic examination should be performed to identify any abnormality in level of consciousness or mental status as well as any focal deficits.

Diagnostic studies are largely useful in ruling out alternative diagnoses and concomitant medical conditions. Patients with mild alcohol withdrawal may not require any laboratory studies or imaging. Those with severe withdrawal may require a more extensive workup, including any or all of the following: complete blood count, electrolytes, renal function tests, glucose, liver enzymes, blood gas, thyroid function studies, cardiac enzymes, urinalysis, urine drug screen, ECG, chest x-ray, computed tomography of the head, and/or lumbar puncture.

Treatment

Treatment of alcohol withdrawal serves several purposes, including symptomatic relief and calming of the patient to allow an adequate evaluation and prevention of progression of symptoms. **The mainstay of treatment is benzodiazepines, most commonly chlordiazepoxide, diazepam, or lorazepam.** These medications are titrated to control the patient's agitation, and high dose or continuous infusion may be required. Neuroleptics such as haloperidol or ziprasidone may be considered for patients who do not respond adequately to benzodiazepines. In addition, a continuous propofol infusion may be beneficial in intubated patients with severe withdrawal who are refractory to high-dose benzodiazepines. The alpha-agonist clonidine may be a useful adjunct to counteract the autonomic hyperactivity associated with alcohol withdrawal. **Beta-blockers may also help control tachycardia and hypertension;** however, they may mask some of the earlier signs of impending DTs. Depending on the patient's fluid and nutrition status, IV hydration and repletion of electrolytes (eg, potassium, magnesium, and phosphorus) may be needed. These patients are often at risk of hypoglycemia if they have not had sufficient nutritional intake. Malnourished patients should also be given thiamine and folate replacement.

The disposition of patients with alcohol withdrawal depends on the severity of symptoms, response to treatment, and availability of outpatient support. If the patient responds well to therapy in the ED, he/she may be discharged with an oral benzodiazepine taper, abstinence from alcohol, and participation in a rehabilitation program. Patients who require high doses of benzodiazepines, have more severe symptoms or DTs, or have comorbid diagnoses requiring hospitalization should be admitted.

CASE CORRELATION

- See also Case 56 (Cocaine Intoxication), Case 57 (Acetaminophen Toxicity), and Case 59 (Anti-muscarinic Toxicity).

COMPREHENSION QUESTIONS

58.1 A 25-year-old woman has been taking clonazepam every day for 3 years for generalized anxiety disorder. She is in town on vacation but forgot her medication at home. When is she most likely to start showing symptoms of withdrawal?

    A. 12 hours

    B. 2 days

    C. 6 days

    D. 10 days

58.2 A 50-year-old man is admitted for a femur fracture following a motor vehicle collision. Two days after admission, he becomes very agitated, tremulous, diaphoretic, tachycardic, and hypertensive. Which of the following is the neurotransmitter receptor governing the substance withdrawal?

    A. GABA

    B. Acetylcholine

    C. Norepinephrine

    D. Serotonin

58.3 A 60-year-old homeless man presents to the ED with acute alcohol withdrawal. He has been given 2 mg of lorazepam IV but still appears very agitated and anxious. What is the most appropriate next step?

    A. Clonidine 0.2 mg PO

    B. Haloperidol 5 mg IV

    C. Lorazepam 2 mg IV

    D. Propanolol 100 mg PO

ANSWERS

58.1 **C. Clonazepam is a long-acting benzodiazepine.** Abrupt discontinuance of short-acting benzodiazepines may be symptomatic after 2-3 days, while withdrawal from long-acting agents may present up to 7 days after cessation. Treatment of benzodiazepine withdrawal involves reinstitution of a benzodiazepine followed by a gradual taper.

58.2 **A.** The agitation, tremor, and autonomic hyperactivity point toward alcohol withdrawal. Both alcohol and benzodiazepines activate the inhibitory GABA-A receptor, producing increased GABA inhibition. During withdrawal from alcohol or benzodiazepines, the loss of GABA-A receptor stimulation occurs, leading to the withdrawal signs and symptoms. All patients admitted to the hospital for medical or traumatic conditions should be asked about drug and alcohol use. After admission, they may not have access to the drugs and/or alcohol they regularly use and may present with withdrawal syndromes.

58.3 **C.** While all are appropriate treatments for alcohol withdrawal, benzodiazepine dosing is tapered to the patient agitation. It may be re-dosed at 10-30 minute intervals for patients in severe withdrawal. Very high doses may be required, especially if the patient has DTs.

CLINICAL PEARLS

▶ Alcohol is a CNS depressant. Withdrawal leads to CNS stimulation and autonomic hyperactivity.

▶ The differential diagnosis of alcohol withdrawal includes infections, other seizure disorders, endocrine disorders, trauma, metabolic abnormalities, psychiatric disorders, drug intoxications, and other types of withdrawal syndromes.

▶ The mainstay of treatment for alcohol withdrawal is benzodiazepines.

REFERENCES

Kelly JF, Renner JA. Alcohol-related disorders. In: Stern TA, Rosenbaum JF, Fava M, Biederman J, Rauch SL, eds. *Stern: Massachusetts General Hospital Comprehensive Clinical Psychiatry*. 1st ed. Philadelphia, PA: Mosby Elsevier; 2006:2858-2882.

Kosten TR, O'Connor PG. Management of drug and alcohol withdrawal. *N Engl J Med*. 2003; 348(18):1786-1795.

Marx JA, Hockberger RS, Walls RM, eds. *Rosen's Emergency Medicine: Concepts and Clinical Practice*. 8th ed. Philadelphia, PA: Saunders; 2014.

Tintinalli JE, Stapczynski JS, Ma OJ, et al, eds. *Emergency Medicine: A Comprehensive Study Guide*. 8th ed. New York, NY: McGraw-Hill; 2016.

An 18-year-old man presents to the emergency department (ED) agitated, confused and hallucinating. The patient's friends state that the group was walking around in the woods looking for some "weeds to smoke" in order to get "high." The patient was first to smoke one of the weeds and subsequently became agitated. His friends decided to bring him to the ED for evaluation. On arrival to the ED, the patient's vital signs are blood pressure 180/100 mm Hg, heart rate 120 beats per minute, respiratory rate 18 breaths per minute, temperature 101°F, and pulse oximetry 98% on room air. On physical examination, his pupils are 6 mm, skin is erythematous and warm to the touch, axillae are dry, abdomen has decreased bowel sounds, and the patient is grabbing at things that are not there.

▶ What is the most likely diagnosis?
▶ What is the next step in treatment?

ANSWERS TO CASE 59:

Anti-Muscarinic Toxidrome

Summary: This is a case of an unknown plant ingestion in a patient who presents with several signs of toxicity. The key features of this case include recognizing signs and symptoms of a toxidrome and knowing how to stabilize and manage poisoned patients. The patient presents with anti-muscarinic toxicity after smoking jimson weed, which contains belladonna alkaloids. These alkaloids possess strong anti-muscarinic properties.

- **Most likely diagnosis:** Jimson weed (anti-muscarinic) toxicity.

- **Best initial treatment:** Benzodiazepines and possibly physostigmine.

ANALYSIS

Objectives

1. Develop an initial approach to the poisoned patient.

2. Learn the five basic classes of toxidromes.

3. Understand how to classify a patient into a toxidrome.

4. Understand the initial steps for stabilization of a symptomatic overdose.

5. Review the basic treatment for each of the toxidromes.

Considerations

This patient has several classic features of an anti-muscarinic toxidrome. The primary treatment efforts for the poisoned patient are the same as any other patient: maintenance and stabilization of the airway, breathing, and circulation (ABCs) systems. For **any intentional overdose, levels of acetaminophen and salicylate levels should be checked** due to their ubiquity in medications and great potential for morbidity and mortality.

In this case, the patient is febrile. Fever in the setting of a toxicologic problem is a predictor of increased morbidity and mortality. The cause of the fever is usually secondary to increased muscle activity. Initial treatment should include administration of benzodiazepines (eg, diazepam and lorazepam) and intravenous fluids for hydration.

In general, symptomatic poisoned patients require hospital admission for continued monitoring. However, the majority does well with simple supportive care.

The local poison control center should be contacted early in the workup of all symptomatic overdoses. This is critical both for epidemiologic purposes as well as for management of complex patients and continuity of care. The national phone number for the nearest **poison control center is 1-800-222-1222.**

APPROACH TO:
Toxidromes

DEFINITIONS

TOXIDROME: A clinical syndrome that is essential for the successful recognition of poisoning patterns. A toxidrome is the constellation of signs and symptoms that suggests a specific class of poisoning.

DECONTAMINATION: Prevention of the continued absorption of a toxicant.

DRUG ABSORPTION: The movement of drug from its site of administration into the bloodstream.

ADSORPTION: The binding of a chemical (eg, drug or poison) to a solid material, such as activated charcoal.

ANTIDOTE: A remedy to counteract a poison or injury.

OPIATE: A compound found in opium poppies (eg, morphine, codeine, thebane, etc) that binds to the opiate receptor.

OPIOID: A synthetic (eg, fentanyl, methadone, tramadol, etc) or semi-synthetic (eg, heroin, oxycodone, hydrocodone, etc) compound that binds to the opiate receptor.

BODY PACKER: An individual who ingests wrapped packets of illicit drugs such as cocaine, heroin, amphetamines, ecstasy, marijuana, or hashish to transport them.

BODY STUFFER: Someone who admits to or is strongly suspected of ingesting illegal drugs in order to escape detection by authorities, and not for recreational purposes or to transport the drug across borders. Cocaine is the drug most commonly involved in the body stuffer syndrome.

CLINICAL APPROACH

General Overdose Management

Airway and Breathing The general approach to the overdose patient is to start with an initial assessment that includes evaluation of the patient **ABCs**. The most easily correctable cause of toxicologic death is airway support. Sedated patients may have a partially obstructed airway due to a relaxed tongue. In addition, obtunded patients may lose their gag reflex. Understand also that breathing consists of both oxygenation and ventilation. A hypoxic patient with a suspected overdose and no history of known medical problems is also at risk for poor ventilation. Masking this hypoventilation and hypoxia by applying supplemental oxygen may actually decrease the patient intrinsic respiratory drive and lead to further hypoventilation. **Definitive airway management includes endotracheal or nasotracheal intubation.**

Circulation Toxidromes can lead to both extreme hypertension and hypotension. Extreme hypertension (sympathomimetics) may require the use of a direct alpha$_1$-receptor antagonist, such as phentermine. Hypotension should first be treated with intravenous fluids. Other agents such as vasopressors (norepinephrine and dopamine) may be required. Often, cardiac function is also affected in toxidromes. Tachy- and bradydysrhythmias are both common. Treatment depends on the underlying etiology of the dysrhythmia.

Decontamination In addition to the ABCs, it is also essential to consider **decontamination** and **elimination** (or ABCDE) in the management of a poisoned patient. Decontamination involves preventing further absorption into the system. For topical contaminations, removing the patient's clothing, as well as washing off the affected area, may be all that is required. Another way of preventing absorption into the system is the administration of activated charcoal. **Activated charcoal** comes in two forms: with and without sorbitol. Sorbitol is thought to facilitate the movement of activated charcoal through the gastrointestinal (GI) tract. It is, however, a GI irritant, and more than one dose of activated charcoal with sorbitol is not recommended. Patients who have the greatest benefit from activated charcoal include those who present early in their ingestion (<1 hour), are awake and can drink the activated charcoal without risk of aspiration, and whose ingested chemicals are well absorbed by activated charcoal.

One main concern with the administration of activated charcoal is the potential for aspiration and subsequent charcoal pneumonitis. This risk can be decreased by administering activated charcoal only to patients who are awake and protecting their airway. In addition to this complication, activated charcoal poorly adsorbs certain chemicals (Table 59–1), and therefore has little benefit in these ingestions. Moreover, patients with caustic injuries often undergo endoscopy. Prior administration of activated charcoal may complicate the procedure.

Another method of decontamination is **gastric lavage**. This is accomplished by inserting a large oral gastric tube (eg, 40 French) into the stomach for the rapid administration and removal of large volumes (several liters) of fluid in an attempt to try to remove whole pills before they are dissolved and absorbed. One potential adverse effect is lavaging the lungs instead of the stomach. This can be avoided by intubating the patient prior to lavage. In addition, given the increasing number of bariatric surgery patients, a complication can occur if the tube gets stuck in the gastric band or causes gastric perforation. Given the large number of treatment options that are available for a wide variety of ingestions, gastric lavage should only be performed on patients who present early (<1 hour) and have a potentially life-threatening ingestion for which there are limited treatment options. This technique

Table 59–1 • POORLY ADSORBED COMPOUNDS BY ACTIVATED CHARCOAL
Ethanol
Methanol
Isopropyl alcohol
Ethylene glycol
Hydrocarbons
Caustics (acid and base)
Lithium and other salts

is not to be confused with nasogastric lavage (the administration and subsequent removal of fluid from an NG tube), which has **not** been shown to substantially alter the course of *any* substantially poisoned patient and usually ends at just removing some of the excipients (starches, waxes, and binding agents).

Another method of decontamination is **whole bowel irrigation.** In this method, a large amount of polyethylene glycol-electrolyte lavage solution (PEG-ELS) is administered through an NG tube at a rate of approximately 1 L an hour. The goal of this therapy is to push whole pills through the GI tract to prevent absorption. This method is especially helpful in treatment of body packers and body stuffers and in cases of sustained release medications.

Elimination   Once the drug is absorbed into the body, there are options that may help to increase elimination from the body. These options include multidose charcoal, hemodialysis, charcoal hemoperfusion, and urinary alkalinization. **Multidose charcoal** has been shown to be effective with certain drugs, namely dapsone, carbamazepine, phenobarbital, quinine, and theophylline. While the first dose of charcoal with these patients can be given with sorbitol, subsequent doses should not contain sorbitol, as it is a GI irritant and can lead to dehydration and GI upset.

Hemodialysis is effective for certain drugs that have a **low volume of distribution** (ie, water soluble) and may be used if there is no better antidote or if the patient is critically ill. Examples of these drugs include lithium, methanol, and aspirin. Acetaminophen technically is also amenable to dialysis, but there is a noninvasive antidote that is more commonly used.

Charcoal hemoperfusion is similar to arterial venous hemodialysis, except that the drug is passed through a charcoal filter prior to systemic return. This is particularly effective in phenobarbital and theophylline overdoses, as they adsorb well to charcoal.

Urinary alkalinization is a treatment regimen that increases poison elimination by the administration of intravenous sodium bicarbonate to produce urine with a pH >7.5. Alkaline urine facilitates ion trapping and excretion. This method is particularly useful for aspirin and phenobarbital toxicities.

Supplemental Testing

For any intentional overdose, an acetaminophen and salicylate level should be obtained. These medications are readily accessible and carry a high morbidity and mortality while being fairly easy to treat if caught early.

For **acetaminophen**, if the time of ingestion is known and it is a single acute ingestion, use of the **Rumack-Matthew nomogram** for acetaminophen toxicity can determine if the patient requires treatment. If the time of ingestion is unknown and any detectable acetaminophen level is found, then strong consideration should be given toward treatment. Consideration should also be made with unexplained elevations in transaminases.

For **salicylates**, levels above 30 mg/dL should be treated with bicarbonate infusion and potassium supplementation to increase urinary elimination (prevent reabsorption). Certain patients may require dialysis. These include but are not limited to salicylate-induced pulmonary edema, salicylate-induced encephalopathy, severe acidosis, and levels greater than 80 mg/dL in the correct clinical setting.

Twelve-lead ECG may be helpful in early identification of **sodium channel blocking drugs** (eg, tricyclic antidepressants, diphenhydramine, and various other antidepressants and antipsychotics). Sodium channel blockade is manifested by a prolonged QRS complex. The first manifestation of this may be in lead aVR, where it is possible to see an R-R-prime pattern and slurring of the terminal 30 msec of the QRS complex. Administering intravenous sodium bicarbonate until the QRS complex narrows helps treat this condition.

Patients with a wide QRS may also have QT prolongation. One should be careful to distinguish QRS prolongation from QT prolongation. Drugs that affect potassium efflux or influx or drugs that affect calcium influx will also cause QT prolongation. Treatment with sodium bicarbonate for a prolonged QRS can worsen a prolonged QT interval by pushing potassium into cells, which may lead to torsade de pointes.

Routine urine drug screen testing is not necessary for treatment of an acute overdose. Most urine drug screen testing is an immunoassay that tests for the presence of drug metabolites and are tailored to a specific core molecule. They do not necessarily detect the presence of the active compound, and they do not tell you if the patient is under the effects of that particular compound. There are many false positives and false negatives in any given class of drugs tested on the urine drug screen. Treatment of an overdose should not wait until the return of the urine drug screen.

Toxidromes

Sedative Hypnotic This is a large class of drugs that includes alcohols, benzodiazepines, barbiturates, chloral hydrate, propofol, carisoprodol, and many others. In general, the sedative hypnotic toxidrome is characterized by relatively **normal vital signs** (Table 59–2) and a relatively normal examination, except for a markedly **decreased level of consciousness**. The patient may be hypothermic, but this would be due to environmental heat loss and loss of the shiver response. Treatment for this toxidrome is largely **support of airway and breathing**. In the undifferentiated sedative hypnotic patient, administration of **flumazenil, a benzodiazepine antagonist, is not indicated because it may precipitate a benzodiazepine-resistant seizure.**

Opioid/Opiate This class of drugs includes synthetics and semi-synthetics such as fentanyl and meperidine, as well as compounds found in nature and close derivatives such as morphine and codeine. These agonize the opiate receptors in the body. Agonism at these receptors induces **euphoria, analgesia, antidepressant effects, and sedation** as well as **respiratory depression, miosis, decreased GI motility, and dependence.**

Vital signs in these patients may demonstrate decreased respirations and a **low pulse oximetry**. In severe overdoses the patient may be hypotensive or bradycardic or both. On physical examination the pupils will be small **(miotic)**, **bowel sounds are decreased**, reflexes are decreased, and overall level of consciousness is decreased. Unless the patient has hypotension or bradycardia, the focus is maintaining ventilation and oxygenation. Treatment for hypoxia in the opiate or opioid overdose patient is either **naloxone** (Narcan) administration or **endotracheal intubation**. In the non-critically ill patient, the amount of naloxone administered should be based on the patient response. The goal of treatment is to get the patient breathing again,

Table 59–2 • PHYSICAL EXAMINATION CHARACTERISTICS SEEN IN TOXIDROMES					
	Sedative Hypnotic	Opiate	Sympathomimetic	Anti-Muscarinic	Cholinergic
Vital signs	+/− (usually relatively normal, maybe hypotensive, bradycardic in severe overdoses; sometimes hypothermic if prolonged exposure)	↓ (decreased respiratory rate and pulse oximetry, sometimes hypotensive or bradycardic, sometimes hypothermic if prolonged exposure)	↑ (febrile, tachycardic, hypertensive, tachypneic)	↑ (febrile, tachycardic, hypertensive, tachypneic)	↓ (bradycardic, sometimes tachypneic or bradypneic, sometimes hypotensive, sometimes hypoxic)
Bowel sounds	+/−	↓	↓	↓	↑
Skin moisture (axillae)	+/−	+/−	↑	↓	↑
CNS	↓	↓	↑	↑	↓
Treatment	Airway and breathing	Airway and breathing (consider naloxone)	Benzodiazepines	Benzodiazepines and consider physostigmine	Atropine and pralidoxime

not necessarily to make the patient awake and conversant. Naloxone administration should be avoided in an intubated patient with opiate or opioid overdose since this will lead to significant vomiting.

Sympathomimetic This class of drugs includes stimulants such as cocaine, ecstasy and methamphetamine, but it may also include therapeutic medications such as albuterol, pseudoephedrine, and many others. Their mechanisms of action may vary, but the end result is increased **stimulation of the α- and β-adrenergic receptors**. This alpha and beta stimulation results in **tachycardia, hypertension**, and **hyperthermia**. Physical examination often reveals dilated pupils (**mydriasis**), increased CNS activity (**hallucinations or seizures**), increased reflexes, and **diaphoretic skin**. This toxidrome can look very similar to the anti-muscarinic toxidrome but is usually distinguished by the presence of diaphoresis.

Mortality in these patients is typically from **hyperthermia**, so it is critical to **keep them cool**. Physically restraining a patient who is agitated or delirious without a sedative medication may lead to rhabdomyolysis and a dangerous increase in temperature. The mainstay in treatment includes the administration of benzodiazepines and intravenous fluids. If the patient is still agitated after receiving large doses of benzodiazepines, **consideration should be given to administering barbiturates or paralysis and intubation.**

Anti-Muscarinic There are a large variety of drugs that fall under the anti-muscarinic toxidrome. These may also be referred to as **anticholinergic drugs**, but very few medications have anti-nicotinic activity, and thus we should correctly refer to this as the anti-muscarinic toxidrome. Antagonism at the muscarinic receptors leads a physical examination that is **very similar to the sympathomimetic toxidrome**. The area in which the sympathomimetic toxidrome differs from the anti-muscarinic toxidrome is that the **anti-muscarinic toxidrome will have dry skin**, while the sympathomimetic toxidrome will have wet skin. Patients tend to be tachycardic, hypertensive, and febrile. On physical examination they will have mydriatic pupils, an altered level of consciousness (hallucinating or seizing), **urinary retention**, and decreased bowel sounds. There is a mnemonic for this toxidrome: mad as a hatter (hallucinations), dry as a bone (anhydrosis), red as a beet (increased agitation and fever), and blind as a bat (mydriasis).

Treatment of the anti-muscarinic toxidrome varies depending on the severity of effects and whether the effects are acting more peripherally (anhydrosis) or centrally (seizure, heart rate, and blood pressure). Peripheral anti-muscarinic toxicity can be treated with benzodiazepines. Central anti-muscarinic toxicity should also be treated with benzodiazepines and consideration should be given to a medication that increases levels of acetylcholine, such as **physostigmine**, an **acetylcholinesterase inhibitor.**

Cholinergic Cholinergic drugs are drugs that increase the level of acetylcholine. This is usually through inhibition of acetylcholinesterase. Examples of these medications include edrophonium and physostigmine. Other sources for cholinergic toxicity include **insecticides**, such as carbamates and organophosphates. Organophosphates are notable in that they have the potential to irreversibly bind and inhibit acetylcholinesterase—this process is called aging and is highly dependent upon the type of organophosphate, such that significant aging varies between 2 and 36 hours after initial binding.

Excess acetylcholine can cause effects at both muscarinic and nicotinic receptors, and its effects depend on the time course and severity of toxicity. Classically, it is associated with **bradycardia** and hypoxia secondary to either increased fluid in the lungs or diaphragmatic paralysis. Other findings on physical examination include **miotic pupils** (pinpoint), **hyperactive bowel sounds, and excessive secretions from the mouth, GI tract, and skin.**

The mnemonic SLUDGE (Salivation, Lacrimation, Urination, Defecation, GI upset, and Emesis) covers some but not all aspects of this toxidrome. It does not account for the bradycardia, bronchospasm, bronchorrhea, or miotic pupils that are noted on physical examination. An alternative mnemonic is **DUMBBELLS** (Defecation, Urination, Miosis, Bradycardia, Bronchorrhea/Bronchospasm, Emesis, Lacrimation, Lethargy, and Salivation).

Treatment involves the administration of anticholinergic medication such as **atropine** as well as **pralidoxime (2-PAM)**. Atropine should be administered to help **control bronchorrhea.** Pralidoxime should be administered to prevent binding and aging of the acetylcholinesterase in the case of organophosphate poisoning.

CASE CORRELATION

- See also Case 56 (Cocaine Intoxication), Case 57 (Acetaminophen Toxicity), and Case 58 (Ethanol Withdrawal).

COMPREHENSION QUESTIONS

59.1 A farmer presents to the ED with difficulty in breathing. His vitals are blood pressure 85/55 mm Hg, heart rate 50 beats per minute, temperature 97.8°F, respiratory rate 28 breaths per minute, and pulse oximetry 91% room air. His examination reveals wheezing; excessive perspiration, vomiting, tearing, and 1 mm pupils. Which is the best treatment for this patient toxicity?

    A. Benzodiazepines

    B. Physostigmine

    C. Pyridoxine

    D. Pralidoxime

    E. Naloxone

59.2 A teenager comes home after visiting his grandmother who is sick with cancer. His parents call 911 because he is minimally responsive. They find him with a blood pressure 90/60 mm Hg, heart rate 65 beats per minute, temperature 98.5°F, respiratory rate 6 breaths per minute, and pulse oximetry 89% on room air. His examination includes 2 mm pupils, decreased bowel sounds, hyporeflexia, and responsiveness only to noxious stimuli. The paramedics check his blood sugar, which is normal, and administer which of the following?

A. Charcoal

B. Naloxone

C. Flumazenil

D. Lorazepam

E. Atropine

59.3 A college student with a history rhinorrhea comes in after being found by her roommate with an altered mental status. Her vitals are blood pressure 160/90 mm Hg, heart rate 120 beats per minute, respiratory rate 18 breaths per minute, temperature 100.5°F, and pulse oximetry 100%. On examination she is picking at the air, has decreased bowel sounds, 6-mm pupils and no moisture in her axillae. Her blood sugar is normal. Which medication should they give her?

A. Atropine

B. Pralidoxime

C. Physostigmine

D. Flumazenil

E. Fomepizole

59.4 A 55-year-old homeless woman presents to the ED by ambulance. The police found her seizing in the street. Her vital signs are blood pressure 220/150 mm Hg, heart rate 140 beats per minute, temperature 101°F, respiratory rate 16 breaths per minute, and pulse oximetry 100% on room air. On examination she has 6 mm pupils, very wet skin, decreased bowel sounds and uncontrollable limb movements. A check of her blood sugar is normal. What medication should this patient be administered?

A. Physostigmine

B. Lorazepam

C. Labetalol

D. Atropine then pralidoxime

E. Phytonadione

ANSWERS

59.1 **D.** This patient is exhibiting a **cholinergic toxidrome.** The mnemonic for this is **DUMBBELLS** (**D**efecation, **U**rination, **M**iosis, **B**radycardia, **B**ronchorrhea, **E**mesis, **L**acrimation, **L**ethargy, and **S**alivation). The treatment is to prevent the patient from drowning in his or her own saliva by administering atropine 1 mg at a time until the secretions dry up. In addition, **pralidoxime (2-PAM)** is administered to increase acetylcholinesterase availability and reduce acetylcholine. Benzodiazepines would not help with this patient. Physostigmine is a treatment for anti-muscarinic toxicity and would worsen this patient condition. Pyridoxine is vitamin B6 and can be useful in treating seizures if they are caused by isoniazid (INH). Naloxone is an opiate antagonist and while this presentation has some overlap with the opiate toxidrome, this patient is tachypneic and has excessive secretions that are not seen in the opiate toxidrome. His exposure was from the **pesticides** on the farm.

59.2 **B.** This patient is exhibiting an **opiate toxidrome.** He has miotic pupils and decreased respirations, GI motility, and mental status. The treatment for this is patient should include **a trial of naloxone, enough to increase his oxygenation.** This patient likely stole opiate medication from his grandmother. Charcoal would not help this patient, as he is already severely symptomatic. Additionally, **charcoal would be contraindicated** in this patient because of the risk of aspiration. Flumazenil is a benzodiazepine antagonist. Lorazepam is a benzodiazepine. Atropine is a strong anti-muscarinic drug and would not be helpful in treating this patient.

59.3 **C.** This patient is exhibiting an **anti-muscarinic toxidrome.** This is characterized by **tachycardia, fever, hallucinosis, dilated pupils, hypoactive bowel sounds, and dry axillae.** The mnemonic is: **mad as a hatter (hallucinations), dry as a bone (anhydrosis), red as a beet (increased agitation and fever), and blind as a bat (mydriasis).** Treatment should be either decreasing the agitation and temperature through benzodiazepines or increasing acetylcholine by preventing its metabolism (physostigmine, an acetylcholinesterase inhibitor). Atropine is an anti-muscarinic drug and would worsen this patient toxidrome. Pralidoxime is a drug which makes acetylcholinesterase work again after exposure to an organophosphate. This patient does not have signs of cholinergic excess, so pralidoxime would not be helpful. Flumazenil should not be given to adult patients because, as an acting benzodiazepine antagonist, it may precipitate seizures that are not responsive to benzodiazepines. Fomepizole is an inhibitor of alcohol dehydrogenase and is helpful in the treatment of patients poisoned with ethylene glycol, methanol or other toxic alcohols. This patient had an accidental overdose of her **diphenhydramine** for her seasonal allergies.

59.4 **B.** This patient is exhibiting a **sympathomimetic toxidrome.** Her presentation is very similar to the patient in question 3. However, the key difference is that this patient has wet skin, while the patient in question 3 has dry skin. **The patient should receive as much lorazepam as needed to stop the seizure and allow the temperature to fall.** Physostigmine is a treatment for anti-muscarinic toxicity and would not be helpful in this patient. Labetalol is a β-blocker. This patient has signs of active sympathomimetic excess. Treatment with a **β-blocker may lead to unopposed α-1 agonism and potentially may worsen a patient tissue perfusion.** While this patient is wet, she has none of the other signs of a cholinergic toxicity. Therefore, atropine and pralidoxime are not recommended. Phytonadione is vitamin K and is the treatment for warfarin toxicity. This patient recently used crack cocaine.

CLINICAL PEARLS

▶ Patients who are hypoxic from an overdose typically will require a definitive airway, such as endotracheal or nasotracheal intubation.

▶ Fever from an overdose is a poor prognostic indicator and should usually be addressed with large doses of benzodiazepines and intravenous fluids.

▶ Symptomatic patients require observation or admission until they are asymptomatic.

▶ In the undifferentiated altered mental status patient, blood sugar level should immediately be checked.

▶ The nearest poison control center should be contacted (1-800-222-1222) for overdoses, accidental ingestions, and adverse drug effects.

REFERENCES

Aaron CK, Bora KM. Toxin ingestions in children. *BMJ Point-of-Care.* 2010. Available at: https://online.epocrates.com/u/2911885/Toxic+ingestions+in+children. Accessed March 24, 2017.

Chyka PA, Seger D, Krenzelok EP, Vala JA. American Academy of Clinical Toxicology, European Association of Poisons Centres, Clinical Toxicologists. Position paper: single-dose activated charcoal. *Clin Toxicol (Phila).* 2005;43:61-87.

Goldfrank L, Flomenbaum N, Lewin N, et al. *Goldfrank's Toxicologic Emergencies.* 10th ed. New York, NY: McGraw-Hill; 2014.

Roberts DM, Aaron CK. Management of acute organophosphorus pesticide poisoning. *BMJ.* 2007;334:629-634.

Wu AH, McKay C, Broussard LA, et al. National academy of clinical biochemistry laboratory medicine practice guidelines: recommendations for the use of laboratory tests to support poisoned patients who present to the emergency department. *Clin Chem.* 2003;49:357-379.

Review Questions

The following are strategically designed review questions to assess whether the student is able to integrate the information presented in the cases. The explanations to the answer choices describe the rationale, including which cases are relevant.

REVIEW QUESTIONS

R-1.   A 60-year-old female presents to the Emergency Department (ED) with chest pain, jaw pain, and diaphoresis. She has a history of hypertension, hyperlipidemia, COPD, and Type 2 diabetes. Which of the following is the most important next step in management?

    A.   Collect arterial blood gas

    B.   Stat chest CT

    C.   Check blood glucose level and administer insulin accordingly

    D.   Perform ECG

    E.   Give morphine for pain

R-2.   A 72-year-old man with a history of hypertension, atrial fibrillation, and seizures, arrives to the ED via ambulance with left-sided weakness and slurred speech. EMS reports they found him at a park, where bystanders witnessed him collapse while walking and called 911. Vital signs are as follows: BP 150/90 mm Hg, pulse 92 bpm, respirations 22 breaths/min, and temperature 97.9°F. The patient's O_2 saturation is 99% on room air. The patient's condition is most likely a complication originating from which of the following?

    A.   Concussion from his fall

    B.   Atrial fibrillation

    C.   Overdose of seizure medication

    D.   Thromboembolism

    E.   Hypoglycemia

R-3.   An 8-month-old male infant is brought to the ED by his parents, who are visibly distraught and tearful. The parents state that their son is usually very mild-tempered but has been irritable and refusing to eat for 2 days. Vital signs show respirations at 30 breaths/min, HR 144 beats/min, temperature 102°F rectally, and BP 86/54 mm Hg. Physical examination is normal except for crying and resistance to the log roll test. What is the best next step in treatment?

A.   Reassure the parents the infant is healthy and likely has FWS (fever without a source)

B.   Lumbar puncture

C.   Labs, imaging, and possibly arthrocentesis

D.   Report the parents for suspected child abuse

R-4.   A 55-year-old man presents to the ED with nausea, weakness, and malaise. He reports he has a history of chronic back pain, end stage renal failure, hypertension, and gall stones. He tells you, "I missed my last dialysis day because my niece was getting married, but it was just 1 day." His Hgb is 9.7 g/dL, Hct is 35%, serum potassium 6.6 mEq/L, serum sodium 126 mEq/L, BUN 52 mg/dL, and serum creatinine 3.7 mg/dL. What is the most appropriate treatment for this patient?

A.   Administer 2 units PRBC and recheck hemoglobin and hematocrit 1 hour after infusion

B.   Give 30 g kayexalate PO stat, and then scheduled BID

C.   Emergent dialysis

D.   Start a bolus of 1 L hypertonic saline

E.   Administer 40 mg furosemide IV

R-5.   A 22-year-old man arrives to the ED via ambulance after a mountain climbing accident in which he fell 50 feet to a rocky ledge. The patient's right arm is immobilized, and he has multiple abrasions to his abdomen. He received 2 L Lactated Ringer's solution in the ambulance. His vitals are as follows: BP 86/40 mm Hg, pulse rate 123 bpm, respirations 22 breaths/min, temperature 97.9°F, and oxygen saturation 92% on 4 L O_2 via non-rebreather mask. Which of the following is the best next step in management?

A.   Order imaging of the patient's right arm

B.   Assess the patient's alertness and Glasgow Coma Score (GCS)

C.   CT imaging of the abdomen

D.   Type and cross-match blood, and transfuse 2 units PRBC

R-6. A 14-year-old African-American girl with a history of sickle cell disease and asthma is brought to the hospital by her mother. The patient is complaining of pain level of 9 on a 0-10 scale. The patient has dyspnea. Oxygen saturation is 89% on room air. A chest radiograph shows multiple infiltrates of the right and left lungs. Which of the following is the best treatment for this condition?

A. Exchange transfusion

B. IV heparin

C. IV furosemide

D. IV Antibiotics

E. Nebulized beta-agonist

R-7. An 80-year-old woman is brought from a nursing home for a fever of 102°F. She has a Foley catheter in and has been taking oral cephalexin for a urinary tract infection (UTI). Her vital signs are significant for BP 88/45 mm Hg and pulse rate 108 bpm. Labs show WBC 14,000 cells/mL and lactic acid of 2.3 mmol/L. Which of the following is the best management of this patient?

A. CT imaging of the brain

B. IV fluid bolus of 50 mL/kg

C. Ultrasound of the abdomen

D. Maintain glucose level at 140-180 mg/dL

R-8. A 34-year-old woman complains of lower abdominal pain and vaginal spotting. Her last menstrual period was 6 weeks ago. BP is 110/60 mm Hg, HR 80 beats/min and temperature 98.7°F. The abdomen is nontender, and pelvic examination is unremarkable. The pregnancy test is positive. Which of the following is the best next step?

A. FAST examination to assess for free fluid in abdomen

B. Follow-up in 48 hours

C. Prescribe prenatal vitamins and ask patient to follow up with an obstetrician

D. Prescribe macrodantin antibiotics

R-9. A 66-year-old man presents with a cough, pitting edema in his legs, and dyspnea on exertion. He has a history of hypertension, diabetes, a myocardial infarction 5 years ago, and congestive heart failure. He states he recently went on a trip to see his grandchildren out of state and has not been able to find his "water pills" after returning home. Which of the following is the best initial treatment for this patient?

A. Immediate cardiac catheterization

B. Vasopressor use (ie, norepinephrine)

C. High-flow oxygen via noninvasive positive-pressure ventilation (NIPPV)

D. Diuresis with furosemide or bumetanide

R-10. A 20-year-old woman is brought to the ED by a friend who states they were at a party when the patient began having a seizure. The patient is anxious and somewhat combative. BP is 160/100 mm Hg, HR is 120 bpm, and temperature is 98.2°F. That patient's urine drug screen returns positive for cocaine. Which class of medication is best for this patient?

A. Benzodiazepines

B. Calcium channel blockers

C. Phenothiazines

D. Beta blockers

R-11. A 46-year-old male electrician was electrocuted while working on a power line. The patient is alert and oriented and has evidence of minor burns on his hands, but his physical examination is otherwise unremarkable. He is complaining of cramping and muscle aches. Which of the following is appropriate in management?

A. Order cardiac enzymes

B. Discharge patient after a bolus of fluid

C. Aggressive fluid administration and monitor urine output

D. Inspect burns for Lichtenberg figure

E. Prepare for fasciotomy

R-12. A 45-year-old woman arrives to the ED complaining of chest pain. Troponin levels are normal, and ECG shows concave ST elevation with PR depression. Pulse rate is 124 beats/min, BP is 138/78 mm Hg, respirations are 20 breaths/min, and oxygen saturation is 97% on room air. The patient says she has had a bad cold and just wants to sleep, but her chest pain is excruciating when she lays down, and she feels better when she's sitting up straight and leading forward. What will likely be included in the treatment plan for this patient?

A. Percutaneous coronary intervention

B. NSAIDs and colchicine

C. Proton pump inhibitor, H2 blocker, and antibiotics

D. IV Tylenol

R-13. A 50-year-old woman reports she has been having bloody stools all day. She appears pale but denies any abdominal pain. Which of the following is accurate regarding gastrointestinal bleeds?

A. Octreotide is helpful for variceal bleeding

B. A proton pump inhibitor decreases rebleeding rates in lower GI bleeds

C. Patients with lower GI bleeds often go into hypovolemic shock

D. Tagged RBC scans are helpful in unstable patients

R-14. A 17-year-old male was raking leaves in his front yard when he accidentally disturbed a copperhead snake. The patient presents to the hospital with two puncture bites to his right ankle, which is edematous and red. Care for pit viper bites includes which of the following?

A. Hyperbaric oxygen therapy

B. Surgical debridement

C. X-ray of the affected area

D. Blood cultures

ANSWERS

R-1. **D.** This patient is highly suspicious for myocardial infarction (MI). Even prior to stat ECG, the patient should have aspirin to chew and nitroglycerin to relieve the pain. Answer A is important if the patient is suspected of having hypoxemia or was in respiratory distress. Answer B (chest CT) is important if there is suspicion of a pulmonary embolism. Though the other steps are appropriate in managing MI, an ECG is the priority next step for diagnosis and treatment. See Case 7 (Chest Pain/Acute Myocardial Infarction) and Case 8 (Noncardiac Chest Pain).

R-2. **B.** This patient with hemiparesis and slurred speech is likely having a stroke. The most common long-term complication of atrial fibrillation is stroke. Typically concussions (A) and overdose of seizure medications (B) do not manifest in this way. Overdose of seizure medication can lead to lethargy or ataxia (phenytoin), but the history is not suggestive. Thromboembolism (Answer D) would present with hypoxemia and respiratory distress. Hypoglycemia usually manifests as tremor, palpitations and diaphoresis. (Answer E). However, it is important to consider the differential diagnosis of Todd's paralysis, which can occur after seizure and manifests as one-sided weakness and speech and vision impairments. See Case 26 (Syncope), Case 28 (Stroke/TIA), and Case 30 (Seizure in Adult).

R-3. **C.** This patient likely has septic arthritis. On physical examination the child will likely appear ill, and the position of maximum comfort will be with the hip flexed, abducted, and externally rotated. Passive range of motion examination will be resisted and painful. Appropriate initial laboratory studies include complete blood count (CBC), blood cultures, erythrocyte sedimentation rate (ESR), and C-reactive protein (CRP). Plain radiographs are key to rule out several alternative diagnoses, and bedside ED ultrasound may identify a hip effusion. The definitive diagnosis of septic arthritis is made by examination of synovial fluid obtained by arthrocentesis. See Case 32 (Fever in Infant), Case 33 (Child with Limp/Septic Arthritis), and Case 34 (Febrile Seizure).

R-4.   **C.** Emergency dialysis the best treatment for this patient with end stage renal disease (ESRD) who has symptoms of uremia and abnormal laboratory levels. This is likely due to his missed dialysis day. Though answer B (kayexalate), D (hypertonic saline), and E (IV furosemide) are appropriate interventions to address singular electrolyte abnormalities, they will not solve the underlying problem. Emergent dialysis will clear the extra potassium and will remove the extra fluid causing dilutional hyponatremia. ESRD patients often have chronic anemia due to decreased erythropoietin production by the kidneys, and hemoglobin and hematocrit levels should be compared to baseline before administering blood products. See Case 23 (Hyperkalemia due to Renal Failure).

R-5.   **B.** Assess alertness and GCS. The Emergency Medicine approach to every critically ill patient begins with evaluation and stabilization of the airway, breathing, and circulation (ABCs). Although the patient's arm and circulatory status do need to be addressed, a quick assessment of the patient's GCS will determine if he can properly protect his airway or if he needs to be intubated. After the airway is secured, resuscitation for hemorrhagic shock is indicated since the patient is still in shock after the 2 L bolus. When possible, typed and cross-matched blood is optimal; however, in the acute setting, this is often unfeasible. Type-specific unmatched blood is the next best option, followed by O-negative blood in females and O-positive blood in males. See Case 2 (Hemorrhagic Shock), Case 44 (Extremity Fracture), and Case 45 (Trauma at Extremes of Age).

R-6.   **A.** Acute chest syndrome (ACS) is a complication of sickle cell disease that usually manifests on hospital day 3-5, best treated by exchange transfusion. ACS is defined in the literature as the presence of two of the following: a new lobar or segmental pulmonary infiltrate or focal abnormality on CXR, fever higher than 38.5°C (101.3°F), respiratory symptoms, hypoxemia, or chest pain. Clinically, ACS is differentiated from pneumonia when patients continue to deteriorate despite antibiotics and supportive care. See Case 13 (Asthma), Case 14 (Pulmonary Embolism), Case 15 (Bacteria Pneumonia), and Case 50 (Sickle Cell Crisis).

R-7.   **D.** This patient is likely septic due to UTI. In sepsis management, most clinicians target blood glucose levels between 140 and 180 mg/dL (7.7-10 mmol/L). Initial broad-spectrum therapy against both gram-positive and gram-negative bacteria is recommended, as there is evidence that inappropriate antibiotic selection is associated with worsened mortality. A fluid bolus of 30 mL/kg (2-4 L in adults) crystalloid should be administered, but fluids should be given more judiciously in the presence of a fluid overload condition (eg, CHF and advanced renal failure). Thus, answer choice B of 50 mL/kg is excessive. See Case 3 (Septic Shock).

R-8. **A.** This patient has a possible ectopic pregnancy and should have quantitative hCG and transvaginal ultrasound to assess for possible viable vs nonviable vs ectopic pregnancy. Pending these studies, a FAST examination of the abdomen may be performed, and if significant free fluid is seen in the abdomen, then a ruptured ectopic pregnancy is highly suspected. See Case 36 (Ectopic Pregnancy).

R-9. **D.** Diuresis is appropriate. A mild CHF exacerbation with trace pulmonary edema and fluid overload from medication or dietary noncompliance may only require diuresis. A patient with hypotension and poor perfusion (cardiogenic shock) may require inotropic support (dobutamine or milrinone to enhance myocardial contractility), vasopressor support (norepinephrine to increase coronary diastolic perfusion), and possibly a small fluid bolus to increase preload. An unstable patient with ischemia may need to undergo cardiac catheterization for emergent reperfusion. If the patient is in respiratory distress, high-flow oxygen via NIPPV with continuous or biphasic positive airway pressure can be considered. See Case 11 (Congestive Heart Failure).

R-10. **A.** Benzodiazepines are useful in controlling agitation, sympathomimetics, atrial dysrhythmias, and seizures in patients with cocaine intoxication. Calcium channel blockers may be used to treat atrial dysrhythmias. Phenothiazines should be avoided because they may lower the seizure threshold, contribute to hyperthermia, and have dysrhythmic effects. The use of β-blockers is controversial due to the risk of an unopposed α-adrenergic effect, leading to increased hypertension and coronary vasoconstriction. See also Case 56 (Cocaine Intoxication) and Case 58 (Ethanol Withdrawal).

R-11. **C.** This patient likely has rhabdomyolysis, which is common after electrical injuries (but rare after lightning strike). Treatment for rhabdomyolysis focuses on preventing acute kidney injury. Fluids should be titrated to a targeted urine output of 1-2 mL/kg/h in patients with rhabdomyolysis. Head CT should be ordered if patients present with neurological findings or loss of consciousness, and cardiac enzymes if the patient has chest pain. The Lichtenberg figure is a fern-like pattern in burns due to lightning strike, and fasciotomy is only indicated in cases of compartment syndrome. See Case 53 (Lightning and Electrical Injury).

R-12. **B.** NSAIDs and colchicine are the best treatment for pericarditis. The findings of concave ST elevation with PR depression, tachycardia, pain alleviation when sitting up, and viral etiology are all consistent with pericardial disease. Other findings may include a rough scratchy sound (pericardial friction rub) upon auscultation. Echocardiography can be used to evaluate for pericardial effusion and rule out the potentially lethal complication of pericardial tamponade. If the troponin level had been elevated, myocarditis would have been suspected. Proton pump inhibitor, H2 blocker, and antibiotics are appropriate management for peptic ulcer disease and GERD. Percutaneous coronary intervention is used to address atherosclerosis. IV Tylenol is not indicated. See Case 7 (Chest Pain) and Case 8 (Noncardiac Chest Pain).

R-13.   **A.** In patients with variceal bleeding, a somatostatin analog such as octreotide or vasopressin can be helpful. However, vasopressin has fallen out of favor because of the side effects and the risk of end-organ ischemia. A proton pump inhibitor should be given to patients with upper GI bleeding to decrease rebleeding rates. In general, patients with lower GI bleeding rarely exhibit hemodynamic instability unless the process has gone on unrecognized for some time. Tagged red blood cell (RBC) scans are used for stable patients. See Case 17 (Acute Upper and Lower GI Bleeding).

R-14.   **C.** Radiographs should be performed to evaluate for retained teeth. Asymptomatic patients who were bit by a pit viper should be observed for 8-12 hours after the bite. This should be extended to 24 hours for coral snakebites because of the absence of early symptoms. Surgical debridement or fasciotomy in the setting of envenomation should not be done, as this may lead to further bleeding. Blood cultures are not indicated, but laboratory studies should be ordered, including clotting studies, liver enzymes, and CBC with platelets. The mainstay in treatment in venom-induced coagulopathy is antivenom, preferably type specific.

Page numbers followed by *f* indicate figures; *t* indicate tables.